Nutritional Care of the Patient with Gastrointestinal Disease

Nutritional Care of the Patient with Gastrointestinal Disease

Alan L Buchman, MD, MSPH
Visiting Clinical Professor of Surgery and Medical Director,
Intestinal Rehabilitation and Transplant Center,
the University of Illinois at Chicago

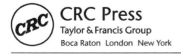

CRC Press
Taylor & Francis Group
Boca Raton London New York

CRC Press is an imprint of the
Taylor & Francis Group, an **informa** business

CRC Press
Taylor & Francis Group
6000 Broken Sound Parkway NW, Suite 300
Boca Raton, FL 33487-2742

First issued in paperback 2021

© 2016 by Taylor & Francis Group, LLC
CRC Press is an imprint of Taylor & Francis Group, an Informa business

No claim to original U.S. Government works

Version Date: 20150731

ISBN 13: 978-1-03-209841-8 (pbk)
ISBN 13: 978-1-4822-2603-4 (hbk)

Library of Congress Cataloging-in-Publication Data

Nutritional care of the patient with gastrointestinal disease / editor, Alan L. Buchman.
p. ; cm.
Includes bibliographical references and index.
ISBN 978-1-4822-2603-4 (hardcover : alk. paper)
I. Buchman, Alan, editor.
[DNLM: 1. Gastrointestinal Diseases--diet therapy. 2. Nutrition Assessment. 3. Nutrition Disorders--diet therapy. 4. Nutrition Therapy--methods. WI 140]

RC806
616.3'30654--dc23   2015003516

Visit the Taylor & Francis Web site at
http://www.taylorandfrancis.com

and the CRC Press Web site at
http://www.crcpress.com

Contents

Preface

Food enters the body and leaves the body primarily through the gastrointestinal tract. This organ system is the site for nutrient digestion, absorption, and assimilation into the body. Questions on nutrition are probably the most frequent inquiries a physician, especially an internist, gastroenterologist, or surgeon receives from patients. Unfortunately, most are ill-equipped to provide correct answers, if at all. Most physicians are unable to correctly identify and intervene in patients considered nutritionally at risk. It is scandalous that the teaching of nutritional science education has actually decreased in medical schools since a congressional requirement for such education. It is well established that both under- and overnutrition result in significant morbidity and mortality. The incidence of food allergies, celiac disease, and obesity are increasing at alarming rates yet the knowledge base with regard to specialized nutritional support of these patients is abysmal. Physicians are demanding more education on nutrition to meet the needs and desires of their patients. As examples in an ever-evolving field, recent studies have found nutrition, via specific carbohydrates, plays a substantial role in irritable bowel syndrome, and the so-called elimination diets are useful in the therapy of eosinophilic esophagitis. Nutrition plays a very important role in the management of several serious gastrointestinal disorders both through the correction of specific nutritional deficiencies, and also in regard to the prevention of nutritional deficiencies due to enhanced nutrient losses, intake, or malabsorption. Pharmacologic nutrition, through the use of specific nutrients in larger than usual doses, has come into practice not only by medical professionals, but also by patients themselves. Additionally, there are many contemporary concerns regarding the use of probiotics: Are they effective, and if so, which ones, in what combination, and for what disease? *Nutritional Management of Gastrointestinal Disease* is designed to provide clinicians with contemporary practical and reference tools to help enhance the nutritional care of their patients. Illustrative cases should help to provide practical examples of nutritional problems encountered in the clinic.

Alan L. Buchman, MD, MSPH
Visiting Clinical Professor of Surgery
Medical Director, Intestinal Rehabilitation and Transplant Program
Department of Surgery
University of Illinois at Chicago

Editor

Dr. Alan L. Buchman is a practicing gastroenterologist. He is the director of the Center for Gastroenterology and Nutrition and visiting clinical professor of surgery at the University of Illinois at Chicago where he is the medical director of the Intestinal Rehabilitation and Transplant Program. Dr. Buchman also serves as a medical director for Blue Cross Blue Shield of Illinois. Dr. Buchman is a former professor of medicine and surgery at the Feinberg School of Medicine, Northwestern University in Chicago where he established the Inflammatory Bowel Disease Center and Intestinal Rehabilitation Center. Dr. Buchman took his undergraduate training at Northwestern and earned his medical degree at The Chicago Medical School. After a residency at Cedars Sinai Medical Center in Los Angeles, he completed a fellowship in clinical nutrition at UCLA and also received his Master of Science in public health. Following this, he completed a fellowship in gastroenterology at Emory University and then served on the faculties of the Baylor College of Medicine and the University of Texas at Houston Medical School.

Dr. Buchman has served on 21 peer-reviewed journal editorial boards in such capacities as associate editor and section editor and has authored nearly 250 peer-reviewed articles, editorials, book chapters, and four books. He has been the recipient of numerous national awards from several different societies including the American Gastroenterology Association (AGA), American Society for Nutrition, American College of Nutrition, American Society for Enteral and Parenteral Nutrition, and the Southern Medical Society. He is the former president of the American Federation for Medical Research (AFMR) and has served on numerous national committees, including the FDA's Gastrointestinal Drugs Advisory Committee, where he has served as acting chair; the AGA's Education and Manpower and Training Committees; the Council of the Central Society for Clinical Research; and the National Commission on Digestive Diseases. He is a past chair of the AGA's Nutrition and Obesity Section.

Dr. Buchman's research has focused on complications and treatment of inflammatory bowel disease as well as on the complications of intestinal failure and long-term parenteral nutrition, and he has published seminal manuscripts in these areas. Dr. Buchman is considered a world authority in nutrition, intestinal failure, and inflammatory bowel disease and has had numerous television, radio, and print media appearances.

Contributors

Eslam Ali
Division of Gastroenterology,
    Hepatology, and Nutrition
Brody School of Medicine
East Carolina University
Greenville, North Carolina

Anil K. Asthana
Department of Gastroenterology
Monash University and Alfred
    Health
Melbourne, Victoria, Australia

Mara Lee Beebe
Department of Nutrition
Medical University of South Carolina
Charleston, South Carolina

Mandy L. Corrigan
Nutrition Support Clinician/
    Consultant
St Louis, Missouri

Sheila E. Crowe
Division of Gastroenterology
University of California
San Diego, California

Mark H. DeLegge
Division of Gastroenterology
Medical University of South Carolina
Charleston, South Carolina

Aaron M. Dickstein
Division of Gastroenterology
Tufts Medical Center and Tufts
    University School of Medicine
Boston, Massachusetts

Bethany Doerfler
Division of Gastroenterology and
    Hepatology
Northwestern University—The
    Feinberg School of Medicine
Chicago, Illinois

Martin Floch
Department of Internal Medicine
Yale University School of
    Medicine
New Haven, Connecticut

Peter R. Gibson
Department of Gastroenterology
Monash University and Alfred
    Health
Melbourne, Victoria, Australia

Nirmala Gonsalves
Division of Gastroenterology and
    Hepatology
Northwestern University—The
    Feinberg School of Medicine
Chicago, Illinois

Khursheed N. Jeejeebhoy
Department of Medicine
University of Toronto
Toronto, Ontario, Canada

Hossam M. Kandil
Division of Gastroenterology,
    Hepatology, and Nutrition
Brody School of Medicine
East Carolina University
Greenville, North Carolina

Nitin Kumar
Division of Gastroenterology,
    Hepatology, and Endoscopy
Brigham and Women's Hospital
Harvard Medical School
Boston, Massachusetts

John Leung
Departments of Gastroenterology,
    Pediatric Gastroenterology, and
    Allergy and Immunology
Food Allergy Center at Tufts Medical
    Center and Floating Hospital for
    Children
Boston, Massachusetts

Joel B. Mason
Division of Gastroenterology
Tufts Medical Center and Tufts
    University School of Medicine
and
USDA Human Nutrition Research
    Center at Tufts University
Boston, Massachusetts

Laura E. Matarese
Division of Gastroenterology,
    Hepatology, and Nutrition
Brody School of Medicine
and
Department of Nutrition Science
East Carolina University
Greenville, North Carolina

Travis J. McKenzie
Department of Surgery
Mayo Clinic
Rochester, Minnesota

Jane G. Muir
Department of Gastroenterology
Monash University and Alfred Health
Melbourne, Victoria, Australia

Joseph A. Murray
Division of Gastroenterology and
    Hepatology
Department of Immunology
Mayo Clinic
Rochester, Minnesota

S.J. O'Keefe
Division of Gastroenterology,
    Hepatology, and Nutrition
University of Pittsburgh School of
    Medicine
Pittsburgh, Pennsylvania

Eamonn M.M. Quigley
Department of Medicine and
    Division of Gastroenterology and
    Hepatology
Houston Methodist Hospital
Houston, Texas
and
Weill Cornell Medical College
New York, New York

Jacalyn A. See
Division of Endocrinology,
    Diabetes, Metabolism, and
    Nutrition
Mayo Clinic
Rochester, Minnesota

Joseph H. Sellin
Section of Gastroenterology and
    Hepatology
Baylor College of Medicine
Houston, Texas

Scott A. Shikora
Department of Surgery
Brigham and Women's Hospital
Harvard Medical School
Boston, Massachusetts

Robert Shulman
Division of Pediatric Gastroenterology
Texas Children's Hospital
Baylor College of Medicine
Houston, Texas

Vladimir Stanisic
Department of Medicine and
    Division of Gastroenterology and
    Hepatology
Houston Methodist Hospital
Houston, Texas
and
Weill Cornell Medical College
New York, New York

Ezra Steiger
Department of Surgery
Cleveland Clinic
Cleveland, Ohio

Zhouwen Tang
Section of Gastroenterology and
    Hepatology
Baylor College of Medicine
Houston, Texas

Kelly A. Tappenden
Department of Food Science and
    Human Nutrition
University of Illinois at
    Urbana-Champaign
Champaign, Illinois

Christopher C. Thompson
Division of Gastroenterology,
    Hepatology, and Endoscopy
Brigham and Women's Hospital
Harvard Medical School
Boston, Massachusetts

Kishore Vipperla
Division of General Internal
    Medicine
University of Pittsburgh Medical
    Center
Pittsburgh, Pennsylvania

Seema Mehta Walsh
Division of Pediatric
    Gastroenterology
Baylor College of Medicine
Houston, Texas

1 Nutritional Assessment

Khursheed N. Jeejeebhoy

CONTENTS

1.1 INTRODUCTION

Nutritional health is maintained by a state of equilibrium in which nutrient intake and requirements balance.

Malnutrition occurs when net nutrient intakes (nutrient intake corrected for abnormally large fecal or urinary losses) is less than requirements. Recently, the following definition has been given. "Malnutrition includes both the deficiency or excess (or imbalance) of energy, protein, and other nutrients. In practice, undernutrition or inadequate intake of energy, protein, and nutrients is the focus."[1]

Malnutrition of macronutrients namely protein, carbohydrates, and fats as energy sources leads to a succession of metabolic abnormalities, physiological changes, reduced organ and tissue function, and loss of body mass. Concurrent stress such as trauma, sepsis, inflammation, and burns accelerates loss of tissue mass and function. Ultimately, critical loss of body mass and function occur and result in death. Traditionally, the recognition of the end stage phenotype reduced weight, muscle wasting, loss of body fat, reduced plasma proteins, and immune dysfunction were the features that defined malnutrition.[2] At this point it is important to realize why we want to determine the presence of malnutrition: It is to identify persons who will benefit from nutritional support. The simple recognition of these features as a mark of malnutrition while intuitively obvious has several pitfalls. First there is a range of normal weights, muscle, and fat mass among the population so it is not easy to define the early stages of abnormal deficiency. Second, if we use the presence of this phenotype to start nutritional care, then we fail to prevent malnutrition because we will not recognize it before it becomes extreme nor will we recognize persons who would ultimately develop the complications of malnutrition before they occur. Third, there are conditions such as cachexia[3] in which the same phenotype occurs without lack of nutrition and nutritional support has no benefit.

On the contrary there are micronutrients, namely, trace elements and vitamins, which can become deficient without altering the macronutrient status. For example, patients on parenteral nutrition, who had been provided with adequate amounts of protein and energy developed rash and became immune deficient due to lack of zinc in the infused mixture.

Hence, theoretically ideal way to determine the nutritional status of a person would include assessment of both macro- and micronutrient status. Furthermore, in order for nutritional assessment to be clinically useful it is necessary to examine each of the proposed methods by asking the following questions:

1. Does the method specifically assess the risk of morbidity and mortality resulting from malnutrition?
2. Does it identify and separate the causes and consequences of malnutrition and disease in the individual patient?
3. Can the technique determine whether the patient will clinically benefit from nutritional support?

1.2   TRADITIONAL PARAMETERS OF NUTRITIONAL STATUS

The assessment of nutritional status has previously been focused on the fact that the obvious effect of protein–energy deficiency was weight loss, loss of body fat and muscle bulk, circulating proteins and immune competence. Unfortunately, this phenotype of the thin muscle and fat wasted person can be due to factors other than a simple deficiency of nutrients.[3]

1.2.1   BODY WEIGHT AND WEIGHT LOSS

Body weight is a simple measure of the total mass of body components and is compared to an ideal or desirable weight. This comparison can be made by using methods such as the Hamwi formula or tables. However, a simple approach, which provides as much information is the calculation of the body mass or Quetelet index (BMI). BMI is calculated as weight in kilograms divided by height in meters squared. A BMI of below 15 is associated with significant mortality. However, measurements of body weight in patients in hospitals, ICUs, those with liver disease, cancer, and renal failure are confounded by changes in body water due to underhydration, edema, ascites, and dialysate in the abdomen. Two studies, one conducted in a German hospital and the other in India concluded that BMI did not predict the development of complications and increased hospital length of stay (LOS).[4,5]

Unintentional weight loss greater than 10% is a good prognosticator of clinical outcome.[6,7] However, it may be difficult to determine true weight loss. Morgan et al.[8] have shown that the accuracy of determining weight loss by history was only 0.67 and the predictive power was 0.75. Hence, 33% of patients with weight loss would be missed and 25% of those who have been weight stable would be diagnosed as having lost weight. Furthermore, the nutritional significance of changes in body weight can again be confounded by changes in hydrational status. In addition with aging there is loss of muscle mass which results in infirmity and susceptibility to pneumonia despite the fact that there may be increased body fat making the BMI normal or even within the obese range called sarcopenic obesity.

1.2.2 ANTHROPOMETRY

Triceps and subscapular skinfold thicknesses provide an index of body fat and midarm muscle circumference provides a measure of muscle mass. Although these measurements seem to be useful in population studies their reliability in individual patients is less clear. The most commonly used standards for triceps skinfold thickness and midarm muscle circumference are based on measurements of white male and female individuals participating in NHANES data. The use of these standards to identify malnutrition in many patients is problematic because of the absence of correction factors for ethnicity, age, hydration status, and physical activity on anthropometric parameters. Several studies have demonstrated that 20%–30% of healthy control subjects would be considered malnourished based on these standards.[9,10] Another factor is the variability in measurement. Hall et al.[11] found considerable inconsistencies when anthropometric measurements were performed by three different observers. The coefficient of variation was 4.7% for arm circumference and 22.6% for triceps skin fold thickness. Therefore, a change in arm muscle circumference (arm circumference minus triceps skinfold thickness) of at least 2.68 cm was needed to demonstrate a true change in a given patient. These considerations in particular apply to patients in ICUs, and those with liver and renal disease where edema is a major problem in assessing skin folds and arm circumference.

1.2.3 CREATININE–HEIGHT INDEX

This is the 24-h creatinine excretion normalized for height. It is often an unreliable measurement because it is dependent upon complete 24-h urine collections and urinary losses or oliguria may result in an inappropriate diagnosis of malnutrition. Patients on diuretics such as those with cardiac and liver failure and those with renal disease are especially likely to have low excretions of creatinine.

1.3 MEASUREMENT OF BODY COMPOSITION

A more sophisticated way of determining the loss of body weight, fat, and muscle is by a formal evaluation of body components.

The body consists of compartments or components. There are over 35 well-recognized components and these are organized into five levels of increasing complexity: atomic, molecular, cellular, tissue system, and whole body. In healthy weight stable subjects there are relatively constant relationships between these components which are correlated with each other. For example, the atomic level component nitrogen is 16% of the molecular level component protein.

1.3.1 ISOTOPE DILUTION

Total-body water, measured by isotope dilution, is usually the largest molecular level component. Water maintains a relatively stable relationship to fat-free body mass and thus measured water isotope dilution volumes allow prediction of fat-free body mass and fat (i.e., body weight minus fat-free body mass). The relationship between total-body water and other body composition components may change with disease and this should be considered when interpreting data from hospitalized or chronically ill patients. The usual approach is to measure a dilution volume using one of the three isotopes, tritium, deuterium, or ^{18}O labeled water. This first step allows estimation of a dilution volume of one of the three isotopes. In the second step, it is assumed that the proportion of fat-free body mass as water is constant at 0.732. This allows calculation of fat-free body mass and fat. The relationship of this measurement to outcome has not been studied.

1.3.2 BIOIMPEDANCE ANALYSIS

Bioimpedance analysis (BIA) is a method of estimating body fluid volumes by measuring the resistance to a high frequency, low amplitude alternating electric current (50 kHz at 500–800 mA).[12] The amount of resistance measured (R) is inversely proportional to the volume of electrolytic fluid in the body and to a lesser extent on the proportions of this volume. A regression equation is then developed based on a reference measurement of fat-free body mass (i.e., isotope dilution) and the measured R, height, and other variables. Recently, the difference in the conductive properties of extra and intracellular fluid has resulted in the development of bioimpedance spectroscopy (BIS). Direct current will pass through extracellular fluid but will not traverse the lipid membrane of cells. As the frequency of the applied current increases the cell membranes, act as the dielectric of capacitors and the alternating current will pass partly and easily through the extracellular fluid and with greater resistance through the cells. The total impedance to the current is defined by an equivalent circuit of a resistance and a reactance through a capacitor. As the frequency of the alternating current increases, the reactance at first increases and then decreases until at very high frequencies there is little impedance to the passage of the current through cells. An analysis of the reactance to different frequencies is used to calculate extra- and intracellular water. BIS has been applied to measure changes of extra- and intracellular fluid in clinical situations.[13] In healthy adults, it is possible to predict total-body water within 2–3 L. Much more variable results are observed in diseased patients, owing in part to the population-specific nature of BIA. From body water and body weight, the lean and fat masses can be calculated[14] easily at the bedside.

A recent paper by Pichard et al.[15] showed that patients who had a low fat-free mass defined as being <17.4 and <15.0 kg/m² in men and women, respectively, were more likely to have longer LOS in hospital. However, malnutrition by SGA also predicted an increased LOS in the same study.

1.3.3 DUAL-ENERGY X-RAY ABSORPTIOMETRY

Dual-energy absorptiometry (DXA) is a method developed originally for the measurement of bone density and mass. Systems today also quantify soft-tissue composition, and it is possible to measure total and regional fat, bone mineral, and bone mineral-free lean components with DXA. The method is based on the attenuation characteristics of tissues exposed to x-rays at two peak energies. Mathematical algorithms allow calculation of the separate components using various physical and biological models. Software can be used to measure regions separately if desired. A typical whole body scan takes approximately 30 min and exposes the subject to ~1 mrem radiation. The method provides the first accurate and practical means of measuring bone mineral mass and offers a new opportunity to study appendicular muscle mass. Again there is no data indicating whether DXA can predict outcome in hospital patients unrelated to treatment.

1.3.4 WHOLE-BODY COUNTING/NEUTRON ACTIVATION

Potassium, nitrogen, phosphorus, hydrogen, oxygen, carbon, sodium, chloride, and calcium can be measured with a group of techniques referred to as whole-body counting/*in vivo* neutron activation analysis. Shielded whole body counters can count the gamma-ray decay of naturally occurring ${}^{40}K$. The method is safe and can be used in children and pregnant women. The ${}^{40}K$ counts can be used to estimate total-body potassium, which in turn can be used to calculate body cell mass and fat-free body mass. Prompt gamma neutron activation analysis can be used to measure total-body N and H. Nitrogen can be used to calculate total-body protein. Delayed gamma neutron activation measures total-body Ca, Na, Cl, and P. These elements can be used to calculate bone mineral mass and extracellular fluid volume. Finally, inelastic neutron scattering methods measure total-body 0 and C Carbon is useful in models designed to quantify total-body fat. Whole-body counting-neutron activation methods are important because they provide a means of estimating all major chemical components *in vivo*. These methods are considered the standard for evaluating the body composition components of nutritional interest, including body cell mass, fat, fat-free body mass, skeletal muscle mass, and various fluid volumes. Refeeding the malnourished subject by mouth or by total parenteral nutrition (TPN) results in a rapid increase in total body potassium (TBK) but not total body nitrogen (TBN). In animal studies, it has been shown that this increase in TBK is the result of improved membrane voltage and an increase in the intracellular ionic potassium. The findings are consistent with improved cell energetics as demonstrated by nuclear magnetic resonance (NMR) spectroscopy as well as improved muscle function shown concurrently. Loss of TBK is a good predictor of poor outcome in a variety of conditions associated with malnutrition.[16–19]

1.3.5 COMPUTERIZED AXIAL TOMOGRAPHY AND MAGNETIC RESONANCE IMAGING

These methods measure components at the tissue-system level of body composition, including skeletal muscle, adipose tissue, visceral organs, and brain. Computerized axial tomography (CT) systems measure x-ray attenuation as the source and detector rotate in a perpendicular plane around the subject. Magnetic resonance imaging (MRI) systems measure nuclear relaxation times from nuclei of atoms with a magnetic moment that are aligned within a powerful magnetic field. Clinical systems are based on hydrogen, although it is possible to create images and spectrographs from phosphorus, sodium, and carbon. The collected data is transformed into high-resolution images, and this allows the quantification of whole or regional body composition. A large number of studies in phantoms, cadavers, and *in vivo* validate these methods. There are no studies of imaging methods in relation to outcome.

1.3.6 BODY COMPOSITION AND OUTCOMES

Although the above methods of body composition can accurately assess different components, they are difficult to apply in the clinical setting except in specialized units. The only method that can be available for wide clinical application in nutritional assessment is BIA or BIS, which shows that reduced fat-free mass increases LOS in hospital patients, but unlike composite clinical evaluation described later in the chapter called subjective global assessment (SGA) has not been shown to predict complications except in cancer patients.[20]

1.3.7 SERUM ALBUMIN

Several studies have demonstrated that a low serum albumin concentration correlates with an increased incidence of medical complications.[21–23] In practice, it is not an index of malnutrition as exemplified by the fact that prolonged protein–calorie restriction induced experimentally in human volunteers[24] or observed clinically in patients with anorexia nervosa,[25] causes marked reductions in body weight but little change in plasma albumin concentration. A protein-deficient diet with adequate calories in elderly individuals causes a decrease in lean body mass and muscle function without a change in plasma albumin concentration.[26]

1.3.8 PREALBUMIN

Prealbumin is a transport protein for thyroid hormones and exists in the circulation as a retinol-binding prealbumin complex. The turnover rate of this protein is rapid with a half-life of 2–3 days. It is synthesized by the liver and is catabolized partly in the kidneys. Protein–energy malnutrition reduces the levels of prealbumin and refeeding restores levels. However, prealbumin levels fall without malnutrition in infections[27,28] and renal failure increases[29] while liver failure may cause decreased levels. Although, prealbumin is responsive to nutritional changes, it is influenced by several disease-related factors making it unreliable as an index of nutritional status in patients.

1.3.9 IMMUNE COMPETENCE

Immune competence, as measured by delayed cutaneous hypersensitivity (DCH), is affected by severe malnutrition. While it is true that immune competence as measured by DCH is reduced in malnutrition, several diseases[30] and drugs influence this measurement making it a poor predictor of malnutrition in sick patients. The following factors nonspecifically alter DCH in the absence of malnutrition: (1) infections (viral, bacterial, and granulomatous); (2) uremia, cirrhosis, hepatitis, trauma, burns, and hemorrhage; (3) steroids, immunosupressants, cimetidine, warfarin, and perhaps aspirin; and (4) general anesthesia and surgery. Hence in critically sick patients many factors can alter DCH and render it useless in assessing the state of nutrition. Meakins et al.[31] have shown that simply draining an abscess can reverse anergy. Immunity is therefore neither a specific indicator of malnutrition nor is it easily studied.[32]

1.3.10 SERUM CHOLESTEROL

Low levels are seen in malnourished patients. However, very low levels are seen in patients with liver disease, renal disease, and malabsorption. In addition, low levels correlate with mortality.[33]

1.3.11 FUNCTIONAL CHANGES

Malnutrition is associated with changes in muscle performance and Klidjian et al.[34] showed that reduced grip strength was predictive of postoperative complications.

Reduced hand grip strength (HGS) has been shown to predict LOS in hospital[35] and is associated with reduced food intake.[36] In cancer patients reduced HGS was correlated with increased LOS, but this correlation was also observed by the degree of malnutrition assessed by SGA and Nutrition Risk Screening (NRS). Unfortunately, while there are trends seen as indicated above there was a wide range of grip strengths described in different studies and it was difficult to assign a cutoff value in an individual patient.[37] Furthermore, while feeding protein supplements to frail elderly patients in a randomized trial improved physical performance and leg extension strength, there was no change in HGS.[38] An attractive test of function HGS is not practically applicable to an individual patient like the clinical methods (SGA) described below.

1.3.12 EXPERIMENTAL STUDIES OF NUTRITION AND FUNCTION

There are more sophisticated diagnostic methods that hold promise in detecting malnutrition and studying response to feeding.

Russell et al. showed a direct relationship of hypocaloric feeding to muscle function before change in body composition.[39] There is a restitution of function before a significant rise in body mass in anorexic wasted patients as well.[40] Hence, functional changes may be a more sensitive marker of malnutrition also showing the benefits of refeeding. In addition, muscle function can predict the likelihood of surgical complications.[41] However, muscle function is difficult to test at the bedside and needs patient cooperation. Thirty-one P-NMR studies have correlated changes in muscle function with altered rates of ATP synthesis[42] indicating an abnormality of the mitochondria. Recently, we have shown that mitochondrial complex I activity in peripheral blood lymphocytes is reduced in malnutrition, not altered by inflammation and restored before body mass after short-term refeeding[43] and further improved after a month of refeeding in human subjects. These findings may lead to the development of an objective and specific way of assessing malnutrition and the effects of nutritional support.

1.4 CLINICAL ASSESSMENT OF NUTRITIONAL STATUS

1.4.1 SUBJECTIVE GLOBAL ASSESSMENT

It is clear from the above that traditional parameters do not meet the needs of identifying patients at risk, have large errors of measurement especially in a busy clinical service, have a wide range of normal values and are also influenced by disease. In a critical assessment of various techniques traditionally used to measure nutritional status, it was clear that these techniques were inadequate,[44] and an alternative method, which identifies the interacting clinical factors that resulted in malnutrition, would have to be used. These factors are shown in Figure 1.1.

In this figure, the initial nutritional and functional status is shown as a blue square that is positively (+, increases size of square) or negatively (−, decreases size of square) influenced by nutrient intake, gastrointestinal disease (which impedes intake and/or prevents absorption), and disease status, which increases energy and nutrient requirements.

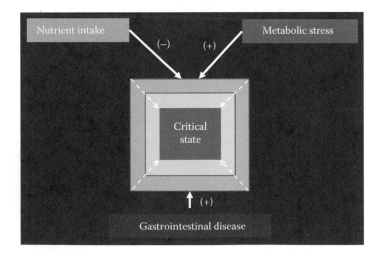

FIGURE 1.1   **(See color insert.)** Interaction of factors influencing nutritional status.

We hypothesized that a composite evaluation of these parameters together with their effect on the direction and rapidity of change in body mass and function evaluated at the bedside would identify outcome without identifying a measured value of weight BMI, arm muscle circumference, fat in skin fold thickness, and albumin levels. We showed that it correctly predicted nutrition-associated complications.[45] Detsky et al.[46] subsequently showed it had better sensitivity and specificity than individual traditional parameters in predicting outcome.

A clinical method for evaluating nutritional status, termed SGA, encompasses historical, symptomatic, and physical parameters.

The history used in SGA focuses on five areas.

1. The loss of body weight in the previous 6 months and continuing in the last 2 weeks. The direction of change rather than absolute weight is recorded. The pattern of loss is also important, and it is possible for a patient to have significant weight loss but still be considered well-nourished if body weight (without edema or ascites) recently increased. For example, a patient who has had a 10% body weight loss but regained 3% of that weight over the past month would be considered well-nourished.
2. Dietary intake is classified as normal or abnormal as judged by a change in intake and whether the current diet is nutritionally adequate.
3. The presence of persistent gastrointestinal symptoms, such as anorexia, nausea, vomiting, diarrhea, and abdominal pain, which have occurred almost daily for at least 2 weeks, is recorded.
4. The patient's functional capacity is defined as bedridden, suboptimally active, or full capacity.
5. The last feature of the history concerns the metabolic demands of the patient's underlying disease state. Examples of high-stress illnesses are burns, major trauma, and severe inflammation, such as acute colitis. Moderate-stress diseases might be a mild infection or limited malignant tumor.

The features of the physical examination are noted as normal, mild, moderate, or severe alterations. They are

1. Loss of subcutaneous fat measured in the triceps region and the midaxillary line at the level of the lower ribs
2. Muscle wasting in the temporal areas and in the deltoids and quadriceps, as determined by loss of bulk and tone detectable by palpation
3. The presence of edema in the ankle and sacral regions and the presence of ascites
4. Mucosal and cutaneous lesions as well as changes in color and appearance of the patient's hair

The findings of the history and physical examination are used as a global composite to categorize patients as being well nourished (category A) having no abnormal features, moderate or suspected malnutrition (category B), or having severe malnutrition (category C). The rank is assigned on the basis of subjective weighting.

Detsky et al.[47] found that the use of SGA in evaluating hospitalized patients gives reproducible results and there was more than 80% agreement when two blinded observers assessed the same patient.

Since the publication of SGA in 1982,[45] a number of similar techniques were published to identify hospital malnutrition. In 1995, Lennard-Jones et al.[48] recommended that all patients at admission answer four questions, unintentional weight loss, unintentional reduced food intake, height, and weight. A screening tool was later developed based on these questions.[49] In 1994, a mini nutritional assessment (MNA) for geriatric patients was described.[50] This lengthy assessment was later shortened to mini nutritional assessment short form (MNA-SF) and validated as compared with the full MNA.[51]

Kondrup et al.[52] described the nutritional risk screening finalized in the year 2002 (NRS-2002). This method used parameters from controlled clinical trials to select those which were associated with response to nutritional support. NRS-2002 assessed the risk for malnutrition by assigning a score to each of the following:

1. Degree of weight loss
2. BMI
3. Food intake
4. Severity of disease
5. Age

The malnutrition universal screening tool (MUST)[53] developed by the British Association for Parenteral and Enteral Nutrition (BAPEN) used the following parameters:

1. BMI graded as obese, normal, reduced
2. Weight loss <5%, 5%–10%, >10%
3. If disease would reduce food intake

Examination of these different methods show that they all use the same parameters first described for SGA namely progressive weight loss, reduced food intake, loss of function (mobility in MNA-SF), stress of disease. Unlike SGA, the others include anthropometric parameters such as BMI or limb muscle circumference (Table 1.1).

1.4.2 Comparison of Different Methods in Predicting Outcome

A comparison of medical inpatients showed excellent agreement between MUST and SGA[53] despite the fact that SGA did not use BMI. In another study[54] in elderly ICU patients it was shown that MNA-SF, MNA(full), SGA, NRS (using only the nutrition score and eliminating the points for age and disease) were in excellent agreement with each other (κ 0.91–0.96). The ICU patients' NRS however if used in its complete form, falsely elevated the incidence of malnutrition in the elderly and sick due to scores given for age and acute illness, resulting in the loss of specificity. They all showed that hospital LOS was increased in patients identified as malnourished. In addition, all methods showed that malnutrition significantly reduced the proportion discharged home and increased the proportion hospice or those who died (Figure 1.2).

TABLE 1.1
Distribution of Parameters Used to Assess Malnutrition

Parameter	SGA	MUST	MNA-SF	NRS	BAPEN
Age[a]	−	−	−	+	−
Weight loss	+	+	+	+	+
Food intake	+	+	+	+	+
Gastrointestinal disease	+	−	+	−	−
Function	+	−	+	−	−
Disease stress	+	+	+	+	−
BMI	−	+	+	+	+
Arm or calf circumference	−	−	+	−	+

Note: +, use; −, not used. For abbreviations, see text.

[a] The age score weights patients to be misclassified as malnourished if applied to elderly acutely sick patients.

The fact that the predictability of outcome by SGA, which does not need to evaluate BMI or limb circumference, is comparable to other techniques in which BMI or limb circumference needs to be evaluated indicates that it is unnecessary to use any anthropometric measurements to complement SGA which remains as simpler and as effective a tool to assess malnutrition clinically.

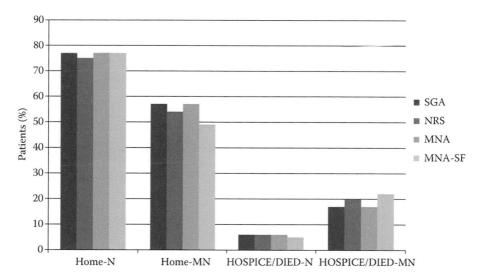

FIGURE 1.2 Malnutrition significantly reduced the proportion discharged home and increased the proportion hospice or those who died. Home-N versus home-MN adjusted for APACHE II: SGA = p 0.001; NRS = p 0.011; MNA = p 0.189; MNS-SF = p 0.189. Hospice/dead-N versus MN adjusted for APACHE II: SGA = p 0.003; NRS = p 0.026; MNA = p 0.090; MNA-SF = p 0.004. N = normal nutrition, MN = malnourished. (Adapted from Sheean, P.M. et al. *Clinical Nutrition* 2013;32(5):1–6.)

REFERENCES

1. McKinlay, A.W. Malnutrition: The spectre at the feast. *Journal of the Royal College of Physicians Edinburgh* 2008;38:317–321.
2. Blackburn, G.L., Bistrian, B.R., Maini, B.S., Schlamm, H.T., and Smith, M.F. Nutritional and metabolic assessment of the hospitalized patient. *Journal of Parenteral and Enteral Nutrition* 1977;1:11.
3. Jeejeebhoy, K.N. Malnutrition, fatigue, frailty, vulnerability, sarcopenia and cachexia: Overlap of clinical features. *Current Opinion in Clinical Nutrition and Metabolic Care* 2012;15:213–219.
4. Pirlich, M., Schutz, T., Norman, K. et al. The German hospital malnutrition study. *Clinical Nutrition* 2006;25:563–572.
5. Shirodkar, M. and Mohandas, K.M. Subjective global assessment: A simple and reliable screening tool for malnutrition among Indians. *Indian Journal of Gastroenterology* 2005;24:246–250.
6. Stanley, K.E. Prognostic factors for survival in patients with inoperable lung cancer. *Journal of the National Cancer Institute* 1980;65:25.
7. DeWys, W.D., Begg, C., Lavin, P.T. et al. Prognostic effect of weight loss prior to chemotherapy in cancer patients. *American Journal of Medicine* 1980;69:491.
8. Morgan, D.B., Hill, G.L., and Burkinshaw, L. The assessment of weight loss from a single measurement of body weight: The problems and limitations. *American Journal of Clinical Nutrition* 1980;33:2101.
9. Harries, A.D., Jones, L.A., Heatley, R.V., and Rhodes, J. Malnutrition in inflammatory bowel disease: An anthropometric study. *Human Nutrition-Clinical Nutrition* 1982;36C:307.
10. Thuluvath, P.J. and Triger, D.R. How valid are our reference standards of nutrition? *Nutrition* 1995;11:731.
11. Hall, J.C.H., O'Quigley, J., Giles, G.R., Appleton, N., and Stocks, H. Upper limb anthropometry: The value of measurement variance studies. *American Journal of Clinical Nutrition* 1980;33:1846.
12. Lukaski, H.C., Johnson, P.E., Bolonchuk, W.W., and Lykken, G.I. Assessment of fat-free mass using bioelectrical impedance measurements of the human body. *American Journal of Clinical Nutrition* 1985;41:810–817.
13. Fagugli, R.M., Pasini, P., Quintaliani, G. et al. Association between extracellular water, left ventricular mass and hypertension in haemodialysis patients. *Nephrology Dialysis Transplantation* 2003;18:2332–2338.
14. Kyle, U.G., Genton, L.C., Slosman, D.O., and Pichard, C. Fat-free and fat-mass percentiles in 5225 healthy subjects aged 15 to 98 years. *Nutrition* 2001;17:534–541.
15. Pichard, C., Kyle, U.G., Morabia, A., Perrier, A., Vermeulen, B., and Unger, P. Nutritional assessment: Lean body mass depletion at hospital admission is associated with an increased length of stay. *American Journal of Clinical Nutrition* 2004;79:613–618.
16. Kotler, D.P., Tierney, A.R., Wang, J., and Pierson, R.N. Jr. Magnitude of body-cell-mass depletion and the timing of death from wasting in AIDS. *American Journal of Clinical Nutrition* 1989;50:444–447.
17. Halliday, A.W., Benjamin, I.S., and Blumgart, L.H. Nutritional risk factors in major hepatobiliary surgery. *Journal of Parenteral and Enteral Nutrition* 1988;12:43–48.
18. Lehr, K., Schober, O., Hundeshagen, H., and Pichlmayr, R. Total body potassium depletion and the need for preoperative nutritional support in Crohn's disease. *Annals of Surgery* 1982;196:709–714.
19. Mann, M.D., Bowie, M.D., and Hansen, J.D. Total body potassium and serum electrolyte concentrations in protein energy malnutrition. *South African Medical Journal* 1975;49:76–78.

20. Fritz, T., Hollwarth, I., Romaschow, M., and Schlag, P. The predictive role of bioelectrical impedance analysis (BIA) in postoperative complications of cancer patients. *European Journal of Surgical Oncology* 1990;16:326–331.
21. Anderson, C.F. and Wochos, D.N. The utility of serum albumin values in the nutritional assessment of hospitalized patients. *Mayo Clinic Proceedings* 1982;57:181.
22. Reinhardt, G.F., Myscofski, J.W., Wilkens, D.B., Dobrin, P.B., Mangan, J.E. Jr., and Stannard, R.T. Incidence and mortality of hypoalbuminemic patients in hospitalized veterans. *Journal of Parenteral Enteral Nutrition* 1980;4:357.
23. Apelgren, K.N., Rombeau, J.L., Twomey, P.L., and Miller, R.A. Comparison of nutritional indices and outcome in critically ill patients. *Critical Care Medicine* 1982;10:305.
24. Keys, A., Brozek, J., Henschel, A., Mickelsen, O., and Taylor, H.L. *The Biology of Human Starvation*. Minneapolis, Minnesota: Minnesota Press; 1950.
25. Russell, D.McR., Prendergast, P.J., Darby, P.L., Garfinkel, P.E., Whitwell, J., and Jeejeebhoy, K.N. A comparison between muscle function and body composition in anorexia nervosa: The effect of refeeding. *American Journal of Clinical Nutrition* 1983;38:229–237.
26. Castenada, C., Charnley, J.M., Evans, W.J., and Crim, M.C. Elderly women accommodate to a low-protein diet with losses of body cell mass, muscle function, and immune response. *American Journal of Clinical Nutrition* 1995;62:30.
27. Hedlund, J.U., Hansson, L.O., and Ortqvist, A.B. Hypoalbuminemia in hospitalized patients with community-acquired pneumonia. *Archives of Internal Medicine* 1995;155:1438.
28. Feitelson, M., Winkler, M.S., Gerrior, S.A. et al. Use of retinol-binding protein and pre-albumin as indicators of response to nutrition therapy. *JADA* 1989;89:684–687.
29. Cano, N., Costanzo-Dufetel, J., Calaf, R. et al. Pre-albumin retinol binding protein-retinol complex in hemodialysis patients. *American Journal of Clinical Nutrition* 1988;47:664–667.
30. Dowd, P.S. and Heatley, R.V. The influence of undernutrition on immunity. *Clinical Science and Molecular Medicine* 1984;66:241–248.
31. Meakins, J.L., Christou, N.V., Shizgal, H.M., and MacLean, L.D. Therapeutic approaches to anergy in surgical patients. *Annals of Surgery* 1979;190:286–296.
32. Dominioni, L. and Diogini, R. Immunological function and nutritional assessment. *Journal of Parenteral and Enteral Nutrition* 1987;11(suppl 5):70S–72S.
33. Degoulet, P., Legrain, M., Reach, I. et al. Mortality risk factors in patients treated by hemodialysis. *Nephron* 1983;31:103–110.
34. Klidjian, A.M., Foster, K.J., Kammerling, R.M., Cooper, A., and Karran, S.J. Relation of anthropometric and dynamometric variables to serious post-operative complications. *British Medical Journal* 1980;2:899–901.
35. Roberts, H.C., Syddall, H.E., Cooper, C., and Sayer, A.A. Is grip strength associated with length of stay in hospitalised older patients admitted for rehabilitation? Findings from the Southampton grip strength study. *Age and Ageing* 2012;41:641–646.
36. Di Trifiletti, A.A., Misino, P., Giannantoni, P., Giannantoni, B., Cascino, A., Fazi, L., Fanelli, F.R., and Laviano, A. Comparison of the performance of four different tools in diagnosing disease-associated anorexia and their relationship with nutritional, functional and clinical outcome measures in hospitalized patients. *Clinical Nutrition* 2013;31:527–532.
37. Roberts, H.C., Denison, H.J., Martin, H.J., Patel, H.P., Syddall, H., Cooper, C., and Sayer, A.A. A review of the measurement of grip strength in clinical and epidemiological studies: Towards a standardised approach. *Age and Ageing* 2011;40:423–429.
38. Tieland, M., Ondine van de Rest, O., Dirks, M.L., van der Zwaluw, N., Mensink, M., van Loon, L.J.C., and de Groot, L.C.P.G.M. Protein supplementation improves physical performance in frail elderly people. *Journal of the American Medical Directors Association* 2012;13:720–726.

39. Russell, D.McR., Leiter, L.A., Whitwell, J., Marliss, E.B., and Jeejeebhoy, K.N. Skeletal muscle function during hypocaloric diets and fasting: A comparison with standard nutritional assessment parameters. *American Journal of Clinical Nutrition* 1983;38:229–237.
40. Rigaud, D., Moukaddem, M., Cohen, B., Malon, D., Reveillard, V., and Mignon, M. Refeeding improves muscle performance without normalization of muscle mass and oxygen consumption in anorexia nervosa patients. *American Journal of Clinical Nutrition* 1997;65:1845–1851.
41. Windsor, J.A. and Hill, G.L. Weight loss with physiologic impairment: A basic indicator of surgical risk. *Annals of Surgery* 1988;207:290.
42. Mijan de la Torre, A., Madapallimattam, A., Cross, A., Armstrong, R.L., and Jeejeebhoy, K.N. Effect of fasting, hypocaloric feeding, and refeeding on the energetics of stimulated rat muscle as assessed by nuclear magnetic resonance spectroscopy. *Journal of Clinical Investigation* 1993;92:114–121.
43. Briet, F., Twomey, C., and Jeejeebhoy, K.N. Effect of malnutrition and short period of refeeding on human peripheral blood mononuclear cell mitochondrial complex I activity. *American Journal of Clinical Nutrition* 2003;77:1304–1311.
44. Jeejeebhoy, K.N., Baker, J.P., Wolman, S.L., Wesson, D.E., Langer, B., Harrison, J.E., and McNeill, K.G. Critical evaluation of the role of clinical assessment and body composition studies in patients with malnutrition and after total parenteral nutrition. *American Journal of Clinical Nutrition* 1982;35(suppl 5):1117–1127.
45. Baker, J., Detsky, A.S., Wesson, D.E., Wolman, S.L., Stewart, S., Whitwell, J., Langer, B., and Jeejeebhoy, K.N. Nutritional assessment: A comparison of clinical judgment and objective measurements. *New England Journal of Medicine* 1982;306:969–972.
46. Detsky, A.S., Baker, J.P., Mendelson, R.A., Wolman, S.L., Wesson, D.A., and Jeejeebhoy, K.N. Evaluating the accuracy of nutritional assessment techniques applied to hospitalized patients: Methodology and comparisons. *Journal of Parenteral and Enteral Nutrition* 1984;8:153.
47. Detsky, A.S., McLaughlin, J.R., Baker, J.P., Johnston, N., Whittaker, S., Mendelson, R.A., and Jeejeebhoy, K.N. What is subjective global assessment of nutritional status? *Journal of Parenteral Enteral and Nutrition* 1987;11:8.
48. Lennard-Jones, J.E., Arrowsmith, H., Davison, C., Denham, A.F., and Micklewright, A. Screening by nurses and junior doctors to detect malnutrition when patients are first assessed in hospital. *Clinical Nutrition* 1995;14:336–340.
49. Weekesa, C.E., Eliab, M., and Emery, P.W. The development, validation and reliability of a nutrition screening tool based on the recommendations of the British Association for Parenteral and Enteral Nutrition (BAPEN). *Clinical Nutrition* 2004;23:1104–1112.
50. Guigos, Y., Vallas, B.J., and Garry, P.J. Mini nutritional assessment: A practical tool for grading the nutritional state of elderly patients. *Facts and Research in Gerontology* 1994;4(suppl 2):15–59.
51. Kaiser, M.J., Bauer, J.M., Ramsch, C. et al. For The Mna-International Group. Validation of the mini nutritional assessment short-form (Mna®-Sf): A practical tool for identification of nutritional status. *The Journal of Nutrition, Health and Aging* 2009;13:782–788.
52. Kondrup, J. Rasmussen, H.H., Hamberg, O., Stanga, Z., and an ad hoc ESPEN Working group. Nutritional Risk Screening (NRS 2002): A new method based on an analysis of controlled clinical trials. *Clinical Nutrition* 2003;22(3):321–336.
53. Stratton, R.J., Hackston, A., Longmore, D., Dixon, R., Price, S., Stroud, M., King, C., and Elia, M. Malnutrition in hospital outpatients and inpatients: Prevalence, concurrent validity and ease of use of the 'malnutrition universal screening tool' ('MUST') for adults. *British Journal of Nutrition* 2004;92:799–808.
54. Sheean, P.M., Peterson, S.J., Chen, Y., Liu, D., Lateef, O., and Braunschweig, C.A. Utilizing multiple methods to classify malnutrition among elderly patients admitted to medical and surgical intensive care units. *Clinical Nutrition* 2013;32(5):1–6.

2 Macronutrient Digestion and Absorption

Kelly A. Tappenden

CONTENTS

2.1 INTRODUCTION

The primary site of macronutrient absorption is the small intestine. Given the diversity of the human diet, the ability for a single layer of specialized epithelial cells to impede the passage of ingested toxins and pathogens, while digesting and subsequently absorbing the ingested nutrients required for life is nothing short of monumental. Absorption of dietary nutrients across the epithelium of the gastrointestinal (GI) tract relies on the coordinated activities of specialized digestive enzymes, the products of which are then transported into the specialized absorptive cells lining the intestinal tract via transport proteins. The digestion of macronutrients into their basic units—monosaccharides, amino acids and peptides, and fatty acids, cholesteryl esters, and phospholipids—permits the absorptive enterocytes of the small intestine to employ specialized transporter proteins that mediate the transfer of these products from the lumen of the intestine into the enterocyte and eventually throughout the body.

2.2 CARBOHYDRATE DIGESTION AND ABSORPTION

2.2.1 Dietary Carbohydrate

Mankind's quest for sugar has been proposed as a driving force for our diversification[1] and one, among many, of the current culprits contributing to obesity and metabolic syndrome.[2] However, dietary carbohydrates also include whole grains and dietary fiber which are associated with important health advantages. The average dietary intake of carbohydrates is roughly 200–300 g, accounting for approximately 50% total energy intake.[3] Given the role of glucose as the primary source of cellular energy, it is fitting that our knowledge of intestinal carbohydrate processing is well developed.

2.2.2 Dietary Carbohydrate Digestion

Initial carbohydrate digestion begins with salivary α-amylase digestion in the mouth. However, salivary amylase function is short-lived due to its rapid degradation when exposed to the low pH environment of the stomach. Upon entrance into the duodenum, pancreatic α-amylase proceeds to digest starches to shorter-chain lengths and disaccharides. Final digestion of dietary carbohydrates occurs at the epithelial brush-border (BB) with membrane-bound disaccharidases that cleave specific bonds to release the monosaccharides—glucose, galactose, and fructose (Table 2.1). Disaccharidase activity is highest among mature enterocytes in the villus tip of the proximal jejunum.[4] The BB location of these disaccharidases creates a microclimate of concentrated monomeric sugars that are readily available for transport across the epithelium.

Only upon digestion to a monosaccharide can carbohydrates be transported across the brush-border membrane (BBM) of the enterocyte. Intact or partially digested oligosaccharide chains are not absorbed making the complete digestion of dietary

TABLE 2.1
Enzymatic Digestion of Dietary Carbohydrates

Enzyme	Target	Product	Source
α-amylase	Starch	Di- and trisaccharides	Saliva Pancreatic secretions
Sucrase	Sucrose	Fructose Glucose	Enterocyte BB
Maltase	Maltose	Glucose	Enterocyte BB
Lactase	Lactose	Glucose Galactose	Enterocyte BB

Note: Various enzymes expressed in the intestinal tract assist in the hydrolysis of polysaccharides to monosaccharides.

carbohydrate vital for the absorption of dietary carbohydrates. To determine a treatment for a defect in carbohydrate assimilation, one must first determine if the defect is primarily the result of insufficient absorptive surface area, defective enzymatic digestion, and/or defective monosaccharide transporter activity.

2.2.3 Intestinal Monosaccharide Absorption

The enterocyte proteins involved in monosaccharide transport across the epithelium are GLUT2, SGLT-1, and GLUT5. The transport of fructose is mediated primarily through a high affinity, low-volume facilitative transporter GLUT5, the product of gene SLC2A5 that mediates the transport of fructose down a concentration gradient.[5] The salient protein involved in glucose and galactose transport across the BB is the sodium glucose/galactose-linked cotransporter 1 (SGLT-1), also called SLC5A1.[6] SGLT-1 is a secondary active transporter that harnesses the inward driving force of sodium created by the sodium potassium ATPase enzyme (Na^+, K^+-ATPase) on the basolateral membrane (BLM), to transfer glucose from the lumen to the cytosol. SGLT-1 transports its solutes with a stoichiometric ratio of 2 sodium molecules: 1 glucose/galactose molecules: 320 water molecules,[7] making it a vital transporter for the absorption of water and explaining the effectiveness of oral rehydration solutions containing appropriate concentrations of sodium, glucose, and water.[8]

Once these monosaccharides—glucose, galactose, and fructose—enter the enterocyte cytoplasm, they are transported down their concentration gradient through the low-affinity, high-volume facilitative hexose transporter GLUT2 (SLC2A2).[9] GLUT2 is a multisolute facilitative transporter that transports glucose, galactose, and fructose across the BLM and into the intracellular space where the nutrients diffuse into the portal circulation. Also important is the fact that this process is normally carried out by enterocytes occupying the upper one-third of the villus. Figure 2.1 illustrates the various carrier-mediated pathways which dietary monosaccharides can be transported across the absorptive enterocyte.

While the plasticity of the described hexose transport system is capable of effective glucose uptake from the lumen when glucose concentrations are between

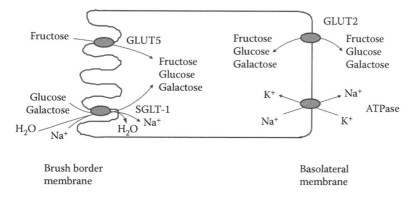

FIGURE 2.1   Monosaccharide transport across the enterocyte BB and BLMs are facilitated via SGLT-1, GLUT5, and GLUT2, and sodium potassium ATPase.

40 and 80 mM, a number of additional hexose transport pathways are implicated to occur in other circumstances. Solvent drag is a process that allows for enormous absorptive capacity through the absorption of solutes, such as the monosaccharides and amino acids, via paracellular channels with water flow driven by the osmotic gradients induced by carrier-mediated absorption. Postabsorptive nutrient concentration in the intracellular space beneath the tight junctional complex can create a microclimate reaching 600–1000 mOsm, which creates an enormous osmotic gradient across the epithelium.[10] In addition, the entrance of glucose has been shown to stimulate a contraction of the actin–myosin fibers in the terminal web cytoskeletal array, which supports the BB and tight junction complex, resulting in a reduction of the enterocyte circumference.[11] As such, the paracellular water flow is facilitated by the contraction of the terminal web within the intestinal epithelium resulting in tight junction dilation and increased pore size between adjacent enterocytes and subsequent flow of nutrients down the osmotic gradient to dilute the intracellular space.

An additional monosaccharide transport pathway is hypothesized to allow for high-volume glucose transport following meal consumption. The classic facilitative glucose transporter, GLUT2, was initially believed to be sequestered to the BLM.[12] However, translocation of GLUT2 to the BBM is postulated to assist SGLT-1 in handling the microclimate of high monosaccharide concentration produced by membrane-bound dissacharidases. This model requires glucose to initially be transported by SGLT-1, whose activity triggers protein kinase-C (PKC) and mitogen-activating protein kinase (MAP-K), the end effect being the rapid translocation of GLUT2 from the BLM into the BBM.[12] The rapid insertion of GLUT2 into the BBM provides a high-volume facilitative hexose transporter capable of handling the microclimate of high monosaccharide concentrated by BB dissacharidases.

2.2.4 REGULATION OF MONOSACCHARIDE TRANSPORT

The intestinal epithelium has an innate capacity for increasing transport volume in response to numerous stimuli.[13] Glucose itself has been shown to elicit rapid increases in active glucose transport mediated via SGLT-1, as have other clinically relevant conditions such as prior exercise, surgical anesthetics, heat-shock injury, epinephrine, and various hormones such as epidermal growth factor and glucagon-like peptide-2 over a longer time.[14] In addition to expression patterns changing in accordance with circadian rhythm, changes in dietary intake of carbohydrates, leading to alterations in the luminal hexose load, have been shown to alter the expression of SGLT-1.[15] Similarly, resection of a significant length of small intestine, which reduces the total absorptive surface area of the remaining gut, stimulates the remnant intestine to mount a number of adaptive responses including enhanced nutrient transport capacity.[16] Conversely, removal of enteral nutrition and provision of nutrients by parenteral route has been shown to induce atrophy of the intestinal tract. The corresponding reduction in absorptive surface with total parenteral nutrition (TPN)-induced the intestinal atrophy area also influences transporter expression and subsequent carbohydrate absorptive capacity.[17] Natural age progression and inhibition of the metabolic enzyme ornithine decarboxylase[18] have been linked to a decrease in intestinal glucose transport indicative of decreased expression of the hexose transporters.[19]

2.2.5 DIETARY FIBER

Fiber is an important dietary carbohydrate which provides an important component of the human diet that escapes enzymatic digestion in the human intestine. Instead, some forms of dietary fiber, termed fermentable fiber, undergo fermentation in the large intestine by the resident microbiota. Similarly, resistant starches and glycoproteins, such as mucins, resist digestion in the small intestine and are fermented by the microbiota.[20]

The fermentation of resistant carbohydrate in the large intestine leads to the production of short-chain fatty acids (SCFAs), with the major forms—acetate (60%–75%), propionate (15%–25%), and butyrate (10%–15%)—produced in fairly consistent ratios across a wide range of species.[20] In an elegant example of symbiosis, these fermentation products, butyrate in particular, serve as the primary metabolic energy source for the colonocytes of the large intestine and can also be readily utilized by the epithelium of the small intestine.

To enter the colonocyte for metabolism or transfer to the portal blood, SCFA must first cross the BBM. The lumen of the colon is generally neutral (pH 7.0), and at this proton concentration, butyrate, and the other SCFA species dissociate to anionic form and cannot readily pass across the colonocyte BB. However, the presence of sodium proton exchange (mediated by NHE3) in the BBM of colonocytes and small intestinal enterocytes acts to acidify the microclimate overlaying these cells that aid in the diffusion of SCFA across the BBM.[21]

In addition, evidence for a carrier-mediated process transporting SCFA across the intestinal BBM also exists. A sodium-dependent SCFA cotransporter, termed sodium-coupled monocarboxylate transporter (SMCT), also called SLC5A8, transports SCFA in a sodium-dependent manner with a stoichiometric ratio of 4:1.[22] In the distal ileum, and throughout the colon, an anion–monocarboxylate exchanger known as MCT1, also as SLC16A1, has been implicated as an important mediator of SCFA uptake from the lumen.[22] MCT1 mediates the exchange of bicarbonate with SCFA, a process that is heightened when the microclimate overlying the BBM is slightly acidic. Studies have also indicated the presence of a chloride/SCFA exchange mechanism in both surface and crypt colonocytes that transports fewer molecules of SCFA when compared to MCT1.[23]

Once across the BBM, SCFA are either rapidly metabolized or transported out of the epithelial cells and into the circulation. Because cytoplasmic pH is neutral, SCFA transported into the epithelial cells undergo dissociation to, or remain in, anionic form. Consequently, the transfer of SCFA across the BLM is likely carrier mediated. There is evidence for bicarbonate/butyrate exchange on the BLM that is functionally distinct from MCT1 located on the BBM.[24]

2.3 PROTEIN DIGESTION AND ABSORPTION

2.3.1 DIETARY PROTEIN

The recommended daily allowance (RDA) for dietary protein intake by an adult is 0.8 g/kg/day.[25] The average daily intake of protein is roughly 70–100 g/day. When coupled in the intestinal lumen with 50–60 g protein/day in the form of digestive enzymes, carrier proteins, antibodies and cellular debris, a large digestive and absorptive load is placed on the intestinal tract.[26] Contained among dietary proteins are the 20 amino acids (AA) utilized by the human body, nine of which are considered essential because they cannot be made endogenously. Physiological AA are those in the L-isomeric configuration, as D-stereoisomers are generally bacterially derived.[27] The intestinal tract has the ability to absorb proteins as AA and peptides resulting from digestion in the lumen by luminal and BB peptidases. It is important to remember the concept of solvent drag and how a portion of the protein assimilation might also occur by noncarrier-mediated passage across the tight junction complex in response to the increased osmotic load and terminal web contraction.

2.3.2 DIETARY PROTEIN DIGESTION

Dietary protein digestion occurs in the following three locations: (1) stomach/intestinal lumen; (2) enterocyte BBM; and (3) enterocyte cytosol. The process begins in the acid environment of the stomach, where the low pH initiates protein hydrolysis, in addition to activating the chief cell-derived pepsinogen, into the protease, pepsin. Gastric pepsin acts to cleave proteins into oligopeptides but is inactivated in the alkaline environment of the duodenum. Next, upon activation by the BBM-bound enterokinase, activated pancreatic zymogens—trypsin, chymotrypsin, elastase, and carboxypeptidase—continue digestion of oligopeptides within the lumen of the small intestine. Luminal digestion of oligopeptides results in the liberation of peptides and free AA. Subsequent BB peptidase digestion of di- and tripeptides yields monomeric AA; however, a significant portion of di- and tripeptides are absorbed intact across BBM. Evidence indicates that di- and tripeptide transport comprise the primary mechanism for protein assimilation in the proximal small intestine and that AA transport comprise the primary transport mechanism that increases qualitatively from the jejunum into the ileum.[26] The gradient of preferential peptide versus AA transport along the length of the small intestine is likely related to the gradual digestion of protein wherein the composition of protein products results in a shift from peptides to free AA as the chyme proceeds down the intestinal tract. Similarly, BB peptidase activity is highest in the villus tip region and demonstrates a decreasing activity gradient along the length of the small intestine.[4]

2.3.3 INTESTINAL PEPTIDE ABSORPTION

The absorption of di- and tripeptides is mediated primarily through the proton-driven peptide transporter PEPT1 (SLC15A1), regardless of their net charge or size. PEPT1 cotransports hydrogen with peptides across the BB in a 1:1 stoichiometric ratio, and the hydrogen is recycled out of the enterocyte by the sodium–hydrogen exchanger 3. Once in the cytoplasm of enterocytes, peptides can either be rapidly digested to monomeric AA by cytoplasmic proteases or transported across the BLM through a peptide transporter distinct from PEPT1 and whose molecular identity is not clearly established.[28] The capacity to transport the intact peptides is particularly important for patients with Hartnup disease, where patients cannot absorb histidine, tryptophan, and phenylalanine, and also for patients with cystinuria type 1, where cytosine transport is defective. These conditions are due to genetic defects in two different AA transporters[28]; however, these patients can assimilate these AA if they are delivered in di- and tripeptide form.[29] Certain oral angiotensin-converting enzyme inhibitors and antibiotics can be transported across the intestinal epithelium via PEPT1.[28] In the case of prodrugs, subsequent proteolytic digestion in the cytoplasm of the enterocyte activates the compound before its release into the circulation.

Normal expression of PEPT1 also follows a distinct circadian rhythm, with maximal daily expression observed during peak feeding times.[30] In accordance with its role in luminal peptide absorption, PEPT1 has been localized to the BBM of villus enterocytes in the small intestine, with very little expression in crypt cells or the colon; this expression follows an increasing expression pattern as one proceeds toward the villus tip.[26] Despite this, PEPT1 expression in the colon is stimulated in patients with inflammatory bowel disease. This latter response is interesting because PEPT1 can also transport the bacterial toxin formyl-Met-Leu-Phe (fMLP), which acts as a chemoattractant for neutrophil recruitment.[31]

2.3.4   INTESTINAL AMINO ACID ABSORPTION

The absorption of AA involves a process that is conceptually similar to monosaccharide absorption. Given that AA do not readily diffuse across cell membrane, membrane-spanning transporter proteins are necessary to traverse the enterocyte BBM. Similarly, the ensuring process involves the following three steps: (1) the substrate (AA, in this case) attaches to the specific transporter binding site; (2) a conformational change in the protein is evoked which exposes the substrate to the opposite membrane face through its central pore; and (3) the substrate is released and the transporter protein returns to its initial conformation. Transport of amino acids across the BBM makes use of sodium-dependent transporters, but also uses the proton-motive force and the gradient of other amino acids to absorb amino acids efficiently from the lumen. In the BLM, AA transporters cooperate with facilitators, such as Na^+/K^+-ATPase, that allow for the necessary movement of ions, including Na^+, H^+, K^+, and/or Cl^-, preventing depletion of cellular nutrients during AA transport. However, in contrast to the monosaccharide absorption, this AA absorption is more complex given differences in the size, polarity, and configuration of the different AA. As such, there is a far greater number of AA transport proteins identified, in addition to those whose activity has only been characterized to date. Furthermore, AA transporters in the human intestine often accept a range of structurally similar AA, such that transport of a given AA may be mediated by multiple transporters with overlapping substrate specificities. With very few exceptions, individual amino acids are transported by more than one transporter, providing backup capacity for absorption in the case of mutational inactivation of a transport system.

Classically, AA transporters have been grouped into systems, based on substrate requirements and kinetic analysis (Table 2.2). However, in recent years, the identification of the specific transport proteins comprising these systems has resulted in a shift to classification based on the sequence similarity into SLC (solute carrier) families (Table 2.2). The biochemistry of each of these AA carriers is beyond the

TABLE 2.2
Intestinal Amino Acid Transporter Classification Systems

Functional Nomenclature		SLC (Solute Carrier) Families	
B⁰/ASC	Na⁺-dependent neutral AA, including alanine, serine, and cystine	SLC1	Excitatory AA transporters
B⁰,⁺	Na⁺-dependent neutral and dibasic AA	SLC6	Neurotransmitter AA transporters
X⁻_AG	Na⁺- and K⁺-dependent anionic AA	SLC7	Glycoprotein-associated AA transports Cationic AA transporters
IMINO or PAT	Proline, betaine	SLC16	Monocarboxylate transporters
b⁰,⁺	Na⁺-independent neutral and dibasic AA	SLC36	Proton-coupled AA transporters
Y⁺	Cationic AA	SLC38	Proton-coupled AA transporters
Gly	Glycine	SLC43	Small neutral AA transporters

scope of this chapter; however, additional details can be found in a comprehensive review by Bröer.[32]

2.3.5 REGULATION OF PEPTIDE/AMINO ACID TRANSPORT

Recent evidence indicates that GI–endocrine interactions actively regulate amino acid and peptide transporter expression and activity. Through functioning as AA sensor–signal–effector pathways, these important transporters in the intestine are becoming the targets of therapeutic strategies ranging from protein–anabolic signals for muscle accretion, upregulated nutrient transport in malabsorption, obesity-related insulin sensitivity, and a wide range of drug delivery innovations.[27]

2.4 LIPID DIGESTION AND ABSORPTION

2.4.1 DIETARY LIPIDS

The essentiality of specific FAs in the human diet was not described until 1963, when a large trial revealed that infants receiving <0.1% of energy as linoleic acid (18:2 n-6) had unsatisfactory growth and developed dry thickened skin. Notably, these problems were reversed when linoleic acid in adequate quantities was added to these infants' diets.[33] Research advances over the past 30 years have shifted our focus from the essentiality of linoleic and linolenic acid (18:3 n-6) to that of the optimal FA composition of the diet. Infant formulas now contain docosahexaenoic acid (22:6 n-3) and arachidonic acid (22:4 n-6) for enhanced neurological, retinal, membrane, and immunological development.[34] Americans adults are encouraged to reduce energy consumed by solid fats in an effort to keep trans FAs as low as possible and limit saturated FAs to <10% of energy consumed.[3]

The predominant form of lipid in the human diet is triglycerides, with other forms including sterols, phospholipids, and free FA. Compared to dietary carbohydrate or protein digestion, dietary lipid digestion is complicated by the aqueous nature of the digestive milieu. As a result, dietary lipids undergo a complex process wherein they "shift" from aqueous to nonaqueous environment in directions opposite to that of their carbohydrate and protein counterparts. As such, several distinguishing processes in the basic digestion and absorption of dietary lipids include their emulsification, hydrolysis, micellization, and uptake by the enterocyte.

2.4.2 DIETARY TRIGLYCERIDE DIGESTION

Dietary triglycerides are digested by lipase enzymes produced in the mouth, stomach, and pancreas to yield diglycerides (2,3-diacylglycerols), monoglycerides (2-monoacylglycerols), and free FA.[35] Lingual lipase is frequently viewed as an auxiliary enzyme for digestion of dietary triglycerides in adults; however, the lipolysis envoked in the oral cavity is postulated to allow for orosensory detection of triglycerides and thereby assist in humankind's evolutionary quest to find nutritive lipids in food.[36] Conversely, in preterm infants, lingual lipase activity is closely coupled with the digestion of approximately 50% of ingested dietary triglycerides prior to exiting the stomach—a phenomenon facilitated by sucking, a high fat diet, and developmental insufficiency in gastric and/or pancreatic lipase activity.[37] Consistent with a compensatory upregulation during triglyceride malabsorption, lingual lipase is also noted to be of particular importance in patients with cystic fibrosis and exocrine pancreatic insufficiency who exhibit varying degrees of steatorrhea because of the lack of pancreatic lipase activity.[38]

In adults, approximately 25% of dietary triglyceride digestion is completed by human gastric lipase, an acid-stable lipolytic enzyme synthesized primarily by the chief cells of the fundic mucosa and secreted into the gastric lumen.[39] However, the vast majority of triglyceride digestion is initiated and completed in the small intestine where emulsification of these lipid molecules is essential for effective digestion. Emulsification is initiated by lipolysis products of dietary lipid and the shearing produced during the passage of chyme through the pyloric sphincter; however, the emulsion is stabilized by interfacing with bile in the duodenum. With the alkalizing action of bicarbonate contained within pancreatic secretions, the pH of the chyme is raised to 6–7, at which point pancreatic lipase becomes quantitatively important in lipid digestion.[39]

Even with emulsified lipid molecules, lipases face a challenge similar to that of other proteins involved in lipid metabolism and intracellular signaling mechanisms. Specifically, these water-soluble enzymes are charged with catalyzing reactions involving water and the water-insoluble target.[40] Further, impairing the action of pancreatic lipase, both structurally and functionally, is the dominating presence of phospholipids, protein, and bile salts at the micelle surface. The efficiency of human pancreatic lipase despite the antagonistic environment of the intestinal lumen is facilitated by colipase. Colipase is secreted from the pancreas as procolipase and activated by trypsin. By binding to lipase in a 1:1 ratio, colipase provides an anchor within the two-dimensional phase by binding to the triglyceride/aqueous interface and facilitates lipase action.[41] The importance of colipase in facilitating human pancreatic lipase absorption is supported by the reported manifestation of severe steatorrhea in two young Assyrian brothers with a confirmed genetic deficiency of colipase.[42]

2.4.3   DIETARY PHOSPHOLIPID AND CHOLESTERYL ESTER DIGESTION

The small intestinal lumen also serves as the venue for digestion of phospholipids and cholesterol esters. Found within the mixed micelle, phosphatidylcholine (lecithin)—the predominant phospholipid—is hydrolyzed by phospholipase A_2, which is secreted from the pancreas as prophospholipase A_2 and then activated by trypsin. The resulting products are lysolecithin (lecithin without the C-2 FA) and a free FA.[43]

Between 10% and 15% of cholesterol present in the diet is found as a cholesteryl ester, necessitating the cleavage of the associated FA prior to being absorbed as free cholesterol by the intestinal epithelium. Cholesterol esterase is secreted by the pancreas as an active enzyme that is stimulated by interaction with bile salts within the mixed micelles. This bile salt stimulation also causes self-aggregation of the enzyme into polymeric forms, which protect the enzyme from proteolytic inactivation. Cholesterol esterase exhibits activity across many lipid molecules, such as triglycerides, phosphoglycerides, esters of fat-soluble vitamins and monoglycerides, and is, therefore, also referred to as carboxyl ester hydrolase and nonspecific esterase.[44]

2.4.4   INTRALUMINAL FORMATION OF MIXED MICELLES

The formation of mixed micelles during intestinal lipid digestion is important to facilitate absorption of lipid substances across the BBM.[45] At a diameter of ~5 nm, the mixed micelle structure allows these monomeric lipid particles to access the intramicrovillus spaces (50–100 nm) of BBM. In addition, the polar bile salts that serve as the foundation for the mixed micelle provide the water solubility necessary for the digested lipid particles to penetrate the unstirred water layer bathing small intestinal epithelium. The unstirred water layer is reported to be the rate limiting uptake of long-chain FA, but not of short or medium-chain FA, whose limiting step occurs at the BBM.[46] The slightly acidic microclimate (pH 5–6) at the unstirred water layer, resulting from actions of the sodium–hydrogen exchanger, decreases FA solubility within the mixed micelle allowing for FA liberation and subsequent absorption across the BBM.

2.4.5   INTESTINAL LIPID ABSORPTION

The cellular mechanism(s) whereby FA traverse the BBM include both passive diffusion and carrier-mediated uptake. Traditionally, the absorption of lipid was thought to be passive wherein lipid molecules would solubilize through the cell membrane in a manner driven by diffusion down the concentration gradient into the enterocyte. The inwardly directed concentration gradient is maintained in the fed state by the high concentration of FA within the intestinal lumen and the rapid scavenging of free FA for triglyceride reformation once inside the enterocyte.

Shaking the long held dogma that FA absorption occurs via passive diffusion, evidence has revealed that enterocyte lipid uptake is saturable, implicating an active transport process.[47] Multiple FA transport proteins that have been identified including plasma membrane-associated FA-binding protein,[48] the fatty acid transport protein 4 (FATP4),[49] and the fatty acid transporter (CD36).[50] Current theories indicate that both passive diffusion and carrier-mediated mechanisms contribute to lipid absorption. At low FA concentrations, carrier-mediated mechanisms take precedence with little passive diffusion occurring. However, when free FA concentration in the intestinal lumen is high, absorption of FA via passive diffusion becomes quantitatively important.[51]

Members of the ATP-binding cassette (ABC) protein family are implicated in the transport of phospholipids, sterols, sphingolipids, bile acids, and related lipid conjugates. These proteins are also important in cell signaling, membrane lipid asymmetry, and metabolite clearance. The importance of these ABC lipid transporters is evident given that mutations in the genes encoding many of these proteins are responsible for severe inherited diseases, such as Tangier disease (defective efflux of cholesterol and phosphatidylcholine from the plasma membrane to the lipid acceptor protein apoA1 [apolipoprotein A1]), neonatal surfactant deficiency, and Stargardt macular degeneration (reduced clearance of retinoid compounds from photoreceptor cells), among others.[52]

Following resynthesization in the enterocyte, components of dietary lipids collect in the enterocyte endoplasmic reticulum as large fat particles. While in the endoplasmic reticulum, a layer of protein is added to enable these lipids to enter the aqueous environment of circulation. The particles pinch off as lipid vesicles and fuse with the Golgi apparatus where carbohydrate is attached to the protein coat—the final step in chylomicron formation. Chylomicrons, a specific class of lipoprotein ranging in diameter from 750 to 6000 nm, are exocytosed into lymphatic circulation. The chylomicron core is comprised of triglycerides, whereas cholesterol ester and phospholipids form more than 80% of the surface coat. Also contained within the surface is the essential apolipoprotein, ApoA. ApoA, synthesized in the small intestine and found in bile, is important for all lipoproteins, including chylomicrons, very low-density lipoproteins (VLDL), and high-density lipoproteins (HDL).[53] Apolipoprotein B (ApoB) is essential for synthesis and secretion of chylomicrons, however, does not appear to be a rate-limiting step.[54]

REFERENCES

1. Hladik CM, Pasquet P, Simmen B. New perspectives on taste and primate evolution: The dichotomy in gustatory coding for perception of beneficent versus noxious substances as supported by correlations among human thresholds. *Am J Phys Anthropol* 2002;117(4):342–348.
2. Soechtig S, Olson S, Marson E, Lazure K, Gibson S, Couric K (Producers), Soechtig, S. (Director). *Fed Up*. United States: Atlas Films; 2014.
3. U.S. Department of Agriculture and U.S. Department of Health and Human Services. *Dietary Guidelines for Americans*, 2010, 7th Edition. Washington, DC: U.S. Government Printing Office.

4. Fan MZ, Stoll B, Jiang R, Burrin DG. Enterocyte digestive enzyme activity along the crypt-villus and longitudinal axes in the neonatal pig small intestine. *J Anim Sci* 2001;79(2):371–381.

5. Jones HF, Butler RN, Brooks DA. Intestinal fructose transport and malabsorption in humans. *Am J Physiol Gastrointest Liver Physiol* 2011;300(2):G202–G206.

6. Hediger MA, Coady MJ, Ikeda TS, Wright EM. Expression cloning and cDNA sequencing of the Na+/glucose co-transporter. *Nature* 1987;330(6146):379–381.

7. Zeuthen T. Molecular water pumps. *Rev Physiol Biochem Pharmacol* 2000;141:97–151.

8. Gagnon MP, Bissonnette P, Deslandes LM, Wallendorff B, Lapointe JY. Glucose accumulation can account for the initial water flux triggered by Na+/glucose cotransport. *Biophys J* 2004;86(1 Pt 1):125–133.

9. Kellett GL, Brot-Laroche E, Mace OJ, Leturque A. Sugar absorption in the intestine: The role of GLUT2. *Annu Rev Nutr* 2008;28:35–54.

10. Pappenheimer JR. On the coupling of membrane digestion with intestinal absorption of sugars and amino-acids. *Am J Physiol* 1993;265(3 Pt 1):G409–G417.

11. Keller TC, 3rd, Conzelman KA, Chasan R, Mooseker MS. Role of myosin in terminal web contraction in isolated intestinal epithelial brush-borders. *J Cell Biol* 1985;100(5):1647–1655.

12. Kellett GL. The facilitated component of intestinal glucose absorption. *J Physiol* 2001;531(Pt 3):585–595.

13. Steyermark AC, Lam MM, Diamond J. Quantitative evolutionary design of nutrient processing: glucose. *Proc Natl Acad Sci USA* 2002;99(13):8754–8759.

14. Shirazi-Beechey SP, Moran AW, Batchelor DJ, Daly K, Al-Rammahi M. Glucose sensing and signalling; regulation of intestinal glucose transport. *Proc Nutr Soc* 2011; 70(2):185–193.

15. Pan X, Terada T, Okuda M, Inui K. The diurnal rhythm of the intestinal transporters SGLT1 and PEPT1 is regulated by the feeding conditions in rats. *J Nutr* 2004; 134(9):2211–2215.

16. Ray EC, Avissar NE, Sax HC. Methods used to study intestinal nutrient transport: Past and present. *J Surg Res* 2002;108(1):180–190.

17. Tappenden KA, McBurney MI. Systemic short-chain fatty acids rapidly alter gastrointestinal structure, function, and expression of early response genes. *Dig Dis Sci* 1998;43(7):1526–1536.

18. Johnson LR, Brockway PD, Madsen K, Hardin JA, Gall DG. Polyamines alter intestinal glucose transport. *Am J Physiol* 1995;268(3 Pt 1):G416–G423.

19. Drozdowski L, Woudstra T, Wild G, Clandinin MT, Thomson AB. The age-associated decline in the intestinal uptake of glucose is not accompanied by changes in the mRNA or protein abundance of SGLT1. *Mech Ageing Dev* 2003;124(10–12):1035–1045.

20. Puertollano E, Kolida S, Yaqoob P. Biological significance of short-chain fatty acid metabolism by the intestinal microbiome. *Curr Opin Clin Nutr Metab Care* 2014; 17(2):139–44.

21. Astbury SM, Corfe BM. Uptake and metabolism of the short-chain fatty acid butyrate, a critical review of the literature. *Curr Drug Metab* 2012;13(6):815–21.

22. Halestrap AP. Monocarboxylic acid transport. *Compr Physiol* 2013;3(4):1611–1643.

23. Rajendran VM, Binder HJ. Characterization and molecular localization of anion transporters in colonic epithelial cells. *Ann N Y Acad Sci* 2000;915:15–29.

24. Sellin JH. SCFAs: The enigma of weak electrolyte transport in the colon. *News Physiol Sci* 1999;14:58–64.

25. Food and Nutrition Board, Institute of Medicine. *Dietary Reference Intakes for Energy, Carbohydrate, Fiber, Fat, Fatty Acids, Cholesterol, Protein, and Amino Acids.* Washington, DC: National Academies Press, 2005.

26. Daniel H. Molecular and integrative physiology of intestinal peptide transport. *Annu Rev Physiol* 2004;66:361–384.
27. Poncet N, Taylor PM. The role of amino acid transporters in nutrition. *Curr Opin Clin Nutr Metab Care* 2013;16:57–65.
28. Daniel H, Kottra G. The proton oligopeptide cotransporter family SLC15 in physiology and pharmacology. *Pflugers Arch* 2004;447(5):610–618.
29. Kleta R, Romeo E, Ristic Z et al. Mutations in SLC6A19, encoding B0AT1, cause Hartnup disorder. *Nat Genet* 2004;36(9):999–1002.
30. Pan X, Terada T, Irie M, Saito H, Inui K. Diurnal rhythm of H+-peptide cotransporter in rat small intestine. *Am J Physiol Gastrointest Liver Physiol* 2002;283(1):G57–G64.
31. Buyse M, Charrier L, Sitaraman S, Gewirtz A, Merlin D. Interferon-gamma increases hPepT1-mediated uptake of di-tripeptides including the bacterial tripeptide fMLP in polarized intestinal epithelia. *Am J Pathol* 2003;163(5):1969–1977.
32. Bröer S. Amino acid transport across mammalian intestinal and renal epithelia. *Physiol Rev* 2008;88:249–286.
33. Hansen AE, Wiese HF, Boelsche AN, Haggard ME, Adam JD, Davis H. Role of linoleic acid in infant nutrition. *Pediatrics* 1963;312:171–192.
34. Tai EK, Wang XB, Chen ZY. An update on adding docosahexaenoic acid (DHA) and arachidonic acid (AA) to baby formula. *Food Funct* 2013;4(12):1767–1775.
35. Moreau H, Laugier R, Gargouri Y, Ferrato F, Verger R. Human preduodenal lipase is entirely of gastric fundic origin. *Gastroenterology* 1988;95(5):1221–1226.
36. Kawai T, Fushiki T. Importance of lipolysis in oral cavity for orosensory detection of fat. *Am J Physiol: Regul Integr Comp Physiol* 2003;285(2):R447–R454.
37. Lindquist S, Hernell O. Lipid digestion and absorption in early life: An update. *Curr Opin Clin Nutr Metab Care* 2010;13(3):314–320.
38. Abrams CK, Hamosh M, Hubbard VS, Dutta SK, Hamosh P. Lingual lipase in cystic fibrosis. Quantitation of enzyme activity in the upper small intestine of patients with exocrine pancreatic insufficiency. *J Clin Invest* 1984;73(2):374–382.
39. Carriere F, Barrowman JA, Verger R, Laugier R. Secretion and contribution to lipolysis of gastric and pancreatic lipases during a test meal in humans. *Gastroenterology* 1993;105(3):876–888.
40. Entressangles B, Desnuelle P. Action of pancreatic lipase on aggregated glyceride molecules in an isotropic system. *Biochim Biophys Acta* 1968;159(2):285–295.
41. Brownlee IA, Forster DJ, Wilcox MD, Dettmar PW, Seal CJ, Pearson JP. Physiological parameters governing the action of pancreatic lipase. *Nutr Res Rev* 2010;23(1):146–54.
42. Hildebrand H, Borgstrom B, Bekassy A, Erlanson-Albertsson C, Helin I. Isolated co-lipase deficiency in two brothers. *Gut* 1982;23(3):243–246.
43. Bakala N'Goma JC, Amara S, Dridi K, Jannin V, Carrière F. Understanding the lipid-digestion processes in the GI tract before designing lipid-based drug-delivery systems. *Ther Deliv* 2012;3(1):105–124.
44. Ghosh S. Early steps in reverse cholesterol transport: Cholesteryl ester hydrolase and other hydrolases. *Curr Opin Endocrinol Diabetes Obes* 2012;19(2):136–41.
45. Hofmann AF, Borgstrom B. Physico-chemical state of lipids in intestinal content during their digestion and absorption. *Fed Proc* 1962;21:43–50.
46. Thomson AB, Schoeller C, Keelan M, Smith L, Clandinin MT. Lipid absorption: passing through the unstirred layers, brush-border membrane, and beyond. *Can J Physiol Pharmacol* 1993;71(8):531–555.
47. Phan CT, Tso P. Intestinal lipid absorption and transport. *Front Biosci* 2001;6:D299–D319.
48. Stremmel W, Lotz G, Strohmeyer G, Berk PD. Identification, isolation, and partial characterization of a fatty acid binding protein from rat jejunal microvillous membranes. *J Clin Invest* 1985;75(3):1068–1076.

49. Schaffer JE, Lodish HF. Expression cloning and characterization of a novel adipocyte long chain fatty acid transport protein. *Cell* 1994;79:427–436.
50. Abumrad NA, el-Maghrabi MR, Amri EZ, Lopez E, Grimaldi PA. Cloning of a rat adipocyte membrane protein implicated in binding or transport of long-chain fatty acids that is induced during preadipocyte differentiation. Homology with human CD36. *J Biol Chem* 1993;268:17665–17668.
51. Frohnert BI, Bernlohr DA. Regulation of fatty acid transporters in mammalian cells. *Prog Lipid Res* 2000;39(1):83–107.
52. Quazi F1, Molday RS. Lipid transport by mammalian ABC proteins. *Essays Biochem* 2011;50(1):265–290.
53. Go MF, Schonfeld G, Pfleger B, Cole TG, Sussman NL, Alpers DH. Regulation of intestinal and hepatic apoprotein synthesis after chronic fat and cholesterol feeding. *J Clin Invest* 1988;81(5):1615–1620.
54. Hayashi H, Fujimoto K, Cardelli JA, Nutting DF, Bergstedt S, Tso P. Fat feeding increases size, but not number, of chylomicrons produced by small intestine. *Am J Physiol* 1990;259(5 Pt 1):G709–G719.

3 Malabsorption

Zhouwen Tang and Joseph H. Sellin

CONTENTS

The diagnosis and therapy of malabsorption should ideally be a logical integration of recognizing clinical symptoms and signs, understanding physiology and pathophysiology, utilizing appropriate laboratory testing, and choosing a specific treatment. However, the ideal is not frequently reached because of vagaries in history and physical exam along with difficulties in obtaining or interpreting tests for malabsorption. This chapter will discuss: (1) the clinical presentation of malabsorption, (2) classification of malabsorption, and (3) a logical approach for evaluation of suspected malabsorption.

Malabsorption syndromes are characterized by three discrete, but interrelated, factors: (1) weight loss and fatigue due to a failure to absorb an adequate amount of calories; (2) symptoms due to deficiency of specific nutrients and vitamins; (3) diarrhea caused by the effect of malabsorbed molecules on intestinal function. Although diarrhea frequently accompanies malabsorption, malabsorption may occur without diarrhea. Diarrhea, which is much more common than malabsorption, is usually not associated with malabsorption. Although the workups for the two often overlap, it is important for the clinician to keep in mind the specific goals of testing for one or the other.

3.1   CLASSIFICATION OF MALABSORPTION

A first step in understanding the spectrum of malabsorption is an accurate classification scheme which will guide the differential diagnosis and result in a parsimonious utilization of appropriate testing.

3.1.1   GLOBAL VERSUS NUTRIENT SPECIFIC

Global malabsorption refers to the condition where there is a generalized impairment of the processes of assimilation of a broad range of carbohydrates, fat, and protein. The clinical consequences of global malabsorption therefore are protean, including weight loss, nutritional deficiencies, and diarrhea.

Nutrient-specific malabsorption, in contrast, involves a very discrete defect in the intestinal capacity to absorb a single molecule (or family of molecules) without impairment of the absorption of the wider spectrum of fat, protein, and carbohydrates. The most common example of nutrient specific malabsorption is lactase deficiency/lactose intolerance. The presentation of nutrient-specific malabsorption will obviously be dependent on the potential development of a specific nutritional deficiency or the effect of the malabsorbed substance on the gastrointestinal tract. Diarrhea may or may not occur depending on the interaction of the malabsorbed molecule with the intestine and the colon. Nutrient specific malabsorption is rarely associated with weight loss. Given the spatial specificity of the absorption of some nutrients, one might be able to predict whether a disease affecting a specific region of the small intestine may lead to malabsorption of a specific nutrient.

3.1.2 GLOBAL MALABSORPTION: MALDIGESTION VERSUS MALABSORPTION

Although somewhat arbitrary, distinguishing between maldigestion and malabsorption is a useful heuristic strategy in better understanding the interpretation of diagnostic studies. It is probably more accurate to think of maldigestion as a discrete subcategory of malabsorption. Many of the diagnostic studies utilized in a malabsorption workup are designed to determine whether the problem exists because of a failure within the lumen of the intestine (maldigestion) or at the intestinal mucosa (malabsorption). However, clinical realities often make it impossible to make such clear distinctions. Other factors may come into play such as intraluminal consumption of nutrients and altered motility that do not fit neatly into these categories.

3.1.2.1 Maldigestion

Nutrients are broken down, hydrolyzed, and/or solubilized within the intestinal lumen to simpler components that can be transported by the intestinal mucosa. Bile acids solubilize dietary fat, forming micelles that are then subject to enzymatic digestion. Pancreatic amylase hydrolyzes starches and complex carbohydrates into mono- and disaccharides. Lipase is responsible for metabolizing triglycerides into monoglycerides and fatty acids. Clinically, chronic pancreatitis is the most common etiology of maldigestion; however, additional pancreatic diseases including cystic fibrosis, pancreatic duct obstruction secondary to tumors, and pancreatic resections may also lead to maldigestion. Deficiencies in luminal bile acids, generally associated with cholestatic diseases, may also lead to maldigestion.

3.1.2.2 Intraluminal Consumption of Nutrients

The normal small intestine is relatively sterile, certainly compared to the colon. An increase in bacteria in the small intestine may lead to a competition within the intestine between the intestinal mucosa and the luminal bacteria for nutrients entering the small bowel. Bacteria frequently are the winners. They are not very picky eaters and may digest intraluminal carbohydrate and protein before they reach the intestinal lumen. The increase in small bowel bacteria may also induce a nonspecific mucosal inflammation in the duodenum and jejunum which may impair villus absorption.

The classic case of intraluminal consumption is infection with *Diphyllobothrium latum*, a fish tapeworm that avidly consumes vitamin B_{12}. Although cited in almost every textbook, it is incredibly uncommon, at least in the United States.

3.1.2.3 Mucosal Malabsorption

In contrast, mucosal malabsorption occurs when the problem lies specifically in the small bowel epithelium. Brush border enzymes are responsible for breaking down peptides and disaccharides into smaller molecules, for example, monosaccharides and amino acids. The most common example of mucosal malabsorption is celiac sprue.

3.1.2.4   Postmucosal Malabsorption (Defective Chylomicron Transport)

Impaired lymphatic transport prevents the movement of dietary fat into the systemic circulation. This may occur with congenital disease (e.g., primary intestinal lymphangiectasia) or acquired disease such as a lymphoma, small bowel metastases, Whipple's disease, retroperitoneal fibrosis, and rarely, Crohn's disease. Additionally very rare congenital diseases that block intraepithelial trafficking of lipids may be included in this category, such as abetalipoproteinemia and chylomicron retention disease.

3.1.2.5   Altered Motility/Decreased Mixing

Appropriate digestion requires both (i) an adequate time for nutrients to mix with digestive enzymes and bile acids and (ii) sufficient contact time with the intestinal mucosa for brush border enzymes to accomplish their tasks. If there is rapid gastric emptying or intestinal transit, then neither of these may occur. Clinical conditions that may be associated with decreased mixing include gastric surgery, autonomic neuropathy, and hyperthyroidism. Pancreaticocibal asynchrony refers to a condition in which pancreatic digestive enzymes never catch up with nutrients that rapidly transit through the upper small intestine, therefore never providing the opportunity for intraluminal digestion.

3.2   CLINICAL PRESENTATION

There is a long list of diseases that may cause malabsorption. Many of them are quite rare (Table 3.1). We will focus on the presentation and diagnosis of the more common malabsorption syndromes including celiac disease, pancreatic insufficiency, Crohn's disease, and bacterial overgrowth.

Weight loss and fatigue are hallmarks of global malabsorption syndromes. These are due to calorie depletion and a resulting catabolic state. Anemia may be a contributing factor and may be secondary to either deficiencies of iron or vitamin B_{12}/folate. Calorie deprivation may lead to some constitutional symptoms such as amenorrhea and infertility. The weight loss in malabsorption, in contradistinction to other diseases associated with weight loss, may be seen with a good appetite and even hyperphagia. Perhaps the only other clinical entity combining weight loss with hyperphagia is hyperthyroidism. However, an increased appetite is far from universal. Some individuals may actually decrease oral intake because of an exacerbation of symptoms such as diarrhea or abdominal pain. In children, growth retardation may be an important clue to the presence of calorie deprivation and malabsorption.

Diarrhea is the other cardinal symptom associated with global malabsorption. There are many factors that may lead to diarrhea. Diffuse inflammatory diseases of the small bowel and/or surgical resection decrease the effective absorptive area. Unabsorbed carbohydrates can lead to an osmotic diarrhea. Unabsorbed bile acids and fatty acids that pass through the ileocecal valve into the colon can stimulate chloride secretion, leading to a secretory diarrhea. Bile acid malabsorption occurs most commonly in diseases that interrupt the enterohepatic circulation such as ileal Crohn's disease.

TABLE 3.1

Causes of Malabsorption

Systemic and autoimmune diseases	Primary immunodeficiency
	Scleroderma
	Systemic lupus erythematosus
	Mixed connective tissue disease
Neuroendocrine diseases	Diabetes mellitus
	Addison disease
	Hyperthyroidism
	Neuroendocrine tumors (carcinoids)
	Pancreatic neuroendocrine tumors (glucagonoma, somatostatinoma, Zollinger–Ellison)
Gastric diseases	Autoimmune atrophic gastritis
Pancreatico-biliary diseases	Pancreatic exocrine insufficiency (chronic pancreatitis, cystic fibrosis)
	Congenital pancreatic enzyme deficiencies
	Pancreatic and biliary cancers
Liver diseases	Cirrhosis
	Portal hypertension
	Sclerosing cholangitis
Intestinal diseases	Crohn's disease
	Celiac disease
	Small intestinal bacterial overgrowth
	Bile acid malabsorption
	Amyloidosis
	Sarcoidosis
	Ischemic injury
	Eosinophilic enteritis
	Intestinal lymphoma
Infectious diseases	HIV enteropathy
	Protozoan infections (cryptosporidiosis, giardiasis)
	Helminthic infections (strongyloidiasis)
	Tropical sprue
	Whipple's disease
	Tuberculosis
Other	Drug induced
	Gastric and intestinal bypass or resection

Although global malabsorption may not necessarily present with additional abdominal symptoms beyond diarrhea, abdominal pain, and flatulence are frequent and may result from gas production from colonic bacterial metabolism of carbohydrates. Foul smelling stool is thought to be a tell-tale sign of malabsorption although the reliability of this finding has never been truly tested. The "flushability" of a bowel movement is more a reflection of the air content of the stool or the quality of plumbing rather than the amount of steatorrhea.

Nutrient deficiencies may occur in either global or nutrient specific malabsorptive states. Although there is a wide gamut of potential deficiencies that might suggest malabsorption, the most common ones are fairly nonspecific and the uncommon ones are so rare as to prompt a case report. For example, the fat soluble vitamin D is frequently low with steatorrhea, but it is also a common finding in the general population with no malabsorption. Although those rare occurrences of niacin deficiency and subsequent pellagra may occur because of malabsorption, they may just as frequently be a result of drug induced side effects (e.g., hydralazine). (Lisa Sanders. Dizzying symptoms, *NYT* June 3, 2010.)

The disaccharide lactose, the major carbohydrate in milk, must be hydrolyzed to glucose and galactose by lactase prior to absorption. Because mammals do not ingest milk after weaning, the natural state of evolutionary affairs is down regulation of lactase in adulthood. However, two distinct enzymes in the lactase promoter have occurred that appear to prevent this normally occurring down regulation, one appearing first in northwest Europe, the other in southern Africa. In that sense, adult lactase persistence is the abnormality, not lactase deficiency.

Lactose is a frequent suspect for many gastrointestinal symptoms, although it is not clear if it is actually at fault. Diarrhea is likely to be due to lactose intolerance only if the patient ingests >12 g/day (240 mL of milk or its equivalent in other dairy foods).[1] Milk ingested in large volumes which may empty rapidly into the small intestine is more likely to cause symptoms than when it is incorporated into solid foods[2] (see Tables 3.2 through 3.4).

More subtle gastrointestinal symptoms and extraintestinal findings not specifically associated with nutrient deficiencies may provide the astute clinician with some clues as to the etiology of malabsorption.

3.3 DIAGNOSTIC STUDIES

Most reviews and chapters on malabsorption describe multiple studies that promise the capability to come to an accurate and speedy diagnosis. However, in the real world of a practicing clinician, things are not quite as simple as might appear from the literature. There are several reasons for this. Some tests are simply no longer available (or not available in the United States) because the necessary materials, usually

TABLE 3.2
Malabsorbed Nutrients

Nutrient	Defect	Symptoms
Lactose	Lactase	Diarrhea, bloating
Lactulose	Naturally nondigestible	Diarrhea, bloating
Fructose/sucrose	Congenital sucrase–isomaltase deficiency; incomplete fructose absorption	Diarrhea, bloating, exacerbation of IBS symptoms
FODMAPs	Limited mucosal absorptive capacity	Diarrhea, bloating, IBS
Trehalose	Trehalase	Diarrhea or vomiting after ingestion of mushrooms
Vitamin B_{12}	Autoimmune gastritis, atrophic gastritis, pancreatic insufficiency, bacterial overgrowth	Paresthesias, peripheral neuropathy, macrocytic anemia

TABLE 3.3

Clinical Presentations of Nutrient Deficiencies

Nutrient Deficiency	Clinical Presentation
Vitamin D, calcium	Osteopenia (osteomalacia and osteoporosis) (common)
	Tetany, muscle weakness, paresthesias (rare)
Vitamin B complexes	Glossitis, cheilosis, stomatitis
Zinc	Acrodermatitis
Niacin	Hyperpigmented dermatitis, pellagra, diarrhea, neurological symptoms
Vitamin C	Scurvy, perifollicular hemorrhage
Vitamin A	Night blindness
Vitamin B_{12}	Paresthesias, peripheral neuropathy
	Macrocytic anemia
Folate	Macrocytic anemia
	Neurologic symptoms
Thiamine	Peripheral neuropathy
Iron	Microcytic anemia, angular cheilitis, koilonychia, glossitis

TABLE 3.4

Extraintestinal Manifestations of Malabsorption Syndromes

Celiac disease	Dermatitis herpetiformis
	Iron deficiency anemia
	Peripheral neuropathy
	Ataxia
	Elevated liver enzymes
Crohn's disease	Erythema nodosum
	Pyoderma gangrenosum
	Axial and polyarticular peripheral arthritis
Addison's disease	Hyperpigmentation

radioisotopic tracers, are not obtainable. The prime example of this is the Schilling test. It is technically simple and safe to do and can provide important information. But the lack of the Cobalt-59 intrinsic factor makes it no longer possible to routinely do this test. Other tests are only done by a limited number (or sometimes only a single investigator) in a few academic medical centers. Examples of this include fecal bile acids or a 13 D-xylose breath test. Finally, there are tests that are done so rarely that it is impossible to assess the accuracy and reproducibility of the results, with the secretin stimulation test for pancreatic function as an example. In addition, both patients and laboratory personnel find tests involving stool collections somewhat odious. In our review of studies below, we will mention the availability of specific tests.

3.3.1 ENDOSCOPY IN THE WORKUP OF MALABSORPTION

Historically, endoscopy in the evaluation of malabsorption was generally relegated to the end of a long list of tests, almost as an afterthought. However, recognizing the central role of the gastroenterologist/endoscopist in the work up of malabsorption, it is reasonable to understand clearly both well-defined and possible roles of upper gastrointestinal (GI) endoscopy (EGD). The role of EGD has been studied in the diagnosis of celiac disease, probably the most common cause of malabsorption amenable to small bowel biopsy. However, these studies usually involve preselected individuals with positive celiac serologies and therefore do not address the more generalized issue of the utility of EGD, specifically, in the work up for suspected malabsorption. Although there may be endoscopic findings that suggest a specific etiology, for example, scalloping (see below), the true value of EGD is that it is a safe, easy, and reliable method to obtain small bowel biopsies (see Section 3.3.1.1) Endoscopic clues may suggest additional uncommon causes of diarrhea, such as aphthous ulcers (Crohn's) or white punctate lesions (primary or secondary lymphangiectasia). Endoscopy may also provide some novel diagnostic opportunities beyond visualization and biopsy, including duodenal aspiration for Giardia infection, endoscopy-assisted pancreatic function tests, and quantitative bacterial culture for the diagnosis of small bowel bacterial overgrowth. These may not be commonly performed, but may provide another diagnostic avenue in difficult cases that may have eluded diagnosis by other means.

3.3.1.1   Small Bowel Biopsies

Over the last 50 years, the role of small bowel biopsies in the diagnosis of malabsorption has changed greatly. Adequate sampling of the small bowel for histologic diagnosis has evolved from a laborious task to a quick and easy 5-min procedure. A variety of complex tubes with ingenious devices at the tip were passed orally under fluoroscopic guidance beyond the duodenal bulb. Most of them "sucked up" a bit of the mucosal surface into a small orifice of a capsule (Crosby capsules, Rubin capsules), detached the section by a sharp knife blade, and withdrew it into the capsule. With some experience, a small bowel biopsy could be obtained within 30–60 min in >50% of the time.[3,4] One of the first studies to demonstrate clinical usefulness of small bowel biopsies was a cohort study of 41 Peace Corps volunteers with a history of frequent diarrhea and weight loss while in service in Pakistan. Five patients with inflammatory changes on jejunal biopsies obtained in Pakistan received follow up jejunal biopsies within 44 months of return. All five subjects demonstrated normal histology on follow up biopsies, including two subjects with continued diarrhea.[5]

Today, a small bowel biopsy is a simple endoscopic procedure with a 100% technical success rate. A normal endoscopic appearance of the small bowel mucosa should never deter one from obtaining biopsies for histologic examination. The dilemma in determining the effectiveness of EGD in this evaluation is that there are many rare or uncommon causes that may only be diagnosed by small bowel biopsies.

The most common diagnosis made on small bowel biopsies is celiac disease. In a large data base study evaluating the diagnostic value of duodenal biopsies in 28,000 patients, there was a significant histologic finding in 8.6% of the 5197 patients in whom the primary indication for endoscopy was diarrhea. These findings were all related to a spectrum of celiac disease, including intraepithelial lymphocytosis (5.6%), variable villous atrophy (1.4%), and celiac disease (1.6%).[6] For the

TABLE 3.5
Diagnoses by Small Bowel Biopsy

Diffuse lesions	Whipple's disease
	Mycobacteria avium intracellulare
	Abetalipoproteinemia
Patchy lesions	Lymphoma
Definitive diagnosis by biospy	Lymphangectasia
	Amyloidosis
	Crohn's
	Giardiasis
Suggestive but not diagnostic	Celiac disease
	Olmesartan
	Refractory sprue
	Tropical sprue
	Megaloblastic anemias

976 patients in this database whose primary indication was suspected or confirmed sprue, intraepithelial lymphocytosis was found in 8.9%, variable villous atrophy in 11.2%, and overt sprue in 12%. No nonsprue-related histopathology was identified.

Nevertheless, because accurate diagnosis of uncommon diseases such as Whipple's disease or eosinophilic gastroenteritis may only be achieved with endoscopy and small bowel biopsy, it is reasonable to include EGD earlier rather than later in the diagnostic workup. Dialog between the clinician and the pathologist is usually necessary to consider these rare diagnoses and pursue the appropriate histologic techniques, for example, Congo red staining for amyloidosis, polymerase chain reaction for Tropheryma whipplei, immunohistochemical staining for lymphoma (see Table 3.5).

3.3.1.2 Endoscopic Diagnosis of Celiac Disease

Serological testing for celiac disease has advanced to impressive levels of sensitivity and specificity. Antitissue transglutaminase antibodies improve significantly upon the diagnostic accuracy of traditional antigliadin antibodies as well as the cost and reliability of endomysial antibody testing.[7] Though antitissue transglutaminase IgA assay, with the addition of immunoglobulin A levels, is now recommended as initial screening in low risk populations, histological examination remains mandatory for confirmation of disease and is the recommended initial test in patients with high suspicion for celiac disease.[8]

Histological evidence of celiac disease include increasing numbers of duodenal intraepithelial lymphocytes (IEL) and abnormalities of villous and crypt architecture. Because these changes are dynamic, several classifications schemes, including the Marsh,[9] Marsh-Oberhuber,[10] and Corazza[11] classifications, have been developed to capture the continuum of histological changes in celiac disease. A common histologic dilemma is the significance of intraepithelial lymphocytosis in isolation. Other relatively common causes of increased duodenal IELs include *Helicobacter pylori* infection and nonsteroidal anti-inflammatory drug (NSAID) use.[12] Other causes of villous atrophy include small intestine bacterial overgrowth (SIBO) and malnutrition. Although much has been made of the fact that histological evidence may not be diagnostic in isolation, combined histological and serological evidence is very strong evidence of celiac disease.[8]

The effectiveness of EGD in diagnosing celiac disease may depend on the biopsy protocols employed. The most recent expert consensus has settled upon 4–6 duodenal biopsies for the highest diagnosis yield. Undersampling of the duodenal mucosa invites missed diagnoses due to inadequate sample orientation as well as the sometimes patchy nature of villous atrophy. At least four regular forceps biopsies should be taken from the distal duodenum. In a retrospective study of 93 patients with histologically confirmed celiac disease, only 86% would have been diagnosed with a single duodenal biopsy and yield improved to the ideal 100% only after at least four biopsies.[13] Recent studies demonstrating isolated villus atrophy may occur in the duodenal bulb alone in celiac disease suggest that strategies for adequate biopsy sampling should be modified to include biopsies from the bulb as well as the second and third portion of the duodenum, totaling at least six tissue samples.[14,15] Despite guidelines suggesting that screening for celiac disease is more effective with more than four biopsies, this occurs in <40% of cases.[16] It may reasonable to take one biopsy/pass to better preserve the architecture and simplify the pathologist's tasks of accurately orienting the specimen and identifying villus/crypt changes.

3.3.1.3   Endoscopic Diagnosis of Pancreatic Insufficiency

The practical role of endoscopy in the diagnosis of chronic pancreatitis is evolving from endoscopic retrograde cholangiopancreatography (ERCP) to endoscopic ultrasound (EUS). This is driven by the limitation of traditional invasive and noninvasive pancreatic imaging. Trans-abdominal ultrasound does not reliably demonstrate the pancreas. Multidetector computed tomography (CT) may demonstrate gland atrophy and calcifications but is not reliable for small duct disease or early chronic pancreatitis. Magnetic resonance imaging (MRI) and magnetic resonance cholangiopancreatography (MRCP) are much more reliable and accurate but similarly limited in detection of early disease. Secretin-enhanced MRCP improves sensitivity to early chronic pancreatitis.[17] ERCP may be more sensitive to early chronic pancreatitis but is associated with complications and imaging is limited to the pancreatic ductal system without being able to directly assess the parenchyma.[18] ERCP is rarely performed purely for diagnosis due to these limitations.

EUS has been established as a useful test for diagnosis of early small duct or "minimal change" chronic pancreatitis. Findings of early parenchymal changes on EUS may predict eventual development of ductal abnormalities on ERCP[19] and both parenchymal and ductal features have been incorporated into the Rosemont criteria for diagnosis of chronic pancreatitis, a consensus diagnostic system.[20] Thus far, validation studies of the Rosemont criteria have not shown increased interobserver agreement when compared to traditional diagnostic criteria despite the Rosemont criteria being more complex and more nuanced. Further validation studies are needed, especially those that correlate with pancreatic histology.[21–23] A number of advanced imaging techniques, including digital image analysis and elastography has been investigated as potential adjuncts to EUS but these studies have so far been preliminary in scope, small in size, and predominantly focused on identification of malignancy rather than early parenchymal changes of chronic pancreatitis.[24,25] Steatorrhea does not occur until the pancreas has lost the majority of its exocrine reserve.[26] Similarly, imaging evidence of chronic pancreatitis may not correlate with exocrine function insufficiency. There can be a significant amount of discordance between EUS findings of chronic pancreatitis and exocrine insufficiency as measured by secretin pancreatic function testing.[21,27] This implies that parenchymal changes and exocrine insufficiency may occur concurrently or that there is a significant reserve capacity for absorption that is still adequate in early parenchymal disease.

Endoscopic variations of traditional gold standard direct pancreatic function tests have also been developed. The traditional secretin test of pancreatic function is performed by placing a double lumen "Dreiling" tube under fluoroscopy so that the distal port is in the duodenum and the proximal port in the stomach. After aspiration of gastric contents, duodenal secretions are stimulated by secretin or cholecystokinin (CCK) and collected for upwards of 1 h in serial increments. The duodenal fluid is then analyzed for bicarbonate or pancreatic enzyme content. The test is traditionally performed without sedation and suffers from poor patient tolerance and lack of routine expertise. Endoscopic pancreatic function testing (EPFT) maintains the same principles of Dreiling tube testing, but has the advantage of improved patient tolerance and operator convenience by performing the test under sedation during EUS or routine upper endoscopy.[28,29] However, specimen collection time remains up to 1 h with attempts at a more "rapid" EPFT yielding less accurate results.[30] Performing concurrent EPFT and EUS or at least utilizing results of both modalities may improve sensitivity for diagnosis of early chronic pancreatitis.[31]

3.3.2 COMMON DIAGNOSTIC STUDIES

3.3.2.1 Fecal Fat

Fecal fat, rather than fecal carbohydrate or fecal protein, is the measure of global malabsorption. Both carbohydrate and protein are subject to significant breakdown by colonic bacteria and rarely survive intact in the feces. In contrast, a minimal amount of fat is metabolized in the colon and therefore it can serve as an accurate indicator of overall nutrient malabsorption.

Quantitative fecal fat analysis is performed after amassing a 72 h stool collection while the patient maintains intake of 100 g of fat/day and subsequent titration to yield fecal fat/24 h. The upper limit of normal fat excretion in the stool is considered 7 g/day. But an otherwise healthy patient with induced diarrhea can have as much as 14 g fat in the stool/day.[32]

Stool may also be stained and examined under microscopy in a qualitative test as a screen for fat malabsorption. Acetic acid and Sudan III stain is added to a sample of stool on a slide. The mixture is heated and examined for orange stained fat globules. Acidification allows staining of both split fats (fatty acids) and neutral fats (triglycerides). The test can be performed without acidification which results in preferential staining of neutral fats.[33] Increased staining for neutral fats only implies a disorder of digestion such as pancreatic enzyme synthesis or function, while increased staining for split fats implies malabsorption at the brush border.

TABLE 3.6

Laboratory Tests for Fat Malabsorption

	Pros	Cons
Quantitative	Gold standard test with best sensitivity and specificity; can be used to follow and monitor treatment	Prolonged stool collection; adherence to strict diet during collection
Qualitative (Sudan)	Ease of collection and use	Subject to daily variability of fat excretion; reduced accuracy
Steatocrit	Ease of collection and use	Subject to daily variability of fat excretion

For aficionados of stool testing, there are additional nuances that may aid in the differential diagnosis. In general, very high fecal fats (>30 g/day) are associated with pancreatic insufficiency. A further calculation is the steatocrit, that is, the fat concentration, rather than the absolute amount of fat. A steatocrit >9.5% implies maldigestion, while a lower value implies malabsorption. In general, mucosal disease is associated with intestinal fluid secretion secondary to a higher level of free fatty acids that stimulate colonic chloride secretion and a greater degree of osmotic diarrhea from malabsorption of disaccharides. Both these factors lead to an increase in stool water and thus, a lower steatocrit. In comparison, in pancreatic insufficiency, lipase deficiency impairs the hydrolysis of dietary triglycerides to free fatty acids, leading to a higher steatocrit[34] (Table 3.6).

3.3.2.2   Hydrogen Breath Tests for Carbohydrate Malabsorption

The recognition that hydrogen (H_2) is produced in mammals only as result of bacterial metabolism of carbohydrate has led to the development of novel technologies to detect malabsorption of carbohydrates and/or small bowel bacterial overgrowth. Bacterial metabolism of carbohydrate may occur under two circumstances: (a) if a carbohydrate normally absorbed by the small intestine is not absorbed and passes into the colon, where bacteria ferment the carbohydrate to short-chain fatty acids, carbon dioxide (CO_2), methane (CH_4), and H_2 and (b) if there is a significant increase in luminal bacteria in the small intestine that degrades nutrients before they can be absorbed, again producing short-chain fatty acids, CO_2, and H_2. Under either scenario, CH_4 and H_2 diffuse across the mucosa into the blood stream and ultimately are excreted by the lungs. Hydrogen and CH_4 in the exhaled breath can be easily quantified by a mass spectrometer.[2,35]

The first clinical application of breath hydrogen tests was to diagnose malabsorption of lactose.

Lactase deficiency leads to the failure to hydrolyze lactose into its component monosaccharides: glucose and galactose, with passage of lactose into the colon and generation of H_2 or CH_4 by colonic bacteria.

Other sugars and sugar alcohols, such as fructose, lactulose, or sorbitol, can be used as substrates and yield information about malabsorption or small bowel transit time. Technical issues include the type of substrate given, the dose of substrate, time course of sampling, and criteria for a positive test.[2]

Many factors may affect the accuracy of hydrogen breath tests (HBT). In addition to carbohydrate malabsorption, increased oral bacterial flora or failure to adhere to a low fiber diet can result in false positive tests. A false negative result may also occur either because of recent or concurrent antibiotic treatment or because of the lack of H_2 producing bacteria in an individual's microbiome. Variables in the test protocols, such as the dosage of carbohydrate administered, the method of collection, and the amplitude of increase in H_2 considered as positive test, can all affect the results.[2,36]

3.3.3 ADDITIONAL DIAGNOSTIC STUDIES

3.3.3.1 Breath Tests for SIBO

Breath testing also can be used to assess SIBO. These tests rely on bacterial digestion of a carbohydrate substrate to produce either hydrogen or radiolabeled CO_2, which is then absorbed and measured in exhaled breath. Substrates include glucose, lactulose, and D-xylose.

HBT using glucose or lactulose substrates operate on the same principles as carbohydrate malabsorption testing and are the most commonly used tests for SIBO. Though relatively convenient and noninvasive, these breath tests uniformly suffer from lack of sensitivity and are confounded by many intestinal and extraintestinal factors similar to HBT for carbohydrate malabsorption. HBT for SIBO are falsely low in the roughly 15% of the population colonized by methane producing bacteria which shunt hydrogen into methane production, away from absorption and excretion into the lungs. Local acidic environment in the colon may also inhibit bacterial digestion and both fast and slow intestinal transit time may affect accuracy. Furthermore, patient-dependent factors such as recent diet, smoking, and exercise also affect baseline hydrogen excretion.

As with the noninvasive pancreatic function tests (see Section 3.3.3.4), improved convenience of noninvasive breath testing comes at the cost of worsened diagnostic certainty. Sensitivity of glucose and lactulose breath tests for SIBO ranged from 17% to 93% while specificity ranged from 34% to 100%. 14C-D-xylose breath testing appears to be slightly less variable, with sensitivity of 42%–100% and specificity 40%–100%.[37]

Rapid intestinal transit is the most important confounding variable in applying either glucose or lactulose HBT to the diagnosis of SIBO. Because lactulose is a nonabsorbable disaccharide, it normally passes into the colon where it is quickly fermented. The rise in exhaled H_2 concentration signals the arrival of lactulose in the cecum and the time from ingestion of lactulose represents the oral–cecal transit time (OCTT). If the lactulose encounters bacteria in the small intestine an "early" or "double" peak pattern may be recognized and has been interpreted as indicating the presence of SIBO. The reliability of that interpretation has been questioned.[36] A combined study, linking a glucose or lactulose breath hydrogen test with a scintigraphic intestinal transit scan that provides an independent measure of OCTT, may improve the diagnostic accuracy of HBTs for SIBO.[38] Such an approach improved the specificity of a lactulose HBT from 70% to 100%, although the sensitivity was still limited.[39,40] Therefore, the combination of a breath test and scintigraphy may make it feasible to improve the reliability of the H_2 breath test, with either lactulose or glucose. At this point in time, lactulose HBT by itself should not be used to diagnose SIBO.

The 14C-D-xylose breath test, with measurement of radioactive CO_2 in the breath, has been the most rigorously tested and performs fairly well, but it is only available in selected academic centers. Its cousin, the 13C-D-xylose breath test may be used in children because of the lack of radioactivity.

3.3.3.2   D-xylose

The D-xylose absorption test, not to be confused with 14C-D-xylose breath testing for SIBO, is a simple but nonspecific assessment of carbohydrate malabsorption. In the most common method, 25 g of D-xylose is ingested and the amount of xylose is measured either in urine collected over 5 h or in serum collected at 1 h. Though D-xylose is a monosaccharide, the small amount administered is absorbed by passive diffusion alone; therefore, the amount of D-xylose measured reflects global small bowel carbohydrate absorption capacity, rather than specific to xylose malabsorption, and pancreatic insufficiency does not affect the test. Measuring serum D-xylose at 1 h preserves the simplicity of the test and is more specific to intestinal absorption, but results are more vulnerable to differing rates of intestinal transit and metabolic clearance. Urine D-xylose collection over 5 h is more sensitive but is affected by renal insufficiency and bacterial overgrowth. When discrepancy exists between serum and urine results, the greater sensitivity of urine testing seems to capture more cases of malabsorption.[41]

3.3.3.3   Schilling Test

The Schilling test is an elegant assay for both the existence and etiology of vitamin B_{12} malabsorption. An oral dose of radiolabeled B_{12} is given simultaneously with a large dose of nonradiolabeled intramuscular B_{12} injection. The intramuscular injection saturates B_{12} carriers allowing measurement of radiolabeled B_{12} in the urine which directly reflects B_{12} absorption. The diagnosis of vitamin B_{12} malabsorption is confirmed if <10% of oral B_{12} is recovered in the urine within 24 h. Further steps in testing can narrow down distinct etiologies of malabsorption. In the classic two step test, intrinsic factor is then administered with radiolabeled B_{12}. If malabsorption corrects, then pernicious anemia is diagnosed. The elegance of this test lies within its use of simple deductive reasoning and its reflection of pathophysiology. For example, coadministration of oral radiolabeled B_{12} with pancreatic enzymes and antibiotics can, respectively, diagnose pancreatic insufficiency and small bowel bacterial overgrowth as causes of B_{12} malabsorption.

Though the Schilling test remains an exemplar of syllogistic reasoning and a sophisticated demonstration of the physiology of B_{12} absorption, it is unavailable in the United States for clinical use because of the lack of radiolabeled B_{12}.[42]

3.3.3.4   Tests to Diagnose Pancreatic Insufficiency:
Indirect Pancreatic Function Tests

In addition to direct Dreiling tube and endoscopic secretin testing for pancreatic insufficiency as discussed previously, various tubeless or indirect pancreatic function tests have been developed and are so named because they avoid the inconvenience of duodenal intubation with either a catheter or endoscope and subsequent direct collection of pancreatic secretions after stimulation with secretagogues such as secretin or CCK. They include fecal chymotrypsin or elastase assays, bentiromide (N-benzoyl-L-tyrosyl-para-aminobenzoic acid [NBT-PABA]), or fluorescein dilaurate testing. Unfortunately, several of these once promising assays remain unavailable for common clinical use.

3.3.3.4.1   Fecal Chymotrypsin or Elastase

Fecal chymotrypsin or elastase testing have the advantage of convenient testing on random stool collections but are hampered by being insensitive-to-mild-to-moderate pancreatic exocrine insufficiency, though they are very sensitive for severe disease causing steatorrhea. Fecal chymotrypsin activity assays are also affected by exogenous pancreatic enzyme supplementation which must be stopped beforehand. In addition, fecal elastase ELISA assays are more sensitive than fecal chymotrypsin and the antibody test is specific for human elastase and not affected by pancreatic enzyme supplementations. However, fecal elastase testing is also insensitive for mild-to-moderate pancreatic insufficiency. Both tests may produce false positive results if the submitted stool sample is unformed and dilute.[43,44]

3.3.3.4.2   NBT-PABA (Bentiromide)

Bentiromide or NBT-PABA testing is another indirect test of pancreatic function. NBT-PABA is cleaved by chymotrypsin, forming para-aminobenzoic acid (PABA), which is absorbed, conjugated in the liver, and excreted in the urine. Subsequent measurement of PABA in either serum or urine is proportional to chymotrypsin activity. The Bentiromide test is sensitive for severe pancreatic insufficiency and malabsorption but, as with other indirect tests of pancreatic dysfunction, it is not sensitive to mild or moderate pancreatic impairment. Additionally, the test is hampered by being nonspecific for pancreatic exocrine dysfunction as any limitation in enterocyte absorption, liver conjugation, or renal secretion may result in false positive results.[43,45] By the same logic, intestinal resections, certain foods, and medications may also interfere with the study. Finally, the substrate necessary to perform the test is currently not available in the United States.

3.3.3.4.3   Fluorescein Dilaurate

Another indirect test operating on the same principles as the bentiromide test is the fluorescein dilaurate assay. It too relies on hydrolysis of the substrate by specific pancreatic arylesterases to yield fluorescein, which is then absorbed, conjugated in the liver, and secreted in the urine and measured. This is then compared to urine fluorescein measured after free fluorescein ingestion on another day and reported as a ratio.[46] As with bentiromide testing, fluorescein dilaurate is not sensitive for mild-or-moderate pancreatic exocrine dysfunction and is also not available in the United States.[43]

3.3.3.4.4   Empiric Trial of Pancreatic Enzymes

Because diagnostic tests are cumbersome and inaccurate, it may be reasonable to initiate patients with steatorrhea on a trial of pancreatic enzymes rather than embark on cumbersome diagnostic testing for exocrine pancreatic insufficiency.

Modern pancreatic enzyme formulations predominantly consist of pH sensitive enteric-coated microspheres, microtablets, or microbeads. These enteric-coated formulations are designed to release enzymes in the duodenum, escaping the deactivating action of gastric acidity. Patients should be initiated on at least 30,000 USP (or 10,000 IU) of lipase/meal. Expert opinion recommends administration of at least a portion of the dose with the first bite to promote mixing in the stomach and simultaneous gastric emptying. The remainder of the dose may be taken during the meal.[47]

As with any empiric therapy, efficacy should be monitored and treatment altered or abolished should there be no therapeutic response. This is especially important because the Food and Drug Administration in the United States has mandated new drug applications for all pancreatic enzyme products. Since the mandate, only six enzyme products have been approved with resultant increase in prescription costs.[48]

Strategies for treatment failure include coadministration with a proton pump inhibitor and antacid or with nonenteric-coated pancreatic enzymes. Dose escalation is often futile.[49]

3.3.4   FECAL ALPHA 1 ANTITRYPSIN FOR PROTEIN LOSING ENTEROPATHY

Alpha 1 antitrypsin is a small protein synthesized in the liver that, due to its antiprotease activity, is resistant to luminal proteolysis. Once alpha 1 antitrypsin leaks into the intestinal lumen, it exits unmolested in feces. Fecal alpha 1 antitrypsin clearance (mL/day), as derived from a 72 h stool collection and serum alpha 1 antitrypsin concentration, is therefore a test for protein losing enteropathy. A mild increase in clearance rate may be due to diarrhea per se as demonstrated in measurements in normal subjects with laxative induced diarrhea.[50] Occult gastrointestinal bleeding may also cause a mildly elevated alpha 1 antitrypsin clearance. Its utility in assessing for malabsorption is limited, since the differential diagnosis of luminal protein loss is multitude and includes the broad categories of conditions with increased lymphatic and interstitial pressure, conditions with increased mucosal permeability, and conditions with mucosal ulcerations. In a series of 87 patients referred for chronic diarrhea, suspected malabsorption, or hypoalbuminemia, only 19 had elevated alpha 1 antitrypsin clearance. Of these 19, six subjects had Crohn's disease or microscopic colitis and two had heart failure.[50] Therefore, it is much more logical to utilize fecal alpha 1 antitrypsin testing as a test for protein losing enteropathy rather than a first line test for malabsorption.

3.3.4.1   Serum Carotene

Beta carotene is a fat soluble provitamin which is chiefly incorporated into vitamin A. Evidence suggests that beta carotene is not stored in large amounts in the body as is evidenced by the quick response in serum levels after a change in dietary intake. Therefore, serum beta carotene is used as a screening test for fat malabsorption and decreased serum beta carotene is well correlated with increased fecal fat in patients with severe malabsorption but not in mild malabsorption.[51] Interpretation should be made with further care since elevated levels of serum beta carotene may also be seen in hypothyroidism, diabetes, hyperlipidemia, high fever, and liver disease.[52]

3.3.4.2   Bile Acid Malabsorption Tests

3.3.4.2.1   Fecal Bile Acid

The gold standard for diagnosing diarrhea due to bile acid malabsorption is quantitative assay of fecal bile acids by gas chromatography—mass spectrometry, the test is expensive, time consuming, and not available for clinical use.[53] Enzymatic assays for quantifying stool bile acids are available but yield falsely low values in the setting of steatorrhea.[54]

3.3.4.2.2 ^{14}C Glycocholate Breath Test

The ^{14}C glycocholate breath test was one of the first breath tests for small intestinal bacterial overgrowth. It depends on the ability for small bowel bacterial to deconjugate bile acids, releasing ^{14}C glycerine which is then metabolized to $^{14}CO_2$ and detected in the breath. The assay is insensitive for bacterial overgrowth and fails to distinguish between SIBO and ileal malabsorption of bile acids, leading it to fall out of favor as an assay for either condition.[37,55]

3.3.4.2.3   Selenium-75-Homocholic Acid Taurine

In Great Britain and Canada, the measurement of whole body retention of a radioactive bile acid, 75SeHCAT (selenium-75-homocholic acid taurine), is the most widely available test for bile acid diarrhea (BAD). The radiolabeled bile acid is absorbed and then excreted at the same rate as native bile acids. Following oral administration of the tracer, whole body counting using a standard gamma camera is done after 3 h to establish a baseline and again at 7 days to measure retention in the body. The results usually are expressed as percentage retained at 7 days, although half-life also can be calculated. Experts suggest that patients with chronic diarrhea who have SeHCAT retention of <5% at 7 days (indicating severe bile acid malabsorption) often respond to bile acid binding drugs, whereas patients with retention of >10% at 7 days (indicating more normal ileal bile acid absorption) are less likely to respond to those drugs.[56-60] In evaluating the results of SeHCAT in clinical studies, we would recommend using a benchmark of <5% as providing the most reliable data.

SeHCAT testing has been found to have a sensitivity of 100% and a specificity of 94% for bile acid loss.[61] Retention of <10% corresponds with clinical response to bile acid chelators in patients with unexplained chronic diarrhea[62] and retention of <15% with clinical response to cholestyramine in patients with diarrhea predominant irritable bowel syndrome (IBS).[63] Unfortunately, due to its radioactivity, SeHCAT testing is not approved in the United States and is predominantly used in the United Kingdom.

3.4   CHANGING FACE OF MALABSORPTION

There has been an evolution of what may be considered malabsorption syndromes over the last several decades. These new conditions include iatrogenic causes such as bariatric surgery while others are the results of more sophisticated testing now available such as idiopathic bile acid diarrhea (BAD). Still other "new" syndromes, such as the concept of FODMAP (fermentable oligosaccharides, disaccharides, monosaccharides and polyols) intolerance, represent a reevaluation and synthesis of common

TABLE 3.7

Bile Acid Malabsorption

Type 1	Secretory diarrhea resulting from resection of terminal ileum or loss of bile acid reabsorption
Type 2	Idiopathic bile acid malabsorption in patients with histologically normal terminal ileum
Type 3	Associated with a variety of disorders, including postcholecystectomy and celiac disease

symptoms to form new entities. Finally, recently recognized side effects of some medications may lead to an explanation and straightforward treatment of previously difficult and challenging cases (shown in Table 3.7).

3.4.1 Bile Acid Malabsorption

In normal subjects, >95% of the bile acids secreted by the liver are reabsorbed in the ileum before reaching the cecum. When the enterohepatic circulation is disrupted, diarrhea may occur due to reduction of absorption or stimulation of secretion by excess bile acid in the colon.

Classically, three types of bile acid malabsorption (BAM) have been recognized as listed in Table 3.7.

Type 1 BAM typically occurs in diseases of the ileum, most commonly Crohn's disease, or after surgical resection of the ileum. In general, >50 cm of the ileum needs to be lost before clinically significant malabsorption will occur. In this situation, malabsorbed dihydroxy bile acids, such as chenodeoxycholic acid and deoxycholic acid, inhibit colonic sodium absorption and stimulate chloride secretion causing diarrhea.[64] Malabsorbed bile salt may also increase colonic permeability and motility, thereby providing another mechanism for diarrhea.

Type 2 BAM is also known as idiopathic bile acid diarrhea (BAD); its prevalence is controversial. BAD was thought to be a rare cause of chronic diarrhea, but has been reported much more frequently since the introduction of SeHCAT as a diagnostic tool (see above). The prevalence of BAD in patients with chronic diarrhea ranges from 33%–60% in several reports.[60,65–69] In trying to sort out cause and effect, it is important to recognize that diarrhea induced in normal subjects can cause mild bile acid malabsorption, so some degree of BAD might result from just the presence of diarrhea.[70]

Type 3 BAM is a grab bag of diagnoses that have been associated with bile salt-induced diarrhea. Of these, the most common is postcholecystectomy diarrhea, occurring in 10%–20% of individuals after removal of the gallbladder. Sometimes this may be described as a loosening of stool consistency or an improvement in constipation rather than diarrhea. The pathophysiology is unclear. Because bile acids are no longer stored in the gallbladder, they may reside in the gut for a greater time and may be more subject to bacterial dehydroxylation that would increase production of diarrheogenic bile acids. Alternatively, altered motility may play a role. Colonic transit time has been shown to be decreased after cholecystectomy.[71] The migrating motor complex may sweep intestinal content including bile acids rapidly through the ileum into the colon, leading to type III BAM. However, it is unclear how frequently BAM actually occurs after cholecystectomy.[72–74]

As detailed previously, specific diagnostic tests for BAM are limited in most settings and therefore a confident diagnosis may be difficult to obtain. The 14 C-glycocholate breath test has been abandoned because it is laborious, and neither very sensitive nor specific.[75] Direct measurement of fecal bile acid output involves complicated research methods not applicable to clinical use and does not predict response to bile acid binders in patients with chronic diarrhea.[70] The true frequency of BAM in IBS and functional diarrhea remains to be determined (shown in Table 3.8).

Given that BAM may be a manifestation of diarrhea instead of the cause, it is important to recognize that SeHCAT cannot delineate primary and secondary BAM related to diarrhea.[70] Nevertheless, it has gained widespread acceptance in Europe. Unfortunately, the radioisotope is not available in the United States and consequently American physicians have no experience with this test.

The development of a simple blood test for bile acid malabsorption would be a major advance. Normally serum bile acid levels are very low due to efficient clearance of bile acid from portal blood by the liver and so it would be impossible to detect lower than normal levels that might result from bile acid malabsorption. When bile acid is malabsorbed by the ileum, however, the liver compensates by increasing synthesis, which is reflected by increased serum levels of C4 (7α-hydroxy-4-cholesten-3-one), a precursor in the bile acid synthetic pathway and a reliable reflection of CYP7A1 activity, the rate limiting step in bile acid synthesis. While increased serum C4 is consistent with ileal bile acid malabsorption, this assay needs further validation before it can be accepted for widespread use as a measure of BAM.[75]

For physicians outside of Great Britain and Canada, response to empiric treatment with bile acid-binding drugs, such as cholestyramine, colestipol, or colesevelam, may be a simpler "diagnostic" test. Failure to respond to a therapeutic trial of bile acid binders makes BAM an unlikely cause of diarrhea. However, if patients respond only to a large amount of bile acid-binder (e.g., >12 g of cholestyramine), it

TABLE 3.8
Diagnosis of BAM

Glycocholate breath test	Fails to distinguish between SIBO and ileal malabsorption of bile acids, leading it to fall from favor
Quantitative stool bile acids	Gold standard but expensive, time consuming, and not routinely available
SeHCAT	Widely accepted in Great Britain and Canada but is a radioactive test over several days and not available in the United States and not able to differentiate between primary BAD and secondary BAD related to diarrhea
C4 (7α-hydroxy-4-cholesten-3-one)	Indicator of bile acid pool size. Convenience factor of serum testing but requires specialized lab expertise and needs further validation
Empiric trial of bile acid binding resins	Relatively cheap and easy but subject to significant false positive and false negative results

is unclear whether this should be considered a positive or a negative trial.[60] One must recognize the possibility of falsely concluding that BAM is present because of the well-recognized constipating effect of bile acid-binders.

3.4.2   Bacterial Overgrowth

SIBO is associated with anatomic, functional or motility abnormalities of the intestine such as strictures, achlorhydria, neuromuscular diseases, and scleroderma (Table 3.9). Patients are typically elderly and symptoms related to SIBO include diarrhea, bloating, weight loss, malabsorption, and anemia. The diagnostic "gold standard" is quantitative culture of luminal fluid from the small intestine. However, this test is not commonly performed in clinical practice. Otherwise, testing for bacterial overgrowth is limited to various breath testing methods detailed above. Breath testing, regardless of substrate, suffers from insensitivity and is subject to multiple patient and intestinal confounding factors, such as intestinal transit time, recent diet, smoking, and exercise.

Treatment of bacterial overgrowth should begin with treating the predisposing disease, if possible. Rifaximin at doses of 600–1600 mg/day may be used either for a short course or as part of cyclical therapy, though high cost is a major factor that limits its use. Other antibiotics used for overgrowth include tetracycline, norfloxacin, ciprofloxacin, amoxicillin clavulanate, and metronidazole.[76–78]

3.4.3   Fermentable Oligosaccharides, Disaccharides, Monosaccharides, and Polyols

Beginning with lactose malabsorption, there has been an effort to link carbohydrate malabsorption with multiple gastrointestinal symptoms including diarrhea, bloating, and abdominal pain. Fructose/sucrose malabsorption has been suspected as an etiologic factor in diet-induced diarrhea and abdominal symptoms; however, it has been a challenge to establish a reliable causal relation because there are

---

TABLE 3.9
Causes of Bacterial Overgrowth

Old age
Achlorhydria
Reduced intestinal motility
Small bowel diverticulosis
Previous intestinal surgery
Liver cirrhosis
Diabetes mellitus
HIV infection
Scleroderma
Celiac disease
Pancreatitis
Radiation enteritis

---

many individuals who may malabsorb fructose and sucrose without developing any clinically significant symptoms. More recently, the development of the concept of FODMAPs (fermentable oligosaccharides, disaccharides, monosaccharides and polyols) has significantly advanced our understanding of malabsorption. Rather than focusing on a single abnormality, that is, lactose or fructose, FODMAPs basically embraces a multiple hit hypothesis that implicates a wide spectrum of carbohydrates that are poorly absorbed and together may lead to significant gastrointestinal symptoms.

The recognition that food processing may lead to the introduction of a variety of novel carbohydrates has led to a refocusing of the link between diet and diarrhea. Gibson et al.[79] introduced the term FODMAPs to include fermentable oligosaccharides, disaccharides, monosaccharides and polyols. Fructans (fructooligosaccharides and inulins) are nonabsorbable polymers of fructose frequently added during the commercial production of a variety of foods. Prebiotics such as inulin and mannitol, which have become increasingly popular dietary supplements, may also be classified as FODMAPs. Because they deliver carbohydrate to the colon, they are necessarily associated with the occurrence of an osmotic diarrhea.

Sucrose is a disaccharide of fructose and glucose and is the sweetest of natural sugars. High fructose corn syrup (HFCS) is frequently added to processed foods as a sweetener and has become a dietary villain. The recent increase in fructose intake is striking. Intake in adolescents is significantly higher. Three quarters of fructose consumption came from foods and beverages other than whole fruits and vegetables.[80,81]

Sorbitol is the most common of the sugar alcohols. It can be found in small amounts in fruits and has limited intestinal absorption. Although there are apocryphal case reports of diarrhea associated with sugar-free gum, the actual frequency of sorbitol-induced diarrhea is unknown.[82,83]

Although there are limitations to the clinical studies of the frequency of fructose and/or sorbitol as the specific cause of diarrhea, there is reasonable circumstantial evidence.[84] A combination of increasing dietary intake of fructose and limited intestinal absorptive capacity can lead to an osmotic diarrhea.

Fructose sorbitol malabsorption occurs frequently in both individuals with d-IBS and healthy controls thereby, raising the possibility that malabsorption itself is not abnormal, but that the intestinal reaction including luminal events, bacteria, and motility, may be more of the problem.

The FODMAP hypothesis was validated in a rigorous, randomized, quadruple-arm, placebo-controlled rechallenge trial performed in a community setting, in which adherence to a FODMAP restricted diet alleviated intestinal symptoms in approximately 75% of IBS patients. The general applicability in an unselected population remains to be determined, but the initial results with a FODMAP restricted diet serves to emphasize the subtlety and complexity of diet in evaluating diarrhea and carbohydrate malabsorption.[85,86]

3.4.4 MALABSORPTION AFTER BARIATRIC SURGERY

Bariatric surgery is an increasingly common and successful management strategy for morbid obesity that not only results in reliable long-term weight loss[87] but also in reversal or prevention of comorbidities such as diabetes mellitus, cardiovascular disease, cancer, and mortality.[87–89]

The most common bariatric surgery procedures can be categorized by increasing potential for malabsorption and postoperative nutritional deficiencies. Restrictive operations such as sleeve gastrectomy and band gastroplasty do not cause malabsorption. Roux en Y gastric bypass (RYGB) is the predominant bariatric surgery performed in the United States[90] and is a combined restrictive and malabsorptive method, as reduced caloric intake is shunted directly to the distal jejunum via anastomosis. Pancreaticobiliary diversion (PBD) and pancreaticobiliary diversion with duodenal switch (BPD-DS) are also combined restrictive and malabsorptive procedures. The anatomical alteration in BPD-DS and BPD are analogous to RYGB but result in a bypass of a greater length of small intestine and therefore harbor a greater potential for malabsorption and nutritional deficiency.[90]

The most common vitamin deficiencies after gastric bypass are vitamin B_{12}, thiamine, and vitamin D. Vitamin B_{12} deficiency may be due to decreased intake of animal protein, lack of intrinsic factor after partial gastrectomy, and bacterial overgrowth in the de-functionalized small intestine.[91,92] Additional supplementation with oral vitamin B_{12} at 1–2 mg/day is as effective as intramuscular administration likely due to adequate absorption due to sufficient passive diffusion even in the postdiversion state.[93] Nasal vitamin B_{12} may also be used. Folate deficiency is uncommon after bariatric surgery.

Due to limited total body storage, thiamine deficiency may manifest acutely in the postoperative state as Wernicke's encephalopathy (WE), often within 3 months of surgery and as soon as 3 weeks. Persistent vomiting was the dominant risk factor and postoperative glucose load without concomitant thiamine replacement may precipitate cases of WE.[94] Thiamine deficiency has also been linked to SIBO. While thiamine supplementation should be included within the standard multivitamin regimen, routine screening is not recommended in asymptomatic patients. Acutely symptomatic patients should be treated initially with intravenous thiamine and antibiotics for SIBO can be considered in recalcitrant cases.[95]

The influence of bariatric surgery on calcium and vitamin D homeostasis are complex. Vitamin D and calcium deficiency with secondary hyperparathyroidism are already apparent in obese patients before bariatric surgery.[96,97] Postsurgical absorption is further decreased by bypass of sites of absorption and by fat malabsorption from duodenal bypass leading to decreased CCK signal for biliary and pancreatic secretions. This potential for malabsorption may be balanced by release of fat-stored vitamin D as weight is lost,[98] though evidence for sustained increase in vitamin D in the postoperative patient is lacking.[99] In addition to vitamin D insufficiency, calcium absorption is partially dependent on acidity and is decreased after partial gastrectomy. Calcium citrate appears to have improved bioavailability and suppresses parathyroid hormone to a greater extent than compared to calcium carbonate.[100] After bariatric surgery, patients should ingest at least 1.2–1.5 g of calcium citrate and 3000 IU of vitamin D daily. Further supplementation with 50,000 IU of intramuscular vitamin D with or without concurrent oral supplementation may be needed in patients with severe deficiency.[95]

The remaining fat soluble vitamins: A, E, and K, are less commonly deficient after bariatric surgery. Iron is the most common mineral deficiency in the postoperative state, followed by copper deficiency. As with vitamin D, iron stores are decreased even in preoperative obese patients as a pro-inflammatory response to adiposity possibly via up regulation of the antimicrobial peptide and acute phase reactant hepcidin.[101] Postoperative iron malabsorption may be due to several mechanisms. The most obvious is the bypass of the duodenum, which is the primary area of iron absorption (see Figure 3.1). Partial gastrectomy and achlorhydria also decreased reduction of ferric to ferrous iron, which is the preferentially absorbed form. Prophylactic ferrous sulfate supplementation prevents iron deficiency when compared with a placebo[91] with increasing doses of oral iron used for patients already deficient in iron. Vitamin C coadministration, as demonstrated in a internally controlled trial, may improve iron stores over oral iron alone.[102] Vitamin C coadministration as well as parenteral iron repletion has been recommended for severe deficiency.[95,103]

Copper, like other divalent cations such as calcium, zinc, and iron, are dependent on acidity for solubilization and are predominantly absorbed in the duodenum. As such, the postgastrectomy state with achlorhydria and bypass of the duodenum can result in malabsorption after bariatric surgery. Because copper is essential for iron mobilization,[104] copper deficiency may result in microcytic anemia, though leukopenia and pancytopenia are also encountered.[105] Copper deficiency may also cause a myelopathy resulting in subacute combined degeneration manifested by peripheral neuropathy, posterior column dysfunction, gait disorders, and cognitive dysfunction akin to vitamin B_{12} deficiency.[104] Because copper deficiency may mimic both iron deficiency anemia and vitamin B_{12} deficiency, copper malabsorption should be suspected when typical symptoms are not supported by laboratory evidence, especially since the neurological sequelae of copper deficiency may not be completely reversible.[104] Routine screening for copper deficiency is not recommended in the

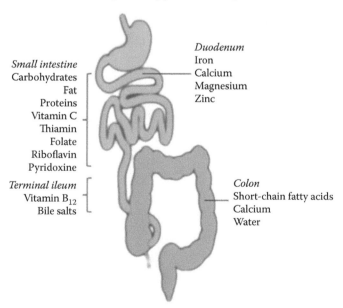

FIGURE 3.1   Sites of nutrient absorption.

postoperative patient as long as copper supplementation is included in routine multi-vitamin supplementation.

Zinc deficiency has also been described. Malabsorption is likely due to the same mechanisms as that of other divalent cations, including decreased acidity and bypass of the duodenum. Symptoms of zinc deficiency are nonspecific and include hair loss, delayed wound healing, diarrhea, and hypogonadism.[106,107] Because zinc supplementation may lead to enterocyte copper sequestration and thus precipitate copper deficiency, 1 mg of copper should be given for each 8–15 mg of zinc.[95]

Several recent comprehensive reviews and consensus guidelines on this topic are available.[95,103,106–108]

3.4.5 DRUG-INDUCED MALABSORPTION

Drug-induced diarrhea is very common. Among that long list of medications, there are several that cause diarrhea via malabsorption (Table 3.10).

Certain common oral antibiotics, such as neomycin, polymixin, and bacitracin, may cause malabsorption by acting as membrane detergents, dissolving the apical membrane and leading to the reduction of enterocyte enzyme activity.[109–111] Paromomycin, another aminoglycoside, has been linked to xylose and sucrose malabsorption if not to steattorrhea.[112]

In 10%–53% of patients, biguanide oral antihyperglycemic metformin may cause malabsorption by reducing disaccharidase activity.[113,114] Severe cases may be managed by dose reduction. Metformin may also cause late onset chronic diarrhea, which resolves after discontinuation of the drug.[115,116]

Cholestyramine in doses of 24–30 g/day may cause steatorrhea.[117]

Auranofin (previously used for rheumatoid arthritis) and colchicine may both cause diarrhea via inhibition of the Na/K ATPase. In addition, colchicine stimulates

---

TABLE 3.10

Drug-Induced Malabsorption

Aminoglycosides
Auranofin
Biguanides
Cholestyramine
Colchicine
Highly active antiretroviral therapy[a]
Laxatives
Methyldopa
Octreotide
Olestra
Olmesartan (ARBS)
Orlistat (lipase inhibitor)[b]
Polymixin, bacitracin
Tetracyclines

[a] ≥20% incidence of diarrhea.
[b] >10% incidence of diarrhea.

---

intestinal motility and long term use has been associated with steatorrhea and lactose malabsorption.[117]

Highly active antiretroviral therapy (HAART) may also cause steatorrhea. Of the nucleoside analog reverse transcriptase inhibitors (NRTI), didanosine and abacavir may induce diarrhea within 1–4 weeks after initiation of therapy, but the condition usually resolves after drug discontinuation. Rechallenging with the same medication may lead to return of symptoms with increased severity. Protease inhibitors are commonly associated with chronic diarrhea. Ritonavir, often used for pharmacological boosting of other protease inhibitors, can cause diarrhea in up to 52% of patients.[118] The mechanism may be related to inhibition of lipase; coadministration of pancreatic enzymes may partially reverse the effect in vitro.[119]

The somatostatin analog octreotide is associated with fatty diarrhea which may be mediated by concomitant decrease in secretion of bile acids, pancreatic lipase, and bicarbonate after administration.[120,121]

Colchicine can cause not only secretory and inflammatory diarrhea, but also villous atrophy and malabsorption when taken in large doses.[109]

The common nonabsorbable fat substitute olestra may theoretically cause fatty diarrhea from over consumption. However, an randomized controlled trial (RCT) using higher than consumption doses did not show an increase in stool frequency, but showed a modest stool softening effect in subjects compared to the controls.[122]

The gastrointestinal lipase inhibitor orlistat is now available over the counter under the name Alli and is associated with fatty diarrhea from malabsorption in 60% to >80% of patients in a dose-dependent fashion. Symptoms typically resolve when fat intake is reduced to <15 g/day.[123] Increased doses of orlistat may also result in malabsorption of fat-soluble vitamins.

The antihypertensive methyldopa has been described to cause malabsorption manifesting as chronic diarrhea and weight loss. In one case report, D-xylose testing was abnormal and recovered in association with resolution of diarrhea upon discontinuation of the drug. Rechallenge resulted in renewed symptoms and worsened D-xylose absorption. Partial villous blunting and chronic inflammation were seen on jejunal biopsy and also reversed after discontinuation of the drug.[124]

Olmesartan is a commonly used angiotensin II receptor antagonist that has been associated with a sprue-like enteropathy causing chronic diarrhea. Histological findings are often similar to celiac disease with villous blunting and inflammatory infiltrate. A subset of patients may have histology analogous to collagenous enteropathy. Both symptoms and histology are reversed with cessation of omesartan.[125]

3.4.5.1 Clinical Case

A 64-year-old woman was referred for painless diarrhea and weight loss occurring over the last 6 months. There was no prior history of diarrhea nor was there a family history of diarrhea. She described the diarrhea as watery, occurring 6–8 times daily, occasionally waking her up from sleep. She had lost 21 lbs, from 143 to 122, over this time period. There was no abdominal pain or blood in the stool.

She had no significant dietary changes over that time period. She drank one cup of coffee daily, no milk and no sodas. There were no new medicines prescribed over that time. Loperamide, taken up to six tablets daily, slowed the diarrhea, but did not eliminate it. Her primary care physician referred her to a gastroenterologist who recommended a colonoscopy.

The colonic and ileal mucsoa appeared endoscopically normal. However, the biopsies demonstrated mild microscopic colitis. The gastroenterologist recommended discontinuation of both her proton pump inhibitor and NSAIDs. He prescribed budesonide for 8 weeks. It did not provide any benefit. He then followed this with an 8-week course of bismuth subsalicylate which also did not have any significant effect. Cholestyramine was tried, empirically for possible bile acid diarrhea, to no avail. The patient continued to lose weight.

Because of an association between microscopic colitis and celiac disease, an EGD was performed. There was scalloping of the small bowel folds. Small bowel biopsies, two from the bulb and four from the second portion of the intestine, were done. They revealed subtotal villous atrophy and a presumptive diagnosis of celiac disease. A gluten-free diet was started and celiac serologies obtained. Curiously, the serologies were negative although the patient was HLA DQ2 positive. Despite strict adherence to a gluten-free diet there was no improvement in the diarrhea and the patient continued to lose weight, now down to 110 lbs.

At this point, a thorough review of her history revealed that she had been taking olmesartan for hypertension for the last 5 years. There had been no change in dosage. However, another antihypertensive was substituted for olmesartan and, over the next 3 weeks, the diarrhea stopped and the patient began to gain weight.

3.4.5.2 Commentary

This case highlights some of the complexities of discovering the etiology of malabsorption. This patient had watery diarrhea, consistent with the microscopic colitis, but weight loss was a clue that there may be more involved. Given a lack of easily obtained diagnostic studies for bile acid diarrhea, an empiric trial was reasonable. Recognition of the association between microscopic colitis and celiac disease led to the upper GI endoscopy and small bowel biopsies. It was clearly unusual, but possible, to have a case of celiac disease with negative serologies (antitissue transglutaminase IgA and IgG). HLA DQ2/DQ8 may reasonably rule out celiac disease, but positivity does not make a diagnosis since up to 25% of the general (nonceliac) population may be positive. The lack of response to a gluten-free diet again called into question the diagnosis of celiac disease. At that point, probably in desperation, the physicians reviewed all the details of the patient's history, labs and clinical course. As discussed above, the angiotensin receptor blocker olmesartan has recently been recognized as a cause of nonresponsive "Celiac disease."[125] There may also be colonic changes suggestive of microscopic colitis. The etiology of the small bowel damage has not been elucidated.

3.5 CONCLUSION/SUMMARY

The recognition, diagnosis and treatment of malabsorption remain a clinical challenge. However, the astute clinician may achieve success through a consideration of the classifications of diarrhea, a careful history and a judicious use of testing.

Recently, there has been an expansion of clinical entities associated with malabsorption. This ongoing evolution of the field requires continued recalibration of the clinical approach to malabsorption.

REFERENCES

1. Hammer HF, Hammer J. Diarrhea caused by carbohydrate malabsorption. *Gastroenterol Clin North Am* 2012;41(3):611–627.
2. Lomer MCE, Parkes GC, Sanderson JD. Review article: Lactose intolerance in clinical practice—Myths and realities. *Aliment Pharmacol Ther* 2008;27(2):93–103.
3. Smith RB, Sprinz H, Crosby WH, Sullivan BH. Peroral small bowel mucosal biopsy. *Am J Med* 1958;25(3):391–394.
4. Shwachman H, Khaw KT, Antonowicz I. Diagnosis and treatment: Peroral intestinal biopsy. *Pediatrics* 1969;43(3):460–462.
5. Lindenbaum J, Gerson CD, Kent TH. Recovery of small-intestinal structure and function after residence in the tropics. I. Studies in Peace Corps volunteers. *Ann Intern Med* 1971;74(2):218–222.
6. Carmack SW, Genta RM. The diagnostic value of the duodenal biopsy: A clinico-pathologic analysis of 28,000 patients. *Dig Liver Dis* 2010;42(7):485–489.
7. Leffler DA, Schuppan D. Update on serologic testing in celiac disease. *Am J Gastroenterol* 2010;105(12):2520–2524.
8. Rubio-Tapia A, Hill ID, Kelly CP, Calderwood AH, Murray JA. ACG clinical guidelines: Diagnosis and management of celiac disease. *Am J Gastroenterol* 2013;108(5):656–676; quiz 677.
9. Marsh MN. Gluten, major histocompatibility complex, and the small intestine. A molecular and immunobiologic approach to the spectrum of gluten sensitivity ('celiac sprue'). *Gastroenterology* 1992;102(1):330–354.
10. Oberhuber G. Dossier: Gastroenterology-histopathology of celiac disease. *Biomedicine* 2000:368–372.
11. Corazza GR, Villanacci V, Zambelli C et al. Comparison of the interobserver reproducibility with different histologic criteria used in celiac disease. *Clin Gastroenterol Hepatol* 2007;5(7):838–843.
12. Owens SR, Greenson JK. The pathology of malabsorption: Current concepts. *Histopathology* 2007;50(1):64–82.
13. Pais WP, Duerksen DR, Pettigrew NM, Bernstein CN. How many duodenal biopsy specimens are required to make a diagnosis of celiac disease? *Gastrointest Endosc* 2008;67(7):1082–1087.
14. Evans KE, Aziz I, Cross SS et al. A prospective study of duodenal bulb biopsy in newly diagnosed and established adult celiac disease. *Am J Gastroenterol* 2011;106(10):1837–1742.
15. Gonzalez S, Gupta A, Cheng J et al. Prospective study of the role of duodenal bulb biopsies in the diagnosis of celiac disease. *Gastrointest Endosc* 2010;72(4):758–765.
16. Lebwohl B, Kapel RC, Neugut AI, Green PHR, Genta RM. Adherence to biopsy guidelines increases celiac disease diagnosis. *Gastrointest Endosc* 2011;74(1):103–109.
17. Sai J-K. Diagnosis of mild chronic pancreatitis (Cambridge classification): Comparative study using secretin injection-magnetic resonance cholangiopancreatography and endoscopic retrograde pancreatography. *World J Gastroenterol* 2008;14(8):1218.
18. Bozkurt T, Braun U, Leferink S, Gilly G, Lux G. Comparison of pancreatic morphology and exocrine functional impairment in patients with chronic pancreatitis. *Gut* 1994;35(8):1132–1136.

19. Kahl S, Glasbrenner B, Leodolter A, Pross M, Schulz H, Malfertheiner P. EUS in the diagnosis of early chronic pancreatitis: A prospective follow-up study. *Gastrointest Endosc* 2002;55(4):507–511.
20. Catalano MF, Sahai A, Levy M et al. EUS-based criteria for the diagnosis of chronic pancreatitis: The Rosemont classification. *Gastrointest Endosc* 2009;69(7):1251–1261.
21. Stevens T. Update on the role of endoscopic ultrasound in chronic pancreatitis. *Curr Gastroenterol Rep* 2011;13(2):117–122.
22. Kalmin B, Hoffman B, Hawes R, Romagnuolo J. Conventional versus Rosemont endoscopic ultrasound criteria for chronic pancreatitis: Comparing interobserver reliability and intertest agreement. *Can J Gastroenterol* 2011;25(5):261–264.
23. Del Pozo D, Poves E, Tabernero S et al. Conventional versus Rosemont endoscopic ultrasound criteria for chronic pancreatitis: Interobserver agreement in same day back-to-back procedures. *Pancreatology* 12(3):284–287.
24. Irisawa A, Mishra G, Hernandez LV, Bhutani MS. Quantitative analysis of endosonographic parenchymal echogenicity in patients with chronic pancreatitis. *J Gastroenterol Hepatol* 2004;19(10):1199–1205.
25. Janssen J, Schlörer E, Greiner L. EUS elastography of the pancreas: Feasibility and pattern description of the normal pancreas, chronic pancreatitis, and focal pancreatic lesions. *Gastrointest Endosc* 2007;65(7):971–978.
26. DiMagno EP, Go VL, Summerskill WH. Relations between pancreatic enzyme ouputs and malabsorption in severe pancreatic insufficiency. *N Engl J Med* 1973;288(16):813–815.
27. Conwell D, Zuccaro G. Cholecystokinin-stimulated peak lipase concentration in duodenal drainage fluid: A new pancreatic function test. *Am J Gastroenterol* 2002;97(6):2–7.
28. Conwell DL, Zuccaro G, Vargo JJ et al. An endoscopic pancreatic function test with synthetic porcine secretin for the evaluation of chronic abdominal pain and suspected chronic pancreatitis. *Gastrointest Endosc* 2003;57(1):37–40.
29. Stevens T, Conwell DL, Zuccaro G et al. A prospective crossover study comparing secretin-stimulated endoscopic and Dreiling tube pancreatic function testing in patients evaluated for chronic pancreatitis. *Gastrointest Endosc* 2008;67(3):458–466.
30. Raimondo M, Imoto M, Dimagno EP. Rapid endoscopic secretin stimulation test and discrimination of chronic pancreatitis and pancreatic cancer from disease controls. *Clin Gastroenterol Hepatol* 2003;1(5):397–403.
31. Albashir S, Bronner MP, Parsi MA, Walsh RM, Stevens T. Endoscopic ultrasound, secretin endoscopic pancreatic function test, and histology: Correlation in chronic pancreatitis. *Am J Gastroenterol* 2010;105(11):2498–2503.
32. Fine KD, Ogunji F. A new method of quantitative fecal fat microscopy and its correlation with chemically measured fecal fat output. TL - 113. *Am J Clin Pathol* 2000;113 VN - (4):528–534.
33. Khouri MR, Huang G, Shiau YF. Sudan stain of fecal fat: New insight into an old test. TL - 96. *Gastroenterology* 1989;96 VN - r(2 Pt 1):421–427.
34. Bo-Linn GW, Fordtran JS. Fecal fat concentration in patients with steatorrhea. *Gastroenterology* 1984;87(2):319–322.
35. Knudsen CD, Di Palma JA. Carbohydrate challenge tests: Do you need to measure methane? *South Med J* 2012;105(5):251–253.
36. Ghoshal UC. How to interpret hydrogen breath tests. *J Neurogastroenterol Motil* 2011;17(3):312–317.
37. Rana SV, Bhardwaj SB. Small intestinal bacterial overgrowth. *Scand J Gastroenterol* 2008;43(9):1030–1037.
38. Sellin JH, Hart R. Glucose malabsorption associated with rapid intestinal transit. *Am J Gastroenterol* 1992;87(5):584–589.

39. Riordan SM, McIver CJ, Walker BM, Duncombe VM, Bolin TD, Thomas MC. The lactulose breath hydrogen test and small intestinal bacterial overgrowth. *Am J Gastroenterol* 1996;91(9):1795–1803.
40. Yu D, Cheeseman F, Vanner S. Combined oro-caecal scintigraphy and lactulose hydrogen breath testing demonstrate that breath testing detects oro-caecal transit, not small intestinal bacterial overgrowth in patients with IBS. *Gut* 2011;60(3):334–340.
41. Peled Y, Doron O, Laufer H, Bujanover Y, Gilat T. D-xylose absorption test. Urine or blood? *Dig Dis Sci* 1991;36(2):188–192.
42. Oh R, Brown DL. Vitamin B$_{12}$ deficiency. *Am Fam Physician* 2003;67(5):979–986.
43. Chowdhury RS, Forsmark CE. Pancreatic function testing. *Aliment Pharmacol Ther* 2003;17(6):733–750.
44. Lankisch PG. Now that fecal elastase is available in the United States, should clinicians start using it? *Curr Gastroenterol Rep* 2004;6(2):126–131.
45. Glasbrenner B, Kahl S, Malfertheiner P. Modern diagnostics of chronic pancreatitis. *Eur J Gastroenterol Hepatol* 2002;14(9):935–941.
46. Malfertheiner P, Büchler M, Müller A, Ditschuneit H. Fluorescein dilaurate serum test: A rapid tubeless pancreatic function test. *Pancreas* 1987;2(1):53–60.
47. Sikkens ECM, Cahen DL, Kuipers EJ, Bruno MJ. Pancreatic enzyme replacement therapy in chronic pancreatitis. *Best Pract Res Clin Gastroenterol* 2010;24(3):337–347.
48. Gardner TB, Munson JC, Morden NE. The FDA and prescription pancreatic enzyme product cost. *Am J Gastroenterol* 2014;109(5):624–625.
49. Toskes PP, Secci A, Thieroff-Ekerdt R. Efficacy of a novel pancreatic enzyme product, EUR-1008 (Zenpep), in patients with exocrine pancreatic insufficiency due to chronic pancreatitis. *Pancreas* 2011;40(3):376–382.
50. Strygler B, Nicar MJ, Santangelo WC, Porter JL, Fordtran JS. Alpha 1-antitrypsin excretion in stool in normal subjects and in patients with gastrointestinal disorders. *Gastroenterology* 1990;99(5):1380–1387.
51. Evans WB, Wollaeger EE. Incidence and severity of nutritional deficiency states in chronic exocrine pancreatic insufficency: Comparison with nontropical sprue. *Am J Dig Dis* 1966;11(8):594–606.
52. Wenger J, Kirsner JB, Palmer WL. Blood carotene in steatorrhea and the malabsorptive syndromes. *Am J Med* 1957;22(3):373–380.
53. Johnston I, Nolan J, Pattni SS, Walters JR. New insights into bile acid malabsorption. TL - 13. *Curr Gastroenterol Rep* 2011;13 VN - r(5):418–425.
54. Porter JL, Fordtran JS, Santa Ana CA et al. Accurate enzymatic measurement of fecal bile acids in patients with malabsorption. *J Lab Clin Med* 2003;141(6):411–418.
55. Ferguson J, Walker K, Thomson AB. Limitations in the use of 14C-glycocholate breath and stool bile acid determinations in patients with chronic diarrhea. *J Clin Gastroenterol* 1986;8(3 Pt 1):258–262.
56. Fellous K, Jian R, Haniche M et al. Measurement of ileal absorption of bile salts with the selenium 75 labelled homotaurocholic acid test. Validation and clinical significance. *Gastroentérol Clin Biol* 1994;18(10):865–872.
57. Van Tilburg AJ, de Rooij FW, van den Berg JW, Kooij PP, van Blankenstein M. The selenium-75-homocholic acid taurine test reevaluated: Combined measurement of fecal selenium-75 activity and 3 alpha-hydroxy bile acids in 211 patients. *J Nucl Med* 1991;32(6):1219–1224.
58. Nyhlin H, Merrick M V, Eastwood MA, Brydon WG. Evaluation of ileal function using 23-selena-25-homotaurocholate, a-gamma-labeled conjugated bile acid. Initial clinical assessment. *Gastroenterology* 1983;84(1):63–68.
59. Thaysen EH, Orholm M, Arnfred T, Carl J, Rødbro P. Assessment of ileal function by abdominal counting of the retention of a gamma emitting bile acid analogue. *Gut* 1982;23(10):862–865.

60. Williams A, Merrick M, Eastwood M. Idiopathic bile acid malabsorption—A review of clinical presentation, diagnosis, and response to treatment. *Gut* 1991;32(9):1004–1006.

61. Sciarretta G, Fagioli G, Furno A et al. 75Se HCAT test in the detection of bile acid malabsorption in functional diarrhoea and its correlation with small bowel transit. TL - 28. *Gut* 1987;28 VN - r(8):970–975.

62. Williams A, Merrick M, Eastwood M. Idiopathic bile acid malabsorption—A review of clinical presentation, diagnosis, and response to treatment. *Gut* 1991;32(9):1004–1006.

63. Wedlake L, A'Hern R, Russell D, Thomas K, Walters JRF, Andreyev HJN. Systematic review: The prevalence of idiopathic bile acid malabsorption as diagnosed by SeHCAT scanning in patients with diarrhoea-predominant irritable bowel syndrome. *Aliment Pharmacol Ther* 2009;30(7):707–717.

64. Mekjian HS, Phillips SF, Hofmann AF. Colonic secretion of water and electrolytes induced by bile acids: Perfusion studies in man. *J Clin Invest* 1971;50(8):1569–1577.

65. Sinha L, Liston R, Testa HJ, Moriarty KJ. Idiopathic bile acid malabsorption: Qualitative and quantitative clinical features and response to cholestyramine. *Aliment Pharmacol Ther* 1998;12(9):839–844.

66. Sciarretta G, Furno A, Morrone B, Malaguti P. Absence of histopathological changes of ileum and colon in functional chronic diarrhea associated with bile acid malabsorption, assessed by SeHCAT test: A prospective study. *Am J Gastroenterol* 1994;89(7):1058–1061.

67. Rössel P, Sortsøe Jensen H, Qvist P, Arveschoug A. Prognosis of adult-onset idiopathic bile acid malabsorption. *Scand J Gastroenterol* 1999;34(6):587–590.

68. Fernández-Bañares F, Esteve M, Salas A et al. Systematic evaluation of the causes of chronic watery diarrhea with functional characteristics. *Am J Gastroenterol* 2007;102(11):2520–2528.

69. Luman W, Williams AJ, Merrick MV, Eastwood MA. Idiopathic bile acid malabsorption: Long-term outcome. *Eur J Gastroenterol Hepatol* 1995;7(7):641–645.

70. Schiller LR, Hogan RB, Morawski SG et al. Studies of the prevalence and significance of radiolabeled bile acid malabsorption in a group of patients with idiopathic chronic diarrhea. *Gastroenterology* 1987;92(1):151–160.

71. Fort JM, Azpiroz F, Casellas F, Andreu J, Malagelada JR. Bowel habit after cholecystectomy: Physiological changes and clinical implications. *Gastroenterology* 1996;111(3):617–622.

72. Hearing SD, Thomas LA, Heaton KW, Hunt L. Effect of cholecystectomy on bowel function: A prospective, controlled study. *Gut* 1999;45(6):889–894.

73. Fromm H, Tunuguntla AK, Malavolti M, Sherman C, Ceryak S. Absence of significant role of bile acids in diarrhea of a heterogeneous group of postcholecystectomy patients. *Dig Dis Sci* 1987;32(1):33–44.

74. Breuer NF, Jaekel S, Dommes P, Goebell H. Fecal bile acid excretion pattern in cholecystectomized patients. *Dig Dis Sci* 1986;31(9):953–960.

75. Vijayvargiya P, Camilleri M, Shin A, Saenger A. Methods for diagnosis of bile acid malabsorption in clinical practice. *Clin Gastroenterol Hepatol* 2013;11(10):1232–1239.

76. Bures J. Small intestinal bacterial overgrowth syndrome. *World J Gastroenterol* 2010;16(24):2978.

77. Attar A, Flourié B, Rambaud JC, Franchisseur C, Ruszniewski P, Bouhnik Y. Antibiotic efficacy in small intestinal bacterial overgrowth-related chronic diarrhea: A crossover, randomized trial. *Gastroenterology* 1999;117(4):794–797.

78. Di Stefano M, Miceli E, Missanelli A, Mazzocchi S, Corazza GR. Absorbable vs. nonabsorbable antibiotics in the treatment of small intestine bacterial overgrowth in patients with blind-loop syndrome. *Aliment Pharmacol Ther* 2005;21(8):985–992.

79. Gibson PR, Newnham E, Barrett JS, Shepherd SJ, Muir JG. Review article: Fructose malabsorption and the bigger picture. *Aliment Pharmacol Ther* 2007;25(4):349–363.

80. Vos MB, Kimmons JE, Gillespie C, Welsh J, Blanck HM. Dietary fructose consumption among US children and adults: The Third National Health and Nutrition Examination Survey. *Medscape J Med* 2008;10(7):160.
81. Park YK, Yetley EA. Intakes and food sources of fructose in the United States. *Am J Clin Nutr* 1993;58(5 Suppl):737S–747S.
82. Bauditz J, Norman K, Biering H, Lochs H, Pirlich M. Severe weight loss caused by chewing gum. *BMJ* 2008;336(7635):96–97.
83. Breitenbach RA. Halloween diarrhea. An unexpected trick of sorbitol-containing candy. *Postgrad Med* 1992;92(5):63–66.
84. Fernández-Bañares F, Esteve M, Viver JM. Fructose-sorbitol malabsorption. *Curr Gastroenterol Rep* 2009;11(5):368–374.
85. Shepherd SJ, Gibson PR. Fructose malabsorption and symptoms of irritable bowel syndrome: Guidelines for effective dietary management. *J Am Diet Assoc* 2006;106(10):1631–1639.
86. Shepherd SJ, Parker FC, Muir JG, Gibson PR. Dietary triggers of abdominal symptoms in patients with irritable bowel syndrome: Randomized placebo-controlled evidence. *Clin Gastroenterol Hepatol* 2008;6(7):765–771.
87. Sjöström L, Narbro K, Sjöström CD et al. Effects of bariatric surgery on mortality in Swedish obese subjects. *N Engl J Med* 2007;357(8):741–752.
88. Sjöström L, Peltonen M, Jacobson P et al. Bariatric surgery and long-term cardiovascular events. *JAMA* 2012;307(1):56–65.
89. Sjöström L, Gummesson A, Sjöström CD et al. Effects of bariatric surgery on cancer incidence in obese patients in Sweden (Swedish obese subjects study): A prospective, controlled intervention trial. *Lancet Oncol* 2009;10(7):653–662.
90. Buchwald H, Oien DM. Metabolic/bariatric surgery worldwide 2011. *Obes Surg* 2013;23(4):427–4.
91. Brolin RE, Gorman JH, Gorman RC et al. Are vitamin B_{12} and folate deficiency clinically important after roux-en-Y gastric bypass? *J Gastrointest Surg* 1998;2:436–442.
92. Gasteyger C, Suter M, Gaillard RC, Giusti V. Nutritional deficiencies after Roux-en-Y gastric bypass for morbid obesity often cannot be prevented by standard multivitamin supplementation. *Am J Clin Nutr* 2008;87(5):1128–1133.
93. Butler CC, Vidal-Alaball J, Cannings-John R et al. Oral vitamin B_{12} versus intramuscular vitamin B_{12} for vitamin B_{12} deficiency: A systematic review of randomized controlled trials. *Fam Pract* 2006;23(3):279–285.
94. Aasheim ET. Wernicke encephalopathy after bariatric surgery: A systematic review. *Ann Surg* 2008;248(5):714–720.
95. Mechanick JI, Youdim A, Jones DB et al. Clinical practice guidelines for the perioperative nutritional, metabolic, and nonsurgical support of the bariatric surgery patient—2013 update: Cosponsored by American Association of Clinical Endocrinologists, The Obesity Society, and American Society. *Obesity (Silver Spring)* 2013;21(Suppl 1):S1–S27.
96. Ybarra J, Sánchez-Hernández J, Gich I et al. Unchanged hypovitaminosis D and secondary hyperparathyroidism in morbid obesity after bariatric surgery. *Obes Surg* 2005;15(3):330–335.
97. Ducloux R, Nobécourt E, Chevallier J-MM, Ducloux H, Elian N, Altman J-JJ. Vitamin D deficiency before bariatric surgery: Should supplement intake be routinely prescribed? TL - 21. *Obes Surg* 2011;21 VN - r(5):556–560.
98. Wortsman J, Matsuoka LY, Chen TC, Lu Z, Holick MF. Decreased bioavailability of vitamin D in obesity. *Am J Clin Nutr* 2000;72(3):690–693.
99. Lin E, Armstrong-Moore D, Liang Z et al. Contribution of adipose tissue to plasma 25-hydroxyvitamin D concentrations during weight loss following gastric bypass surgery. *Obesity (Silver Spring)* 2011;19(3):588–594.

100. Tondapu P, Provost D, Adams-Huet B, Sims T, Chang C, Sakhaee K. Comparison of the absorption of calcium carbonate and calcium citrate after Roux-en-Y gastric bypass. TL - 19. *Obes Surg* 2009;19 VN - r(9):1256–1261.
101. McClung JP, Karl JP. Iron deficiency and obesity: The contribution of inflammation and diminished iron absorption. *Nutr Rev* 2009;67(2):100–104.
102. Rhode BM, Shustik C, Christou NV, MacLean LD. Iron absorption and therapy after gastric bypass. *Obes Surg* 1999;9(1):17–21.
103. Decker GA, Swain JM, Crowell MD, Scolapio JS. Gastrointestinal and nutritional complications after bariatric surgery. *Am J Gastroenterol* 2007;102(11):2571–2580; quiz 2581.
104. Jaiser SR, Winston GP. Copper deficiency myelopathy. *J Neurol* 2010;257(6):869–881.
105. Halfdanarson TR, Kumar N, Li C, Phyliky RL, Hogan WJ. Hematological manifestations of copper deficiency: A retrospective review. *Eur J Haematol* 2008;80(6):523–531.
106. Gletsu-Miller N, Wright BN. Mineral malnutrition following bariatric surgery. *Adv Nutr* 2013;4(5):506–517.
107. Shankar P, Boylan M, Sriram K. Micronutrient deficiencies after bariatric surgery. *Nutrition* 2010;26(11–12):1031–1037.
108. Saltzman E, Karl JP. Nutrient deficiencies after gastric bypass surgery. *Annu Rev Nutr* 2013;33:183–203.
109. Ratnaike RN, Jones TE. Mechanisms of drug-induced diarrhoea in the elderly. *Drugs Aging* 1998;13(3):245–253.
110. Andersson K-E. Current concepts in the treatment of disorders of micturition. *Drugs* 1988;35(4):477–494.
111. Price AB. Pathology of drug-associated gastrointestinal disease. *Br J Clin Pharmacol* 2003;56(5):477–482.
112. Keusch GT, Troncale FJ, Buchanan RD. Malabsorption due to paromomycin. *Arch Intern Med* 1970;125(2):273–276.
113. Berchtold P, Dahlqvist A, Gustafson A, Asp N-G. Effects of a biguanide (metformin) on vitamin B 12 and folic acid absorption and intestinal enzyme activities. *Scand J Gastroenterol* 1971;6(8):751–754.
114. Czyzyk A, Tawecki J, Sadowski J, Ponikowska I, Szczepanik Z. Effect of biguanides on intestinal absorption of glucose. *Diabetes* 1968;17(8):492–498.
115. Foss MT, Clement KD. Metformin as a cause of late-onset chronic diarrhea. *Pharmacotherapy* 2001;21(11):1422–1424.
116. Bytzer P, Talley NJ, Jones MP, Horowitz M. Oral hypoglycemic drugs and gastrointestinal symptoms in diabetes mellitus. *Aliment Pharmacol Ther* 2001;15(1):137–142.
117. Chassany O, Michaux A, Bergmann JF. Drug-Induced Diarrhoea. *Drug Saf* 2000;22(1):53–72.
118. Cameron DW, Heath-Chiozzi M, Danner S et al. Randomised placebo-controlled trial of ritonavir in advanced HIV-1 disease. *Lancet* 1998;351(9102):543–549.
119. Wignot TM, Stewart RP, Schray KJ, Das S, Sipos T. *In vitro* studies of the effects of HAART drugs and excipients on activity of digestive enzymes. *Pharm Res* 2004;21(3):420–427.
120. Ho PJ, Boyajy LD, Greenstein E, Barkan AL. Effect of chronic octreotide treatment on intestinal absorption in patients with acromegaly. *Dig Dis Sci* 1993;38(2):309–315.
121. Nakamura T, Kudoh K, Takebe K et al. Octreotide decreases biliary and pancreatic exocrine function, and induces steatorrhea in healthy subjects. *Intern Med* 1994;33(10):593–596.
122. McRorie J, Zorich N, Riccardi K et al. Effects of olestra and sorbitol consumption on objective measures of diarrhea: Impact of stool viscosity on common gastrointestinal symptoms. *Regul Toxicol Pharmacol* 2000;31(1):59–67.

123. Sjöström L, Rissanen A, Andersen T et al. Randomised placebo-controlled trial of orlistat for weight loss and prevention of weight regain in obese patients. *Lancet* 1998;352(9123):167–172.

124. Shneerson JM, Gazzard BG. Reversible malabsorption caused by methyldopa. *Br Med J* 1977;2(6100):1456–1457.

125. Rubio-Tapia A, Herman ML, Ludvigsson JF et al. Severe spruelike enteropathy associated with olmesartan. *Mayo Clin Proc* 2012;87(8):732–738.

4 Food Allergy and Food Intolerance

John Leung and Sheila E. Crowe

CONTENTS

4.1 INTRODUCTION

Patients often associate foods with various gastrointestinal (GI) symptoms such as abdominal pain or discomfort, bloating, acid reflux, nausea, vomiting, and altered bowel movements. It is estimated that one-fifth of the population restricts their diet because of perceived adverse reactions to food (ARF).[1] Dietary restrictions resulting

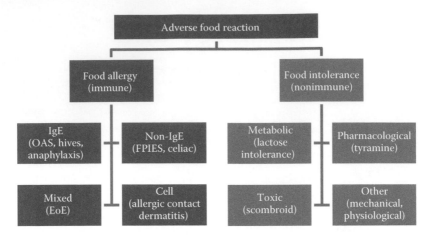

FIGURE 4.1 Adverse reaction caused by either food allergy or food intolerance. (Adapted from Sampson HA et al. *J Allergy Clin Immunology* 2014;135(5):1016–1025.)

from ARF can lead to nutritional deficiency without appropriate supervision and monitoring. Adverse reaction to foods can be caused by either food allergy or food intolerance (Figure 4.1). Food allergy is an abnormal immunological response to a food protein while food intolerance typically involves nonimmunological mechanisms. Contrary to the common belief that most adverse food reactions are allergic/immunological in nature, less than a fifth are actually due to food allergy. In clinical practice, it is of paramount importance to distinguish food allergy from food intolerance because their nutritional management is rather different. For instance, while patients with cow's milk allergy (CMA) are advised to strictly avoid all dairy products as it can cause potentially life-threatening anaphylaxis, patients with lactose intolerance are often encouraged to consume tolerable amounts of lactose-containing dairy products to achieve their nutritional goals. In this chapter, we will provide an overview of various types of food allergies and food sensitivities, and corresponding management strategies.

4.2 FOOD ALLERGY

Fifteen million Americans are estimated to have food allergy (4% of adults and 8% of children), and the prevalence is increasing.[2-6] The economic cost of food allergies exceeds 25 billion US dollars per year.[7] Approximately 200,000 emergency room visits and 300,000 ambulatory-care visits annually in the United States are related to food allergy.[6,8] Eight foods account for 90% of all food allergic reactions in North America: milk, eggs, peanuts, tree nuts, soy, wheat, fish, and shellfish.[9] Early childhood allergies to milk, eggs, soy, and wheat usually resolve by school age (approximately 80% of the time).[10] Adults are more likely to have allergies to shellfish, peanuts, tree nuts, and fish.[11] Immune-mediated reactions to food are very complex and may involve multiple components of the immune systems.[12] IgE-mediated reactions are the most studied and best characterized. Other forms of food allergy can involve pathological T cells, generation of immune complexes, and/or activation of eosinophils.

4.2.1 IgE-Mediated Food Allergy

IgE-mediated food allergic reactions are typically rapid in onset and occur within minutes to 2 h after ingestion, with few exceptions. IgE-mediated food allergy has a wide spectrum of clinical manifestations.[13] They can range from self-limited urticaria/angioedema to life-threatening anaphylaxis. GI, cutaneous, cardiovascular, and/or respiratory systems can be involved. These reactions develop when food allergens bind the food-specific IgE antibodies residing on the mast cells and basophils in sensitized individuals, leading to degranulation and release of potent mediators and cytokines.

4.2.1.1 Clinical Manifestations of IgE-Mediated Food Allergy

Acute urticaria and angioedema are the most common cutaneous manifestations of IgE-mediated food allergy, generally appearing within minutes of ingestion of the food allergen. Acute urticaria is the most common symptom in patients experiencing food-induced anaphylaxis.[14–16] Often urticaria is associated with angioedema in food-induced allergic reactions.[17] Although urticaria and angioedema are amongst the most common symptoms of anaphylaxis, their absence does not exclude a food allergic reaction. Indeed, cases of anaphylaxis proving to be fatal have been reported to occur in the absence of any cutaneous reactions.[6]

Urticaria can also develop upon direct skin contact with the food allergen.[18] These reactions are confined to the site of skin contact and do not progress to systemic reactions unless the food is also ingested.[19] In addition to the "big eight" allergens, raw meats, seafood, raw vegetables and fruits, mustard, and rice are among the foods that have been implicated in this form of reaction.[18,20,21]

Allergic reactions to foods are now the leading cause of anaphylaxis treated in emergency departments.[22] The onset is rapid and even minute amounts of the allergen can trigger anaphylactic reactions.[23–26] Multiple organ systems can be affected and may culminate in hypotension, respiratory distress, arrhythmia, and cardiac arrest. Such reactions are responsible for 150–200 deaths annually in North America.[27] Failure to promptly administer epinephrine is a risk factor for a fatal outcome.[28] Biphasic reactions are the recurrence of symptoms 4–12 h after the initial anaphylactic reaction and occur in up to 20% of cases of anaphylaxis.[29] Half of these reactions are severe and potentially life threatening. The potential for such biphasic reactions is one of the reasons why patients successfully treated with epinephrine in the acute setting should be admitted to the hospital for continued monitoring.[30]

4.2.1.2 Examples of IgE-Mediated Food Allergy

4.2.1.2.1 Oral Allergy Syndrome

The oral allergy syndrome, or pollen-food allergy syndrome, is a form of contact hypersensitivity confined almost exclusively to the oropharynx.[31] Symptoms include the rapid onset of pruritus and swelling of the lips, tongue, palate, and throat. It rarely involves other organs and symptoms and usually subsides within minutes. It is commonly seen in patients with seasonal allergic rhinitis to birch or ragweed pollens when they consume uncooked fruits and vegetables.[32–35] For example, ingestion of watermelons or bananas may trigger the oral allergy syndrome in up to 50% of patients with ragweed-induced allergic rhinitis.[36] The reactions are caused by heat-labile proteins present in these uncooked fruits and vegetables that cross-react with pollen proteins.[37] Cooking often destroys these cross-reacting heat-labile proteins, allowing some patients to tolerate cooked form of the trigger foods. For example, patients with symptoms limited to oral pruritus due to raw apple ingestion can usually tolerate cooked apples in apple pie. Patients are advised to only avoid foods that trigger their symptoms, and they do not necessarily have to avoid fruits that cross-react. For instance, as depicted in Table 4.1, cantaloupe, honeydew, watermelon, and banana all share heat-labile proteins with ragweed. A patient with ragweed allergy and oral allergy syndrome from cantaloupe may tolerate watermelon and other cross-reacting fruits.

4.2.1.2.2 GI Anaphylaxis

GI anaphylaxis is a relatively common manifestation of IgE-mediated food allergy.[1] It is reported in more than 50% of patients experiencing food allergy. It generally occurs in conjunction with other extraintestinal allergic manifestations such as respiratory and/or cutaneous reactions.[38,39] GI symptoms usually develop within minutes to 2 h after ingestion and typically consist of moderate-to-severe nausea, vomiting, diarrhea, and abdominal pain.[40]

4.2.1.2.3 Food-Dependent Exercise-Induced Anaphylaxis

Food-dependent exercise-induced anaphylaxis is a rare type of anaphylaxis. A given food only triggers an anaphylactic reaction when the individual exercises within 2–4 h of ingesting the offending food.[41] The problem is food can be ingested without consequences in the absence of exercise. Although, the prevalence of this condition is unknown, it seems to be most prevalent in female adolescents.[42] Wheat is the most implicated food, although an array of foods has been reported, including fruits, vegetables, seeds, legumes, various meats, cow's milk, and egg.[43–46]

4.2.1.2.4 Latex–Food Allergy Syndrome

Appropriately 30%–50% of individuals allergic to latex may be clinically reactive to one or more fresh fruits and/or nuts.[47] This results from a cross-reaction between

---

TABLE 4.1

Cross-Reactivity between Pollens and Fruits and Vegetables in Oral Allergy Syndrome

Birch	Almond, aniseed, apple, apricot, carrot, celery, cherry, hazelnut, parsley, peach, peanut, pear, plum
Ragweed	Banana, cantaloupe, cucumber, honeydew, watermelon, and zucchini
Mugwort	Aniseed, bell pepper, broccoli, cabbage, caraway, cauliflower, celery, fennel, garlic, mustard, onion, parsley
Orchard	Cantaloupe, honeydew, peanut, tomato, watermelon, white potato
Timothy	Swiss chard, orange

the food antigens and various latex antigens.[48] Symptoms can range from pruritus, eczema, oral–facial swelling, asthma to life-threatening anaphylaxis. Banana, avocado, chestnut, kiwi, peach, tomato, white potato, and bell pepper are common causes of latex–food allergy syndrome.[49]

4.2.1.2.5 Meat Allergy

Meat allergy is uncommon, and its prevalence is not known. Allergy to mammalian flesh is more prevalent than allergy to poultry. Beef is the most common meat allergy. It is estimated that as many as 20% of children with CMA also have beef allergy.[50] Clinical manifestations of meat allergy are variable. In children with meat allergy, ingestion of meat can exacerbate their atopic dermatitis although other symptoms such as hives, asthma, and pruritus can develop. Unlike other IgE-mediated food allergy (e.g., peanut), reaction to meat may be delayed up to 6 h after ingestion.[51] These individuals are sensitized to a carbohydrate component in meat (galactose-α-1,3-galactose), rather than the protein component which causes immediate reactions. Studies suggest that these patients are sensitized to the carbohydrate component of meat through the bite of lone star ticks, most commonly found in the Southeastern United States.[52]

4.2.2 Diagnosis of IgE-Mediated Food Allergy

The diagnosis of IgE-mediated food allergy begins with a detailed history and physical examination. With few exceptions such as meat allergy and food-dependent exercise-induced anaphylaxis, most IgE-mediated food allergic reactions occur within minutes after ingestion of the food allergen. A detailed clinical history will reveal whether the timing and nature of the reaction are compatible with an IgE-mediated reaction, allowing the physician to estimate the likelihood of a true IgE-mediated reaction. This information will be used to guide subsequent testing and interpretation of the results. To evaluate IgE-mediated food allergies, skin prick test (SPT) and immunoassay (a blood test for detecting specific IgE antibodies against a specific food) are commonly used.[53–56] In general, both tests have high negative predictive values (reliable in ruling out IgE-mediated diseases when they are negative) but low positive predictive values (abnormal test results are not sufficient to confirm the diagnosis of food allergies). Because of its modest positive predictive value, it is important to interpret the results of allergy testing in the context of the patient's clinical history and physical examination. In patients who report a delayed systemic reaction to red meat, or unexplained anaphylaxis, we recommend testing for IgE specific for the galactose-α-1,3-galactose (α-gal), which is a carbohydrate component of meat, as discussed previously.

An oral challenge and/or empirical trial of an elimination diet are often prescribed by an experienced allergist as part of an evaluation for food allergy when the clinical history is ambivalent.[10] Component-resolved diagnostics (CRD) is a blood test that measures specific IgE antibodies to individual allergen components of the food protein, rather than the total extract. It has been postulated that level of specific IgE against individual components of the food protein is more predictive than that to total extract in predicting severe allergic reactions. It has recently become available for clinical use in the United States, but its exact role in the diagnosis and management of food allergy remains to be defined.[57,58]

In our experience, patients can present in clinic with results of allergy tests that have not been validated. These include food-specific IgG and IgG_4 tests, which typically yield multiple positive results and do not reliably indicate food allergy or intolerance.[59] These tests are widely available in commercial laboratories across the country. Both the American Academy of Allergy and Immunology as well as the European Academy of Allergy and Clinical Immunology have independently issued position statements that recommend against the use of IgG4 or IgG in general for routine clinical diagnostic purposes.[59,60]

It should be noted that in vitro testing and SPT have no role in diagnosing reactions to food that are not mediated by IgE antibodies (e.g., eosinophilic esophagitis [EoE], celiac disease, and food protein-induced enterocolitis syndrome [FPIES]). Food allergy patch testing, T cell cytokine assays, and measurements of eosinophil activation markers have shown promise, but they are not standardized and cannot be recommended outside of research or specialized clinical settings. As discussed in other chapters, mucosal biopsies are required to establish the diagnosis of celiac disease, EoE, and eosinophilic GI disorders.[61]

Guidelines for the evaluation and management of food allergies have been published by the American Gastroenterological Association,[62] National Institute of Allergy and Infectious Diseases,[63] Joint Task Force on Practice Parameters (representing the American Academy of Allergy, Asthma and Immunology, the American College of Allergy, Asthma and Immunology, and the Joint Council of Allergy, Asthma and Immunology)[61] and various organizations at local or national levels.

4.2.2.1   Emerging Role of Dietitians in Oral Food Challenge

The role of dietitians in food allergy has been evolving and expanding over the years. Dietitians play an important role, not only in the management, but also in the diagnosis of food allergy. Double-blind, placebo-controlled food challenge (DBPCFC) is the gold standard for diagnosing food allergy. At specialized food allergy centers, the dietitian plays a key role in conducting the DBPCFC. It is often difficult to conceal the identity of food being given in the challenge (because of the texture, color, smell, and taste), and this is where expertise of a dietitian comes into play. They are often involved in the preparation of foods for the trial. In DBPCFC, the allergenic food is hidden either in another food or in opaque capsules. Opaque capsules pose several potential problems: (1) inability of younger children to swallow the capsule; (2) capsules can bypass oral contact, which would normally provide the earliest clues of an allergic reaction; (3) slow degradation of capsules may result in overlapping doses resulting in unintended administration of a higher than needed dose to elicit symptoms. Therefore, mixing allergenic foods into masking foods is preferable in clinical practice. Common masking foods include baby foods (squash, carrot, and potato), applesauce, corn meals, oats, mashed potatoes, and juices. In patients with multiple food allergies, use of hypoallergenic formula or amino acid-based formula as the masking vehicles can be considered. Recipes for masking common food allergens have been published and validated.[64,65] Knowledge of preparing challenge foods and placebos for oral challenge has become a critical part of training for dietitians in specialized food allergy centers.

4.2.3   Management of IgE-Mediated Food Allergy

The management of an IgE-mediated food allergy consists of the 3Es: elimination, education, and epinephrine.

Elimination: Currently, there is no cure for food allergy. Oral immunotherapy is promising but cannot be recommended outside of research settings.[66] Strict avoidance is the cornerstone of management.[67] Elimination of food protein is easy in theory but difficult in practice.[68–70] In many countries including the United States, Canada, European Union, and China, food labeling laws require food manufacturers to declare in plain language the presence of common allergens (including egg, milk, wheat, soy, fish, crustacean, peanut, and tree nuts) in a food product.[71] Educational materials related to the eight most common food allergens and general approaches to avoidance in different settings are available through resources such as the Food Allergy Research and Education (http://www.foodallergy.org) and the Consortium of Food Allergy Research (http://www.cofargroup.org).[72]

Education: Family members and other caretakers must be taught to recognize the early signs and symptoms of food allergy, and to promptly administer the necessary medications if an allergic reaction occurs.[73,74] Delayed recognition of allergic reactions and administration of epinephrine are associated with fatal allergic reactions.[28] The authors recommend wearing an alert bracelet for all patients with food allergy. It is important to educate patients about cross-reaction and cross-contact. For example, an estimated 25%–40% of people who have peanut allergy also are allergic to tree nuts (cross-reaction). In addition, peanuts and tree nuts often come into contact with one another (cross-contact) during manufacturing and serving processes. For these reasons, allergists often advise young children with peanut allergy to avoid tree nuts as well.

Epinephrine: Most food-triggered allergic reactions are accidental and occur in foods that are thought to be safe.[75] It is often due to mislabeling, cross-contact or cross-contamination. Intramuscular (IM) epinephrine is the first-line treatment in all cases of anaphylaxis. Given the difficulty in preventing accidental exposure to the offending allergen, all patients with food allergy must carry two self-injectable epinephrine devices (EpiPen®, Twinject®, or Auvi-Q™) with them at all times.[76] All patients with food allergy should have a clear and simple written action plan for the treatment of allergic reactions to food. A template of food allergy action plan can be downloaded from http://www.foodallergy.org/.

4.2.3.1   Tips for Managing Specific IgE-Mediated Food Allergy

4.2.3.1.1   Peanuts and Tree Nuts

Up to 50% of peanut-allergic patients are also allergic to tree nuts.[77] Avoidance of all tree nuts by young peanut-allergic children is recommended, given the concerns about cross-contamination and challenges in reliably identifying specific tree nuts.[78] For older children and motivated individuals, supervised oral challenge may be prescribed before introducing tree nuts in the diet.

4.2.3.1.2 Milk

IgE-mediated CMA is one of the most common food allergies. While avoidance is the cornerstone of management, there are unique challenges in the nutrition management of adults and pediatric patients with CMA.

Cow's milk (CM) is a common ingredient in baked goods, cereals, chocolate, candy, custard, pudding, sherbet, luncheon meats, hot dogs, sausages, margarine, salad dressing, breaded foods, casseroles, soups, potato, pasta, and vegetable dishes. It is a good source of protein, fat, calcium, vitamin D, vitamin B_{12}, vitamin A, pantothenic acid, and riboflavin. Since it is so ubiquitous, eliminating CM from the diet can be difficult and can pose nutritional as well as quality of life concerns.[79]

For adults, most nutrients found in CM can easily be replaced from alternative dietary sources (Table 4.2). Calcium and vitamin D may be an exception because it is difficult to meet calcium needs through nondairy sources without careful substitution.[80,81] Patients with CMA are at risk of vitamin D and calcium deficiency leading to increased risk of osteoporosis and fracture. Calcium and vitamin D supplement are generally recommended for adult patients with CMA.

There are unique aspects in the nutrition management of breastfed infants, formula infants, and toddlers with CMA.[79] For breastfed infants, continuation of breast feeding is encouraged provided that the mother can eliminate dairy products from her diet reliably. A mother on a milk-free diet is advised to take calcium supplement (1000 mg/day) and a milk-free prenatal vitamin supplement.[82]

For formula-fed infants with CMA, extensively hydrolyzed formula (eHF) is recommended (e.g., Similac® Alimentum®, Enfamil Nutramigen®, Enfamil Nutramigen® with Enflora™ LGG, and Pregestimil®) over soy formula or partially hydrolyzed CM formula (e.g., Nestle Good Start® and Enfamil Gentlease®).[79]

At 1 year of age, most infants transition from a complete formula to whole milk. Enriched alternative milk beverages (EAMB) such as rice milk, soymilk, and potato milk generally do not provide comparable nutrition to whole CM or formula (Table 4.3). Breast milk and/or eHF remain very good options. For older toddlers, enriched soymilk is an appropriate alternative if they tolerate soy. For toddlers with concomitant milk and soy allergy, enriched oat milk is a viable option. It is important to meet

---

TABLE 4.2

Alternative Dietary Source of Milk Nutrients

Calcium	EAMB[a], calcium-fortified juices and tofu
Protein	Meat, eggs, fish, poultry, peanut, tree nuts, seeds, soy, and legumes
Fat	Meat, fish, poultry, peanuts, tree nuts, seeds, vegetable oils, margarine
Vitamin D	EAMB, fortified margarine, salmon, and other fatty fish
Vitamin B_{12}	Meat, fish, poultry, eggs, and EAMB
Vitamin B_5	Eggs, meat, vegetables, legumes, whole grains
Vitamin A	Dark green leafy vegetables, egg yolk, fortified margarine, EAMB
Riboflavin	Dark green leafy vegetables, whole grain products

[a] EAMB = enriched alternative milk beverages (soy, rice, oat, almond, hemp, and potato).

TABLE 4.3

Nutritional Comparison of Enriched Alternative Milk Beverages

8 oz of:	Kcal	Protein (g)	Fat (g)	Calcium (g)	Vitamin D (units)
Cow's milk (whole)	150	8	8	300	100
Enriched soy milk	100	7	4	350	100
Enriched rice milk	120	1	2.5	300	100
Enriched oat milk	120	4	3	300	100
Enriched almond milk	50	1	2.5	300	100
Enriched potato milk	70	0	0	300	100

Note: Nutritional contents may vary depending on the individual brand and formulation.

the entire protein requirement through solid foods in the diet prior to switching to EAMB because of their lower protein contents. Additional fat in the form of vegetable oils may be warranted.

In general, plant-based EAMB are preferred to mammalian milk because of their wide availability and concern of clinically relevant cross-reactivity between CM and milk from other mammals.[83] For example, most patients with CMA do not tolerate milk from sheep and goats.[84,85] Milk from donkeys and mares may be better tolerated in some cases, but they are generally not commercially available.[86]

The majority of patients (~75%) with CMA tolerate extensively heated or baked forms of milk (such as muffins, cookie, cake, etc.)[87] For those who tolerate extensively heated milk, regular ingestion seems to accelerate the development of CM tolerance as compared to those who avoid all dairy products.[88] However, skin testing or immunoassays are not helpful in identifying these patients. Roughly a quarter of the patients with CMA react to extensively heated milk and of those who react, a third of them can develop anaphylaxis. Therefore, a supervised oral challenge to extensively heated milk is required to document the tolerance before baked milk products can be added to the diet of individuals with CMA.

4.2.3.1.3 Seafood

There is considerable risk of clinical cross-reactivity between crustaceans,[11] and avoidance of all members of the crustacean family is generally recommended for a patient who has crustacean allergy.[89] Crustaceans do not cross-react with vertebrate fish. It is not necessary to avoid fish in patients with crustacean allergy and vice versa. Cross-reactivity between vertebrate fish is highly variable. Patients with a specific vertebrate fish allergy may tolerate vertebrate fish of a different species. For example, a patient who is allergic to salmon may tolerate tuna. In highly motivated patients, oral challenge may be prescribed to determine clinical tolerance to various vertebrate fish. Many other foods can supply the nutrients found in seafood and substitution can easily be made.

Contrary to popular belief, seafood or shellfish allergy is NOT an independent risk factor for intravenous (IV) contrast hypersensitivity.[90] This misconception stems from the fact that both seafood and IV contrast have a high iodine content. However, iodine does not cause an allergic reaction. It is the tropomyosin protein in the seafood that triggers allergic reactions.

4.2.3.1.4 Wheat

Wheat is present in many processed foods such as crackers, cookies, cakes, pasta, bread, and cereal. As a minor ingredient, it can be found in condiments, marinades, cold cuts, soy sauce, hard candies, low-fat products, and so on. The major product of wheat, wheat flour, is a great source of carbohydrates, iron, thiamine, riboflavin, niacin, folic acid, vitamin B_6, magnesium, and fiber. Alternative dietary sources of these macro- and micronutrients are shown in Table 4.4. In addition, there is a wide variety of wheat-free and gluten-free products made from alternative flours (rice, corn, oat, barley, buckwheat, rye, amaranth, millet, and quinoa). These alternative flours are widely available, but few of them are fortified. A fortified infant cereal (made from grains that the patient is not allergic to) can be added to the alternative flours to enhance its nutritional value. It is important to note that up to 20% of the individuals with an allergy to one grain will have allergies to other grains.[35] Use of these alternative grain products should be individualized and based upon tolerance as determined by an allergist. Note that celiac disease is not considered a grain allergy in this context.

4.2.3.1.5 Egg

Individuals with egg allergy should avoid eggs from duck, turkey, goose, quail, and other species as they cross-react with chicken egg. Elimination of egg from the diet is unlikely to cause nutritional deficiency as many foods supply the nutrients found in eggs (protein, vitamin B_{12}, riboflavin, pantothenic acid, biotin, and selenium). Egg is a common ingredient in the Western diet, and one major challenge is to learn how to replace eggs as an ingredient in cooking/baking. Eggs serve two major roles in baking: (1) as a binder and (2) leavening agent. For recipes that use eggs as a binder (such as drop cookie), possible substitutes for one egg include 1/2 of a mashed banana,

---

TABLE 4.4

Alternative Dietary Source of Wheat Nutrients

Fiber	Fruits, vegetables, alternative whole grains
Carbohydrates	Products made with alternative grains or flours: rice, oat, corn, buckwheat, potato, tapioca, chickpea, amaranth, millet, quinoa; fruits, and vegetables
Niacin (vitamin B_3)	Meat, fish, poultry, liver, peanuts, sunflower seeds, legumes, enriched and whole grain alternative grain products
Thiamine (vitamin B_1)	Liver, pork, other meats, sunflower seeds, enriched and whole grain alternative grain products, nuts, and legumes
Riboflavin	Milk, dark green leafy vegetables, enriched and whole grain alternative grain products
Iron	Meat, fish, shellfish, poultry, enriched and whole grain alternative grain products, legumes, and dried fruits
Folic acid	Enriched and whole grain alternative grain products, beef liver, green leafy vegetables, legumes, seeds, orange juice

1/4 cup of applesauce, 3.5 teaspoons of gelatin blend, and 1 teaspoon of ground flax seed mixed with 3 tablespoons warm water. To replace egg as a leavening agent, use 1½ tablespoons of vegetable oil mixed with 1½ tablespoons of water and 1 teaspoon of baking powder per egg replaced. Many egg replacement recipes can be found in the Internet. Commercial egg replacement products are readily available. They are different from egg substitute, which contain egg and are designed for cholesterol-conscious patients, not egg-allergic patients. For those who can tolerate baked eggs (as demonstrated by supervised oral challenge), its regular ingestion may accelerate the development of egg tolerance.[91]

Some vaccines utilize egg proteins during production and/or as an ingredient. Examples include influenza vaccines, yellow fever vaccines, measles, mumps and rubella (MMR) vaccines. Allergic reactions to yellow fever vaccines have been reported.[92] The management of these vaccinations in patients with egg allergy is beyond the scope of this chapter and information can be found in published guidelines.[93]

There are case reports of anaphylaxis due to consumption of lipid emulsion that contain egg (e.g., propofol and intralipids) as well as drugs containing egg lysozyme.[94–96] There are no guidelines on how to approach patients with egg allergy who require propofol or drugs containing lysozyme. We manage these patients on a case-by-case basis with the assistance from an allergist. To note, IV fat emulsion contains egg, and there is currently no egg-free alternative. Given the absolute risk of anaphylaxis is very small, we give IV fat emulsion to egg-allergic patients if clinically indicated.

4.2.3.1.6   Soy

Soy contains protein, thiamine, riboflavin, pyridoxine, folic acid, calcium, phosphorus, magnesium, iron, and zinc. Soy does not appear in large quantities in a Western diet and its elimination usually does not lead to any nutritional deficiency, unless the patient has concomitant allergy (most commonly milk) or other dietary preference (such as vegetarianism). Many vegetarian-based products contain soy proteins, and so do a large assortment of products, including baked goods, cereals, crackers, canned tuna and soups, reduced-fat peanut butter, prebasted meat products, cold cuts, and hot dogs. Most patients with soy allergy can tolerate highly refined soy oil and soy lecithin,[97] which are present in many processed or manufactured foods. On the other hand, soy fibers (a by-product of soybean processing) may contain soy proteins and should be avoided in individuals with soy allergy.

4.2.3.1.7   Meat

Meat allergy is broadly classified into immediate and delayed (a.k.a. α-galactose allergy). Immediate meat allergy is usually triggered by the protein component of meat from one particular species,[98] although cross-reactivity of meats between two closely evolutionarily related species is plausible.[99] For example, patients with immediate beef allergy may react to mutton or pork, but rarely to poultry or fish. Similarly, patients may react to chicken and turkey, but not to mammalian meats. Delayed IgE-mediated reactions are usually triggered by the carbohydrate component of meat, galactose-α-1,3-galactose. Avoidance of all mammalian meats is recommended in delayed meat allergy because galactose-α-1,3-galactose is widely expressed in mammalian tissues.[51]

4.2.3.1.8   Food Additives

Of the thousands of food additives used in the food industry, only a relatively small number have been implicated in causing allergic reactions. The prevalence of allergy to food additives was 0.23%, far less than that from nutritive foods.[100] Examples of food additives that have been reported to cause allergic reactions include sodium benzoate (E211), spearmint, peppermint, menthol, annatto (E160b), carmine (E120), saffron, erythritol, guar gum (E412), psyllium, carrageenan, lupine flour, gelatin, and pectin. Sulfite has been associated with severe asthmatic reactions in as many as 5% of asthmatics. Similar to food allergy, avoidance is the cornerstone of the management.

4.2.3.1.9   Multiple Food Allergies and Dietary Preference

The first step in evaluating a patient who complains of multiple food allergies is to rule out other causes of adverse food reactions (e.g., inflammatory bowel disease [IBD], celiac disease, functional dyspepsia and other functional GI disorders [FGID], and symptomatic gallstones) and to confirm the diagnosis of food allergies. The diagnostic approach should be individualized on a case-to-case basis. In general, few patients have multiple clinically relevant IgE-mediated food allergies. When food allergies are suspected or need to be systematically ruled out, we recommend referring the patient to an allergist with expertise in the evaluation of food allergies/intolerances. Securing a diagnosis is particularly prudent in patients with FGID because they often self-report allergy to multiple foods and treat themselves with a restrictive diet. Multiple food elimination has a negative impact on nutritional status. Serial supervised oral challenges are often needed to rule out their food allergies and to convince patients that it is safe to add the food back into their diet. Some patients refuse to proceed with oral challenge or are reluctant to reintroduce food back to their diet despite negative oral challenge. In other cases, patients with dietary restriction for other reasons can present with food allergy (e.g., a vegetarian child who develops soy allergy). These patients are at higher risk of suffering from nutritional deficiency because many vegetarian foods contain soy proteins and elimination of soy from a vegetarian diet limits the food choices and varieties significantly. Clinicians should be sensitive to a patient's diet preference and understand that changing one's diet might not be acceptable to the individual for cultural, religious or other reasons.

4.2.4   GENETICALLY MODIFIED FOOD AND FOOD ALLERGY

The United States is the largest commercial producer of genetically modified (GM) crops in the world. Since the first GM food, delayed ripening tomato, became commercially available in 1994,[101] production and consumption of GM foods have been steadily increasing. Soybeans, corn, canola, and cottonseed oil are some of the major GM foods consumed today. They gained popularity because of their resistance to pathogens and herbicides, as well as enhanced nutritional values. In the United States, the Food and Drug Administration (FDA) does not mandate labeling of GM foods.[102] Because these foods are genetically altered, there are concerns about their safety and questions whether their consumption contributes to the rising incidences of food allergy. To date, there is no published evidence of adverse human health effects or allergic reactions to any GM food from approved GM crops.[103] There is a broad scientific consensus that GM foods in the market are safe to eat and pose no greater risk than conventional food.[104]

4.2.5 PREVENTION OF FOOD ALLERGY

Dietitians and clinicians are often asked if food allergy can be prevented by manipulation of either the mother's and/or infant's diet. Recent guidelines recommended exclusive breast feeding of all infants for the first 4–6 months of life, regardless of their allergy risks.[10,105] Should breast feeding not be feasible, guidelines have suggested that a hydrolyzed infant formula may be considered as a strategy for the prevention of food allergy (milk allergy specifically) or atopic dermatitis for infants with a family history of atopy.[10,105,106] Maternal avoidance diets during pregnancy or lactation have not been proven to be effective in reducing the risk of developing food allergy.[78] Probiotics or prebiotics have not been conclusively shown to prevent food allergy.[107]

4.2.6 OTHER IMMUNE-MEDIATED GI ADVERSE REACTIONS TO FOOD

Examples of non-IgE mediated food allergy include FPIES, food protein-induced proctocolitis, food protein-induced enteropathy syndrome, celiac disease, EoE, and eosinophilic gastrointestinal disorders (EGID). Similar to IgE-mediated food allergies, the prevalence of these other forms of immune-mediated ARF seems to be on the rise over the past 10–15 years. This is a very heterogeneous group of diseases, and each appears to have very different underlying mechanisms. Multiple components of the immune systems appear to play a role. Each of these conditions has its unique nutritional challenges. The nutritional management of celiac disease, EoE, and EGID will be discussed elsewhere.

4.2.6.1 Food Protein-Induced Enterocolitis Syndrome

FPIES is a rare, severe disorder primarily affecting infants. It is most often triggered by CM or soy protein, but it can also be caused by solid food such as rice.[108] Affected infants present with protracted vomiting, bleeding, diarrhea, anemia, lethargy, failure to thrive, and in some cases, shock. Since this disorder is not IgE-mediated, food-specific IgE antibodies have no value in diagnosing FPIES. The fact that FPIES can mimic the presentation of IBD and a variety of GI infections makes the diagnosis difficult. Given the severity of the immune reaction, provocative food challenges are not always necessary or practical.[109] Diagnosis is based on compatible history and physical examination. Breastfeeding can be continued and should be encouraged if the mother is able to eliminate soy and cow milk from her diet. If breastfeeding is not possible, an extensively hydrolyzed formula is recommended over soy-based formula, due to frequent concomitant cow's milk and soy FPIES.[110] Improvement of symptoms is expected in 3–10 days after the elimination of the food trigger.[111] Up to 20% of the infants do not tolerate extensively hydrolyzed formula and require an elemental amino acids-based formula.[112] With close monitoring, malnutrition is rare in infants fed these alternative milk formulas. One-third of infants with milk or soy FPIES develop solid food FPIES with rice and other grains. Therefore, yellow fruits and vegetables should be introduced at 6 months of age, instead of cereals.[113] Given the high rate of reactions to multiple foods, a delayed introduction of grains, legumes, and poultry is recommended for infants with solid food FPIES, up to 1 year old.[109]

4.2.6.2 Food Protein-Induced Proctitis/Proctocolitis

Food protein-induced proctitis/proctocolitis is a common cause of rectal bleeding in otherwise healthy infants.[114] As its name implies, the disease is limited to the rectum and distal sigmoid colon. The most common food triggers are CM, soymilk, or human breast milk during infancy. Since food protein-induced proctitis/proctocolitis is not mediated by IgE, food-specific IgE and SPT results are typically negative. Diagnosis is made based on clinical history and prompt resolution of symptoms with elimination of food trigger. The mother should be encouraged to continue breast feeding if she is willing to completely eliminate dairy products from her diet, including butter.[115] It may take up to 2 weeks for the rectal bleeding to improve. If there is no improvement, then soy (and possibly egg) should be eliminated from the mother's diet. If breastfeeding is not possible, an eHF should be used. The parents should be warned that many infants have green loose stools when fed with eHF, and it does not indicate ongoing colitis. In rare cases, elemental formula is needed in refractory cases.

4.2.6.3 Food Protein-Induced Enteropathy

Food protein-induced enteropathy is an uncommon disorder that primarily affects the small bowel.[116] A typical presentation is a young infant who presents with chronic diarrhea due to malabsorption, anemia, weight loss, and growth failure.[117] The most common trigger is CM protein, but other foods such as soy, chicken, rice, and fish have also been reported.[118] Skin testing and specific IgE serology is not helpful in identifying the food trigger(s). Diagnosis is based on clinical history, and a biopsy of the small bowel is sometimes needed in equivocal cases to confirm villous injury. Due to malabsorption, affected infants can develop moderate anemia and hypoproteinemia.

4.3 FOOD INTOLERANCE

Most adverse food reactions are not immunological in origin.[10] These nonimmunological food-triggered reactions are commonly referred to as food sensitivity or food intolerance.[10] For our discussion, we will use the term food intolerance to describe food-triggered adverse reaction that is not driven by our immune system. Food intolerance is much more common than food allergy. Clinically, it is important to distinguish food intolerance from food allergy because the prognosis, management, and nutritional implications are different. In this section, we will discuss some key examples of food intolerance that can mimic food allergy.

4.3.1 FOODBORNE DISEASES

Foodborne disease results from microbial contamination of food and typically manifests as a mixture of nausea, vomiting, fever, abdominal pain, and diarrhea.[119] A good history and physical examination are usually sufficient to distinguish such reactions from other forms of food-triggered reactions. Occasionally, the patient can develop irritable bowel syndrome (IBS) or other FGID following a foodborne illness.[120] GI infections affecting the small bowel can also lead to transient lactose intolerance, causing bloating, abdominal pain, and diarrhea with milk ingestion. Since most food poisoning episodes are self-limited, they do not pose a significant risk for malnutrition.

4.3.2 PHARMACOLOGICAL REACTIONS

Ingestion of a tyramine-rich food (such as wine and aged cheese) in an individual taking a class of antidepressant known as monoamine oxidase inhibitors (MAOIs) can lead to hypertensive crisis. MAOIs inhibit the breakdown of tyramine by impairing the function of monoamine oxidase A (MAO_A). If a sufficient quantity of tyramine is ingested in the setting of MAO_A inhibition, a hypertensive crisis can result with the potential to cause a stroke or arrhythmia. Certain individuals develop migraine headaches with ingestion of various foods including those rich in amines. Despite the widespread belief that monosodium glutamate can cause "Chinese restaurant syndrome," a constellation of symptoms including headache, flushing, chest pain, sense of facial numbness and swelling, whether the relationship is causal has recently been challenged.[121,122] Ingestion of foods with high histamine content such as well ripened cheese, pickled cabbage, red wine, and tuna fish can rarely cause a wide range of allergic-like symptoms in susceptible individuals with a genetic defect in the metabolism of exogenous histamine.[123]

4.3.3 LACTOSE INTOLERANCE

Lactose intolerance is the most common food intolerance, with most cases resulting from a genetically regulated reduction of intestinal lactase activity later in childhood or early adolescence.[124] It affects up to 20% of Caucasian adults, 50% Hispanics, 75% African and African Americans, and exceeds 90% in some Asian populations.[125] Congenital lactase deficiency is a rare autosomal recessive disorder, and less than 40 cases have been reported.[126] Lactose intolerance in children younger than 5 years of age of any racial or ethnic group almost always indicates a secondary cause of lactase deficiency such as bacterial overgrowth or mucosal injury of the GI tract (e.g., celiac disease, IBD, and viral gastroenteritis).[127] Clinical symptoms of lactose intolerance include diarrhea, abdominal pain, and flatulence after ingestion of milk or milk-containing products.[128] The lactose breath hydrogen test provides a simple, accurate and noninvasive way to confirm the diagnosis.[129] It is important to confirm the diagnosis in some settings because patients with FGID such as IBS, functional dyspepsia, or functional bloating often complain of GI symptoms after eating most types of dairy products.[130,131]

The majority of individuals with lactose intolerance can tolerate adequate dairy products to achieve their daily calcium requirement (1500 mg/day). Studies have shown most patients with lactose intolerance can tolerate up to 240 mL of milk a day without exacerbation of their symptoms.[132,133] Strict avoidance of dairy products is not necessary and should be avoided, because dairy products are one of the most bio-available sources of ingested calcium and vitamin D. Among dairy products, milk, and ice cream contain the highest concentration of lactose, while cheeses and live culture yogurts contain the least. These low to no lactose dairy products are usually well tolerated by patients with lactose intolerance and are an excellent source of protein and calcium.[134] Commercially available lactase enzymes can be added to lactose-containing food or ingested with meals containing lactose to reduce symptoms. Moreover, lactose-free milk products are readily available in grocery stores. Since patients with lactose intolerance often have significantly lower calcium intake, calcium and vitamin D supplementation should be considered to reduce the risk for osteoporosis and fracture.[135]

4.3.4   OTHER CARBOHYDRATES INTOLERANCE

With the increasingly widespread use of high fructose corn syrups in food processing, there is a growing concern over fructose malabsorption. GI symptoms related to fructose malabsorption appear to be more common in individuals who have an underlying FGIDs such as IBS. Carbohydrate intolerance due to a congenital enzyme deficiency (e.g., sucrase isomaltase, fructose aldolase B and others) or a transport defect (e.g., GLUT5) is very rare and accounts for only a minority of the cases. This topic is discussed in more details in Chapter 2.

4.3.5   PSYCHOLOGICAL ADVERSE REACTIONS TO FOOD

Psychological ARF appear to be more prevalent in patients with FGIDs and/or underlying psychiatric disorders.[136] Patients with psychological ARF often report adverse reactions to multiple foods. They often associate headache, acnes, pain, fatigues, and a variety of nonspecific symptoms to food ingestion. It is not uncommon to see such patients self-treat themselves with a whole array of elimination diets such as VIRGIN, PALEO, anti-yeast diet, and so on. The more foods that are excluded from their diet, the greater the risk of nutritional deficiency. On the other hand, this same group of patients is more likely to supplement their diet with supra-therapeutic amounts of "health food" preparations and nutritional supplements. The dangers of over-supplementation are well described.[137] Some patients may be willing to reintroduce suspect foods into their diet if diagnostic tests fail to confirm a food-related reaction. Targeted skin testing, IgE serology, and/or food challenges may be indicated in selected patients.

4.3.6 Physiological Reactions to Food

Fatty foods, chocolate, peppermint, colas, red wine, orange juice, and excessive alcohol are known to reduce lower esophageal sphincter pressure and worsen symptoms of GERD.[138] Legumes, onions, cabbage, bran fiber, and grains serve as a substrate for gas production by colonic flora and can aggravate bloating symptoms. These physiological reactions to foods are typically noted by patients with FGID, many of whom appear to have heightened sensory responses to normal digestive events. As long as a balanced diet is maintained, avoidance of the specific food items described herein has virtually no impact on nutritional status.

4.3.7 Other Causes of Food Intolerance

Peptic ulcer disease, biliary dyskinesia, hiatal hernia, small bowel bacterial overgrowth, Hirschsprung's disease, gallstone, pancreatic insufficiency, short bowel syndrome, luminal stricture, achalasia, and pseudo-obstruction are just a few examples of GI conditions that patients with such disorders often perceive as a food-triggered adverse reaction.[139]

4.3.8 Fish Poisoning

Fish poisoning can often present with symptoms similar to that of seafood allergy. Examples of fish poisoning that can mimic fish allergy are scombroid, ciguatera fish, and pufferfish poisoning.

Scombroid poisoning is a common seafood-associated disease.[140] It is classically associated with tuna, mackerel, mahi-mahi, bluefish, swordfish, salmon, trout, and so on. Signs and symptoms usually begin within an hour of eating contaminated fish that are improperly stored after being caught, leading to bacterial overgrowth and the accumulation of toxic levels of histamine. Patients may experience flushing, rash, diarrhea, and headache.[141] Perioral burning or itching, dizziness, palpitations, and tachycardia may also be present. Rarely, severe bronchospasm, arrhythmia, and cardiovascular collapse can occur in individuals with underlying asthma or cardiopulmonary disorders. These symptoms mimic allergic reactions and are frequently misdiagnosed as seafood allergy.

Another fish-associated disease that is often confused with fish allergy is ciguateria fish poisoning. Ciguatera fish poisoning accounts for 20% of all fish-related foodborne disease outbreaks in the United States.[142] Ciguatera fish poisoning is caused by consumption of fish contaminated with toxins formed by single-celled algae-like organisms that grow on coral reefs. These toxins are concentrated in the organs and flesh of large, predatory reef fish such as moray eel, barracuda, red snapper, and grouper. Ciguatera toxin-containing fish do not appear, taste, or smell different. Cooking and freezing do not destroy the toxins. Patients can present with various GI symptoms (e.g., vomiting, diarrhea, abdominal pain), neurologic abnormalities (perioral paraesthesias, pruritus, a metallic taste, painful urination, blurred vision), and cardiovascular signs (arrhythmia, heart block, and/or drop in blood pressure).

One specific neurologic finding of ciguatera poisoning is temperature-related dyses-thesias (cold stimuli perceived as hot or producing an abnormal or unpleasant sensation) that occurs in up to 10% of patients.

Sporadic cases of pufferfish (also known as blowfish) poisoning have been reported in the United States.[143] It is more common in Japan where pufferfish is considered a delicacy. It is caused by a neurotoxin, tetrodotoxin, that is produced by microorganisms associated with the fish. Symptoms occur rapidly after ingestion and manifest as paresthesias of the face and extremities, nausea, lightheadedness, weakness, and loss of reflexes. In severe cases, patients can develop cardiopulmonary collapse and generalized paralysis.

All patients with suspected fish poisoning and/or fish allergy should be referred to a physician for further evaluation and management.

4.3.9   NONCELIAC GLUTEN SENSITIVITY

The gluten-free diet (GFD) has been gaining popularity among patients with IBS in whom celiac disease has been excluded. Such patients, as well as others, with FGIDs are thought to have nonceliac gluten sensitivity (NCGS).[144] How gluten might cause symptoms in the absence of celiac disease/gut inflammation, and its exact role in triggering symptoms is a subject of intense interest.[145,146] NCGS may be the one form of food sensitivity in which there is some evidence of immune system activation, but the findings have not been reproducible. However, what exactly constitutes NCGS remains to be defined and as such NCGS is a seemingly heterogeneous condition and is likely to arise from many factors.

Gluten has been shown to cause symptoms in IBS patients in a double-blind, randomized, placebo-controlled trial.[147] However, these same investigators recently showed that after eliminating fermentable oligosaccharides, disaccharides, mono-saccharides and polyols (FODMAPs) for a 2-week washout period, a blinded challenge with gluten showed no difference in symptoms in IBS patients when compared to a placebo challenge suggesting that it may be fermentable carbohy-drates that may lead to perceived gluten intolerance.[146] Low FODMAP diets are discussed below.

A formal nutritional consult is warranted for patients who are counseled to or decide to undergo an empirical trial of GFD. The role of a dietitian is to help patients eliminate gluten effectively and to help the patient to understand the goal and end points of the GFD trial. The end-points of the trial are individualized and negoti-ated among the patient, physician, and the dietitian. Common end points used are: the patient's specific symptoms such as bloating and dyspepsia, bowel movement frequency, texture of stool, and/or ease of passage. If there is no meaningful clinical improvement after a 4-week GFD trial, gluten can be introduced back into the diet to avoid any nutritional deficiency. Long-term avoidance of gluten may be needed for those who find symptom relief from a GFD. Nutritional management of patients with NCGS who avoid gluten completely is not different from that of celiac disease but it is unclear if there is any harm beyond symptoms in those with NCGS who eat small amounts of gluten compared to the immunological damage that could occur in those with celiac disease.

4.3.10 INTOLERANCE TO FERMENTABLE STARCHES INCLUDING WHEAT STARCH

A group in Australia has reported that some patients with IBS are sensitive to foods that can be fermented by the gut microbial flora. These food components are referred to as FODMAPs. The low FODMAP diet has been shown, in a limited number of studies, to benefit patients with IBS.[147] Although the same group reported that gluten caused GI symptoms in patients with IBS (see prior section), recently they showed that gluten had no significant effect compared to a placebo in IBS patients treated with a low FODMAP diet for 2 weeks.[146] This study and others have suggested that NCGS may actually be wheat intolerance since wheat starch is a major member of the FODMAP group in most Western diets. The number of foods that constitute FODMAPS is extensive, and it is strongly recommended that an expert dietitian is involved in counseling and monitoring patients on a low FODMAP diet. The role of dietary factors in patients with IBS is a major area of interest and investigation,[148,149] and is discussed in Chapter 10.

REFERENCES

1. Bischoff S, Crowe SE. Gastrointestinal food allergy: New insights into pathophysiology and clinical perspectives. *Gastroenterology* 2005;128:1089–1113.
2. Sampson HA. Update on food allergy. *J Allergy Clin Immuno* 2004;113:805–819.
3. Anon. QuickStats: Percentage of children aged <18 years with reported food, skin, or hay fever/respiratory allergies—National Health Interview Survey, United States, 1998–2009. Available at: http://www.cdc.gov/mmwr/preview/mmwrhtml/mm6011a7.htm?s_cid+mm6011a7_w. Accessed November 3, 2013.
4. Liu AH, Jaramillo R, Sicherer SH et al. National prevalence and risk factors for food allergy and relationship to asthma: Results from the National Health and Nutrition Examination Survey 2005–2006. *J Allergy Clin Immunol* 2010;126:798–806.e13.
5. Gupta RS, Springston EE, Warrier MR et al. The prevalence, severity, and distribution of childhood food allergy in the United States. *Pediatrics* 2011;128:e9–e17.
6. Sampson HA, Mendelson L, Rosen JP. Fatal and near-fatal anaphylactic reactions to food in children and adolescents. *N Engl J Med* 1992;327(6):380–384.
7. Gupta R, Holdford D, Bilaver L et al. The high economic burden of childhood food allergy in the United States. *J Allergy Clin Immunol* 2013;131:AB223.
8. Clark S, Espinola J, Rudders SA et al. Frequency of US emergency department visits for food-related acute allergic reactions. *J Allergy Clin Immunol* 2011;127:682–683.
9. Sicherer SH. Epidemiology of food allergy. *J Allergy Clin Immunol* 2011;127:594–602.
10. Sampson HA, Aceves S, Bock SA et al. Food allergy: A practice parameter update-2014. *J Allergy Clin Immunol* 2014;135(5):1016–1025.
11. Sicherer SH, Muñoz-Furlong A, Sampson HA. Prevalence of seafood allergy in the United States determined by a random telephone survey. *J Allergy Clin Immunol* 2004;114:159–165.
12. Sicherer SH, Sampson HA. Food allergy: Recent advances in pathophysiology and treatment. *Annu Rev Med* 2009;60:261–277.
13. Sicherer SH, Sampson HA. 10. Food allergy. *J Allergy Clin Immunol* 2009. Available at: http://www.ncbi.nlm.nih.gov.ezproxy.library.tufts.edu/pubmed/20042231. Accessed February 1, 2010.
14. Järvinen KM. Food-induced anaphylaxis. *Curr Opin Allergy Clin Immunol* 2011;11:255–261.
15. Simons FER. Anaphylaxis. *J Allergy Clin Immunol* 2010;125:S161–181.

16. Sampson HA, Muñoz-Furlong A, Bock SA et al. Symposium on the definition and management of anaphylaxis: Summary report. *J Allergy Clin Immunol* 2005;115:584–591.
17. Burks W. Skin manifestations of food allergy. *Pediatrics* 2003;111:1617–1624.
18. Delgado J, Castillo R, Quiralte J et al. Contact urticaria in a child from raw potato. *Contact Dermatitis* 1996;35:179–180.
19. Wainstein BK, Kashef S, Ziegler M et al. Frequency and significance of immediate contact reactions to peanut in peanut-sensitive children. *Clin Exp Allergy J Br Soc Allergy Clin Immunol* 2007;37:839–845.
20. Fisher AA. Contact urticaria from handling meats and fowl. *Cutis* 1982;30:726, 729.
21. Jovanovic M, Oliwiecki S, Beck MH. Occupational contact urticaria from beef associated with hand eczema. *Contact Dermatitis* 1992;27:188–189.
22. Ross MP, Ferguson M, Street D et al. Analysis of food-allergic and anaphylactic events in the National Electronic Injury Surveillance System. *J Allergy Clin Immunol* 2008;121:166–171.
23. Hourihane JO'B, Kilburn SA, Nordlee JA et al. An evaluation of the sensitivity of subjects with peanut allergy to very low doses of peanut protein: A randomized, double-blind, placebo-controlled food challenge study. *J Allergy Clin Immunol* 1997;100:596–600.
24. Jones RT, Squillace DL, Yuninger JW. Anaphylaxis in a milk-allergic child after ingestion of milk-contaminated kosher-pareve-labeled "dairy-free" dessert. *Ann Allergy* 1992;68:223–227.
25. Laoprasert N, Wallen ND, Jones RT et al. Anaphylaxis in a milk-allergic child following ingestion of lemon sorbet containing trace quantities of milk. *J Food Prot* 1998;61:1522–1524.
26. Gern JE, Yang E, Evrard HM et al. Allergic reactions to milk-contaminated "nondairy" products. *N Engl J Med* 1991;324:976–979.
27. Sampson HA. Anaphylaxis and emergency treatment. *Pediatrics* 2003;111:1601.
28. Sampson HA, Mendelson L, Rosen JP. Fatal and near-fatal anaphylactic reactions to food in children and adolescents. *N Engl J Med* 1992;327:380–384.
29. Ellis AK, Day JH. Incidence and characteristics of biphasic anaphylaxis: A prospective evaluation of 103 patients. *Ann Allergy Asthma Immunol Off Publ Am Coll Allergy Asthma Immunol* 2007;98:64–69.
30. Kemp SF. The post-anaphylaxis dilemma: How long is long enough to observe a patient after resolution of symptoms? *Curr Allergy Asthma Rep* 2008;8:45–48.
31. Hofmann A, Burks AW. Pollen food syndrome: Update on the allergens. *Curr Allergy Asthma Rep* 2008;8:413–417.
32. Ortolani C, Ispano M, Pastorello EA et al. Comparison of results of skin prick tests (with fresh foods and commercial food extracts) and RAST in 100 patients with oral allergy syndrome. *J Allergy Clin Immunol* 1989;83:683–690.
33. Groot H de, Jong NW de, Vuijk MH et al. Birch pollinosis and atopy caused by apple, peach, and hazelnut; comparison of three extraction procedures with two apple strains. *Allergy* 1996;51:712–718.
34. Pastorello EA, Incorvaia C, Pravettoni V et al. New allergens in fruits and vegetables. *Allergy* 1998;53:48–51.
35. Sicherer SH. Clinical implications of cross-reactive food allergens. *J Allergy Clin Immunol* 2001;108:881–890.
36. Anderson LB, Dreyfuss EM, Logan J et al. Melon and banana sensitivity coincident with ragweed pollinosis. *J Allergy* 1970;45:310–319.
37. Breiteneder H, Ebner C. Molecular and biochemical classification of plant-derived food allergens. *J Allergy Clin Immunol* 2000;106:27–36.
38. James JM, Burks AW. Food-associated gastrointestinal disease. *Curr Opin Pediatr* 1996;8:471–475.

39. Crowe SE, Perdue MH. Gastrointestinal food hypersensitivity: Basic mechanisms of pathophysiology. *Gastroenterology* 1992;103:1075–1095.
40. Sicherer SH. Clinical aspects of gastrointestinal food allergy in childhood. *Pediatrics* 2003;111:1609–1616.
41. Toit G Du. Food-dependent exercise-induced anaphylaxis in childhood. *Pediatr Allergy Immunol Off Publ Eur Soc Pediatr Allergy Immunol* 2007;18:455–463.
42. Beaudouin E, Renaudin JM, Morisset M et al. Food-dependent exercise-induced anaphylaxis—Update and current data. *Eur Ann Allergy Clin Immunol* 2006;38:45–51.
43. Romano A, Scala E, Rumi G et al. Lipid transfer proteins: The most frequent sensitizer in Italian subjects with food-dependent exercise-induced anaphylaxis. *Clin Exp Allergy J Br Soc Allergy Clin Immunol* 2012;42:1643–1653.
44. Kano H, Juji F, Shibuya N et al. Clinical courses of 18 cases with food-dependent exercise-induced anaphylaxis. *Arerugī Allergy* 2000;49:472–478.
45. Dohi M, Suko M, Sugiyama H et al. Food-dependent, exercise-induced anaphylaxis: A study on 11 Japanese cases. *J Allergy Clin Immunol* 1991;87:34–40.
46. Romano A, Fonso M Di, Giuffreda F et al. Food-dependent exercise-induced anaphylaxis: Clinical and laboratory findings in 54 subjects. *Int Arch Allergy Immunol* 2001;125:264–272.
47. Blanco C. Latex-fruit syndrome. *Curr Allergy Asthma Rep* 2003;3:47–53.
48. Salcedo G, Diaz-Perales A, Sanchez-Monge R. The role of plant panallergens in sensitization to natural rubber latex. *Curr Opin Allergy Clin Immunol* 2001;1:177–183.
49. García Ortiz JC, Moyano JC, Alvarez M et al. Latex allergy in fruit-allergic patients. *Allergy* 1998;53:532–536.
50. Werfel SJ, Cooke SK, Sampson HA. Clinical reactivity to beef in children allergic to cow's milk. *J Allergy Clin Immunol* 1997;99:293–300.
51. Commins SP, Satinover SM, Hosen J et al. Delayed anaphylaxis, angioedema, or urticaria after consumption of red meat in patients with IgE antibodies specific for galactose-alpha-1,3-galactose. *J Allergy Clin Immunol* 2009;123:426–433.
52. Commins SP, James HR, Kelly LA et al. The relevance of tick bites to the production of IgE antibodies to the mammalian oligosaccharide galactose-α-1,3-galactose. *J Allergy Clin Immunol* 2011;127:1286–1293.e6.
53. Sampson HA. Utility of food-specific IgE concentrations in predicting symptomatic food allergy. *J Allergy Clin Immunol* 2001;107:891–896.
54. Celik-Bilgili S, Mehl A, Verstege A et al. The predictive value of specific immunoglobulin E levels in serum for the outcome of oral food challenges. *Clin Exp Allergy J Br Soc Allergy Clin Immunol* 2005;35:268–273.
55. García-Ara C, Boyano-Martínez T, Díaz-Pena JM et al. Specific IgE levels in the diagnosis of immediate hypersensitivity to cows' milk protein in the infant. *J Allergy Clin Immunol* 2001;107:185–190.
56. Sampson HA, Ho DG. Relationship between food-specific IgE concentrations and the risk of positive food challenges in children and adolescents. *J Allergy Clin Immunol* 1997;100:444–451.
57. Lieberman JA, Glaumann S, Batelson S et al. The utility of peanut components in the diagnosis of IgE-mediated peanut allergy among distinct populations. *J Allergy Clin Immunol Pract* 2013;1:75–82.
58. Dang TD, Tang M, Choo S et al. Increasing the accuracy of peanut allergy diagnosis by using Ara h 2. *J Allergy Clin Immunol* 2012;129:1056–1063.
59. Stapel SO, Asero R, Ballmer-Weber BK et al. Testing for IgG4 against foods is not recommended as a diagnostic tool: EAACI Task Force Report. *Allergy* 2008;63:793–796.
60. AAAI Board of Directors. Measurement of specific and nonspecific IgG4 levels as diagnostic and prognostic tests for clinical allergy. *J Allergy Clin Immunol* 1995;95:652–654.

61. Chapman JA, Bernstein IL, Lee RE et al. Food allergy: A practice parameter. *Ann Allergy Asthma Immunol Off Publ Am Coll Allergy Asthma Immunol* 2006;96:S1–S68.
62. American gastroenterological association medical position statement: Guidelines for the evaluation of food allergies. *Gastroenterology* 2001;120:1023–1025.
63. Anon. Clinical practice guidelines for the diagnosis and management of food allergy. Available at: http://www3.niaid.nih.gov/topics/foodAllergy/clinical/. Accessed March 23, 2010.
64. Vlieg-Boerstra BJ, Bijleveld CMA, Heide S van der et al. Development and validation of challenge materials for double-blind, placebo-controlled food challenges in children. *J Allergy Clin Immunol* 2004;113:341–346.
65. Vlieg-Boerstra BJ, Herpertz I, Pasker L et al. Validation of novel recipes for double-blind, placebo-controlled food challenges in children and adults. *Allergy* 2011;66:948–954.
66. Kostadinova AI, Willemsen LEM, Knippels LMJ et al. Immunotherapy—Risk/benefit in food allergy. *Pediatr Allergy Immunol Off Publ Eur Soc Pediatr Allergy Immunol* 2013;24:633–644.
67. Chafen JJS, Newberry SJ, Riedl MA et al. Diagnosing and managing common food allergies: A systematic review. *J Am Med Assoc* 2010;303:1848–1856.
68. Taylor SL, Hefle SL. Food allergen labeling in the USA and Europe. *Curr Opin Allergy Clin Immunol* 2006;6:186–190.
69. Mills ENC, Valovirta E, Madsen C et al. Information provision for allergic consumers—Where are we going with food allergen labelling? *Allergy* 2004;59:1262–1268.
70. Cornelisse-Vermaat JR, Voordouw J, Yiakoumaki V et al. Food-allergic consumers' labelling preferences: A cross-cultural comparison. *Eur J Public Health* 2008;18:115–120.
71. Simons E, Weiss CC, Furlong TJ et al. Impact of ingredient labeling practices on food allergic consumers. *Ann Allergy Asthma Immunol Off Publ Am Coll Allergy Asthma Immunol* 2005;95:426–428.
72. Sicherer SH, Vargas PA, Groetch ME et al. Development and validation of educational materials for food allergy. *J Pediatr* 2012;160:651–656.
73. Gupta RS, Kim JS, Springston EE et al. Development of the Chicago Food Allergy Research Surveys: Assessing knowledge, attitudes, and beliefs of parents, physicians, and the general public. *BMC Health Serv Res* 2009;9:142.
74. Gupta RS, Springston EE, Kim JS et al. Food allergy knowledge, attitudes, and beliefs of primary care physicians. *Pediatrics* 2010;125:126–132.
75. Bock SA, Muñoz-Furlong A, Sampson HA. Further fatalities caused by anaphylactic reactions to food, 2001–2006. *J Allergy Clin Immunol* 2007;119:1016–1018.
76. Lack G. Clinical practice. Food allergy. *N Engl J Med* 2008;359:1252–1260.
77. Ewan PW. Clinical study of peanut and nut allergy in 62 consecutive patients: New features and associations. *BMJ* 1996;312:1074–1078.
78. Burks AW, Tang M, Sicherer S et al. ICON: Food allergy. *J Allergy Clin Immunol* 2012;129:906–920.
79. Fiocchi A, Schünemann HJ, Brozek J et al. Diagnosis and rationale for action against cow's milk allergy (DRACMA): A summary report. *J Allergy Clin Immunol* 2010;126:1119–1128.e12.
80. Jensen VB, Jørgensen IM, Rasmussen KB et al. Bone mineral status in children with cow milk allergy. *Pediatr Allergy Immunol Off Publ Eur Soc Pediatr Allergy Immunol.* 2004;15:562–565.
81. Konstantynowicz J, Nguyen TV, Kaczmarski M et al. Fractures during growth: Potential role of a milk-free diet. *Osteoporos Int J Establ Result Coop Eur Found Osteoporos Natl Osteoporos Found USA* 2007;18:1601–1607.
82. Mannion CA, Gray-Donald K, Johnson-Down L et al. Lactating women restricting milk are low on select nutrients. *J Am Coll Nutr* 2007;26:149–155.

83. Järvinen KM, Chatchatee P. Mammalian milk allergy: Clinical suspicion, cross-reactivities and diagnosis. *Curr Opin Allergy Clin Immunol* 2009;9:251–258.

84. Vita D, Passalacqua G, Pasquale G Di et al. Ass's milk in children with atopic dermatitis and cow's milk allergy: Crossover comparison with goat's milk. *Pediatr Allergy Immunol Off Publ Eur Soc Pediatr Allergy Immunol* 2007;18:594–598.

85. Bellioni-Businco B, Paganelli R, Lucenti P et al. Allergenicity of goat's milk in children with cow's milk allergy. *J Allergy Clin Immunol* 1999;103:1191–1194.

86. Tesse R, Paglialunga C, Braccio S et al. Adequacy and tolerance to ass's milk in an Italian cohort of children with cow's milk allergy. *Ital J Pediatr* 2009;35:19.

87. Nowak-Wegrzyn A, Bloom KA, Sicherer SH et al. Tolerance to extensively heated milk in children with cow's milk allergy. *J Allergy Clin Immunol* 2008;122:342–347.e2.

88. Kim JS, Nowak-Węgrzyn A, Sicherer SH et al. Dietary baked milk accelerates the resolution of cow's milk allergy in children. *J Allergy Clin Immunol* 2011;128: 125–131.e2.

89. Taylor SL. Molluscan shellfish allergy. *Adv Food Nutr Res* 2008;54:139–177.

90. Huang S-W. Seafood and iodine: An analysis of a medical myth. *Allergy Asthma Proc Off J Reg State Allergy Soc.* 2005;26:468–469.

91. Huang F, Nowak-Węgrzyn A. Extensively heated milk and egg as oral immunotherapy. *Curr Opin Allergy Clin Immunol* 2012;12:283–292.

92. Kelso JM, Mootrey GT, Tsai TF. Anaphylaxis from yellow fever vaccine. *J Allergy Clin Immunol* 1999;103:698–701.

93. Kelso JM, Greenhawt MJ, Li JT et al. Adverse reactions to vaccines practice parameter 2012 update. *J Allergy Clin Immunol* 2012;130:25–43.

94. Artesani MC, Donnanno S, Cavagni G et al. Egg sensitization caused by immediate hypersensitivity reaction to drug-containing lysozyme. *Ann Allergy Asthma Immunol Off Publ Am Coll Allergy Asthma Immunol* 2008;101:105.

95. Buchman AL, Ament ME. Comparative hypersensitivity in intravenous lipid emulsions. *J Parenter Enteral Nutr* 1991;15:345–346.

96. Hofer KN, McCarthy MW, Buck ML et al. Possible anaphylaxis after propofol in a child with food allergy. *Ann Pharmacother* 2003;37:398–401.

97. Crevel RW, Kerkhoff MA, Koning MM. Allergenicity of refined vegetable oils. *Food Chem Toxicol Int J Publ Br Ind Biol Res Assoc* 2000;38:385–393.

98. Cahen YD, Fritsch R, Wüthrich B. Food allergy with monovalent sensitivity to poultry meat. *Clin Exp Allergy J Br Soc Allergy Clin Immunol* 1998;28:1026–1030.

99. Restani P, Beretta B, Fiocchi A et al. Cross-reactivity between mammalian proteins. *Ann Allergy Asthma Immunol Off Publ Am Coll Allergy Asthma Immunol* 2002;89:11–15.

100. Young E, Patel S, Stoneham M et al. The prevalence of reaction to food additives in a survey population. *J R Coll Physicians London* 1987;21:241–247.

101. Bruening G, Lyons JM. The case of the FLAVR SAVR tomato. *Calif Agric* 2000; 54:6–7.

102. Nutrition C for FS and A. Labeling & nutrition—Guidance for industry: Voluntary labeling indicating whether foods have or have not been developed using bioengineering; Draft guidance. Available at: http://www.fda.gov/Food/GuidanceRegulation/GuidanceDocumentsRegulatoryInformation/LabelingNutrition/ucm059098.htm. Accessed November 15, 2013.

103. Thomas K, MacIntosh S, Bannon G et al. Scientific advancement of novel protein allergenicity evaluation: An overview of work from the HESI Protein Allergenicity Technical Committee (2000–2008). *Food Chem Toxicol Int J Publ Br Ind Biol Res Assoc* 2009;47:1041–1050.

104. Ronald P. Plant genetics, sustainable agriculture and global food security. *Genetics* 2011;188:11–20.

105. Greer FR, Sicherer SH, Burks AW et al. Effects of early nutritional interventions on the development of atopic disease in infants and children: The role of maternal dietary

restriction, breastfeeding, timing of introduction of complementary foods, and hydro-lyzed formulas. *Pediatrics* 2008;121:183–191.

106. Høst A, Halken S, Muraro A et al. Dietary prevention of allergic diseases in infants and small children. *Pediatr Allergy Immunol Off Publ Eur Soc Pediatr Allergy Immunol* 2008;19:1–4.

107. Osborn DA, Sinn JK. Probiotics in infants for prevention of allergic disease and food hypersensitivity. *Cochrane Database Syst Rev* 2007:CD006475.

108. Mehr S, Kakakios A, Frith K et al. Food protein-induced enterocolitis syndrome: 16-year experience. *Pediatrics* 2009;123:e459–e464.

109. Sicherer SH. Food protein-induced enterocolitis syndrome: Case presentations and management lessons. *J Allergy Clin Immunol* 2005;115:149–156.

110. American Academy of Pediatrics: Committee on Nutrition. Hypoallergenic infant for-mulas. *Pediatrics* 2000;106:346–349.

111. Nowak-Wegrzyn A, Muraro A. Food protein-induced enterocolitis syndrome. *Curr Opin Allergy Clin Immunol* 2009;9:371–377.

112. Boissieu D de, Matarazzo P, Dupont C. Allergy to extensively hydrolyzed cow milk proteins in infants: Identification and treatment with an amino acid-based formula. *J Pediatr* 1997;131:744–747.

113. Nowak-Wegrzyn A, Sampson HA, Wood RA et al. Food protein-induced enterocolitis syndrome caused by solid food proteins. *Pediatrics* 2003;111:829–835.

114. Moon A, Kleinman RE. Allergic gastroenteropathy in children. *Ann Allergy Asthma Immunol Off Publ Am Coll Allergy Asthma Immunol* 1995;74:5–12; quiz 12–16.

115. Lake AM. Food-induced eosinophilic proctocolitis. *J Pediatr Gastroenterol Nutr* 2000;30 Suppl:S58–60.

116. Iyngkaran N, Yadav M, Boey CG et al. Severity and extent of upper small bowel muco-sal damage in cow's milk protein-sensitive enteropathy. *J Pediatr Gastroenterol Nutr* 1988;7:667–674.

117. Savilahti E. Food-induced malabsorption syndromes. *J Pediatr Gastroenterol Nutr* 2000;30 Suppl:S61–66.

118. Verkasalo M, Kuitunen P, Savilahti E et al. Changing pattern of cow's milk intolerance. An analysis of the occurrence and clinical course in the 60s and mid-70s. *Acta Paediatr Scand* 1981;70:289–295.

119. Mead PS, Slutsker L, Dietz V et al. Food-related illness and death in the United States. *Emerging Infect Dis* 1999;5:607–625.

120. Halvorson HA, Schlett CD, Riddle MS. Postinfectious irritable bowel syndrome—A meta-analysis. *Am J Gastroenterol* 2006;101:1894–1899; quiz 1942.

121. Freeman M. Reconsidering the effects of monosodium glutamate: A literature review. *J Am Acad Nurse Pract* 2006;18:482–486.

122. Williams AN, Woessner KM. Monosodium glutamate "allergy": Menace or myth? *Clin Exp Allergy J Br Soc Allergy Clin Immunol* 2009;39:640–646.

123. Maintz L, Novak N. Histamine and histamine intolerance. *Am J Clin Nutr* 2007;85:1185–1196.

124. Schirru E, Corona V, Usai-Satta P et al. Decline of lactase activity and c/t-13910 variant in Sardinian childhood. *J Pediatr Gastroenterol Nutr* 2007;45:503–506.

125. Scrimshaw NS, Murray EB. The acceptability of milk and milk products in populations with a high prevalence of lactose intolerance. *Am J Clin Nutr* 1988;48:1079–1159.

126. Lomer MCE, Parkes GC, Sanderson JD. Review article: Lactose intolerance in clinical practice—Myths and realities. *Aliment Pharmacol Ther* 2008;27:93–103.

127. Montalto M, Curigliano V, Santoro L et al. Management and treatment of lactose mal-absorption. *World J Gastroenterol WJG* 2006;12:187–191.

128. Swagerty DL, Walling AD, Klein RM. Lactose intolerance. *Am Fam Physician* 2002;65:1845–1850.

129. Heyman MB. Lactose intolerance in infants, children, and adolescents. *Pediatrics* 2006;118:1279–1286.
130. Vernia P, Camillo M Di, Marinaro V. Lactose malabsorption, irritable bowel syndrome and self-reported milk intolerance. *Dig Liver Dis Off J Ital Soc Gastroenterol Ital Assoc Study Liver* 2001;33:234–239.
131. Vesa T, Seppo L, Marteau P et al. Role of irritable bowel syndrome in subjective lactose intolerance. *Am J Clin Nutr* 1998;67:710–715.
132. Johnson AO, Semenya JG, Buchowski MS et al. Correlation of lactose maldigestion, lactose intolerance, and milk intolerance. *Am J Clin Nutr* 1993;57:399–401.
133. Suarez FL, Savaiano DA, Levitt MD. A comparison of symptoms after the consumption of milk or lactose-hydrolyzed milk by people with self-reported severe lactose intolerance. *N Engl J Med* 1995;333:1–4.
134. Hove H, Nørgaard H, Mortensen PB. Lactic acid bacteria and the human gastrointestinal tract. *Eur J Clin Nutr* 1999;53:339–350.
135. Stefano M Di, Veneto G, Malservisi S et al. Lactose malabsorption and intolerance and peak bone mass. *Gastroenterology* 2002;122:1793–1799.
136. Kelsay K. Psychological aspects of food allergy. *Curr Allergy Asthma Rep* 2003; 3:41–46.
137. Hathcock J. Vitamins and minerals: Efficacy and safety. *Am J Clin Nutr* 1997;66:427–437.
138. Nocon M, Labenz J, Willich SN. Lifestyle factors and symptoms of gastro-oesophageal reflux—A population-based study. *Aliment Pharmacol Ther* 2006;23:169–174.
139. Zopf Y, Baenkler H-W, Silbermann A et al. The differential diagnosis of food intolerance. *Dtsch Ärztebl Int* 2009;106:359–369; quiz 369–370; 4p following 370.
140. Banks TA, Gada SM. Cross-reactivity and masqueraders in seafood reactions. *Allergy Asthma Proc Off J Reg State Allergy Soc* 2013;34:497–503.
141. Vickers J, Safai B. Scombroid poisoning. *N Engl J Med* 2013;368:e31.
142. Pennotti R, Scallan E, Backer L et al. Ciguatera and scombroid fish poisoning in the United States. *Foodborne Pathog Dis* 2013;10:1059–1066.
143. Centers for Disease Control and Prevention (CDC). Neurologic illness associated with eating Florida pufferfish. *Morb Mortal Wkly Rep* 2002;51:321–323.
144. Ludvigsson JF, Leffler DA, Bai JC et al. The Oslo definitions for coeliac disease and related terms. *Gut* 2013;62:43–52.
145. Gibson PR, Muir JG. Not all effects of a gluten-free diet are due to removal of gluten. *Gastroenterology* 2013;145:693.
146. Biesiekierski JR, Peters SL, Newnham ED et al. No effects of gluten in patients with self-reported non-celiac gluten sensitivity after dietary reduction of fermentable, poorly absorbed, short-chain carbohydrates. *Gastroenterology* 2013;145:320–328.e1–3.
147. Halmos EP, Power VA, Shepherd SJ, Gibson PR, Muir JG. A diet low in FODMAPs reduces symptoms of irritable bowel syndrome. *Gastroenterology* 2014;146(1):67–75.
148. Gibson PR, Shepherd SJ. Evidence-based dietary management of functional gastrointestinal symptoms: The FODMAP approach. *J Gastroenterol Hepatol* 2010;25:252–258.
149. Boettcher E, Crowe SE. Dietary proteins and functional gastrointestinal disorders. *Am J Gastroenterol* 2013;108:728–736.

5 Prebiotics and Dietary Fiber

Martin Floch

CONTENTS

5.1 INTRODUCTION

Prebiotics and dietary fiber are the nutrients and fuels that nurture the microbiota of the intestinal microecology.[1] Although proteins excreted from the gut wall, including mucus are used by the microbiota as fuels, they are supplementary.[2] The intestinal microecology is affected by nutrients, and its makeup can be changed dramatically by various prebiotics and foods.[3] The interplay of these nutrients and the microbiota is a dynamic process that varies from day to day and week to week. The metabolism of the nutrients by the microbiota is also a dynamic process and has variable effects on the host.[4] In this chapter, we will define and go into the details of prebiotics and dietary fiber and review initial research in this area.

5.2 MICROBIOTA

Great interest has been aroused in the dynamics of intestinal microecology based on the awareness of the importance of the microbiota in humans.[5] It was realized that human intestinal microflora contain approximately 10^{14} of anaerobic organisms,[5,6] which is as many cells as exist in the human body. These diverse organisms are also active metabolically.[4–6] Although the intestinal microflora were first identified late in the twentieth century, it was found that anaerobic flora dominates by a factor of somewhere between 100 and 1000 times over aerobic flora.[7] At this same time, theories were formulated and developed regarding the importance of the flora in human microecology.[8]

5.3 INTESTINAL MICROECOLOGY

The intestinal microecology consists of a closed ecologic unit consisting of (1) a different epithelium in different areas of the gastrointestinal tract and (2) secretions entering the tract that interact with the nutrients fed into it. All of this makes up a dynamic ecologic unit. Using standard biochemical identification methods, Neish reviewed the microbiota; both *Bifidobacteria*, and *Lactobacillus* were most common.[9] *Bifidobacteria* and *Lactobacillus* colonize early after normal childbirth.[3] In breastfed infants, *Bifidobacteria* are the primary organisms, but in formula-fed infants, *Bacteroides* and *Bifidobacteria* are found.[3] Once infants are fed regular foods, the flora then equate to that found in adults using standard growth techniques. When disease entities are evaluated, such as inflammatory bowel disease, alterations in the flora or numbers of bacteria, identified as a dysbiosis, may occur.[2] Now that genetic polymerase techniques have been added to the pool of diagnostic testing, it is startling that an organism such as *Faecalibacterium prausnitzii* is found most commonly but was not identified as such by biochemical technology. Changes in the microbiota, as found in obesity and nonalcoholic fatty liver, occur more readily in disease states.[10,11] These studies clearly identify the diverse complexity of the microbiota and the subtle selective changes that occur in cases of disease such as nonalcoholic fatty liver disease (NAFLD).[11] It is clear that the type of microbiota diversity will be identified in many other diseases as well, but it remains to be seen whether alteration in the intestinal flora by the use of prebiotics and probiotics will have an effect on reversal of the disease process. However, one can currently accept that dysbiosis occurs and can be altered by changing the intake of prebiotics and probiotics.[1,2] The new advances in biotechnology provided by 16S genetic identification of organisms within the microbiota has opened up vast horizons for future investigation.[11] Unfortunately, there are all too few laboratories in the world with expertise in this area so new information will come slowly, but it is certain that changes in nutrient intake and alteration in dysbiosis will provide us with a better understanding of disease and human health caused by alterations in microecology.[5,10,12]

5.4 PREBIOTICS

5.4.1 DEFINITION OF PREBIOTICS

In 1995, Roberfroid and Gibson introduced the concept that certain nondigested food ingredients may beneficially affect the host through the stimulation of growth or activity of a limited number of colonic bacteria that could improve the host's health.[13] These substances were called prebiotics. They were not absorbed from the small intestine unless first metabolized by the microbiota.

5.4.2 PREBIOTICS IN USE

Experiments revealed that when either inulin, oligofructose, or sucrose were added to a controlled diet in patients with a conventional ileostomy, there was no effect on either cholesterol absorption or the excretion of cholesterol, bile acids, fat, calcium, magnesium, zinc, or iron.[14] Because the effects of various prebiotics are dependent on the microbiota, the major interactions occur in the distal ileum and colon.[15–17]

Defining a prebiotic was relatively simple when the term was first introduced.[13] Now that our experience in the function of prebiotics and in their relation to the ecosystem in the colon has become more sophisticated, the definition has become more complex. Slavin wrote that Gibson and Roberfroid, in their studies,[13,18] required prebiotics to include the following properties: (1) the ability to be hydrolyzed by mammalian enzymes and resistance to gastric acidity, (2) the ability to be fermented by intestinal microflora, and (3) the ability to selectively stimulate the growth or activity of intestinal bacteria potentially associated with health and well-being.[13,18]

Table 5.1 shows the common prebiotic substances. However, this list is relatively simple and almost naïve when it is related to a review of multifunctional fructans and raffinose family oligosaccharides (RFOs).[19] As the authors of this study pointed out, both fructans and RFOs are the two most important classes with regard to the microbiota of all the soluble carbohydrates and plants. There are many additional

TABLE 5.1
Simple Prebiotic Substances

Disaccharide
Lactulose
Oligosaccharide
Fructooligosaccharide (FOS)
Galactooligosaccharide
Soybean oligosaccharide
Other main digestible oligosaccharides:
Xylooligosaccharide, isomaltooligosaccharide, lactulosesucrose, palatinose
Polycondensats
Inulin
Resistant starch

Source: Adapted from Floch MH. Prebiotics, probiotics and dietary fiber. In: Buchman A, Ed. *Clinical Nutrition in Gastrointestinal Disease.* Thorofare, NJ: Slack Inc.; 2006. pp. 123–138.

TABLE 5.2
Prebiotic Substances

Prebiotic	Manufacturer Country
Fructooligosaccharide	Orafti, Belgium
Inulin	Jarrow, Los Angeles, CA
Fructooligosaccharide	Ross Laboratories, Columbus, OH
Galactooligosaccharides (GOS)	Clasado BioSciences, United Kingdom
Guar	Novartis Nutrition, Minneapolis, MN
Isomaltooligosaccharide	Showa Sangyo, Japan
Lactulose (Duphalac)	Solvay, Marietta, GA
Kristalose	Cumberland Pharmaceuticals, Nashville, TN
Oligomate	Yakult, Japan
Palatinose	Sudzucker, Germany
Pyrodextrin	Matsutani, Japan
Raftiline	Orafti, Belgium
Soybean oligosaccharide	Calpis, Japan
Xylooligosaccharide	Sutory, Japan

Source: Adapted from Floch MH, Hong-Curtiss J. *Curr Treat Op Gastro* 2003;6:283–288; Floch MH. Prebiotics, probiotics and dietary fiber. In: Buchman A, Ed. *Clinical Nutrition in Gastrointestinal Disease*. Thorofare, NJ: Slack Inc.; 2006. pp. 123–138.

substances, including inulin, for example, that can be chemically isolated and called a prebiotic, but many of these may or may not fulfill all of the scientific criteria required of a prebiotic as classified by Gibson and Roberfroid.[13,18]

Food chemists now focus on the classification of short-chain, long-chain, and full-spectrum prebiotics. "Short-chain" prebiotics, such as oligofructose, contain 2–8 links per saccharide molecule and are rapidly fermented in the right side of the colon. Longer-chain prebiotics, such as inulin, contain 9–64 links per saccharide molecule, and tend to be fermented more slowly and in the distal colon.[20] Since prebiotic substances are not digested by human enzymes, there are a large number that can stimulate bacterial growth in the distal ileum and colon.[15,16,18–20]

Prebiotics are now used worldwide. Table 5.2 lists many of the products, their manufacturers, and the countries in which they are marketed or sold.[20–24]

The number of products being sold and marketed around the world is burgeoning, particularly in Japan, China, and the rest of Asia. Recent meetings have emphasized that galactooligosaccharides (GOS) will become the most important prebiotic products worldwide.[20]

5.4.3 PREBIOTIC EFFECTS IN HUMAN DISEASE

The amount of dedicated human experimentation with prebiotics in humans is limited. Furthermore, many investigators have are combined a prebiotic with a probiotic, and therefore render it difficult to evaluate the effect of the prebiotic alone.

5.4.4 CONSTIPATION

5.4.4.1 Lactulose

Lactulose is a disaccharide of D-galactos linked D (1–4) to fructose.

An area in which prebiotics have clinically demonstrated effectiveness is in the treatment of constipation.[25–27] Lactulose is very effective for the treatment of constipation. It also is one of the oldest drugs used for the treatment of hepatic encephalopathy.[26,27] The mechanism of action of lactulose in both of these conditions is not clearly understood. The administration of lactulose results in a change in the intestinal microbiota, with increased *Bifidobacteria* and a decrease in *Bacteroides* and *Clostridia*.[26] The exact mechanism by which it assists in the control of the encephalopathy is not clearly understood.[25,26] The dose may require modifications for efficacy or to prevent diarrhea.

Other investigators have noted that inulin may be effective in producing a softer and more frequent stool.[21–29] Inulin increased log counts of *Bifidobacteria* from 7.9 to 9.2/g of feces and a change in short-chain fatty acid (SCFA) concentrations was detected.

5.4.4.2 The Bifidogenetic Effect of Prebiotics and Effects on Fermentation

Since prebiotics are bifidogenetic, they stimulate production of SCFA via fermentation.[15,16,22] However, there has been no definitive data demonstrating that any prebiotic is clinically effective for the treatment of inflammatory bowel disease, irritable bowel syndrome (IBS), or any other gastrointestinal functional disorders.[25]

A main part of the bifidogenetic effect includes the production of SCFA.[30] The microbiota provide the enzymes that ferment prebiotics into acetic, propionic, and butyric acids. These SCFA provide a vital energy source for human colonic epithelium and are involved in other metabolic processes. Acetic acid is absorbed and used as a building block for cholesterol. Propionic acid is also absorbed and plays a role in the control of lipid metabolism, and butyric acid is the primary fuel for colonocytes.[27,30] SCFA are the most important products of fermentation of nondigestible carbohydrates of prebiotics and dietary fiber.[30] The extent of SCFA production, the rate of fermentation, and the ratios of the different fatty acids can be altered by the type of microbiota and the type and amounts of prebiotics.[30] In addition, there is some interconversion between the SCFA. In a randomized crossover study that investigated the effects of GOS on the fecal microbiota in men and women over 50 years of age, GOS supplementation significantly increased *Bifidobacteria* numbers both *in vivo* and *in vitro*, and the increased butyric acid production and elevated *Bifidobacteria* numbers were suspected to be beneficial in a maturing population.[31]

5.4.4.3 Childhood Diarrhea

In infants and children, prebiotics have been shown to decrease diarrhea duration as well as ameliorate some of the symptoms of diarrhea.[21,32,33] No studies exist for adults.

Except for the aforementioned, treatment of constipation, hepatic encephalopathy, and some diarrheas, there are no significant studies on the use of prebiotics to warrant additional clinical recommendations.[18,21,23,24] This statement holds for the maintenance of general gastrointestinal health, normal blood sugar regulation, colon cancer prevention, inflammatory bowel disease, IBS, and the regulation of immunity. A recent small study has shown that prebiotics may be helpful in treating NAFLD or even obesity, but much more work is needed in this field before making recommendations.[11,12,21]

5.5 DIETARY FIBER

5.5.1 DEFINITION, CLASSIFICATION, AND PROPERTIES

In simple terms, dietary fiber is nonstarch polysaccharide in plant food that is poorly digested by human enzymes.[25] Because it involves all our plant foods, it has become complicated, and there are numerous definitions have evolved.

The surgeon Thomas L. (Peter) Cleave was among the first to recognize the importance of dietary fiber.[34] He believed that almost all the degenerative diseases of western society were due to a substantial increase in simple sugar intake. As food underwent a greater degree of processing during the industrial revolution and more sugar and more starch become available, Cleave thought the marked increase in the availability and consumption of these substances occurred in concert with the observed increase in prevalence of degenerative diseases. This theory was then promulgated further by Burkitt and Trowell in 1975.[35-37] The scientific world began to accept that diverticular disease, colonic polyposis, hiatus hernia, and other degenerative diseases could be attributed to insufficient dietary fiber intake.[35-40]

However, the definition of dietary fiber becomes very complex when evaluated from an analytic or functional point of view. The analytic work done by Englyst and Asp[41,42] is summarized in Table 5.3.

Most clinicians involved with dietary fiber often use a simple categorization of dietary fiber components into either water soluble or insoluble.[25,38,39] Physiologists and clinicians also frequently refer to dietary fiber from a physiological point of view because of the properties that enabled Slavin to develop a classification as outlined in Table 5.4.[18,39] When evaluating water soluble carbohydrates in plants, the definition becomes even further complicated when one evaluates the inclusion of the fructans and RFOs as discussed in detail by van den Ende.[19] Therefore, there exists no definition used for dietary fiber that has gained worldwide acceptance at the present time.[18] Despite the lack of an accepted definition, clinical properties of fiber have been well-defined in order to explain clinical responses of fiber on physiologic properties.

Classification of fiber can be designed based on the unique physical properties of dietary fibers. Essentially, they exist in one of four categories[25,40]:

1. The *particle size* of the fiber will cause variation in some of its properties. Some fiber consists of small particles while others consist of large particles. Smaller particles may combine with ions, and larger ones may cause variation in solubility.
2. The *hydrophilic property* of fiber is extremely important. For example, cellulose is very limited in its ability to swell or take on water, whereas other polysaccharides can swell profusely and take on large amounts of water.

TABLE 5.3

Dietary Fiber Components of Foods

Classical Nomenclature	Solubility Characteristics	Classes of Polysaccharide
Plant Cell Wall Components		
Pectic substances	Water soluble	Galacturonans
		Arabinogalactans
		β-glucans
		Arabinoxylans
Hemicelluloses	Insoluble in water	Arabinoxylans
		Galactomannans
	Soluble in alkali	Xyloglucans
α-cellulose	Insoluble in alkali	Cellulose (glucan)
Lignin	Insoluble in 12 M H_2SO_4	Lignin (Klason)
		Noncarbohydrate
Nonstructural Components		
Gums	Water soluble	Galactomannans
		Arabinogalactans
Mucilages	Dispersible	Wide range of branched and substituted galactans

Source: Adapted from Asp, N-GL. *Am J Clin Nutr* 1995; 61:930S–937S; Cummings JH, Englyst HN. *Am J Clin Nutr* 1995; 61:938S–945S.

This water holding capacity usually defines fiber as either soluble or insoluble. Insoluble fibers are largely not fermented, whereas the soluble ones are fermented by the microflora.

3. *Ion binding* is an important function of fibers. The degree of ion binding varies greatly through the colon and the small bowel where the fiber may bind ions that are then released in the colon. Polysaccharides containing neuronic acid and lignin components have an eosinophilic function that reacts readily with ions. The same ion and calcium are readily bound and readily freed in the intestinal ecology. Bile acids are also bound and free easily. Certain ions are absorbed or removed if they are harmful making for a very dynamic process.

4. Finally, *fermentation* is one of the most important properties of fibers. The soluble fibers are almost completely fermented, as opposed to the insoluble that are not. Soluble fibers are invariably more bifidogenetic resulting in a larger stool that is made up of bacteria.

The three most important SCFA are acetic, propionic, and butyric.[43–45] Fermentation occurs at a rate in soluble fibers 10 times greater than that in insoluble fibers. Acetic, propionic, and butyric acids are in the molecular ratio of 57, 22, and 21. These ratios are the same in the left colon. However, when measured in the portal vein, the ratio of acetic acid rises to 71, propionic acid remains at 21, and butyric acid falls to 8. These SCFA are absorbed into the blood stream. Total

TABLE 5.4

Classification of Fibers Based on Four Characteristics

Fibers	Classification
Dietary fibers	Lignin
	Cellulose
	β-glucans
	Hemicelluloses
	Pectins
	Gums
	Resistant starch
Soluble fibers	β-glucans
	Gums
	Wheat dextrin
	Psyllium
	Pectin
	Inulin
Fermentable fibers	Wheat dextrin
	Pectins
	β-glucans
	Guar gum
	Inulin
Viscous fibers	Pectins
	β-glucans
	Some gums (e.g., guar gum)
	Psyllium
Functional fibers	Resistant dextrins
	Psyllium
	Fructooligosaccharides
	Polydextrose
	Isolated gums
	Isolated resistant starch
Insoluble fibers	Cellulose
	Lignin
	Some pectins
	Some hemicelluloses
Nonfermentable fibers	Cellulose
	Lignin
Nonviscous fibers	Polydextrose
	Inulin

Source: Adapted from Slavin J. *Nutrients* 2013; 5:1417–1435.

SCFA is negligible in the jejunum, higher in the ileum, and more than 10 times the amount in the cecum. The preferred energy for colonocytes is butyrate, from which 70%–80% of the colonic mucosa energy needs is obtained. It is more essential in the distal than the proximal colon.[46,47] SCFA are also necessary and can be controlled by manipulation of intestinal microecology.[48]

It is important to note that wheat bran is 90% insoluble, oat bran 50% soluble and 50% insoluble, and psyllium is 90% soluble. Those that are soluble will ferment more readily. Later in this chapter, when food fiber content is reviewed, it will be noted that fruits are the major contributors of dietary soluble fiber.[43]

5.5.2 FIBER CONTENT IN FOOD AND INTAKE

There is a wide range of dietary fiber intake among different in societies around the world. Initially, when epidemiologists began to study this issue, they found that some groups, notably in Asia and Africa, ingested as much as 60–80 g of dietary fiber daily.[35–38] This occurred because of a very high intake of cereals and grains. In western societies, where raw foods were had been processed to a much greater level, initial studies indicated that dietary fiber intake was as low as 5–10 g per day.[25,49,50] Snack food ingestion is associated with decreased fiber intake in industrialized societies, where so-called bulk foods are often avoided. However, on a worldwide basis, there appears to be more appeal to eat high-fiber foods to correct some of the disorders mentioned following this, and recommendations for dietary fiber are now becoming refined so that it is more closely related to body size and to particular health patterns such as occur with allergies. Table 5.5 has these recommendations for age, gender, and pregnancy. It should be understood that some subjects may require more fiber and others less fiber to elicit similar effects. Some people will require more soluble and other more insoluble depending on their clinical condition. For example, some constipated people require more soluble fiber, and it is assumed that is because they need a greater change in their microbiota, whereas others require more insoluble fiber because they need to hold more water. The clinician will need to prescribe fiber to some degree based on a trial and error approach. Industries have been particularly aggressive in marketing their particular fiber products, but in the absence of supportive and well-controlled clinical trials, it currently falls on the clinician and patient to decide what is better for them.

Table 5.5 refers to the current recommended total fiber intakes, based on age, whereas Table 5.6 refers to the particular foods and their relative fiber composition. It should be understood that most foods have a mixture of fiber types, and consequently when a clinician attempts to prescribe a detailed fiber-containing diet, food tables must be utilized. A simple example is found in Table 5.6, whereas detailed examples are found in the appropriate reference. Many constipation problems can be solved by correct manipulation of dietary fiber. However, it requires careful advice from the clinician when other medical controls, such as control of lipid metabolism are desired.

In general, between 20 and 35 g of daily dietary fiber are sufficient, but that depends on the size of the patient and his or her total energy intake. The individual that ingests twice as many calories will usually also ingest more dietary fiber simultaneously. An individual subject can be trained to eat anywhere from 3–5 g per portion of fiber-containing foods. Fiber recommendations will need to vary depending on whether, for example, the individual eats 3 or 10 food choices that are of fiber-containing typical food choices for northern society and their fiber content are included in Table 5.6. These are largely taken from Pennington.[52]

TABLE 5.5
Recommended Dietary Allowance for Fiber

Age	Carbohydrate (g/day)	Total Fiber (g/day)
Infants		
0–6 months	60	ND
7–12 months	95	ND
Children		
1–3 years	130 (100)	19
4–8 years	130 (100)	25
Males		
9–13 years	130 (100)	31
14–18 years	130 (100)	38
19–30 years	130 (100)	38
31–50 years	130 (100)	38
51–70 years	130 (100)	30
>70 years	130 (100)	30
Females		
9–13 years	130 (100)	26
14–18 years	130 (100)	26
19–30 years	130 (100)	25
31–50 years	130 (100)	25
51–70 years	130 (100)	21
>70 years	130 (100)	21
Pregnancy		
18–50 years	175 (135)	28
Lactation		
18–50 years	210 (160)	29

Source: Adapted from Anderson JW. *Plant Fiber in Foods.* Lexington KY: HCF Diabetes
Research Foundation Inc.; 1986. pp. 10–30; Pennington JAT, Douglass JS, *Bowes
& Church's Food Values of Portions Commonly Use*, 19th Edition, Philadelphia:
Lippincott William & Wilkins, 2010.

Pennington[52] has a listing of dietary fiber (DFIB) in many restaurant foods such as *Bob Evans'* Cobb Salad has 3 DFIB and turkey sandwich 2 DFIB, and *Taco Bell* bean burrito has 7.7 DFIB.

For example, a male that eats approximately 2000 cal per day would have two fruits, two pieces of bread, a portion of cereal, and three vegetables or eight fiber choices, each averaging four each for approximately 32 g of dietary fiber per day. By varying the food selection, one can easily provide for the correct male age-appropriate fiber intake in a regular diet. It is critical that the clinician and patient understand that when specific diets are recommended, it is extremely difficult for them to have

TABLE 5.6
Fiber Content of Some Common Foods

	WT (g)	KCAL	CHO	DFIB
	Cereals			
Cream of rice	244	127	28	0.2
Multigrain oatmeal	234	143	32	5.1
Oatmeal (cooked)	234	166	28	4.0
Rice, brown	195	218	46	3.5
Rice, white	186	242	53	1.0
	Cereals, Ready to Eat			
All bran	31	81	20	9.9
Cheerios	30	110	22	3.0
Corn flakes	30	110	25	1.2
Fiber one	30	60	25	14.2
Granola	55	218	37	6.3
Heart to heart kashi	53	118	25	4.7
Mini-wheats	52	185	43	5.0
Muesli	88	289	66	6.2
Oat bran flakes	47	166	37	6.1
Raisin bran	59	190	44	6.3
Uncle Sam cereal	55	237	36	11.0
Eggs, cheeses, dairy foods	These contain no fiber			0
	Fruits (Raw)			
Apple	138	72	19	3.3
Apricots	3	105	12	3.0
Avocado	146	234	12	9.5
Banana	118	105	27	3.1
Blackberries	144/cup	75	14	4.6
Cherries	117/cup	74	19	2.5
Fig	60/1	37	9	1.4
Grapefruit	118	38	9	1.3
Grapes	92/cup	62	16	0.8
Mango	207	138	35	0.3
Nectarine	136	60	14	2.3
Orange	141	65	16	3.4
Peach	98	38	9	1.5
Pear	166/1	96	26	5.1
Pineapple	155/cup	133	20	2.2
Plum	66/1	30	7	0.9
Prune	16/2	38	10	1.1
Raisins	73	220	58	2.9
Raspberries	123/cup	64	15	8.0
Strawberries	144/cup	46	11	2.9

(Continued)

TABLE 5.6 (Continued)
Fiber Content of Some Common Foods

	WT (g)	KCAL	CHO	DFIB
Vegetables (Cooked unless Noted)				
Artichokes	120	56	13	6.8
Asparagus	180/cup	40	11	3.6
Broccoli	180	63	13	5.9
Cauliflower	100/cup	25	7	2.5
Celery	40	6	2	0.6
Sweet pepper	120	37	7	2.5
Tomato, raw	62	11	2.4	0.7
Tomato, stewed	255/cup	201	33	4.3
Zucchini	180	29	7	2.5
Brussels sprouts	156/cup	56	11	4.1
Cabbage	150/cup	38	8	2.8
Coleslaw, homemade	60	47	7	0.9
Lettuce, iceberg	55	7	1	0.7
Spinach	30	7	1	0.7
Carrots	72	30	7	2.0
Onion	160	64	7	2.7
Potato				
French fries	50/10 pieces	67	12	1.0
Hash browns	156	340	44	3.1
Mashed	240	199	42	3.6
Raw	213	164	37	4.7
Red	213	149	34	3.6
Radish	58/1/2 cup	9	2	0.9
Turnip	156	34	7.9	3.1
Corn	154/cup	132	29	4.2
Beans[a]				
Baked	253	392	54	13.9
Chickpeas	164	269	45	12.5
Kidney	177	225	40	13.1
French	177	228	42	16.6
Green	145	117	21	7.4
Lentils	198	230	40	15.6
Lima	170	209	40	9.0
Navy	182	255	47	19.1
Breads and Snacks				
Bagel	105/3.7 oz.	270	53	2.3
Banana bread	60	196	33	0.7
French bread	32	92	18	0.8
Italian bread	30	81	15	0.8
Rye	32	83	15	1.3
Wheat	36	89	17	1.4
Potato chips	28/1 oz.	157	15	0.9

(Continued)

TABLE 5.6 (*Continued*)
Fiber Content of Some Common Foods

	WT (g)	KCAL	CHO	DFIB
Taco chips	23	115	16	1.7
English muffin	57	129	25	2.0
Baby ruth	7	96	14	0.5
Chocolate fudge	20	88	14	0.4
Party mix	30	150	17	1.0
Drinks				
Club soda	355	0	0	0
Diet coke	366	0	0	0
Grape soda	372	160	42	0
Orange soda	372	166	46	0
Root beer	370	152	45	0
Coffee, brewed	237	0	0	0
Distilled spirits	42	110	0	0
Beer	356	153	126	0
Tea, brewed	240	0.03	0	0
Wine	103	88	3	0
Nuts				
Almonds	28	161	6.0	3.4
Cashews	28	155	8.5	0.9
Pecans	28	193	3.9	2.7
Pistachio	28	156	7.8	2.9
Peanuts	28	158	4.6	2.4

Note: WT = weight, the mass of the serving of food measured in grams; food weights less than 5 g were carried to the first decimal point; weights greater than or equal to 5 g were rounded to the nearest whole number.

KCAL = kilocalories; measures of the energy value of a food when consumed; in nutrition, the term *kilocalories* is used synonymously with *calories* and *Calories*.

CHO = total carbohydrate; sum of mono- and disaccharides (sugars) and polysaccharides (starch); usually includes the weight of dietary fiber; composed of carbon, hydrogen, and oxygen; measured in grams.

DFIB = dietary fiber; includes cellulose, hemicellulose, lignin, pectin, and other nondigestible plant components; measured in grams. The main component of dietary fiber is cellulose $(C_6H_{10}OS)_n$; a nondigestible polysaccharide composed of several hundred to over 10,000 glucose units.

[a] There are a great many varieties and forms of serving beans. These are examples and far more exact information in Pennington[52] should be checked.

pure dietary fiber or prebiotic substances in the diet. They invariably will be mixed with other foods. Although one can attempt to increased dietary content of one substance, this will invariably lead to increased consumption of another component. For example, a diet rich in psyllium will also invariably be rich in β-glucans. This is another reason why some subjects have excellent results with some fiber products and while others will not. Patients and dieticians must be patient with dietary recommendations and outcomes to avoid frustration. For example, Bonsu et al.[53] found that 13 independent studies of fructans diabetes found no significant effect on serum glucose in humans, and they concluded that more studies were needed. This was largely because of the significant difference in fiber intake across the studies, which could well have had an effect on the reported outcomes.

5.5.3 Lipid Control and Prevention of Atherosclerotic Heart Disease

A study published in 1977 in Great Britain showed that higher intakes of dietary fiber resulted in a statistically important risk mitigation for coronary artery disease.[54] Subsequently, Zutphen reported heart disease as a cause of death was three times higher in the lowest quintile of fiber intake in a group of 871 allowed over a 10-year period.[55] Another study, from Sweden, of 17,126 adults showed the risk of cardiovascular events was significantly reduced when a high-quality diet was followed although there were a variety of dietary factors at play.[56] Although there are numerous trials that indicate a decrease in atherosclerotic disease, there is significant variation between studies.[51-57] Of note, is the fact that in men there also is a decrease in stroke disease.[58] This makes the clinician and one interested in preventative medicine adhere to the A1 level of 14 g of fiber intake per 1000 cal of energy consumed. This recommendation is based on a protective mechanism, and there are numerous facts that support it, such as a reduction in low-density fibroprotein levels, C-reactive protein levels, apolipoprotein levels, and blood pressure. All of these markers are consistent with a protective effect of dietary fiber for atherosclerotic disease.[57] A landmark study, the Los Angeles Atherosclerotic Thickness Study reported anatomic evidence that soluble fiber intake was associated with improvement in atherosclerosis.[56]

5.5.4 Control of Type 2 Diabetes

The classic experiments of Jenkins demonstrated the importance of the glycemic index of foods.[59] This, in conjunction with numerous observations by diabetologists, makes recommendations for dietary intake of carbohydrates. Dietary recommendations for patients with diabetes or who are being treated for type 2 diabetes are a daily intake of 55% carbohydrate, 12%–15% protein, and less than 30% of fat, with monosaturated fat being 12%–15%. The appreciation of the importance of dietary fiber goes beyond the glycemic index and conversely includes the glycemic index in dietary fiber recommendations that a diet should provide 14–15 g fiber for anyone eating 1000 cal.[62-64] Numerous studies of type 2 diabetes reveal interesting factors and facts that vary with different risks. Clearly fiber may have a protective effect for type 2 diabetes. For example, one study of 75,000 individuals showed a substantially lower risk of diabetes if more than 15 g of fiber were ingested daily. In addition, those who ate greater amounts of insoluble fiber had a lower risk than those who ate lower intakes of soluble fiber. Many interventional studies, including a seminal study with oats made of glucan, revealed reduced postprandial glucose and insulin responses following fiber supplementation. The literature is replete with selected studies of different foods, but it is clear that the amount of different dietary fibers is extremely important in controlling type 2 diabetes.[39,51,59-64]

5.5.5 Diverticular Disease

One of the most widely held medical epidemiological discoveries revealed that while diverticular disease was extremely rare in African and Asian populations, it was extremely prevalent in westernized societies.[34–37] Burkitt and Walker popularized the fact that individuals in African societies that rarely had diverticular disease ate as much as 40–50 g of dietary fiber daily.[35–37] Burkitt and Walker implicated dietary fiber deficiency as the cause of diverticulosis Painter and Burkett[65] and Parks[66] popularized the theory that decreased fiber intake resulted in decreased colon content and increased intracolonic pressure that produced outpocketings of colonic mucosa (diverticula, which were most prominent in the descending and sigmoid colon).[25,65,66] The penetration of viscera through blood vessel openings represents a point of natural weakness in the colon wall, and increased intracolonic pressure permits the diverticula to form. It is to be noted there are really "pseudo-diverticula" in which they do not contain the complete colon mucosa, only the mucosal wall. This topic has been reviewed many times in recent history. In 2006 Bogardus and the National Diverticular Study Group[67] looked at the relationship to dietary fiber, and this subject was thoroughly rereviewed by Ravikoff and Korzenik.[68] These investigators concluded that dietary fiber deficiency was indeed the cause for diverticulosis and concluded that the theories on fiber deficiency were correct. In the United States, 95% of patients with diverticulosis have had it primarily in the descending and sigmoid colon. For those that require surgery, 95% involved the sigmoid colon.[67,69]

Many challenge the dietary fiber theories. A thorough Veterans Administration Study showed that popcorn and small food particles are not associated with diverticulitis[70] but there are subsequent studies that do support the dietary fiber deficiency theory.[71] Peery and colleagues published the results of their diet and health studies phase III–V, which was a cross-sectional study to assess environmental and life style factors associated with colorectal adenomas.[72] It consisted of patients that had a colonoscopy and then were given specific dietary instructions on increasing their fiber intake. The investigators concluded that fiber did not protect against diverticular formation.[72] This study was then reevaluated by others who challenged the results because the study was based on a colonoscopy finding and follow-up dietary treatment.[73] There have been other recent evaluations, and a large study from Britain also found, based on review of the literature and of new data, that dietary fiber did appear to be protective.[71] Dietary fiber is usually limited in any acute diverticular disease.[74] Surgical therapy may then be necessary and that is limited to surgical indications.[75]

There are many evolving therapies for diverticular disease because of its frequency. The DIVA Study reports some decrease in symptomatology with the use of mesalamine.[76] Other authors have found mesalamine, rifaximin and certain antibiotics, very effective in treating the acute stage of the disease.[77] However, these are limited and vary with each case. The overall picture is that when there is any obstruction, dietary fiber is limited. When there is no obstruction, it is used on a clinical basis as indicated by the practitioner.[78–81]

Certainly there are many subtleties in diverticular disease. One that is emerging is that it may appear to be more frequent in young persons.[82] The subtleties of dietary fiber treatment will remain until more research is done. Nevertheless, there is no question that dietary fiber is related to diverticular disease and that the recommended dietary allowances as discussed above should be followed in all healthy persons.

A prospective study of diet and risk of diverticular disease in British vegetarians and nonvegetarians was conducted in Oxford. The investigation focused on cancer, and the data appeared to be statistically strong which led to the conclusions that consuming a vegetarian diet and a high intake of dietary fiber were both associated with a lower risk of admission to hospitals or death from diverticular disease.[70]

There are numerous subtleties in the natural evolution of diverticular disease which are not discussed in this chapter. However, it is important to note that treatments now include the evaluation of antibiotics, nonabsorbable antibiotics such as rifaximin and probiotics.[77] Evaluation of the life cycle of the disease with recent papers noted that there is the evolution in the elderly, but the young did not appear to have any important differences other than more frequent attacks, though not necessarily more aggressive so that they did not require more surgery.[83]

Fiber is still considered preventive and helpful, but all of the answers on its subtle help appear to relate to the depth of the microbiota effects.[82] Recent further study of the disease indicates that there probably is a low-grade inflammation with motor nerve damage and an associated dysbiosis. The dysbiosis may well be related to an altered microbiota.[82,84,85]

5.5.6 DIETARY FIBER AND IBS

IBS remains a major problem in clinical gastroenterology.[25,27] During the past decade, there have been numerous reviews on the subject.[86–89] Furthermore, Dr. Peter Gibson will be discussing the role of dietary fiber in Chapter 10.

In studying the history of the epidemiology of fiber-deficiency disease, it is clear that gastrointestinal symptomatology is extensive and highly variable in IBS. Constipation, abdominal distention, abdominal pain, and even mild diarrhea are associated with altered dietary fiber intake. The literature on IBS[78–81] is replete with associations between these symptoms and altered dietary fiber altered intake. A review of the older literature clearly reveals that dietary fiber supplementation was used extensively and to some effect.[78–81]

5.5.7 DIETARY FIBER AND CANCER

This is an extensive subject, and it will be reviewed in detail in Chapter 7. The reader is also referred to References 36, 90, and 55 of this chapter. There are numerous other studies, but the debate still rages as to whether increased dietary fiber is preventive of cancers, if so, which ones in particular.[91,92]

5.6 SUMMARY

Prebiotics and dietary fiber are largely nutrients that are not digested by human enzymes. However, they are the most important nutrients for the human intestinal microbiota. As such, they play a vital role in human metabolism as well as in important physiologic processes that occur within the intestinal tract. Very little is known about the microecology and the vast interaction of the ecologic unit, its microbiota, the nutrients, and the host.

REFERENCES

1. Floch MH. Advances in intestinal microecology: The microbiome, prebiotics and probiotics. *Nutr Clin Pract* 2012;2:193–194.
2. Wu GD, Lewis JD. Analysis of the human gut microbiome and association with disease. *Clin Gastroenterol Hepatol* 2013;11:774–777.
3. Floch MH. Intestinal microecology in health and wellness. *J Clin Gastroenterol* 2011;45:S108–S110.
4. Gibson GR, Beatty ER, Wang X et al. Selective stimulations of bifidobacteria in the human colon by oligofructose and inulin. *Gastroenterology* 1995;108:975–982.
5. Turnbaugh PF, Ley RE, Hamady M et al. The human microbiome project. *Nature* 2007;449:804–810.
6. Floch MH. Intestinal microecology. In: Floch MH, Kim A, Eds. *Probiotics: A Clinical Guide*. Thorofare, NJ: Slack Inc; 2010. pp. 3–11.
7. Floch MH, Gorbach SL, Luckey TD. Intestinal microflora. *Am J Clin Nutr* 1970;23:1425–1426.
8. Luckey TD. Introduction to intestinal microecology. *Am J Clin Nutr* 1972;25:1292–1294.
9. Neish AS. Microbes in gastrointestinal health and disease. *Gastroenterology* 2009;136: 65–80.
10. Hansen R, Russell RK, Reiff C et al. Microbiota of de-novo pediatric IBD: Increased Faecalibacterium prausnitzii and reduced bacterial diversity in Crohn's but not in ulcerative colitis. *Am J Gastroenterol* 2012;107:1913–1922.
11. Raman M, Ahmed I, Gillevet PM et al. Fecal microbiome and volatile organic compound metabolome in obese humans with nonalcoholic fatty liver disease. *Clin Gastroenterol Hepatol* 2013;11:868–875.
12. Boursier J, Rawls JF, Diehl AM. Obese humans with nonalcoholic fatty liver disease display alterations in fecal microbiota and volatile organic compounds. *Clin Gastroenterol Hepatol* 2013;11:876–878.
13. Gibson GR, Roberfroid MB. Dietary modulation of the human colonic microbiota: Introducing the concept of prebiotics. *J Nutr* 1995;125:1401–1412.
14. Ellegard L, Andersson H, Bosaeus I. Inulin and oligofructose do not influence the absorption of cholesterol, or the excretion of cholesterol, Ca, Mg, Zn, Fe, or bile acids but increases energy excretion in ileostomy subject. *Eur J Clin Nutr* 1997;51:1–5.
15. Roberfroid MB, Van Loo JAE, Gibson GR. The bifodogenic nature of inulin and its hydrolysis products. *J Nutr* 1998;128:11–19.
16. Cummings JH, Macfarlane GT, Englyst HN. Prebiotics digestion and fermentation. *Am J Clin Nutr* 2001;73:415S–420S.
17. Macfarlane GT, Cummings JH. Probiotics and prebiotics: Can regulating the activities of intestinal bacteria benefit health? *BMJ* 1999;318:999–1003.
18. Slavin J. Fiber and prebiotics: Mechanisms and health benefits. *Nutrients* 2013;5: 1417–1435.

19. den Ende WV. Multifunctional fructans and raffinose family oligosaccharides. *Front Plant Sci* 2013;9(4):247.
20. Sherman PM, Cabana M, Gibson GR et al. Potential roles and clinical utility of prebiotics in newborns, infants, and children: Proceedings from a global prebiotic summit meeting, New York City, June 27–28, 2008. *J Pediatr* 2009;155:S61–S70.
21. Kelly G. Inulin-type prebiotics: A review (Part 2). *Altern Med Rev* 2009;14(1):36–55.
22. Floch MH, Hong-Curtiss J. Probiotics, irritable bowel syndrome, and inflammatory bowel disease. *Curr Treat Op Gastro* 2003;6:283–288.
23. Kumar V, Sinha AK, Makkar HPS et al. Dietary roles of non-starch polysaccharides in human nutrition: A review. *Crit Rev Food Sci Nutr* 2012;52(10):899–935.
24. Douglas LC, Sanders ME. Probiotics and prebiotics in dietetics practice. *J Am Diet Assoc* 2008;108(3):510–521.
25. Floch MH. Prebiotics, probiotics and dietary fiber. In: Buchman A, Ed. *Clinical Nutrition in Gastrointestinal Disease*. Thorofare, NJ: Slack Inc.; 2006. pp. 123–138.
26. Elkington SG, Floch MH, Conn HO. Lactulose in the treatment of chronic portal-systemic encephalopathy. *N Engl J Med* 1960;281:408–411.
27. Floch MH. *Netter's Gastroenterology*. Philadelphia, PA: Saunders Elsevier; 2010. pp. 373–377.
28. Kolida S, Gibson GR. The prebiotic effect: Review of experimental and human data. In: Gibson, GR and Roberfroid MH, Eds. *Handbook of Prebiotics*. London: CRC Press; 2008. pp. 69–92.
29. Kleessen B, Sykura B, Zunft HJ, Blaut M. Effects of inulin and lactose on fecal microflora, microbial activity, and bowel habit in elderly constipated persons. *Am J Clin Nutr* 1997;65:1397–1402.
30. Morrison DJ, Mackay WG, Edwards CA et al. Butyrate production from oligofructose fermentation by the human faecal flora: What is the contribution of extracellular acetate and lactate? *Br J Nutr* 2006;96:570–577.
31. Walton GE, van den Heuvel EG, Kosters MH et al. A randomised crossover study investigating the effects of galactooligosaccharides on the faecal microbiota in men and women over 50 years of age. *Br J Nutr* 2012;107:1466–1475.
32. Brunser O, Gotteland M, Crochet S et al. Effect of a milk formula with prebiotics on the intestinal microbiota of infants after an antibiotic treatment. *Pediatr Res* 2006;59:451–456.
33. Binns CW, Lee AH, Harding H et al. The CUPDAY study: Prebiotic-probiotic milk product in 1–3-year-old children attending childcare centres. *Acta Paediatr* 2007;96:1646–1650.
34. Cleave TL. *The Saccharine Disease*. New Canaan, CT: Keats Publishing, Inc.; 1975.
35. Burkitt DP, Trowell HC. *Refined Carbohydrate Foods and Disease: Some Implications of Dietary Fiber*. London: Academic Press; 1975.
36. Burkitt DP, Walker ARP, Painter NS. Dietary fiber and disease. *JAMA* 1974;229: 1068–1074.
37. Trowell H, Burkitt D, Heaton K. *Dietary Fibre, Fibre-Depleted Foods and Disease*. London: Academic Press; 1985.
38. Spiller GA. *Dietary Fiber in Human Nutrition*, 2nd Edition. Boca Raton, FL: CRC Press, Inc.; 1993.
39. Slavin JL, Savarino V, Parades-Diaz A, Fotopoulos G. A review of the role of soluble fiber in health with specific reference to wheat dextrin. *J Int Med Res* 2009; 37: 1–17.
40. Tannock CW. *Probiotics: A Critical Review*. Wymondham, UK: Horizon Scientific Press; 1999.
41. Asp, N-GL. Classification and methodology of food carbohydrates as related to nutritional effects. *Am J Clin Nutr* 1995;61:930S–937S.

42. Cummings JH, Englyst HN. Gastrointestinal effects of food carbohydrate. *Am J Clin Nutr* 1995;61:938S–945S.
43. Wang YR, Talley NJ, Picco MF. Overlap: Irritable bowel syndrome, inflammatory bowel disease, and diverticular disease. *J Clin Gastroenterol* 2011;45:S36–S42.
44. Cummings JH, Pomare EW, Branch WJ et al. Short chain fatty acids in human large intestine, portal, hepatic and venous blood. *Gut* 1987;28:1221–1227.
45. Hoverstad T. Studies of short-chain fatty acid absorption in man. *Scand J Gastroenterol* 198621:257–260.
46. Roediger WEW. Role of anaerobic bacteria in the metabolic welfare of the colonic mucosa in man. *Gut* 1980;21:793–798.
47. McNeil NI, Cummings JH, James WPT et al. Short chain fatty acid absorption by the human large intestine. *Gut* 1978;19:819–822.
48. Rabassa AA, Rogers AI. The role of short-chain fatty acid metabolism in colonic disorders. *Am J Gastroenterol* 1992;87:419–423.
49. Wolever TMS, Schrade KB, Vogt JA et al. Do colonic short-chain fatty acids contribute to the long-term adaptation of blood lipids in subject with type 2 diabetes consuming a high-fiber diet? *Am J Clin Nutr* 2002;75:1023–1030.
50. Dorfman SH, Ali M, Floch MH. Low fiber content of Connecticut diets. *Am J Clin Nutr* 1976;29:87.
51. Anderson JW. *Plant Fiber in Foods*. Lexington, KY: HCF Diabetes Research Foundation Inc.; 1986. pp. 10–30.
52. Pennington JAT, Douglass JS. *Bowes & Church's Food Values of Portions Commonly Use*, 19th Edition. Philadelphia: Lippincott William & Wilkins; 2010.
53. Bonsu NK, Johnson CS, McLeod KM. Can dietary fructans lower serum glucose? *J Diabetes* 2011;3:58–66.
54. Morris JN, Marr JW, Clayton DG. Diet and heart: A postscript. *Br Med J* 1977; ii: 1307 1314.
55. Kromhout D, Bosschieter EB, de Lezeene Coulander, C. Dietary fiber and 10-year mortality from coronary heart disease, cancer, and all causes. The Zutphen study. *Lancet* 1982;2:518–522.
56. Pereira MA, O'Reilly E, Augustsson K et al. Dietary fiber and risk of coronary heart disease. *Arch Intern Med* 2004;164:370–376.
57. Wu H, Dwyer KM, Fan Z et al. Dietary fiber and progression of atherosclerosis: The Los Angeles Atherosclerosis Study. *Am J Clin Nutr* 2003;78:1085–1091.
58. Gillman MW, Cupples LA, Gagnon D et al. Protective effect of fruits and vegetables on development of stroke in men. *JAMA* 1995;273:1113–1117.
59. Jenkins DJ, Wolever TM, Taylor RH et al. Glycemic index of foods: A physiological basis for carbohydrate exchange. *Am J Clin Nutr* 1981;34:362–366.
60. Jenkins DJA, Netwon AC, Leedes AR, Cummings JH. Effect of pectin, guar gum, and wheat fibre on serum cholesterol. *Lancet* 1975;1:116–117.
61. Olsen BH, Anderson SM, Becker MP et al. Psyllium-enriched cereals lower blood total cholesterol and LDL cholesterol, but not HDL cholesterol, in hypercholesterolemic adults: Results for a meta-analysis. *J Nutr* 1997;127:1973–1980.
62. Anderson JW, Floore TL, Geil PB et al. Hypocholesterolemic effects of different hydrophilic fibers. *Arch Intern Med* 1991;151:1597–1602.
63. Anderson JW, Randles KM, Kendall CWC, Jenkins DJA. Carbohydrate and fiber recommendations for individuals with diabetes: A quantitative assessment and meta-analysis of the evidence. *J Am Coll Nutr* 2004;23:5–17.
64. Brand-Miller JC, Thomas M, Swan V et al. Physiological validation of the concept of glycemic load in lean young adults. *J Nutr* 2003;133:2728–2732.
65. Painter NS, Burkitt DP. Diverticular disease of the colon: A deficiency disease of Western civilization. *Br Med J* 1971;2:450.

66. Parks TG. Natural history of diverticular disease of the colon. *Clin Gastroenterol* 1975;4:53.

67. Bogardus, Jr ST. What do we know about diverticular disease? A brief overview. *J Clin Gastroenterol* 2006;40:S108–S111.

68. Ravikoff JE, Korzenik JR. The role of fiber in diverticular disease. *J Clin Gastroenterol* 2011;45:S7–S11.

69. Rodkey CV, Welch CE. Changing patterns in the surgical treatment of diverticular disease. *Ann Surg* 1984;200:466.

70. Crowe FL, Appleby PN, Allen NE, Key TJ. Diet and risk diverticular disease in Oxford cohort of European prospective investigation into cancer and nutrition (EPIC): Prospective study of British vegetarians and non-vegetarians. *BMJ* 2011;343:d4131. doi: 10.1136/bmj.d4131.

71. Strate LL, Liu YL, Syngal S, Aldoori WH, Giovannucci EL. Nut, corn, and popcorn consumption and the incidence of diverticular disease. *JAMA* 2008;300:907–914.

72. Peery AF, Barrett PR, Park D et al. A high-fiber diet does not protect against asymptomatic diverticulosis. *Gastroenterology* 2012;142:266–272.

73. Strate LL. Diverticulosis and dietary fiber: Rethinking the relationship. *Gastroenterology* 2012;142:205–207.

74. Ravikoff JE, Korzenik. Case presentation; the role of diet-fiber. *J Clin Gastroenterol* 2011;45:S44–S45.

75. Strong SA. Acute diverticulitis. *J Clin Gastroenterol* 2011;45:S62–S69.

76. Stollman N, Magowan S, Shanahan F et al. A randomized controlled study of mesalamine after acute diverticulitis: Results of the DIVA trial. *J Clin Gastroenterol* 2013;47:621–629.

77. Tursi A. Antibiotics and probiotics in the treatment of diverticular disease. *J Clin Gastroenterol* 2011;45:S46–S52.

78. Findlay JM, Smith AN, Mitchell WD et al. Effects of unprocessed bran on colon function in normal subjects and in diverticular disease. *Lancet* 1974;1:146–149.

79. Taylor I, Duthie HL. Bran tablets and diverticular disease. *Br Med J* 1976;1:988–990.

80. Brodribb AJM. Treatment of symptomatic diverticular disease with high-fibre diet. *Lancet* 1977;2:664–666.

81. Painter NS. Bran and the irritable bowel syndrome. *Lancet* 1976;i:540.

82. Floch MH. The microbiota and intestinal microflora in diverticular disease. *J Clin Gastroenterol* 2011;45:S12–S14.

83. Katz LH, Guy, DD, Lahat A, Gafter-Gvili A, Bar-Meir S. Diverticulitis in the young is not more aggressive than in the elderly, but it tends to recur more often. *J Gastroenterol Hepatol* 2013;28:1274–1281.

84. Strate LL, Modi R, Cohen E, Spiegel BM. Diverticular disease as a chronic illness: Evolving epidemiologic and clinical insights. *Am J Gastroenterol* 2012;107:1486–1493.

85. Boynton W, Floch MH. New strategies for the management of diverticular disease: Insights for the clinician. *Ther Adv Gastroenterol* 2013;6:205–213.

86. Johnston JM, Shiff SJ, Quigley EM. A review of the clinical efficacy of linaclotide in irritable bowel syndrome with constipation. *Curr Med Res Opin* 2013;29:149–160.

87. Gibson PR, Barrett JS, Muir JG. Functional bowel symptoms and diet. *Intern Med J* 2013;43:1067–1074.

88. Ruepert L, Quartero AO, de Wit NJ et al. Bulking agents, antispasmodics and antidepressants for the irritable bowel syndrome. *Cochrane Database Syst Rev* 2011;8:CD003460.

89. Khanna R, Macdonald JK, Levesque BG. Peppermint oil for the treatment of irritable bowel syndrome: A systemic review and meta-analysis. *J Clin Gastroenterol* 2014;48:505–512.

90. Bamia C, Lagiou P, Buckland G et al. Mediterranean diet and colorectal cancer risk: Results from a European cohort. *Eur J Epidemiol* 2013;28:317–328.
91. Park Y, Brinton LA, Subar AF, Hollenbeck A, Schatzkin A. Dietary fiber intake and risk of breast cancer in postmenopausal women: The National Institutes of Health-AARP Diet and Health Study. *Am J Clin Nutr* 2009;90:664–671.
92. Daniel CR, Park Y, Chow WH et al. Intake of fiber and fiber-rich plant foods is associated with a lower risk of renal cell carcinoma in a large US cohort. *Am J Clin Nutr* 2013;97:1036–1043.

6 Role of the Intestinal Microbiota and Probiotics in Health and Disease

Vladimir Stanisic and Eamonn M.M. Quigley

CONTENTS

6.1 PART 1: THE MICROBIOTA IN HEALTH

Case: *A 34-year-old woman comes for an annual physical exam. She has no remarkable past medical history and she is otherwise healthy. She is very attentive to her diet and she exercises regularly. She heard from her friends about a new diet based on high fiber and yogurt that is supposed to maintain a healthy body by regulating intestinal bacteria. She would like to hear more about "good" bacteria and their role in health maintenance.*

6.1.1 WHERE DOES OUR INTESTINAL MICROBIOTA COME FROM?

Bacteria colonize our skin and mucosal surfaces and become an integral part of our organism from birth. Because of its sheer size (estimated to exceed 10^{14} cells) and important homeostatic functions, the microbiota is sometimes referred to as "the forgotten" organ.[1,2] It has been estimated that our gut contains 35,000 different microbial species and that our mucosal and skin surfaces contain 10 times more microorganisms than there are cells in our body.[1]

Until recently, it was believed that our gut and our skin are essentially sterile *intra utero*. However, new research indicates that our mucosal surfaces may be exposed to a commensal flora even before birth. Accordingly, commensal bacteria have been detected in the umbilical cords of neonates and bacterial DNA identified in the placenta.[3–5] In addition, the fact that meconium is not sterile further indicates that colonization of the gut begins before the birth. The role of this early exposure of the gut mucosa to bacteria or their DNA may be important in the early developmental stages of the enteric immune system.

Following birth, infants are initially colonized by the mother's flora. Sampling of the microbiota of newborns shows that babies who are born via vaginal delivery have a gut microbiota that is similar to the vaginal microbiota of their mother, whereas those born by cesarean section possess a microbiota more reminiscent of that which inhabits the mother's skin.[6–10] Interestingly, recent studies have shown that breast milk contains viable bacteria of enteric origin indicating that breast feeding may contribute to the colonization of the neonatal gut.[1,6,11] Immediately after birth the microbiota is largely represented by facultative anaerobes.[12] The microbiota of the young infant is very diverse, varies between individuals and is influenced by factors such as mode of feeding (breast versus bottle).[13] By 1–2 years of age, the infant microbiota has become more diverse; as the proportion of *Bifidobacteria* steadily declines, *Firmicutes* and *Bacteroidetes* increase in abundance.[14] By the age of 3, the composition of microbiota stabilizes and now resembles that of an adult.[14,15] Thereafter, and throughout adulthood, its composition remains relatively constant and is shaped predominantly by long-term dietary patterns.[16,17] In old age, diversity decreases, with diminishing numbers of *Firmicutes* and *Bifidobacteria*.[6,18,19]

6.1.2 WHAT IS THE COMPOSITION OF THE GUT MICROBIOTA?

The human enteric microbiota is dominated by phyla *Firmicutes* and *Bacteroidetes*. Phylum *Firmicutes* contains predominantly Gram-positive and spore-forming bacteria and is further divided into anaerobic *Clostridia* and obligate or facultatively anaerobic *Bacilli.*[20] *Bacteroidetes* are Gram-negative obligate anaerobes and are the most abundant and the most variable enteric phylum.[20] Based on large-scale sequencing approaches, three major enterotypes have been identified in the normal human gut microbiome. These adult enterotypes have been identified based on the predominance of particular bacterial genera and do not appear to be nation or continent specific nor do they correlate with age, gender, or body habitus.[14,20] Enterotype type 1 is *Bacteroides* predominant, Enterotype type 2 *Prevotella*, and Enterotype type 3 *Ruminococcus.*[20] The compositional differences between the enterotypes are most likely related to differences in metabolic strategies used to generate energy by the fermentation of proteins and carbohydrates. In a similar manner, compositional differences between enterotypes may represent an adaptation to long-term dietary habits. Studies have shown that a *Bacteroides*-dominant, type 1 enterotype, is associated with a starch- and protein-rich diet (commonly found in the Western world), whereas a *Prevotella*-dominant, type 2 enterotype is most commonly found in those whose diet contains high levels of indigestible fibers (more typical of African diets).[6,16,21]

The gut extends from the mouth to the anus and is functionally and anatomically segregated into distinct units each with its distinctive mucosal morphology, vastly differing luminal pH and contents and varying immune system. It, therefore, comes as no surprise that microbiota of the mouth is substantially different from that found in the stomach or colon. Different microbial communities occupy different intestinal niches depending on nutrient availability, composition, and the nature of the microenvironment they inhabit. The mouth is occupied predominantly by polymicrobial Gram-positive and Gram-negative bacteria including *Streptococci, Lactobacilli, Staphylococci, Corynebacteria, Bacteroides*, and clinically important *Streptococcus viridans*, *Streptococcus mutans*, and *Streptococcus sanguinis.*[22]

The esophagus is largely devoid of a substantial bacterial population given the very rapid transit of food through its lumen. In the upper esophagus, bacterial communities resemble those of the oropharynx with *S. viridans* being the most prominent species.[23] When biopsies from the distal esophagus were examined by pyrosequencing, *Streptococcus, Prevotella, and Veillonellacea* genera were isolated.[23] Moreover, differences were detected between normal subjects and those suffering from Barrett's esophagus. As the contributions of factors such as the use of acid suppressive medications or the secondary effects of gastroesophageal reflux cannot be excluded, a causal relationship between changes in the microbiota and esophageal disease could not be established from these studies.

The stomach has traditionally been considered an inhospitable environment for bacteria because of its highly acidic contents; however; intestinal-type bacteria do occupy the stomach, albeit on a much smaller scale. Estimates suggest that the concentration of the resident bacteria in the stomach falls below 1000 cfu/mL.[23] Despite the harsh acidic environment, acid-resistant bacteria predominate in the gastric juices and the composition of the gastric microbiota is variable and affected by such factors as the composition of the oral microbiome as well as what foods are ingested and medications taken. Nevertheless, several bacterial species normally colonize the gastric mucosa, thereby, furnishing a stable microbiome. Among these, *Lactobacilli*, *Enterococci*, *Catenabacteria*, *Bacilli*, *Veillonella*, *Streptococcus*, *Prevotella* and *Helicobacter pylori* predominate. It is estimated that the prevalence of *H. pylori* among the general population in the United States is 50% and its presence in the stomach is regulated by the presence of other stomach bacteria. For example, a study by Nakagawa et al. showed that germ-free mice are much more susceptible to the colonization by *H. pylori* in the stomach than are mice who possess an intact microbiota.[23]

The duodenum is also characterized by a relative paucity of microbes, given the relatively short transit times through this organ. In addition, due to the technical challenges posed in obtaining samples from this part of the gut and the lack of systematic sequencing studies, not much is known about the bacterial composition of the duodenum.[23] However, it has been estimated that the duodenum and jejunum harbor between 10^3 and 10^4 bacteria/g of luminal content and that duodenal bacterial content is enriched in *Firmicutes* and *Actinobacteria*, in contrast to the *Bacteroidetes* that are enriched in the colon.[1,2,24] The colon has the slowest transit time and the most hospitable environment for the growth of microorganisms. In the colon, bacteria abound and reach an estimated concentration of 10^{12} cells/g of content and encompass a broad range of bacterial phyla.

In addition to the differential distribution of bacteria longitudinally in different compartments along the gut, the composition of the microbiota also varies between the lumen and the mucosal surface. Luminal bacterial contents are dominated, for example, by *Bifidobacteria*, *Bacteroides*, *Prevotella*, *Streptococcus*, *Enterococcus*, *Ruminococcus* spp. Only a very few bacterial species (*Enterococcus*, *Lactobacillus*, *and Clostridium* species) are able to penetrate mucus and establish residence in close proximity to enterocytes.[25]

Studies of the microbiota from different individuals have shown a much greater degree of similarity between the microbiotas of close relatives than between unrelated individuals who happen to share the same living quarters. This indicates that host genetics plays a very significant role in shaping the composition of the gut microbiota.[26]

6.1.3 WHAT IS THE FUNCTION OF THE GUT MICROBIOTA?

6.1.3.1 Development of the Gastrointestinal Tract

Intestinal commensal bacteria play important roles in the morphological and functional maturation of the human gastrointestinal system. The absence of the microbial flora has been shown to result in a decrease in intestinal surface area, villus thickness, and vascular proliferation within the intestinal wall.[1,2,27–29] Furthermore, gut motility and transit times are also influenced by diet and microbial products, such as methane and short-chain fatty acids (SCFAs).[30] The introduction of a normal flora into germ-free mice leads to a greater degree of regularity in the propagation of myoelectrical signals and pressure waves along the gastrointestinal system,[31] and promotes the expression of several key channel proteins involved in the generation of the electrochemical basis of gut peristalsis.[32]

6.1.3.2   Regulation of the Immune System by Resident Microbial Flora

The immune system of the gut is composed of lymphatic tissues such as enteric lymph nodes and Peyer's patches, as well as its own innate and adaptive immune systems. The presence of intestinal commensals affects each of these components of the gut immune system. Gnotobiotic mice that have been reared in a germ-free environment and subsequently exposed to different environmental and microbial conditions exhibit immaturity in the development of the enteric immune system and its responses.[2,33] Under normal, physiologic circumstances, dendritic cells sample the luminal environment and present antigens to the lymphocytes within Peyer's patches. Interactions between antigen presenting cells and T cells determine the nature of the immune response, that is, activation or anergy and tolerance. The immature, underdeveloped Peyer's patches seen in gnotobiotic mice can generate dysregulated immune responses.[33] In addition to influencing the development of the components of the immune system in the gut, the presence of commensal bacteria also affects those components of the innate immune system located in the intestinal mucosa. Toll-like receptors (TLR) on the enterocyte surface and nuclear oligomerization domain (NOD) receptors in enterocyte cytoplasm contribute to innate immunity and act to distinguish innocuous versus pathogenic microorganisms. TLR and NOD receptors, and their interactions with pathogens, are regulated by commensal bacteria. For example, the effect of TLR4 activation may be inhibited by inactivation of its downstream signaling by commensal bacteria.[34] Furthermore, commensal bacteria are involved in the negative regulation of the key inflammatory cascade transcription factor NF-κB via inhibition of degradation of its regulatory protein IκB.[35] The enteric microbiota also influences cellular immunity by affecting the pattern of T cell activation and differentiation as well as the profile of cytokines (pro- versus anti-inflammatory) produced.[2,36] Finally, the humoral immune system is also affected by the presence of a commensal flora as numbers of IgA-producing lymphocytes and production of IgA and IgG have been shown to be reduced in gnotobiotic mice.[37]

Given the immense size of the gut mucosal surface and the consequent amount of exposure that the host immune system has with the external environment, one of the critical functions of the gut microbiota is the development of tolerance. The absence of indigenous microbiota leads to overactivation of the host immune system upon exposure to the usual environmental triggers. One example of this phenomenon is the "hygiene hypothesis" according to which several immune hypersensitivity conditions such as asthma or eczema are thought to be related to the overly sanitized environment of contemporary living. Under such "aseptic" conditions with an associated exposure to a more limited repertoire of bacterial antigens, immune system activation may be exacerbated. Tolerance to bacterial antigens is achieved by a variety of mechanisms including the physical separation of the microbial biofilm from the enterocytes provided by the thick mucus layer and the conditioning of the host immune system by a diverse repertoire of microbial products. For example, mice deficient in the production of mucins quickly develop intestinal inflammation[38,39] and the exposure of the gut mucosa and its associated immune cells to bacterial lipopolysaccharide (LPS) can potentially lead to septic shock. However, several mechanisms have been shown to prevent this latter event, including, firstly, the dephosphorylation of LPS by intestinal alkaline phosphatase induced by the presence of commensal bacteria, secondly, exposure and desensitization to LPS from commensal bacteria during birth or, thirdly, via down-regulation of proinflammatory signaling pathways mediated by NF-κB.[1,40,41]

The presence of commensal bacteria is essential for the protection of the host against pathogenic microorganisms. A thick carpeting of gut mucosal surfaces with commensals provides both a physical and biochemical barrier against pathogenic invaders. Furthermore, multiple studies have shown that resident bacteria play important roles in regulating the expression of proteins involved in the formation and maintenance of junctional complexes, such are desmosomes and tight junctions[32] which are such important components of the intestinal barrier. For example, the expression of barrier protein sprr2a in intestinal villi is increased 280 fold following the introduction of the commensal bacteria indicating the profound effect that bacteria have on host gene expression and barrier integrity.[32]

Commensal bacteria also compete with pathogens and non-commensal bacteria for attachment sites and nutrients. The disappearance of commensals following antibiotic administration opens up an opportunity for the proliferation and colonization of gut surfaces with pathogenic bacteria. As mentioned previously, germ-free mice are more susceptible to colonization with *H. pylori*.[23] Another notable example is the colonization of the gut with *Clostridium difficile* following the administration of broad-spectrum antibiotics with the subsequent development of diarrhea and colitis. In addition, some commensal bacteria secrete peptides (bacteriocins) that can impede the growth of other bacteria while others provoke the host's epithelial cells to produce antimicrobial peptides. For example, *Lactobacilli* stimulate the production of defensins, whereas the pathogen *Shigella flexneri* downregulates their expression.[42]

6.1.3.3   Regulation of Nutrient and Xenobiotic Metabolism

The effect of the microbiota on human metabolism is considerable given that an estimated 10% of our caloric intake comes from intestinal microbial fermentation.[30,43] The microbiota of the human gut contains 150 times more genes that of the human host; thereby, substantially contributing to the host's metabolic and digestive capacities.[44] One way that commensals contribute to increased energy production and assimilation is by making otherwise indigestible plant and animal products such as indigestible starches and plant cells available for intestinal absorption. For example, *Firmicutes* associate with insoluble substrates in the colon and lead to their degradation.[45,46] Furthermore, bacterial species such as *Ruminococcaceae and Bacteroides* possess glycoside hydrolase enzymatic activity which generates metabolic products that can be further metabolized at the brush border. Another major source of energy rich metabolites produced by intestinal bacteria are SCFAs—such as butyrate and acetate produced by fermentation of otherwise indigestible carbohydrates. SCFAs serve, not only as an energy source for the host, but also as signaling molecules that are involved in the regulation of appetite control, food intake, energy expenditure, and intestinal motility.[47–50] Lactic acid is abundant in the gastrointestinal system and its utilization by lactic fermenters is of the great significance for the maintenance of the gut homeostasis.[51] Furthermore, intestinal commensals play important roles in the metabolism of a variety of other compounds, mostly aromatic hydrocarbons produced by digestion and fermentation of food in the lumen. Intestinal bacteria process those compounds and facilitate their elimination in feces. Another example of bacterial metabolite production is the degradation of dietary oxalate by *Oxalobacter formigenes*. This reaction decreases oxalate excretion and has implications for the formation of urinary oxalate stones.[1,52]

6.2 PART 2: THE INTESTINAL MICROBIOTA IN DISEASE

Case: *A 71-year-old male is hospitalized for severe diarrhea following a prolonged course of broad spectrum antibiotics for recurrent urinary tract infections. A stool sample was positive for* C. difficile *toxin and metronidazole was initiated. The family of the patient wants to know why he developed this problem and if probiotics could help?*

6.2.1 Antibiotic-Associated Diarrhea and C. *difficile*-Associated Disease

Given the aforementioned roles of the microbiota in intestinal homeostasis, it is to be expected that its disruption could lead to various different disease states. Antibiotic-associated diarrhea (AAD) and *C. difficile*-associated disease (CDAD) are common and illustrative examples of such disruption with most studies associating the development of *C. difficile* infection with changes in the total number of bacteria in the microbiota as well in its composition and diversity.[53] This infection is characterized by a significant decrease in microbiome diversity and a shift away from the normal dominance of *Bacteroidetes* or *Firmicutes*.[53] Antibiotics suppress commensals and allow already present *C. difficile* to proliferate and become pathogenic. Alternatively, the depletion of a normal microbiota can facilitate de novo colonization by *C. difficile* and the occurrence of overt infection. When compared, the microbiota of asymptomatic *C. difficile* carriers resembled that of healthy individuals, whereas that of symptomatic patients was characterized by decreased microbial diversity.[54] That the status of the resident microbiota is critical to the clinical expression of CDAD is further supported by the study of Antharam et al.[55] who used high-density pyrosequencing to study the microbiota of the distal gut in two groups of patients; a group with CDAD and another with non-*C. difficile* nosocomial diarrhea as well as in a group of healthy subjects. Commensals, including *Ruminococcaceae* and *Lachnospiraceae* and butyrate-producing C2–C4 anaerobic fermenters, were significantly depleted in both patient groups.

6.2.2 Irritable Bowel Syndrome

Irritable bowel syndrome (IBS) is a functional bowel disorder characterized by recurrent abdominal pain or discomfort in association with altered bowel habit. IBS affects as many as 10%–15% of the adult population in Europe and North America.[56] While the cause(s) of IBS is unknown, a variety of factors including dysregulation along the brain–gut axis, dysmotility, visceral hypersensitivity, and altered immune responses manifest in some subjects as low grade inflammation have all been implicated.[57] More recently, attention has focused on a possible role for changes in intestinal microbiome composition in the pathogenesis of IBS. Comparisons of fecal bacterial communities between IBS patients and healthy controls based on cultures showed relative depletion of *Coliforms*, *Lactobacilli*, and *Bifidobacteria*, and a proliferation of *Streptococci*, *Escherichia coli*, and *Clostridium species* in IBS.[58,59] More recent culture-independent analyses of fecal samples again found that the intestinal microbiota of IBS patients differed significantly from healthy controls with a twofold increase in the ratio of *Firmicutes* to *Bacteroidetes* accompanied by a significant increase in *Clostridia* and relative decrease in the numbers of *Bifidobacterium* suggesting that IBS is linked to an excess of Firmicutes and Proteobacteria and loss of Bacteroidetes.[60] Further studies using high-throughput sequencing have been able to distinguish diarrhea-predominant IBS from healthy subjects[61] and to link changes in microbial populations with clinical phenotype.[62]

While few attempts have been made to ascribe causation to these findings or to link specific changes to symptoms, one can speculate on potential roles for bacterial species or strains in dysmotility, impaired integrity of the intestinal barrier and altered intestinal immune responses. Such effects could be mediated by changes in bacterial metabolism that in turn can affect recruitment of inflammatory cells, peristalsis, as well as triggering symptoms such as bloating, flatulence, and abdominal pain.[59] For example, SCFAs, such as butyrate, can change the cytokine profile of helper T cells and promote intestinal epithelial barrier integrity while acetate can down-regulate intestinal inflammation via its interactions with the G protein-coupled receptor, Gpr43. Evidence for potentially relevant interactions between luminal bacteria and the host in IBS is provided by increased expression of TLR-4 and TLR-5 and decreased expression of TLR-7 and TLR-8.[63]

6.2.3 INFLAMMATORY BOWEL DISEASE

The inflammatory bowel diseases (IBDs), Crohn's disease (CD), and ulcerative colitis (UC) are complex, polygenic intestinal disorders whose pathogenesis is linked to both the microbiota and the host immune response. Their phenotypic expression represents a complex interplay between the gut microbiota, host genome, and environmental factors.[64] Many of the multiple genetic polymorphisms associated with IBD involve genes coding for factors such as those engaged in bacterial recognition, mucosal barrier integrity, specific cytokine pathways, or lymphocytic chemotactic mechanisms. The role of the microbiota in the pathogenesis of IBD is more directly suggested by the observation that genetically predisposed animals, such as the IL-10 knockout mouse, do not develop inflammation if raised under germ-free conditions[64] but will develop florid colitis once reconstituted with a normal microbiota.[65–67] Other evidence supporting a critical role for luminal bacteria comes from the ameliorative effect of diversion of the fecal stream on inflammation in CD.[67] Finally, studies have shown that areas of the gastrointestinal system that have greatest exposure to bacterial components are also those most commonly featuring inflammation.[64,66,68] At a molecular level several routes whereby bacteria can activate the immune response in IBD have been identified; such as, through interactions with the NOD2 receptor leading to increased production of proinflammatory cytokines, by promoting a Th1 differentiation profile and, consequently, the production of IL-1, IL-12, and TNF, or by affecting neutrophil chemotaxis and the induction of aberrant T cell activation.[64,68–72]

A number of studies have shown that, in patients with IBD, there are significant changes in the composition of the microbiota; most notably, a decrease in numbers of *Firmicutes* and *Bacteroidetes* species and an increase in *Proteobacteria* and *Actinobacteria*. These shifts will alter SCFA production, leading, in particular, to lower levels of butyrate and acetate; compounds with known anti-inflammatory properties that also enhance the production of mucins and antimicrobial peptides.[68,72–74] Furthermore, parallel changes in the microbiota has been noted among unaffected relatives of patients with CD where, though butyrate-producing bacteria were preserved, bacteria with a capacity to degrade mucus were enhanced.[75]

6.2.4 COLORECTAL CANCER

Colorectal cancer (CRC) is one of the most frequent cancers in the United States with over 130,000 cases being diagnosed in 2010. It is a complex disease that features important contributions from both genetic and environmental factors. CRC has been closely linked with certain chronic dietary habits which, in turn, influence the composition of the gut microbiota.[76] Diets rich in indigestible starches induce higher levels of bacterial fermentation with more production of butyrate and acetate and are, accordingly, thought to contribute to the lower incidence of CRC noted in rural African populations in comparison to North Americans and Europeans.[76–79] The implication of a protein rich diet as a risk factor for CRC may in part be related to the fermentation of proteins in the distal gut into carcinogenic polyamine compounds. In addition, gut microbiota affects overall metabolism and plays a role in the genesis of obesity, that is, of itself, a risk factor for CRC.[78,80] The influence of components of the microbiota on barrier integrity may also be relevant to the development and progression of CRC.[78] Recently, the presence of the gut microbiota has been linked to the expression of the Wnt gene that plays important roles in gut development, homeostasis, and carcinogenesis.[81] The studies from gnotobiotic mice illustrate the importance of a resident bacterial population in tumorigenesis occurring on a background of inflammation.[82,83]

6.3 PART 3: PROBIOTICS

6.3.1 GENERAL PRINCIPLES

Probiotics are preparations of live bacteria that are either incorporated into a food or given as supplements and confer a health benefit to the host. The origin of the probiotic concept is credited to the Russian Nobel Prize winner Eli Metchnikoff who postulated, in the early twentieth century, that intestinal microbes may be related to diet, which could, in turn, be manipulated in order to select for a "beneficial" intestinal flora.[84,85] Around the same time, the French pediatrician Henry Tissier found "bifid" Y shaped bacteria in the stool of children, observed that their numbers were significantly decreased in children with diarrhea[84,85] and suggested that the supplementation of these bacteria could lead to clinical improvement.[84,86] The term "probiotic" (literally, pro-life) first appeared in the literature in the 1950s and 1960s and was initially used to designate "active substances that are essential for a healthy development of life."[87] Over the decades the definition of probiotics has evolved and been the subject of frequent debates and challenges. Attempts to more narrowly define probiotics as those bacteria that are, not only beneficial, but of human origin, acid resistant, able to colonize the gut mucosa and capable of both producing antimicrobial substances and modulating the gut immune system, failed because many commonly used probiotic strains do not fulfill all of these criteria. Currently, definitions of probiotics stress only two essential features for non-pathogenic probiotic bacterial strains—that they must be live microorganisms and that they must, if given in adequate quantities, confer a health benefit to the host.[87]

Probiotics are now a large global market with estimated worth of 15.7 billion dollars in 2008 and increasing at an annual rate of 15%.[88,89] In the United States, probiotics are sold either as nutritional supplements or in foods such as yogurts, breakfast cereals, infant formulas, and even soft drinks.[86–88] The current boom in products that claim to include probiotics is undoubtedly exacerbated by the relatively loose regulation of this market. To address this issue, in 2002 the World Health Organization developed and published "Guidelines for the Evaluation of Probiotics in Food."[85] This guideline specifies an optimal process for the characterization of microbial products that comprises several steps:

1. Precise identification of the microorganism's genus, species, and strain and its deposition in the international culture collection
2. Assessment of safety by *in vitro* animal studies and phase 1 human studies
3. Double-blind, placebo-controlled phase 2 human trials to assess efficacy
4. Phase 3 studies comparing probiotics with current, standard treatments
5. Product labeling that should specify genus, species, and strain, minimum number of viable bacteria at the end of the shelf-life, proper storage conditions, and corporate contact details for further consumer information.

Few products on our shelves today satisfy all of these criteria and many fulfill none. Given that probiotics are not considered as medications from the regulatory standpoint, they do not have to fulfill the stringent standards applied to prescription drugs. As dietary supplements, probiotic product labels can make "qualified health claims" not subject to Food and Drug Administration (FDA) review or endorsement but must carry the disclaimer that the product "is not intended to diagnose, treat, cure, or prevent any disease."[86,90]

Although, there is now a substantial body of basic and translational research on probiotics, the current laxity of regulation has led to a situation aptly described by Caselli et al. as variability: variability in strains studied, doses used (that can range from hundreds of colony forming units in one study to trillions in another) and delivery methods employed (everything from capsules and tablets to yogurts and other foods). Variability extends also to clinical studies where design, duration of treatment, study end points and outcomes vary to such an extent that it is difficult to compare studies, conduct meta-analyses and draw meaningful conclusions about the safety and efficacy of probiotic products and draft reliable clinical recommendations regarding their use in the treatment or prevention of different diseases.[89]

An incomplete understanding of the mechanism(s) of action of all strains,[91] coupled with the fact that individual strains within a given species differ widely in such properties as adherence, antimicrobial activity, or immune engagement yet are all touted as conferring similar health benefits, adds to the challenge that faces the consumer in choosing a product in a particular context.[92]

Given the lax regulatory environment and the ubiquity of probiotic products, the question of safety of probiotics has become important. In theory, problems could arise:

1. As a consequence of bacterial translocation into the systemic circulation and lead to bacteremia and endocarditis
2. Due to gastrointestinal adverse event
3. From transference of antibiotic-resistance genes
4. Arising from poor quality control leading to contamination with pathogenic strains
5. When used in critically ill, hospitalized, and immunosuppressed patients.[93]

However, despite these theoretical concerns, the World Health Organization recommended that probiotics from *Lactobacilli* and *Bifidobacteria* species should be considered safe for human consumption, because of their established use in a number of human foods and supplements worldwide and their presence in commensal mammalian flora.[85] For example, *Lactobacillus GG* has been extensively used in clinical trials in adults of all ages, children, and pregnant women. It has been given to healthy subjects to prevent traveler's diarrhea, as well as to patients with IBD, rheumatoid arthritis, HIV infection, and allergies without significant adverse effects.[91] However, the National Center for Complementary and Alternative Medicine (NCCAM) advises that probiotics should not be used in critically ill patients because most data relating to adverse events comes from severely debilitated patients with multiple comorbidities. For example, in a large double-blind placebo-controlled study, Besselink et al.[94] found in patients critically ill with severe acute pancreatitis "that probiotic prophylaxis with a combination of probiotic strains did not reduce the risk of infectious complications and was associated with an increased risk of mortality." This study used four *Lactobacillus* strains and two *Bifidobacterium* strains, and although the infection rate was similar between groups the mortality rate was significantly higher in the probiotic treated group—16% versus 6% and largely attributable to intestinal ischemia.[94]

So how is the consumer to proceed? Sanders et al. proposed the following approach.[92] In inspecting the label of a probiotic preparation one should seek the following:

1. Name of the species and strain of the microorganism and whether this particular strain has been established as a common ingredient in foods such as yogurts
2. Detailed information about number of bacterial colony forming units

3. Information on the manufacturer and whether further information about the product is available on the manufacturer's web site

Probiotics may be presented as single strain preparations (e.g., *Bifidobacterium infantis* 35624, *Lactobacillus GG, Lactobacillus acidophilus, Saccharomyces boulardii*) or as multistrain or multispecies cocktails which may contain as few as two or as many as 10 individual strains. Despite claims to the contrary and given the strain specificity of bacterial actions, there is currently no data which indicates the superiority of a cocktail over a single strain for a given indication.[95]

6.3.2 INDICATIONS FOR THE USE OF PROBIOTICS

6.3.2.1 Sporadic, Acute Diarrheal Illness

Probiotics are thought to increase host resistance against invading pathogenic species through the production of antimicrobial peptides, competition with pathogenic bacteria for nutrients and binding sites on mucosal epithelial cells, modification of toxins, and toxin receptors, promoting peristalsis and modulating the host's immune system.[96–104]

In 2001, Szajewska et al.[102] analyzed eight double-blind placebo-controlled trials involving 731 children between 1 and 48 months with diarrhea lasting more than 3 days. The probiotic strains studied were *Lactobacillus GG, Lactobacillus reuteri, L. acidophilus LB, S. boulardii, Streptococcus thermophilus lactis, L. acidophilus,* and *Lactobacillus bulgaricus.* Only *Lactobacillus GG* (used in concentrations that ranged from 5×10^{10} to 2×10^{11} cfus [colony-forming units]) significantly reduced the duration of diarrhea compared with placebo; by an average of 18.2 h. This effect was particularly significant in rotavirus-related diarrhea. In addition, they identified one prevention study that showed a reduction in the incidence of diarrhea by pretreatment with *Lactobacillus GG* in children under 2 years of age. Importantly, although these various studies were mostly conducted in children under 2 years of age and employed a variety of bacterial species, no adverse reactions were reported. Authors concluded that there is a modest but clinically significant benefit associated with the use of *Lactobacillus GG* in acute gastroenteritis in infants and children.[102] A further meta-analysis by Huang et al.[105] on the use of probiotics in diarrhea of acute onset in otherwise healthy children under 5 years of age found that treatment with probiotics decreased the duration of diarrhea by 1 day. Finally, a Cochrane review on probiotics in the treatment of acute infectious diarrhea that analyzed 63 trials and 8014 subjects, mostly infants and children, found that use of probiotics decreased the duration of diarrhea by approximately 25 h and decreased stool frequency. Again, no significant adverse effects were noted in the reviewed studies.[106]

6.3.2.2 Antibiotic-Associated Diarrhea, C. difficile-
Associated Diarrhea and Traveler's Diarrhea

With the widespread use of broad-spectrum antibiotics in hospital wards, intensive care units (ICUs) and in outpatient practice, AAD, and CDAD, in particular, have become subjects of significant concern. Based on the known functions of an intact microbiota and on its disruption by antibiotics, considerable interest has been directed on the potential role of probiotics in the treatment and prevention of AAD and CDAD.

A Cochrane review analyzed 16 studies that included 3432 children (from 2 weeks to 17 years of age) that received *Lactobacilli* spp., *Bifidobacterium* spp., *Streptococcus* spp., or *S. boulardii* alone or in combination for treatment durations that ranged from 10 days to 3 months. The authors found that *Lactobacillus rhamnosus GG* and *S. boulardii* may prevent the onset of antibiotic associated diarrhea. Notably, no serious side effects were observed.[107] This review also found that probiotic preparations containing over 5 billion cfus were effective. Another meta-analysis of 31 trials involving 3164 patients and including adults, found that the use of the probiotic strains *S. boulardii* and *L. rhamnosus GG* significantly reduced the risk of development of AAD.[108] Another single-center, randomized, double-blind, placebo-controlled dose-ranging study of 255 adult inpatients assessed the efficacy of 50 or 100 billion cfu. of a probiotic mixture (*L. acidophilus* + *Lactobacillus casei*) or placebo in the prevention of AAD. The higher dose shortened the duration of AAD to just 2.8 days compared to 4.1 days for the lower dose and 6.4 days for placebo.[109]

With regard to CDAD, the most recent Cochrane review of 23 randomized controlled trials including 4213 patients concluded that short-term use of probiotics in patients who are not severely debilitated or immunocompromised is both safe and effective for preventing CDAD.[110] The authors found that if probiotics were administered in conjunction with antibiotics, incidence of CDAD was decreased by 64% with a further 20% decrease in the incidence of other adverse events such as abdominal cramping, flatulence, nausea, and fever. However, the authors cautioned that due to variability among the studies, the strength of their conclusions and recommendations were moderate.[110]

A meta-analysis of double blind placebo controlled trials that included 3326 subjects older than 10 years of age failed to find probiotics (*Lactobacilli* and *S. boulardii*) effective in the prevention of traveler's diarrhea.[111] The 2009 expert review on the topic of traveler's diarrhea found that only *Lactobacillus GG* met the criteria for "moderate evidence to support a recommendation for use" in the prevention of traveler's diarrhea.[112]

Together, these data indicate that the use of probiotics in the treatment of infectious diarrhea, antibiotic-associated diarrhea and *C. difficile* colitis is likely beneficial and safe, and, therefore, should be offered to patient populations at greatest risk for morbidity. When choosing a particular formulation, it appears that preparations with *Lactobacillus GG*, *Saccharomyces boulardii*, *L. reuteri protectis*, and *L. casei* show the most consistent results[95] but it must be emphasized that head-to-head comparisons have not been performed.

6.3.2.3   Irritable Bowel Syndrome

A systematic review of randomized, controlled, blinded trials conducted between 1982 and 2007 and that included 1404 subjects found that the use of probiotics was associated with less abdominal pain. Various strains (*B. infantis, L. acidophilus, L. plantarum, L. reuteri, L. rhamnosu, Saccharomyces boulardii, Streptoccocus faecium*), as well as the probiotic cocktail VSL#3 (a mixture of eight strains), were involved in doses that ranged from 450 to 10^{12} cfu/day and were studied for a median duration of just 4 weeks.[113] However, due to significant variability between the trials no definitive conclusions could be drawn about the relative effectiveness of specific strains or doses.

Another systemic review found evidence of modest improvement in abdominal pain and flatulence with the use of probiotic preparations for up to 8 weeks. Again there were significant limitations related to between-study variability that precluded pooling of the data and subset analysis.[114] It should be stressed that IBS is a chronic disorder with an intermittent and unpredictable course and that longer-term studies are needed in order to provide a true assessment of the impact of probiotics in IBS.

Overall, the data indicate that probiotics may confer modest benefits in IBS, but that it is difficult, due to a lack of comparative studies, to make specific recommendations regarding species or strain or the expected magnitude of benefit.[115]

6.3.2.4   Inflammatory Bowel Disease

Though experimental and human data provide a solid basis for the use of probiotics in IBD,[116] clinical trials have provided much less encouragement. A Cochrane review of randomized clinical trials comparing the impact of probiotics combined with standard therapy to standard therapy alone in the induction of remission in UC failed to detect an additional benefit for probiotics on disease course. Furthermore, they noted that none of the four studies that met inclusion criteria showed a significant impact for probiotics.[117] In addition, another review of probiotics, including 587 subjects, in the maintenance of remission in UC also did not show a significant impact of probiotics on relapse rate which occurred in 40.1% in the probiotic group and 34.1% on mesalazine.[118] Similar conclusions have been reached regarding the use of probiotics in maintenance of remission in CD. A review of seven studies using *Lactobacilli GG*, *Escherichia coli strain Nissle* 1917, VSL#3, or *S. boulardii* for 6–12 months failed to show efficacy for probiotics in the management of CD. No major side effects were recorded.[119] Another meta-analysis of eight randomized placebo-controlled clinical trials from 1966 to 2007 involving *L. rhamnosus GG*, *Lactobacillus johnsonii*, *E. coli*, or *S. boulardii*, over durations of treatment that ranged from 3 to 24 months did not find a significant benefit for probiotics in the maintenance of remission in CD.[120] However, there is evidence that VSL#3 is effective in the prevention of pouchitis.[121]

6.3.2.5   Colorectal Cancer

Experimental studies of the effect of probiotic strains on the development of CRC showed promise. Thus, *Lactobacillus GG* was shown to decrease the production of polyamines in cancer cell lines.[78,122] Other probiotic strains demonstrated antiproliferative effects.[123,124] Yogurt and probiotic preparations containing yogurt bacteria reduced tumor incidence, burden, and size; effects most likely mediated through engagement with the host's acquired and innate immune systems.[78,125–127]

Human data has been more mixed. Thus, a recent randomized trial on the impact of the administration of the yogurt bacterium *L. casei* on CRC recurrence showed that after 4 years of follow-up there was no significant benefit in terms of cancer recurrence but that the level of atypia seen in cancers was lower in the probiotic treated group.[128] In contrast the administration of a synbiotic food comprised of oligofructose-enriched inulin, *L. rhamnosus GG* and *Bifidobacterium lactis* to 37 colon cancer patients and 43 patients following polypectomy reduced proliferation rates.[129] Finally, on an epidemiological basis, yogurt intake has been associated with a decreased risk of CRC.[130] Despite the promise of laboratory experiments, it is clear that further well designed clinical trials are needed before concrete guidelines on the use of probiotics in CRC can be formulated.

6.4 CONCLUSIONS

Commensal bacteria have been clearly demonstrated to play a critical role in the development of the gastrointestinal tract, its functions, and immune responsiveness. It has also been recognized as an important contributing factor in the development of a range of gastrointestinal disorders. Consequently, a number of probiotic preparations have been studied *in vitro* and in clinical trials as a possible treatment strategy for several gastrointestinal disorders. Experimental studies and *in vivo* animal models have provided very promising data on the potential for probiotics to impact on the pathophysiology of various diseases. Clinical studies are less clear-cut and while clinically relevant effects in infectious and antibiotic-associated diarrheas have been demonstrated with some consistency and results in IBS show promise, the role of probiotics in IBD and CRC has not been sufficiently established at this point in time.

6.4.1 CLINICAL SCENARIO

A 42-year-old white female with history of recent complicated urinary tract infection treated with 7 days of broad spectrum antibiotics comes with a complaint of watery diarrhea for 2 days. Her past medical history is significant for irritable bowel syndrome and she has a family history of colon cancer that occurred in her father at the age of 40. She had a negative colonoscopy 2 years ago. We have explained to her that her diarrhea is likely related to the use of antibiotics and that it will subside over time with conservative management. She would like to learn more about probiotics and if probiotics could help her with diarrhea, IBS and potentially prevent the occurrence of colon cancer.

1. Should probiotics be recommended to her, and for what indication?
   Yes. Probiotics are indicated because studies have consistently shown that various probiotic strains can significantly benefit patients at risk for AAD. She can expect a reduction in the duration of AAD as well as in the intensity of symptoms such as stool frequency on probiotics.
2. What probiotic preparation should you recommend?
   While current data are insufficient to permit a confident recommendation for one preparation over another, there are some indications that *Lactobacillus GG* or *Sacharomices boulardii* have shown more positive results. When choosing the product she should be advised to read the label carefully, seek out information on strains and live bacterial numbers and be aware of the reputation of the supplier for high standards of quality control.
3. How much probiotic she should take and for how long?

Currently, given a lack of dose-ranging data, one can only suggest that she follows the manufacturer's recommendation with regard to dose and that the probiotic preparation is consumed until symptoms have resolved or for a total of 5–10 days.

4. She would like to know if she should take probiotics for a longer period of time for the treatment of IBS and prevention of colon cancer.

It is possible that her IBS may be aggravated by the acute diarrheal illness as well as antibiotic use. For these reasons, as well as evidence of efficacy for some probiotic strains in IBS, in general, it seems logical that she continues the probiotic in the longer term. With respect to colon cancer prevention, it should be explained that the evidence for a benefit for probiotics in the prevention of CRC is currently weak.

5. Finally, she would like to know if probiotics are safe and how will they affect her body.

Commonly available probiotic preparations are safe to use. The effect of probiotics on the intrinsic microbiota is transient and the administered organism(s) disappear rapidly from the gastrointestinal tract once consumption ceases. Commonly reported minor side effects include bloating, abdominal discomfort, and diarrhea. However, these effects are usually transient and will usually disappear even if probiotic administration continues.

REFERENCES

1. Sekirov I, Russell SL, Antunes LC, Finlay BB. Gut microbiota in health and disease. *Physiol Rev* 2013;90(3):859–904.
2. O'Hara AM, Shanahan F. The gut flora as a forgotten organ. *EMBO Rep* 2006; 7(7):688–693.
3. Moles L, Gomez M, Heilig H et al. Bacterial diversity in meconium of preterm neonates and evolution of their fecal microbiota during the first month of life. *PLoS One* 2013;8(6):e66986.
4. Jimenez E, Marin ML, Martin R et al. Is meconium from healthy newborns actually sterile? *Res Microbiol* 2008;159(3):187–193.
5. Satokari R, Gronroos T, Laitinen K, Salminen S, Isolauri E. *Bifidobacterium* and *Lactobacillus* DNA in the human placenta. *Lett Appl Microbiol* 2009;48(1):8–12.
6. Flint HJ, Scott KP, Louis P, Duncan SH. The role of the gut microbiota in nutrition and health. *Nat Rev Gastroenterol Hepatol* 2012;9(10):577–589.
7. Dominguez-Bello MG. Delivery mode shapes the acquisition and structure of the initial microbiota across multiple body habitats in newborns. *Proc Natl Acad Sci USA* 2010;107:11971–11975.
8. Karlsson CLJ, Molin G, Cilio CM, Ahrne S. The pioneer gut microbiota in human neonates vaginally born at term—A pilot study. *Pediatr Res* 2011;70:282–286.
9. Penders J, Thijs C, Vink C et al. Factors influencing the composition of the intestinal microbiota in early infancy. *Pediatrics* 2006;118(2):511–521.
10. Dominguez-Bello MG, Costello EK, Contreras M et al. Delivery mode shapes the acquisition and structure of the initial microbiota across multiple body habitats in newborns. *Proc Natl Acad Sci USA* 2010;107(26):11971–11975.
11. Jost T, Lacroix C, Braegger CP, Rochat F, Chassard C. Vertical mother-neonate transfer of maternal gut bacteria via breastfeeding. *Environ Microbiol* 2013;16:2891–2904.

12. Eggesbo M. Development of gut microbiota in infants not exposed to medical interventions. *APMIS* 2011;119:17–35.
13. Palmer C, Bik EM, DiGiulio DB, Relman DA, Brown PO. Development of the human infant intestinal microbiota. *PLoS Biol* 2007;5(7):e177.
14. Yatsunenko T, Rey FE, Manary MJ et al. Human gut microbiome viewed across age and geography. *Nature* 2012;486(7402):222–227.
15. Yatsunenko T. Human gut microbiome viewed across age and geography. *Nature* 2012;486:222–227.
16. De Filippo C. Impact of diet in shaping gut microbiota revealed by a comparative study in children from Europe and rural Africa. *Proc Natl Acad Sci USA* 2010;107: 14691–14696.
17. Costello EK. Bacterial community variation in human body habitats across space and time. *Science* 2009;326:1694–1697.
18. Claesson MJ, Cusack S, O'Sullivan O, Greene-Diniz R, de Weerd H, Flannery E et al. Composition, variability, and temporal stability of the intestinal microbiota of the elderly. *Proc Natl Acad Sci USA* 2011;108:4586–4591.
19. O'Toole PW, Claesson MJ. Gut microbiota: Changes throughout the lifespan from infancy to elderly. *Int Dairy J* 2010;20:281–291.
20. Arumugam M, Raes J, Pelletier E et al. Enterotypes of the human gut microbiome. *Nature* 2011;473(7346):174–180.
21. Wu GD. Linking long-term dietary patterns with gut microbial enterotypes. *Science* 2011;334:105–108.
22. He XS, Shi WY. Oral microbiology: Past, present and future. *Int J Oral Sci* 2009;1(2): 47–58.
23. Wang ZK, Yang YS. Upper gastrointestinal microbiota and digestive diseases. *World J Gastroenterol* 2013;19(10):1541–1550.
24. Frank DN, St Amand AL, Feldman RA, Boedeker EC, Harpaz N, Pace NR. Molecular-phylogenetic characterization of microbial community imbalances in human inflammatory bowel diseases. *Proc Natl Acad Sci USA* 2007;104(34):13780–13785.
25. Johansson ME, Sjovall H, Hansson GC. The gastrointestinal mucus system in health and disease. *Nat Rev Gastroenterol Hepatol* 2013;10(6):352–361.
26. Roberfroid M, Gibson GR, Hoyles L et al. Prebiotic effects: Metabolic and health benefits. *Br J Nutr* 2010;104(suppl 2):S1–S63.
27. Gordon HA, Bruckner-Kardoss E. Effect of normal microbial flora on intestinal surface area. *Am J Physiol* 1961;201:175–178.
28. Banasaz M, Norin E, Holma R, Midtvedt T. Increased enterocyte production in gnotobiotic rats mono-associated with *Lactobacillus rhamnosus* GG. *Appl Environ Microbiol* 2002;68(6):3031–3034.
29. Stappenbeck TS, Hooper LV, Gordon JI. Developmental regulation of intestinal angiogenesis by indigenous microbes via Paneth cells. *Proc Natl Acad Sci USA* 2002; 99(24):15451–15455.
30. Flint HJ. Obesity and the gut microbiota. *J Clin Gastroenterol* 2012;45:S128–S132.
31. Husebye E, Hellstrom PM, Midtvedt T. Intestinal microflora stimulates myoelectric activity of rat small intestine by promoting cyclic initiation and aboral propagation of migrating myoelectric complex. *Dig Dis Sci* 1994;39(5):946–956.
32. Hooper LV, Wong MH, Thelin A, Hansson L, Falk PG, Gordon JI. Molecular analysis of commensal host-microbial relationships in the intestine. *Science* 2001;291 (5505):881–884.
33. Macpherson AJ, Harris NL. Interactions between commensal intestinal bacteria and the immune system. *Nat Rev Immunol* 2004;4(6):478–485.
34. Dubuquoy L, Jansson EA, Deeb S et al. Impaired expression of peroxisome proliferator-activated receptor gamma in ulcerative colitis. *Gastroenterology* 2003;124(5):1265–1276.

35. Kelly D, Campbell JI, King TP et al. Commensal anaerobic gut bacteria attenuate inflammation by regulating nuclear-cytoplasmic shuttling of PPAR-gamma and RelA. *Nat Immunol* 2004;5(1):104–112.
36. Mazmanian SK, Liu CH, Tzianabos AO, Kasper DL. An immunomodulatory molecule of symbiotic bacteria directs maturation of the host immune system. *Cell* 2005;122(1):107–118.
37. Macpherson AJ, Uhr T. Induction of protective IgA by intestinal dendritic cells carrying commensal bacteria. *Science* 2004;303(5664):1662–1665.
38. Koboziev I, Reinoso Webb C, Furr KL, Grisham MB. Role of the enteric microbiota in intestinal homeostasis and inflammation. *Free Radical Biol Med* 2013;68:122–133.
39. Van der Sluis M, De Koning BA, De Bruijn AC et al. Muc2-deficient mice spontaneously develop colitis, indicating that MUC2 is critical for colonic protection. *Gastroenterology* 2006;131(1):117–129.
40. Bates JM, Akerlund J, Mittge E, Guillemin K. Intestinal alkaline phosphatase detoxifies lipopolysaccharide and prevents inflammation in zebrafish in response to the gut microbiota. *Cell Host Microbe* 2007;2(6):371–382.
41. Lotz M, Gutle D, Walther S, Menard S, Bogdan C, Hornef MW. Postnatal acquisition of endotoxin tolerance in intestinal epithelial cells. *J Exp Med* 2006;203(4):973–984.
42. Nuding S, Antoni L, Stange EF. The host and the flora. *Dig Dis* 2013;31(3–4):286–292.
43. McNeil NI. The contribution of the large intestine to energy supplies in man. *Am J Clin Nutr* 1984;39(2):338–342.
44. Qin J, Li R, Raes J et al. A human gut microbial gene catalogue established by metagenomic sequencing. *Nature* 2010;464(7285):59–65.
45. Leitch EC, Walker AW, Duncan SH, Holtrop G, Flint HJ. Selective colonization of insoluble substrates by human faecal bacteria. *Environ Microbiol* 2007;9(3):667–679.
46. Walker AW, Duncan SH, Harmsen HJ, Holtrop G, Welling GW, Flint HJ. The species composition of the human intestinal microbiota differs between particle-associated and liquid phase communities. *Environ Microbiol* 2008;10(12):3275–3283.
47. Pomare EW, Branch WJ, Cummings JH. Carbohydrate fermentation in the human colon and its relation to acetate concentrations in venous blood. *J Clin Invest* 1985;75(5):1448–1454.
48. Sleeth ML, Thompson EL, Ford HE, Zac-Varghese SE, Frost G. Free fatty acid receptor 2 and nutrient sensing: A proposed role for fibre, fermentable carbohydrates and short-chain fatty acids in appetite regulation. *Nutr Res Rev* 2010;23(1):135–145.
49. Hamer HM, Jonkers D, Venema K, Vanhoutvin S, Troost FJ, Brummer RJ. Review article: The role of butyrate on colonic function. *Aliment Pharmacol Ther* 2008;27(2):104–119.
50. Lewis SJ, Heaton KW. Increasing butyrate concentration in the distal colon by accelerating intestinal transit. *Gut* 1997;41(2):245–251.
51. Duncan SH, Louis P, Flint HJ. Lactate-utilizing bacteria, isolated from human feces, that produce butyrate as a major fermentation product. *Appl Environ Microbiol* 2004;70(10):5810–5817.
52. Sidhu H, Allison MJ, Chow JM, Clark A, Peck AB. Rapid reversal of hyperoxaluria in a rat model after probiotic administration of Oxalobacter formigenes. *J Urol* 2001;166(4):1487–1491.
53. Chang JY, Antonopoulos DA, Kalra A et al. Decreased diversity of the fecal Microbiome in recurrent *Clostridium difficile*-associated diarrhea. *J Infect Dis* 2008; 197(3):435–438.
54. Rea MC, O'Sullivan O, Shanahan F et al. *Clostridium difficile* carriage in elderly subjects and associated changes in the intestinal microbiota. *J Clin Microbiol* 2012;50(3):867–875.
55. Antharam VC, Li EC, Ishmael A et al. Intestinal dysbiosis and depletion of butyrogenic bacteria in *Clostridium difficile* infection and nosocomial diarrhea. *J Clin Microbiol* 2013;51(9):2884–2892.

56. Quigley E, Fried M, Gwee KA et al. Irritable bowel syndrome: A global perspective. *World Gastroenterology Organisation Global Guideline* 2009. pp. 1–20. http://www. worldgastroenterology.org/irritable-bowel-syndrome.html (Accessed March 25th 2015).
57. Collins SM. Dysregulation of peripheral cytokine production in irritable bowel syndrome. *Am J Gastroenterol* 2005;100(11):2517–2518.
58. Balsari A, Ceccarelli A, Dubini F, Fesce E, Poli G. The fecal microbial population in the irritable bowel syndrome. *Microbiologica* 1982;5(3):185–194.
59. Hong SN, Rhee PL. Unraveling the ties between irritable bowel syndrome and intestinal microbiota. *World J Gastroenterol* 2014;20(10):2470–2481.
60. Rajilic-Stojanovic M, Biagi E, Heilig HG et al. Global and deep molecular analysis of microbiota signatures in fecal samples from patients with irritable bowel syndrome. *Gastroenterology* 2011;141(5):1792–1801.
61. Kassinen A, Krogius-Kurikka L, Makivuokko H et al. The fecal microbiota of irritable bowel syndrome patients differs significantly from that of healthy subjects. *Gastroenterology* 2007;133(1):24–33.
62. Jeffery IB, O'Toole PW, Öhman L, Claesson MJ, Deane J, Quigley EM, Simrén M. An irritable bowel syndrome subtype defined by species-specific alterations in faecal microbiota. *Gut* 2012;61:997–1006.
63. Kau AL, Ahern PP, Griffin NW, Goodman AL, Gordon JI. Human nutrition, the gut microbiome and the immune system. *Nature* 2011;474(7351):327–336.
64. Sands BE. Inflammatory bowel disease: Past, present, and future. *J Gastroenterol* 2007;42(1):16–25.
65. Sellon RK, Tonkonogy S, Schultz M et al. Resident enteric bacteria are necessary for development of spontaneous colitis and immune system activation in interleukin-10-deficient mice. *Infect Immun* 1998;66(11):5224–5231.
66. de Silva HJ, Millard PR, Soper N, Kettlewell M, Mortensen N, Jewell DP. Effects of the faecal stream and stasis on the ileal pouch mucosa. *Gut* 1991;32(10):1166–1169.
67. D'Haens GR, Geboes K, Peeters M, Baert F, Penninckx F, Rutgeerts P. Early lesions of recurrent Crohn's disease caused by infusion of intestinal contents in excluded ileum. *Gastroenterology* 1998;114(2):262–267.
68. Scaldaferri F, Gerardi V, Lopetuso LR et al. Gut microbial flora, prebiotics, and probiotics in IBD: Their current usage and utility. *Biomed Res Int* 2013;2013:435268.
69. Fuss IJ, Neurath M, Boirivant M et al. Disparate CD4+ lamina propria (LP) lymphokine secretion profiles in inflammatory bowel disease. Crohn's disease LP cells manifest increased secretion of IFN-gamma, whereas ulcerative colitis LP cells manifest increased secretion of IL-5. *J Immunol* 1996;157(3):1261–1270.
70. Mosmann TR, Sad S. The expanding universe of T-cell subsets: Th1, Th2 and more. *Immunol Today* 1996;17(3):138–146.
71. Springer TA. Adhesion receptors of the immune system. *Nature* 1990;346(6283): 425–434.
72. Manichanh C, Borruel N, Casellas F, Guarner F. The gut microbiota in IBD. *Nat Rev Gastroenterol Hepatol* 2012;9(10):599–608.
73. Fava F, Danese S. Intestinal microbiota in inflammatory bowel disease: Friend of foe? *World J Gastroenterol* 2011;17(5):557–566.
74. Sokol H, Pigneur B, Watterlot L et al. Faecalibacterium prausnitzii is an anti-inflammatory commensal bacterium identified by gut microbiota analysis of Crohn's disease patients. *Proc Natl Acad Sci USA* 2008;105(43):16731–16736.
75. Joossens M, Huys G, Cnockaert M et al. Dysbiosis of the faecal microbiota in patients with Crohn's disease and their unaffected relatives. *Gut* 2011;60(5):631–637.
76. Asano TK, McLeod RS. Non-steroidal anti-inflammatory drugs (NSAID) and aspirin for preventing colorectal adenomas and carcinomas. *Cochrane Database Syst Rev* 2004;(2):CD004079.

77. O'Keefe SJ, Ou J, Aufreiter S et al. Products of the colonic microbiota mediate the effects of diet on colon cancer risk. *J Nutr* 2009;139(11):2044–2048.
78. Zhu Y, Michelle Luo T, Jobin C, Young HA. Gut microbiota and probiotics in colon tumorigenesis. *Cancer Lett* 2011;309(2):119–127.
79. O'Keefe SJ, Chung D, Mahmoud N et al. Why do African Americans get more colon cancer than Native Africans? *J Nutr* 2007;137(suppl 1):175S–182S.
80. Kalliomaki M, Collado MC, Salminen S, Isolauri E. Early differences in fecal microbiota composition in children may predict overweight. *Am J Clin Nutr* 2008;87(3):534–538.
81. Neumann PA, Koch S, Hilgarth RS et al. Gut commensal bacteria and regional Wnt gene expression in the proximal versus distal colon. *Am J Pathol* 2014;184(3):592–599.
82. Moran JP, Walter J, Tannock GW, Tonkonogy SL, Sartor RB. Bifidobacterium animalis causes extensive duodenitis and mild colonic inflammation in monoassociated interleukin-10-deficient mice. *Inflammatory Bowel Dis* 2009;15(7):1022–1031.
83. Wu S, Rhee KJ, Albesiano E et al. A human colonic commensal promotes colon tumorigenesis via activation of T helper type 17 T cell responses. *Nat Med* 2009;15(9):1016–1022.
84. World Health Organisation. Health and Nutritional Properties of Probiotics in Food Including Powder Milk with Live Lactic Acid Bacteria: Report of a Joint FAO WHO Expert Consultation on Evaluation of Health and Nutritional Properties of Probiotics in Food Including Powder Milk with Live Lactic Acid Bacteria. 2001, Córdoba, Río Primero; pp. 1–34.
85. World Health Organization. Guidelines for the evaluation of probiotics in food. 2002, pp. 1–11. http://www.fda.gov/ohrms/dockets/dockets/95s0316/95s-0316-rpt0282-tab-03-ref-19-joint-faowho-vol219.pdf. Accessed March 25, 2015.
86. National Center for Complementary and Alternative Medicine (NCCAM). *Oral Probiotics*. URL: http://nccam.nih.gov/health/probiotics/introduction.htm. Published 2014.
87. Guarner F, Perdigon G, Corthier G, Salminen S, Koletzko B, Morelli L. Should yoghurt cultures be considered probiotic? *Br J Nutr* 2005;93(6):783–786.
88. Smith A. Global Probiotics Market Analysis, Size, Share, Growth, Trends and Forecast 2014 to 2020. http://www.benzinga.com/14/09/4874053/global-probiotics-market-analysis-size-share-growth-trends-and-forecast-2014-to-2020#ixzz3VR4Q5YMo. Accessed March 25, 2015. 2014.
89. Caselli M, Cassol F, Calo G, Holton J, Zuliani G, Gasbarrini A. Actual concept of "probiotics": Is it more functional to science or business? *World J Gastroenterol* 2013;19(10):1527–1540.
90. Food and Drug Administration. *Dietary Supplement Labeling Guide: Chapter VI. Claims*. 2005 http://www.fda.gov/Food/GuidanceRegulation/GuidanceDocuments RegulatoryInformation/DietarySupplements/ucm070613.htm#6–41.
91. Sanders ME, Akkermans LM, Haller D et al. Safety assessment of probiotics for human use. *Gut Microbes* 2010;1(3):164–185.
92. Vanderhoof JA, Young R. Probiotics in the United States. *Clin Infect Dis* 2008;46(suppl 2): S67–72; discussion S144–151.
93. Snydman DR. The safety of probiotics. *Clin Infect Dis* 2008;46(suppl 2):S104–111; discussion S144–151.
94. Besselink MG, van Santvoort HC, Buskens E et al. Probiotic prophylaxis in predicted severe acute pancreatitis: A randomised, double-blind, placebo-controlled trial. *Lancet* 2008;371(9613):651–659.
95. Ciorba MA. A gastroenterologist's guide to probiotics. *Clin Gastroenterol Hepatol* 2012;10(9):960–968.
96. Candela M, Perna F, Carnevali P et al. Interaction of probiotic *Lactobacillus* and *Bifidobacterium* strains with human intestinal epithelial cells: Adhesion properties, competition against enteropathogens and modulation of IL-8 production. *Int J Food Microbiol* 2008;125(3):286–292.

97. Matsumoto M, Ishige A, Yazawa Y, Kondo M, Muramatsu K, Watanabe K. Promotion of intestinal peristalsis by Bifidobacterium spp. Capable of hydrolysing sennosides in mice. *PLoS One* 2012;7(2):e31700.
98. Zschuttig A, Zimmermann K, Blom J, Goesmann A, Pohlmann C, Gunzer F. Identification and characterization of microcin S, a new antibacterial peptide produced by probiotic *Escherichia coli* G3/10. *PLoS One* 2012;7(3):e33351.
99. Rund SA, Rohde H, Sonnenborn U, Oelschlaeger TA. Antagonistic effects of probiotic *Escherichia coli* Nissle 1917 on EHEC strains of serotype O104:H4 and O157:H7. *Int J Med Microbiol* 2013;303(1):1–8.
100. Silva M, Jacobus NV, Deneke C, Gorbach SL. Antimicrobial substance from a human *Lactobacillus* strain. *Antimicrob Agents Chemother* 1987;31(8):1231–1233.
101. Wilson KH, Perini F. Role of competition for nutrients in suppression of *Clostridium difficile* by the colonic microflora. *Infect Immun* 1988;56(10):2610–2614.
102. Szajewska H, Mrukowicz JZ. Probiotics in the treatment and prevention of acute infectious diarrhea in infants and children: A systematic review of published randomized, double-blind, placebo-controlled trials. *J Pediatr Gastroenterol Nutr* 2001;33:S17–S25.
103. Pothoulakis C, Kelly CP, Joshi MA et al. *Saccharomyces boulardii* inhibits *Clostridium difficile* toxin a binding and enterotoxicity in rat ileum. *Gastroenterology* 1993; 104(4):1108–1115.
104. Majamaa H, Isolauri E, Saxelin M, Vesikari T. Lactic acid bacteria in the treatment of acute rotavirus gastroenteritis. *J Pediatr Gastroenterol Nutr* 1995;20(3):333–338.
105. Huang JS, Bousvaros A, Lee JW, Diaz A, Davidson EJ. Efficacy of probiotic use in acute diarrhea in children: A meta-analysis. *Dig Dis Sci* 2002;47(11):2625–2634.
106. Allen SJ ME, Gregorio GV, Dans LF. Probiotics for treating acute infectious diarrhoea. *Cochrane Database Syst Rev* 2010;(11):CD003048.
107. Johnston BC, Goldenberg JZ, Vandvik PO, Sun X, Guyatt GH. Probiotics for the prevention of pediatric antibiotic-associated diarrhea. *Cochrane Database Syst Rev* 2011; Nov 9;(11):CD004827.
108. McFarland LV. Meta-analysis of probiotics for the prevention of antibiotic associated diarrhea and the treatment of *Clostridium difficile* disease. *Am J Gastroenterol* 2006;101(4):812–822.
109. Gao XW, Mubasher M, Fang CY, Reifer C, Miller LE. Dose-response efficacy of a proprietary probiotic formula of *Lactobacillus acidophilus* CL1285 and *Lactobacillus casei* LBC80R for antibiotic-associated diarrhea and *Clostridium difficile*-associated diarrhea prophylaxis in adult patients. *Am J Gastroenterol* 2010;105(7):1636–1641.
110. Goldenberg JZ, Ma SS, Saxton JD, Martzen MR, Vandvik PO, Thorlund K, Guyatt GH, Johnston BC. Probiotics for the prevention of *Clostridium difficile*-associated diarrhea in adults and children. *Cochrane Database Syst Rev* 2013;May 31;5:CD006095.
111. Takahashi O, Noguchi Y, Omata F, Tokuda Y, Fukui T. Probiotics in the prevention of traveler's diarrhea: Meta-analysis. *J Clin Gastroenterol* 2007;41(3):336–337.
112. DuPont HL, Ericsson CD, Farthing MJ et al. Expert review of the evidence base for prevention of travelers' diarrhea. *J Travel Med* 2009;16(3):149–160.
113. McFarland LV, Dublin S. Meta-analysis of probiotics for the treatment of irritable bowel syndrome. *World J Gastroenterol* 2008;14(17):2650–2661.
114. Hoveyda N, Heneghan C, Mahtani KR, Perera R, Roberts N, Glasziou P. A systematic review and meta-analysis: Probiotics in the treatment of irritable bowel syndrome. *BMC Gastroenterol* 2009;9:15.
115. Moayyedi P, Ford AC, Talley NJ et al. The efficacy of probiotics in the treatment of irritable bowel syndrome: A systematic review. *Gut* 2010;59(3):325–332.
116. Groeger D, O'Mahony L, Murphy EF et al. *Bifidobacterium infantis* 35624 modulates host inflammatory processes beyond the gut. *Gut Microbes* 2013;4(4):325–339.

117. Mallon P, McKay D, Kirk S, Gardiner K. Probiotics for induction of remission in ulcerative colitis. *Cochrane Database Syst Rev* 2007;Oct 17;(4):CD005573.
118. Naidoo K, Gordon M, Fagbemi AO, Thomas AG, Akobeng AK. Probiotics for maintenance of remission in ulcerative colitis. *Cochrane Database Syst Rev* 2011; Dec 7;(12):CD007443.
119. Rolfe VE, Fortun PJ, Hawkey CJ, Bath-Hextall F. Probiotics for maintenance of remission in Crohn's disease. *Cochrane Database Syst Rev* 2006;Oct 18;(4):CD004826.
120. Rahimi R, Nikfar S, Rahimi F et al. A meta-analysis on the efficacy of probiotics for maintenance of remission and prevention of clinical and endoscopic relapse in Crohn's disease. *Dig Dis Sci* 2008;53(9):2524–2531.
121. Holubar SD, Cima RR, Sandborn WJ, Pardi DS. Treatment and prevention of pouchitis after ileal pouch-anal anastomosis for chronic ulcerative colitis. *Cochrane Database Syst Rev* 2010;6:CD001176.
122. Orlando A, Messa C, Linsalata M, Cavallini A, Russo F. Effects of *Lactobacillus rhamnosus* GG on proliferation and polyamine metabolism in HGC-27 human gastric and DLD-1 colonic cancer cell lines. *Immunopharmacol Immunotoxicol* 2009;31(1):108–116.
123. Lee NK, Park JS, Park E, Paik HD. Adherence and anticarcinogenic effects of *Bacillus polyfermenticus* SCD in the large intestine. *Lett Appl Microbiol* 2007;44(3):274–278.
124. Kim Y, Lee D, Kim D et al. Inhibition of proliferation in colon cancer cell lines and harmful enzyme activity of colon bacteria by *Bifidobacterium adolescentis* SPM0212. *Arch Pharm Res* 2008;31(4):468–473.
125. Pagnini C, Saeed R, Bamias G, Arseneau KO, Pizarro TT, Cominelli F. Probiotics promote gut health through stimulation of epithelial innate immunity. *Proc Natl Acad Sci USA* 2010;107(1):454–459.
126. Perdigon G, Valdez JC, Rachid M. Antitumour activity of yogurt: Study of possible immune mechanisms. *J Dairy Res* 1998;65(1):129–138.
127. Urbanska AM, Bhathena J, Martoni C, Prakash S. Estimation of the potential antitumor activity of microencapsulated *Lactobacillus acidophilus* yogurt formulation in the attenuation of tumorigenesis in Apc(Min/+) mice. *Dig Dis Sci* 2009;54(2):264–273.
128. Ishikawa H, Akedo I, Otani T et al. Randomized trial of dietary fiber and *Lactobacillus casei* administration for prevention of colorectal tumors. *Int J Cancer* 2005; 116(5):762–767.
129. Rafter J, Bennett M, Caderni G et al. Dietary synbiotics reduce cancer risk factors in polypectomized and colon cancer patients. *Am J Clin Nutr* 2007;85(2):488–496.
130. Pala V, Sieri S, Berrino F et al. Yogurt consumption and risk of colorectal cancer in the Italian European prospective investigation into cancer and nutrition cohort. *Int J Cancer* 2011;129(11):2712–2719.

7 Nutrition and Gastrointestinal Cancer

Aaron M. Dickstein and Joel B. Mason

CONTENTS

7.1   NUTRITION IN THE PREVENTION OF GASTROINTESTINAL MALIGNANCIES

7.1.1   INTRODUCTION

Esophageal, pancreatic, gastric, and colorectal cancers account for 17% of all cancers in the United States and lead to approximately 145,000 deaths/year, and globally close to 1.8 million deaths/year.[1] Much effort has been exerted to understand the links between germline genetic defects and cancer but, for the above-mentioned cancers, these genetic changes alone account for only a small percentage of cancer incidence. By contrast, lifestyle factors such as dietary habits, tobacco, and alcohol use, and obesity seem to play a much larger role. Understanding which of these factors can modulate the risk of cancer is thus the subject of intense research and debate. There is little doubt that obesity and being overweight contribute substantially to the risk of colorectal cancer, and probably to the risk of esophageal and pancreatic adenocarcinoma as well. However, despite many years of epidemiological and preclinical studies, consensus has yet to be reached concerning the roles played by a number of specific components of the diet, such as certain vitamins and trace elements.

The first section of this chapter reviews the current literature on dietary and nutritional factors that impact on the risk of developing gastrointestinal malignancies, and thus those factors that can be considered when formulating preventive strategies. Two resources are especially valuable for this purpose: the European Prospective Investigation into Cancer and Nutrition (EPIC) cohort, a multicenter prospective cohort of more than 500,000 individuals being followed in 10 European countries[2] as well as the systematic literature review and analysis by the World Cancer Research Fund and American Institute for Cancer Research.[3] We first discuss the important role played by obesity in determining the risk of gastrointestinal (GI) malignancies, and then focus on the two gastrointestinal malignancies that appear to be particularly responsive to the effects of nutrition: gastric and colorectal cancer, since an exhaustive review of nutrient impact on all gastrointestinal malignancies is beyond the scope of this text. The second section of this chapter examines principles relevant to the nutritional care of patients diagnosed with gastrointestinal malignancy.

7.1.2   OBESITY AND OVERWEIGHTNESS

Excess body weight in both the overweight and obese categories (body mass index [BMI] of 25.0–29.9 and ≥30, respectively) has been convincingly linked to several of the common gastrointestinal malignancies. In particular, a wealth of data indicates conclusively that there are significantly increased risks of esophageal, pancreatic, and colorectal adenocarcinomas in obese patients (see Figures 7.1 and 7.2). In contrast, obesity does not constitute a risk factor for squamous cell carcinoma of the esophagus. Given the remarkably high prevalence of obesity in the United States and worldwide—the U.S. National Health and Nutrition Examination (NHANES) survey found a prevalence of obesity in the United States of over 35% in 2009–2010[4]—targeting weight loss as a strategy for cancer prevention on either an individual or community level would almost certainly yield sizeable benefits.

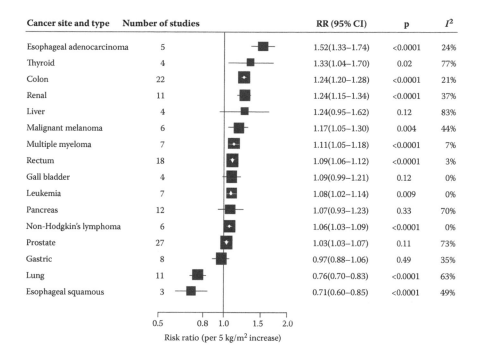

Cancer site and type	Number of studies		RR (95% CI)	p	I^2
Esophageal adenocarcinoma	5		1.52(1.33–1.74)	<0.0001	24%
Thyroid	4		1.33(1.04–1.70)	0.02	77%
Colon	22		1.24(1.20–1.28)	<0.0001	21%
Renal	11		1.24(1.15–1.34)	<0.0001	37%
Liver	4		1.24(0.95–1.62)	0.12	83%
Malignant melanoma	6		1.17(1.05–1.30)	0.004	44%
Multiple myeloma	7		1.11(1.05–1.18)	<0.0001	7%
Rectum	18		1.09(1.06–1.12)	<0.0001	3%
Gall bladder	4		1.09(0.99–1.21)	0.12	0%
Leukemia	7		1.08(1.02–1.14)	0.009	0%
Pancreas	12		1.07(0.93–1.23)	0.33	70%
Non-Hodgkin's lymphoma	6		1.06(1.03–1.09)	<0.0001	0%
Prostate	27		1.03(1.03–1.07)	0.11	73%
Gastric	8		0.97(0.88–1.06)	0.49	35%
Lung	11		0.76(0.70–0.83)	<0.0001	63%
Esophageal squamous	3		0.71(0.60–0.85)	<0.0001	49%

0.5   0.8 1.0   1.5   2.0
Risk ratio (per 5 kg/m² increase)

FIGURE 7.1 Increase in relative risk for cancer per 5 unit increase in BMI (5 kg/m²)—men. (Reprinted from Renehan et al. *Lancet* 2008;371:569–578. With permission.)

The incidence of esophageal and colorectal adenocarcinomas are particularly increased by obesity. A recent review detailing five large meta-analyses noted that approximately 11% of colorectal cancer cases in Europe are attributable to excess weight and obesity, which is also associated with a 30%–70% increased risk of colon cancer in men.[5] The sensitivity of colon cancer risk to this factor is underscored by the fact that even being overweight conveys a significant degree of risk. The incidence of colon and rectal cancers was significantly greater in obese men in all studies with a relative risk ranging from 1.24 to 1.71 for colon cancer and from 1.09 to 1.75 for rectal cancer.[5–7] Interestingly, the magnitude of risk conveyed by obesity in women is substantially less. The relative risk of colon cancer in obese women was 1.12 (1.07–1.18) in one study[7] and for colorectal cancer was 1.15 (1.06–1.24) in another.[8] The reasons behind these gender differences are not clear. Theories to explain this difference include the protective effect of estrogen, differences in age of onset and prevalence of colorectal cancer (CRC) between sexes, and the effects of different patterns of obesity (visceral versus subcutaneous adiposity). When examined individually, the link to colon cancer is much more consistent, and of greater magnitude, than the link to rectal cancer. Indeed, in many studies there is no significant association with the incidence of rectal cancer.[5]

There are three prevailing theories as to how obesity enhances the risk of cancer and they are not mutually exclusive: (1) increases in biologically active insulin and insulin-like growth factors; (2) induction of a chronic low-grade state of

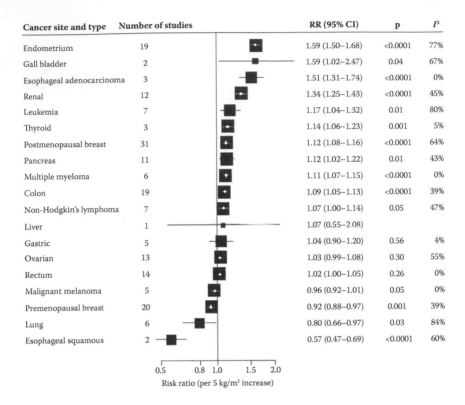

Cancer site and type	Number of studies	RR (95% CI)	p	I^2
Endometrium	19	1.59 (1.50–1.68)	<0.0001	77%
Gall bladder	2	1.59 (1.02–2.47)	0.04	67%
Esophageal adenocarcinoma	3	1.51 (1.31–1.74)	<0.0001	0%
Renal	12	1.34 (1.25–1.43)	<0.0001	45%
Leukemia	7	1.17 (1.04–1.32)	0.01	80%
Thyroid	3	1.14 (1.06–1.23)	0.001	5%
Postmenopausal breast	31	1.12 (1.08–1.16)	<0.0001	64%
Pancreas	11	1.12 (1.02–1.22)	0.01	43%
Multiple myeloma	6	1.11 (1.07–1.15)	<0.0001	0%
Colon	19	1.09 (1.05–1.13)	<0.0001	39%
Non-Hodgkin's lymphoma	7	1.07 (1.00–1.14)	0.05	47%
Liver	1	1.07 (0.55–2.08)		
Gastric	5	1.04 (0.90–1.20)	0.56	4%
Ovarian	13	1.03 (0.99–1.08)	0.30	55%
Rectum	14	1.02 (1.00–1.05)	0.26	0%
Malignant melanoma	5	0.96 (0.92–1.01)	0.05	0%
Premenopausal breast	20	0.92 (0.88–0.97)	0.001	39%
Lung	6	0.80 (0.66–0.97)	0.03	84%
Esophageal squamous	2	0.57 (0.47–0.69)	<0.0001	60%

Risk ratio (per 5 kg/m² increase)

FIGURE 7.2 Increase in relative risk for cancer per 5 unit increase in BMI (5 kg/m²)—women. (Reprinted from Renehan et al. *Lancet* 2008;371:569–578. With permission.)

inflammation; and (3) abnormal activities of adipocytokines such as leptin and adiponectin. These potential pathways are summarized in Figure 7.3.

In addition to colorectal cancer, obesity has also been associated with the precursor of virtually all sporadic CRCs, the colorectal adenoma. A recent meta-analysis showed a dose–response relationship with higher BMIs being associated with increased risk of adenomas.[9] This relationship held in both men and women. Analysis using waist circumference found a significant increase in adenomas in those with greater waist circumference odds ratio (OR) 1.32 (1.17–1.49).[10]

Moreover, though the data at present is limited, obese individuals who lose weight seem to have lower incidences of colorectal cancer than if they had maintained their obesity. An Austrian cohort study, for instance, monitored changes in weight of 28,711 men and 26,938 women over 7 years and then followed these same patients over an approximately 8-year period. Weight loss in these patients reduced the risk of colorectal cancer with a hazard ratio (HR) of 0.50 (0.29–0.87).[11]

Furthermore, accumulating data points toward worse outcomes in obese patients with colorectal cancer. For instance, a cohort study of 4288 patients with Dukes B and C colon cancer showed increased recurrence, increased overall mortality, and increased colon cancer mortality in the very obese.[12,13] Cohort studies have also

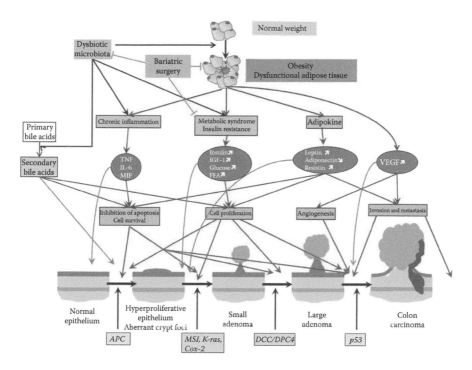

FIGURE 7.3 Proposed mechanistic pathways linking obesity to colorectal cancer. (Reprinted from Bardou M et al. *Gut* 2013;62:933–947. With permission.)

shown those with the metabolic syndrome had increased CRC mortality.[14] Further, small-scale data points to obese patients having a decrease in response to chemotherapy, notably the vascular endothelial growth factor (VEGF) targeting therapies, as well as increased surgical complication rates.[5,15,16]

In addition to colorectal cancer, increased rates of obesity have been linked to the rising incidence of pancreatic cancer and adenocarcinoma of the esophagus. The epidemiologic evidence implicates obesity as a contributor to esophageal adenocarcinoma in up to 40% of cases.[17] A meta-analysis of pooled data in 2006 reported this association in both males and females. Pooled risk for obese males and females, respectively, was 2.4 (95% CI: 1.9–3.2) and 2.1 (95% CI: 1.4–3.2).[18] More recent case-control and cohort data in Europe, North America, and Australia have found even stronger relationships with patients with increased BMIs having markedly higher rates of esophageal adenocarcinoma.[19–30]

In sum, obesity is one of the strongest modifiable risk factors for common gastrointestinal cancers in western countries. The AICR/WCRF estimates in its expert report that up to 35% of pancreatic and esophageal adenocarcinomas and 16% of colorectal cancers are attributable to obesity.[3] With the prevalence of obesity remaining high or increasing worldwide, methods to combat obesity should be entertained as a cornerstone feature of any prevention program intended to diminish the incidence of these cancers.

7.1.3　Gastric Cancer

Gastric cancer is the fourth most common type of cancer worldwide. There are estimated to be 1 million new cases identified globally each year. Of these cases, upwards of two-thirds occur in men. In total, cancers of the stomach are the second most common cause of cancer death. Moreover, there is a marked geographic variability in incidence rates with an estimated 60 cases per 100,000 people in Japan and East Asia versus less than 10 in 100,000 in Africa and North America.[1] Interestingly, age-adjusted gastric malignancy rates have decreased dramatically over the past 30 years in a number of countries, and in most instances this has been attributed to the increased availability of refrigeration. A prevailing hypothesis is that the ability to store food at cold temperatures has led to increased availability and consumption of fresh foods (e.g., fruits and vegetables) and decreased reliance on salt-preserved foods.[31] The merit of this "refrigeration theory" and what accounts for the marked differences in cancer incidence is the subject of this section.

Adenocarcinomas comprise ~95% of all gastric cancers and thus are the focus of this discussion. Of the many nutritional factors that may play a role, the most extensively studied include salt, vitamin C, meat, and nonstarchy and allium vegetables although, as described below, compelling and consistent evidence only exists for salt and to a lesser degree for nonstarchy vegetables. We will highlight the most recent data on the impact of these dietary components on cancer development and on emerging data regarding a particular dietary pattern—"The Mediterranean diet"—and its potential chemoprotective effects.

Some insight into gastric colonization by *Helicobacter pylori* and its carcinogenic effects is essential to understanding the effects of diet and nutrition. This Gram-negative bacteria, which selectively colonizes the gastric epithelium, was identified as a type I carcinogen in 1994.[32] Among infected individuals, 1%–3% will develop gastric adenocarcinoma.[33] It is a ubiquitous organism with a high prevalence that increases with age. In Korea for instance, its prevalence is 50% at 5 years of age and 90% at 20 years. In Japan, the prevalence of *H. pylori* reaches 85% by middle age. Moreover, accumulating data has shown that eradication of the bacterium significantly decreases the progression of premalignant lesions.[34] Moreover, there appears to be some substantial interplay between *H. pylori* and select dietary components in determining the risk of adenocarcinoma. Recent data indicate that infection greatly reduces the bioavailability of vitamin C, which, as described below, feasibly plays a role in cancer development.[3] In addition, a prospective Japanese study has shown that infected subjects consuming high salt diets had increased cancer risk compared to infected subjects with low salt diets.[35] Animal models have also substantiated these concepts.[36] The precise mechanisms of how these interactions effect cancer progression are not clearly understood but they need to be taken into account in future chemoprevention trials.

7.1.3.1　Salt

The dietary component most compellingly linked to the risk of stomach cancer is excessive sodium chloride (table salt). Chronic dietary patterns containing a lot of salt and salty foods have been consistently associated with an increased risk of developing gastric adenocarcinoma, lending credence to the refrigeration theory mentioned earlier. Studies have investigated the contribution of total salt use as well as salt added at the table. Most show an increased risk with increased intake.[3] Indeed, a recent meta-analysis with a sample of nearly 270,000 individuals from seven prospective studies demonstrated a graded positive association between salt consumption and gastric cancer incidence with pooled estimates indicating that those with habitually "high" and "moderately high" salt intake had a 68% and 41% greater risk of gastric cancer, respectively, when compared to "low" salt consumption. The relationship was found in both men and women and was not affected by age.[37] Interestingly, salt was a particularly strong predictor of gastric cancer in the Japanese populations studied. In addition, those reported to be habitual consumers of salt-rich foods were at greater risk, especially those eating increased amounts of pickled foods, salted fish, and processed meats.[37] Salt, in animal studies, has been shown to directly damage the gastric mucosa[38] as well as increase endogenous N-nitroso compound formation.[39] Several of these N-nitroso compounds are recognized human and animal carcinogens.[40] In addition, salt is thought to facilitate *H. pylori* infection and has been shown in molecular studies to increase expression of *H. pylori* virulence factors.[41,42] In sum, restricting salt intake to a modest level will likely have a marked effect on gastric cancer incidence, particularly in those regions that continue to have high rates of gastric adenocarcinoma. In summarizing the existing evidence of the dose–response relationship, the AICR/WCF (American Institute for Cancer Research/World Cancer Fund) report concludes that habitual intake of salt should be kept below 2.4 g/day in order to minimize cancer risk.[3]

7.1.3.2 Nonstarchy Vegetables

A multitude of observational studies have examined the protective effects of vegetables on gastric cancer development and the weight of evidence supports a benefit. Indeed, greater than 20 cohort studies, 100 case-control studies, and 35 ecological studies have looked at the impact of vegetable intake on cancer and these have been stratified to total vegetables, green–yellow vegetables, leafy vegetables, white or pale vegetables, and raw vegetables among others. Most studies show an incremental dose–response relationship with decreasing risk as intake increased. Meta-analysis of prospective cohort data, which eliminates some of the bias inherent to case-control and ecological studies, has shown an approximate 19% decreased risk per 50 g of green/yellow vegetables consumed per day.[3] There is a diverse array of plant constituents that might be contributing to this protective effect (dietary fiber, carotenoids, folate, selenium, glucosinolates, dithiolethiones, indoles, coumarins, ascorbate, chlorophyll, flavonoids, and phytoestrogens, to name just a few). The relative contributions to chemoprevention of these components is very unclear. Indeed, the apparent benefit is more likely due to a combined, synergistic effect of these components rather than the effect of a single agent.

EPIC researchers investigated this potential effect by examining plasma concentrations of carotenoids and tocopherols—as a surrogate measure of vegetable intake—in a nested case-control study. The highest versus lowest quartiles of plasma levels of the carotenoids beta-cryptoxanthin and zeaxanthin as well as retinol and alpha-tocopherol were significantly and negatively associated with gastric cancer risk. This adds further, albeit indirect, evidence to support the protective effects of nonstarchy vegetables.[43]

Identifying the particular class of vegetables that conveys the cancer protective effect has been problematic. Allium vegetables, with garlic being the most studied, have been observed in preclinical studies to decrease the risk of cancer development and progression, including gastric carcinomas, and the effects are usually ascribed to the variety of organic sulfur compounds (OSCs) found in garlic. The potential benefit presumably stems from the promotion of mitotic arrest and increased apoptosis of OSCs, as well as from garlic's antibiotic properties and possible inhibition of *H. pylori* colonization.[44,45] Human studies, however, have not, to date, borne out a protective effect.[46–50] Indeed, an analysis using the Food and Drug Adminstration's review system for scientific claims found no credible evidence to support a protective link between garlic intake and human gastric cancer.[51] The only intervention trial, a double-blind placebo-controlled study in rural China in which aged garlic extract/garlic oil (with, or without, a vitamin supplement containing vitamins E, C, and selenium) was administered for 7 years observed no reduction in gastric cancer incidence.[46,50] At 5 years, the intervention group had a slight, but nonsignificant, reduction in the incidence of gastric cancer but no effect was found at the 10- or 15-year follow-ups. Case-control studies in the Netherlands and Sweden also failed to show significant associations.[47–49]

Another vegetable that has been examined extensively, but for which strong evidence supporting a causal role in the chemoprevention of human gastric cancer is lacking is soy, and soy products. Soy-based foods, and the isoflavones they contain, have frequently been associated with decreased gastric cancer risk in observational studies in East Asian populations[52] but, to date, there is a paucity of convincing interventional data to suggest a role in chemoprevention.

7.1.3.3   Red and Processed Meats

Red meat (typically: beef, pork, and lamb) and processed meat have also been studied as potentially pro-carcinogenic in gastric adenocarcinoma. Small cohort studies have shown an apparent increased risk with higher intake though meta-analyses have shown a nonsignificant relationship.[3] The potential mechanisms leading to increased cancer risk are many. To start, the addition of nitrates to meats is felt to contribute to N-nitroso compound production and exposure and the high content of heme iron in red meat appears to facilitate this conversion process. Processed meats also contain high salt levels that may enhance cancer progression as noted above. Further, red meats cooked at high temperatures (grilling, frying) or over an open flame can contain heterocyclic amines and polycyclic aromatic hydrocarbons that are mutagens and potential carcinogens.

The EPIC investigators have examined the influence of total meat, red meat, and processed meat within their large cohort and found a significant association only with noncardia gastric cancers. The associations were limited to *H. pylori* infected individuals. Of note, the study had a mean follow-up of 6.5 years, which may have limited the findings.[53] A recent meta-analysis of 42 observational studies similarly concluded that red and processed meats each increase the risk of gastric cancer by approximately 50%.[54] Stratification for effect modifiers revealed that the associations were observed in Asian and European populations, but not in North American studies. Moreover, the strength of the effects were equivalent for cancers of the cardia and noncardia. Although the available evidence is somewhat inconsistent the weight of evidence implicates a cancer-promoting effect of red and processed meats, especially in high-risk individuals, such as those infected with *H. pylori*.

7.1.3.4 Vitamin C

The potential for chemoprotective effects of vitamin C on gastric cancer have been studied extensively in preclinical and clinical studies: in balance, the evidence falls far short of a convincing benefit for human populations. Ascorbic acid (vitamin C) is an essential cofactor for many enzymes that has been observed to possess antiproliferative and pro-apoptotic activities under certain cell culture conditions and in animal models[55] and, *in vitro* it can inhibit the growth of *H. pylori*. In a placebo-controlled clinical trial, 5 g of ascorbic acid daily eradicated *H pylori* in a significant minority of subjects,[56] perhaps by modulating the immune response against the organism.[57] Moreover, ascorbic acid has been observed to scavenge free radicals in the human gastric epithelium, which are particularly evident in subjects infected with *H. pylori*.[58] Normally present in gastric secretions, its concentration is lowered in both *H. pylori* colonization and in gastric cancer.[59]

However, a large clinical trial in East Asia did not bear out long-term benefits: although there was initially some evidence of regression in precancerous histology,[60] subsequent follow-up at 6 and 12 years showed no regression of precancerous features of chronic gastritis or of gastric adenocarcinoma.[61,62] A genuine benefit of vitamin C supplementation has yet to be convincingly demonstrated.

7.1.3.5 Mediterranean Diet

Instead of investigating dietary components individually, there is also much to be learned by examining the overall profile of a diet. Long-term adoption of the "Mediterranean diet," with its focus on high intake of olive oil, fruits, vegetables, fiber and legumes, moderate-to-high consumption of fish, and proportionately low consumption of mammalian meats will likely have a sizeable impact on gastric cancer risk, although the evidence is largely observational in nature. In the EPIC cohort, adherence to a traditional Mediterranean diet was associated with a significant reduction of 33% in gastric cancer incidence when comparing subjects with high versus low adherence.[63] A relative Mediterranean score (rMED) was developed, incorporating nine key components of the diet (high intake of fruit and vegetables, cereals, fish, olive oil, legumes, moderate intake of alcohol, and low intake of meat and dairy products), and after adjusting for recognized cancer risk factors, found a 1-unit increase in the rMED score was associated with a decreased risk of GC of 5%.[63] With its many other reported health benefits (a recent observational study using the U.S. Nurses' Health Study database found a 46% greater odds of healthy aging with greater adherence to a Mediterranean diet, see Reference 64) and lack of overt adverse effects, adoption of a Mediterranean diet among individuals at higher risk of gastric adenocarcinoma is a reasonable strategy.

7.1.4 COLORECTAL CANCER

CRC is the third most common type of cancer worldwide in men and the second most common in women. The prevalence is considerably higher in developed countries compared to developing ones. For instance, in men the incidence rate is 37.6/100,000 versus 12.1/100,000, respectively.[1] Dietary patterns almost certainly account for much of these differences. There is little disagreement that a diet modest in calories and alcohol, low in red meat and saturated fat, and high in fiber, fruits, and vegetables is cancer protective but attempts to define the components(s) of this diet that convey the benefits have often been problematic. Indeed, some have argued that this reductive approach is counterproductive since it may be the synergy of all features of this diet that ultimately convey the benefit.[65] Chemoprotective effects conveyed by fiber and by fresh vegetables were widely held to be true for many years, but recent studies have called these assumptions into question. Nevertheless, some dietary components do seem to possess important mechanistic roles unto themselves in determining cancer risk, and this section explores the existing evidence in this regard. Again, we will focus exclusively on adenocarcinoma of the colon and rectum as these comprise 95% of colorectal cancers.

7.1.4.1 Fiber

Although fiber was one of the first dietary components linked to a decreased risk of CRC, there continues to be considerable debate about whether it is genuinely an independent determinant of risk. Almost 100 case-control studies and at least 20 prospective cohort studies have investigated this issue. The precise mechanism for the beneficial effect of fiber has never been fully defined but has been variously ascribed to its pro-motility effects and the subsequent decrease in stool transit time, increases in stool weight, the fermentation products of fiber—short-chain fatty acids, especially butyrate, and changes in the colonic microbiome. Although initial epidemiological studies implicated an effect, subsequent observations in large prospective cohorts containing more rigorous control of confounding factors have not always borne out the earlier studies.[66–69] Indeed, a pooled analysis by Park and colleagues including 13 prospective cohort studies and over 725,000 subjects failed to show a reduction in colon cancer risk after adjusting for other dietary risk factors.[68] Further, large intervention trials with supplementation of different sources of fiber have not shown a reduction in polyp recurrence as a surrogate marker of cancer risk.[70,71]

However, the debate continues since several studies from the EPIC cohort have added more evidence to support a beneficial effect of fiber. Bingham et al. found a significant negative association between dietary fiber and CRC in a dose-related manner with a relative risk of 0.58 between those with the highest intake (mean 35 g/day) to those with the lowest (15 g/day).[72] They later performed a second study with the EPIC cohort correcting for folate intake with a similar outcome.[73] Of note, this study included fiber intake in foods; thus, some component of high fiber foods other than fiber itself might be conveying this protective benefit. After an even longer follow-up (mean of 11 years) investigators examining the EPIC cohort again found that total dietary fiber was inversely associated with colorectal cancer with a hazard ratio per 10 g/day increase in fiber of 0.87 (95% CI 0.79–0.96).[74]

The issue of fiber remains one of debate. However, some practical conclusions can be drawn: if there is a cancer-protective effect of fiber, it exists with foodstuffs containing fiber, not in fiber supplements. The particular type of fiber (soluble versus insoluble) and fiber source providing this benefit has yet to be elucidated. In sum, consuming a diet high in fiber-rich foods, especially when switching from low to high intake, may convey significant benefit in decreasing CRC risk.

7.1.4.2 Fruit and Vegetable Intake

For many years, it was widely accepted that habitually high consumption of fresh fruits and vegetables protected against colorectal cancer. This was a hypothesis that reflected the overwhelming consensus of descriptive, case-control, and cohort studies in the 1990s. Large, prospective cohort studies since that time however, have failed to substantiate significant protection.[75,76] Indeed, evidence to date has revealed a weak inverse association when comparing groups with the highest to lowest intakes.[67]

As opposed to the nonstarchy vegetables, garlic has more consistent data to support a protective effect, although the number of human studies is limited. Animal and cell culture studies have demonstrated effective inhibition of tumor formation and cell growth.[77,78] A small, randomized trial in Japan using aged garlic extract showed a reduction in both size and number of colonic adenomas in those taking high dose aged garlic extract with a prior history of colonic adenomas.[79] Further, a meta-analysis of case-control/cohort studies reported a 30% reduction in CRC relative risk with garlic intake (though this study excluded a large null study in its analysis).[80]

Although the breadth and depth of the evidence is very limited and it is therefore premature to incorporate as a preventive strategy, provocative observations point toward a protective effect of garlic against CRC. The evidence suggesting several other dietary components from plant sources—such as selenium and phytochemicals—can modulate CRC risk resides almost exclusively in animal studies and therefore remains quite inconclusive.

7.1.4.3 Vitamin D and Calcium

Both vitamin D and calcium are thought to be growth retarding as they play a role in apoptosis in intestinal cells as well as in cell differentiation and angiogenesis.[81] Both case-control and cohort studies have investigated the effect of dietary vitamin D, total vitamin D, as well as plasma and serum vitamin D with most showing a decreased risk with increased intake.[82] Indeed, in a nested case-control study from the EPIC cohort, Jenab and colleagues assessed the relationships between serum vitamin D on CRC risk. In this largest European study to date, the authors found a very robust inverse association between prediagnostic circulating vitamin D concentration (25-hydroxy vitamin D) and the risk of CRC: those in the highest quartile having a 40% lower risk of colorectal cancer compared to the lowest quartile of vitamin D. Greater dietary calcium intake was also significantly associated with a lower colorectal cancer risk. Interestingly, dietary vitamin D was not associated suggesting a relevant role of endogenous formation of vitamin D.[83] Randomized trials will be necessary to determine whether true causality exists in the human and to define the dose–response of the effect, that is, whether merely possessing normal physiologic levels of vitamin D conveys optimal protection or whether pushing 25-OH vitamin D levels to supra-physiologic concentrations with supplements is more effective in decreasing the risk of CRC.

In observational studies calcium intake has been consistently shown to be protective against CRC (and its precursor, the adenoma) in a dose-dependent manner. A pooled analysis of 10 cohort studies (with nearly 5000 CRC cases among 530,000 participants) showed a 14% decrease for groups consuming the highest quintile of dietary calcium intakes compared to the lowest; the effect was even more robust when supplemental calcium was included (i.e., a decrease of 22%).[84] Milk intake, as a major source of calcium was similarly protective in this study. Human clinical trials using adenoma recurrence as an endpoint have shown a modest protective effect with a significant reduction of ~15% in the risk of recurrent colorectal adenomas as well as reduced number of adenomas.[85] A revisit of this polyp prevention study years later showed a protective effect of calcium supplementation that extended up to 5 years after cessation of active treatment.[86] The underlying mechanisms for this effect are not clear, but the principle hypothesis is that calcium may precipitate free fatty acids and bile acids, each of which are thought to be cytotoxic to the colorectal epithelium.

In sum, convincing data from clinical trials indicate that 1200 mg of supplemental calcium per day constitutes an effective means of preventing colonic adenomas, and it is likely that it prevents CRC as well. The evidence regarding chemopreventive properties of vitamin D has not matured as far as the calcium literature so it remains speculative as to whether the vitamin offers protection as well.

7.1.4.4   Red Meat/Processed Meat

Red meat consumption has been consistently linked to an elevated risk of CRC development in observational studies although absolute proof from clinical trials is lacking. Epidemiologic studies in both Europe and North America have shown a dose–response relationship with increasing risk with increasing intake. Indeed, a study of the EPIC cohort found a 35% increase in CRC risk in those with over 160 g/day of red and processed meat intake when compared with those consuming less than 20 g/day.[87] In addition, the researchers found that amongst the subjects with high meat intake, those with lower fiber intake had the highest rates of CRC. Fish intake, by contrast, appeared protective. Potential mechanisms for this harmful association of red meat are similar to those mentioned earlier for gastric cancer; consumption may lead to the generation of carcinogenic N-nitroso compounds and cooked meats produce heterocyclic amines and polycyclic aromatic hydrocarbons that are potentially harmful. In addition, it is hypothesized that the heme iron content of red meat can lead to the production of free radicals *in vivo*, which have been hypothesized to accelerate carcinogenesis. In sum, the weight of evidence indicates that limiting ones intake of red meat appears protective against colorectal cancer. Although one must be circumspect when deriving dose–responses from epidemiologic data, observations would suggest that the risk begins to rise with two or more servings of red meat per week, or an average consumption of more than 3 oz/day.[88] Of note, observational studies of white meat intake (including fish and poultry) have not shown an adverse association.[89]

7.1.4.5   Alcohol

Increased alcohol intake has been consistently shown to lead to increased CRC risk. A meta-analysis of cohort data has shown a 9% increased risk/10 g/ethanol/day.[3] Data also suggests a "J" shaped dose–response relationship with low intake being associated with lower risk compared to no intake (Reference 2; low intake is usually defined as one drink per day for women; two for men). Ferrari and colleagues found similar results within the EPIC cohort observing a significant increase of 8% risk/15 g daily increase of alcohol intake. In most studies, the association is highest with rectal cancer. Interestingly, beer intake seemed to lead to higher risk compared to wine intake.[90] Possible mechanisms for alcohol-induced cancer promotion include: the direct toxic effect of metabolites, a solvent effect that enhances penetration of other carcinogens and, more tangentially, the nutrient poor diets of alcoholics may reduce any brake on cancer development.

7.1.4.6   Folate and Selenium

The vast majority of large prospective cohort studies have demonstrated that *adequate* intake of the B-vitamin, folate, is associated with a 40%–60% reduction in the risk of CRC compared to those who habitually consume the lowest quartile or quintile of the vitamin.[91] The cancer-promoting effects of habitually low folate intake has been observed in a number of rodent models of CRC,[92] substantiating a true causal role. The largest prospective cohort to date would suggest that 500 mcgs of total folate per day conveys maximal protection.[91] However, more is not necessarily better: supplemental folic acid has not been shown to convey any benefit, as underscored by a large meta-analysis of clinical trials, encompassing over 47,000 individuals.[93] Indeed, some investigators have even proposed that excessive amounts of supplemental folic acid may paradoxically increase the risk of CRC.[94]

Some initial excitement regarding selenium was generated in the 1990s when a multicenter, randomized trial reported a large reduction in the incidence of colorectal cancer (RR = 0.42) with supplementation of high selenium brewer's yeast.[95] The fact that the study sites were selected in areas of the United States with particularly low soil concentrations of selenium took on particular importance when a subsequent analysis of the data demonstrated that a cancer-protective effect was only observed among those subjects whose baseline selenium status was in the lowest tertile.[96] A similar effect—whereby an apparent benefit is only realized by those who begin with low selenium status—was recapitulated in a recent prostate cancer prevention trial.[97] In a large systematic review of the topic, the Cochrane Database concluded that there is no convincing evidence that selenium supplements can prevent human cancers and, in some circumstances may even promote the risk of cancer.[98]

The roles of selenium and folate in colorectal cancer prevention appear to be consistent with a general principle that is emerging in regard to micronutrients in cancer prevention: although the habitual consumption of an *adequate* amount of some micronutrients appears to be beneficial in regard to cancer prevention, *supraphysiologic* quantities provided by supplements may not convey additional benefit, and may even prove detrimental.[99]

7.1.5 CONCLUSIONS

In summary, there is little question that diet plays a very sizeable role in both the prevention and development of the common gastrointestinal malignancies examined above. Although overall dietary patterns play a paramount role, there is convincing evidence that some individual components of the diet play important roles: excessive dietary salt conveys a distinct risk of gastric cancer and there is a strong suggestion that vegetables play an independently protective role. In colorectal cancer, obesity has an overarching promotional effect (as it does for several other common cancers), and excessive alcohol consumption (particularly for rectal cancer) and habitually inadequate folate intake are both risk factors as well. Calcium intake, both from foodstuffs and supplements is convincingly protective against the colorectal adenoma, and almost certainly CRC itself.

More than individual dietary components, however, it appears that gastrointestinal cancer risk is determined by the interplay of a myriad of components. Supplementation with one particular nutrient at high dosage or avoidance of one particularly detrimental component of a diet is less likely to influence cancer risk than is a larger dietary change with a shift in multiple elements of an individual's diet. Further studies investigating these omnibus dietary patterns, like the Mediterranean diet, may be the most efficacious way forward for chemoprevention.

7.2 NUTRITION IN THE MANAGEMENT OF GASTROINTESTINAL MALIGNANCIES

Protein–calorie malnutrition is a common but not invariable feature of cancer, the most frequent manifestation of which is weight loss. A large, multicenter survey of greater than 3000 patients awaiting initiation of chemotherapy noted weight losses exceeding 4% in one-third of these patients. Half of these patients had weight loss exceeding 10%.[100] This number is of particular importance as a loss of this magnitude in the setting of illness leads to significant increases in morbidity and mortality. The likelihood that an individual will sustain significant weight loss is related to many factors including; the type and extent of cancer, physical impedance of normal intake, and associated emotional issues including depression. For instance, compared to leukemia, sarcomas, and breast cancers which have lower percentages of weight loss (only 4%–7% experience a greater than 10% wt. loss), those with GI malignancies have a much higher likelihood of this degree of weight loss (14% of colon cancer patients, 25%–40% of pancreatic and gastric cancer patients).[101] Moreover, if one uses an indirect measure of muscle mass (the creatinine-height index), significant malnutrition is observed in 90% of hospitalized cancer patients.[102] This malnutrition is particularly important to address as numerous case-control and cohort studies have shown adverse effects including; decreased tolerance and responsiveness to chemotherapy,[100,103] increased perioperative morbidity,[104] worsened quality of life,[103] and shorter survival.[105–107] Section 7.2.1 will describe the mechanisms for malnutrition and wasting in cancer patients, briefly review a simple method for assessing nutritional status, and outline available options for targeted therapy.

7.2.1   Mechanisms for Malnutrition and Wasting

The development of malnutrition in cancer patients is often multifactorial. Factors that contribute to protein–calorie malnutrition include insufficient dietary intake (i.e., appetite suppression related to cytokines, taste changes, nausea, and vomiting), physical impairment of deglutition, and alteration in physiology and metabolism (e.g., malabsorption or increases in catabolism).

The type of tissue that is lost is also a critical factor in the poor outcomes of malnourished cancer patients. Unlike in simple starvation, where the body preferentially uses adipose tissue for energy needs and very little lean mass is lost, in the cancer patient there is a disproportionately large contraction of skeletal muscle mass. For example, in one study of cancer patients who had lost approximately one-fourth of their preillness weight, fat mass, and skeletal muscle mass each decreased to 75%–80% of control values whereas in a comparable degree of weight loss due to starvation nearly all the lost weight would be due to a contraction of the adipose compartment.[108] This *wasting* leads to muscle weakness and worsening functional status.

The mechanisms of wasting are many. Anorexia is a common contributor. With GI tract cancers, the act of eating often incites pain, diarrhea, or vomiting: anorexia develops as a learned means of avoiding these symptoms. In addition, treatment modalities including chemotherapy agents, surgery, and radiotherapy can directly induce anorexia. A prime example is chemotherapy-induced mucositis. Anorexia also appears to be triggered by tumor-associated cytokines: a reproducible and remarkable degree of anorexia is observed with administration of tumor necrosis factor-alpha, IL-1, IL-6, and interferon-gamma.[109–111]

Alterations in metabolism also play a key role in cancer-related wasting. The contraction of skeletal muscle mass, as mentioned above, appears to be due to both a reduction in protein synthesis and an increase in protein degradation.[112] The factors TNF-alpha and IL-6 appear to play major roles in mediating this process as well. The tumor itself may also mediate this cachexia via secretion of a proteolysis inducing factor (PIF) expressed in tumor cells that correlates with weight loss.[113] At the tissue level, activation of an ATP–ubiquitin–proteasome pathway is felt to be a common pathway for protein degradation and preclinical studies using therapeutic agents that target this pathway look promising.[114] Moreover, in cancer-associated wasting, the body continues to use adipose tissue as a major energy source leading to a decrease in fat mass. A notable factor in this process is the diminished activity of lipoprotein lipase, a necessary enzyme for the uptakes of fatty acids. Mediated by cytokines, this decrease explains why cancer patients have a diminished ability to clear an exogenous lipid load and often have elevated plasma triglycerides.[115] In addition, a factor known as lipid mobilizing factor (LMF) has been isolated and is postulated to act by sensitizing adipose tissue to lipolytic stimuli.[116] Lastly, in some instances the presence of cancer tissue induces a state where the host expends more calories per kilogram of lean mass than a normal host. For example, at a molecular level, cancer cells produce lactate that stimulates use of the inefficient Cori cycle, which converts this product back to glucose. Increased activity of the Cori cycle has been observed in some cancer patients with weight loss.[117]

7.2.2 Assessment of Nutritional Status

In order to provide nutritional support in a rational manner, clinicians need an objective means to characterize the nutritional status of a patient. A comprehensive assessment of protein–energy status integrates a dietary history, anthropometric measurements (e.g., weight, midarm muscle circumference, triceps fat fold), biochemical tests (e.g., albumin, prealbumin), and objective measurements of body compartments by tools such as body impedance analysis or dual photon absorptiometry. A simpler and more practical means, and one that has great utility in most circumstances, is to determine the percentage of unintentional weight loss. Among individuals who have lost weight due to illness, a percentage loss of 10% or more of premorbid weight translates into a contraction of 15%–20% of the critical protein-containing compartment of the body. This is the threshold that, when crossed, leads to impaired physiologic function and worsened clinical outcomes.[118]

Body weight, however, can be misleading. A common example is in the patient with cirrhosis and ascites in whom the weight of the ascites masks the loss in lean body mass. Studies using highly accurate means of measuring body compartments have found that nearly all cirrhotics characterized as Child-Pugh class B or C have lost more than 20% of total body protein. One-half of patients in class A have also lost this degree of body protein, which is particularly remarkable because, by definition, such individuals are well nourished.[119] Given this shortcoming, alternate assessment tools are clearly needed in certain settings. Alternative and more sophisticated means of assessing nutritional status are beyond the scope of this chapter; the reader is referred to Chapter 1 of this text for a more comprehensive coverage of nutritional assessment.

7.2.3 Which Groups of Patients Should be Targeted for "Aggressive Nutritional Support"?

Aggressive nutritional support, defined here as *using whatever means is necessary and practical to meet the nutritional needs of the patient*, does not benefit every patient with gastrointestinal cancer. Understanding what can be expected from aggressive nutritional support is therefore quite important in making rational decisions for individual patients. Sections 7.2.3.1 and 7.2.3.2 review some of the more common clinical scenarios where evidence has shown a concrete benefit to the patient from aggressive nutritional support.

7.2.3.1 Malnourished Patients Undergoing Major Surgery

A setting in which nutritional support has been shown to be highly beneficial is in the moderate-to-severely malnourished patient (i.e., those with ≥10% weight loss) who is undergoing major surgery, and this applies to cancer patients as well. Aggressive nutritional support for 5–7 days or more before surgery reduces perioperative complications and in some studies has been shown to reduce mortality. In a Veterans Administration Cooperative Trial of nearly 500 patients comprised largely of patients with cancer, those categorized as "severely" malnourished and who received preoperative total parenteral nutrition (TPN) experienced a nearly 90% decline in noninfectious perioperative complications.[120] Of note, those in the mildly malnourished category did not realize this benefit. Further, a study of 90 patients with gastric or colorectal cancers undergoing surgery demonstrated a 35% decline in overall complications and a decrease in mortality.[121] These benefits are not confined to TPN. Preoperative enteral support trials have shown benefits for those who are moderate-to-severely malnourished.[122,123] These benefits of parenteral and enteral nutrition are not found, however, when deferred until after surgery.

7.2.3.2 Patients with Pharyngoesophageal Cancers Treated with Chemoradiation

Studies examining the utility of aggressive nutritional support in those undergoing radio-therapy have been conducted most often in individuals with head and neck, and esophageal, cancers. There is compelling evidence in such patients that aggressive nutritional support—such as preemptive placement of gastrostomy tubes—prevents deterioration of nutritional status and improves the quality of life,[124] although a reduction in mortality is generally not realized. There is also evidence to suggest that tolerance and responsiveness to chemoradiation may be improved.[103,125,126] This is one scenario where patients do not need to be malnourished in order to realize benefits from aggressive nutritional support. Such benefits—even among those who are not malnourished at the time of initial presentation—are readily understood when one considers the frequent occurrence of severe dysphagia produced by such tumors and the high likelihood of progressing to a state of frank malnutrition. Using the traditional "pull" technique for percutaneous endoscopic gastrostomy (PEG) placement results in an unacceptably high rate of tumor metastases at the site of the PEG stoma, whereas such metastases are avoided by using the "direct" PEG insertion method or by surgical placement of the tube.[127]

There has been a longstanding concern that aggressive nutritional support of cancer patients may accelerate tumor growth. Animal models have shown that nutrient repletion in malnourished tumor bearing animals stimulates tumor growth.[128] Reports in humans showing clinically significant tumor growth with nutritional support, however, are conspicuously lacking. Indeed, some speculate that nutritional support is beneficial in those on active chemotherapy regimens as more cells would theoretically be in the vulnerable DNA synthesis phase. This attractive hypothesis, however, has yet to be proven.

7.2.4 AGENTS TO COMBAT ANOREXIA

Aggressive nutritional support does not invariably require tube feeding or TPN. If anorexia is the primary driver of weight loss, pharmacologic management is often a good starting point. In this section, we will discuss the best studied of these options including progestational agents, cannabinoids, prokinetic agents, and corticosteroids.

The progestational agents megestrol acetate (MA) and medroxyprogesterone acetate (MPA) have been studied and found to be well tolerated options to combat cancer-related anorexia. They were originally discovered when clinical trials investigating their use to treat hormone-responsive breast cancer reported a side effect of increased appetite and weight gain. Subsequent data have shown a dose–response relationship with typical weight gain over several months in the range of 3–6 kg. Accrual of muscle mass or lean body mass has not yet been convincingly shown in cancer patients, unlike in AIDS-related wasting. Although the increase in appetite occurs promptly, the median response time to achieve maximal weight gain is 6–10 weeks.[129] In addition, patients often report an increase in "energy" or a heightened sense of well-being, another beneficial end point.[130] Side effects include male impotence and vaginal spotting. An increased risk of thromboembolic events is linked to this class of drugs but there has been no significant increase of such incidents in clinical trials. The maximal clinical effects for MA are achieved at a dose of 800 mg/day (in adults) and for MPA is 500 mg twice daily.

Another class of drugs that have occasionally been used to improve cancer-related anorexia are the cannabinoids, such as the drug Dronabinol. It has been shown to be an effective antiemetic as well as an appetite stimulant. A regimen of 2.5 mg orally twice daily has been shown to stimulate appetite in cancer patients though beneficial effects against weight loss have not been convincingly demonstrated. When compared with MA, appetite stimulation and weight gain were superior with MA.[131] Side effects include euphoria, dizziness, somnolence, and confusion that may necessitate dose reduction or discontinuation in up to 25% of patients.

Prokinetic agents are also often utilized in the setting of advanced cancer-related gastroparesis and nausea. Metoclopramide (adults: 10 mg orally four times a day), domperidone (10 mg orally three times a day), and cisapride (10 mg orally four times a day) are three agents that have shown benefit for nausea and early satiety related to poor gastrointestinal motility. Cisapride, notably, causes greater colonic motility which is an important benefit given the common constipating effect of opioids on the GI tract. Cisapride and domperidone, however, are currently not available in the United States due to rare but life-threatening prolongation of Q-T intervals and related dysrhythmias.

Although corticosteroids have occasionally been employed as an appetite stimulant, their detrimental side effects seem to far outweigh any beneficial effect they exert on appetite. Dexamethasone (at a combined dose of 4 mg/day), prednisolone, and methylprednisolone have been shown to stimulate appetite though trials have not shown weight gain compared to placebo.[132] Clinical trials that have directly compared corticosteroids with MA have shown similar efficacy but increased toxicity with the former agents[133]: their use for this purpose is therefore not recommended.

7.2.5 Targeted Nutrient Therapy

Another therapeutic avenue for the management of weight loss and cachexia is to utilize supraphysiologic quantities of select nutrients for their pharmacologic effects against the pro-inflammatory cytokines and tumor-elaborated factors that mediate cancer-related malnutrition. For example, omega-3 fatty acids like eicosapentaenoic acid (EPA) have been demonstrated in clinical trials to suppress expression of inflammatory cytokines,[134] and have been shown *in vitro* to counteract the tumor-derived LMF.[135] Similarly, supplementation with three other food components—arginine, RNA, and glutamine—have each been shown to enhance various aspects of immunoresponsiveness. Consequently, specialized enteral formulas containing pharmacologic quantities of RNA, omega-3 fatty acids, arginine, and glutamine (in addition to conventional nutrients) are now commercially available (e.g., Impact®), and have

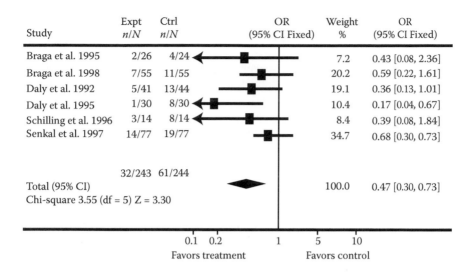

Study	Expt n/N	Ctrl n/N	OR (95% CI Fixed)	Weight %	OR (95% CI Fixed)
Braga et al. 1995	2/26	4/24		7.2	0.43 [0.08, 2.36]
Braga et al. 1998	7/55	11/55		20.2	0.59 [0.22, 1.61]
Daly et al. 1992	5/41	13/44		19.1	0.36 [0.13, 1.01]
Daly et al. 1995	1/30	8/30		10.4	0.17 [0.04, 0.67]
Schilling et al. 1996	3/14	8/14		8.4	0.39 [0.08, 1.84]
Senkal et al. 1997	14/77	19/77		34.7	0.68 [0.30, 0.73]
Total (95% CI)	32/243	61/244		100.0	0.47 [0.30, 0.73]

Chi-square 3.55 (df = 5) Z = 3.30

```
          0.1   0.2          1        5    10
       Favors treatment          Favors control
```

FIGURE 7.4 Effect of immunomodulatory nutritional support on the incidence of major infections in patients with gastrointestinal cancers. Expt = patients receiving immunomodulatory nutrition; Ctrl = patients receiving standard nutrition; n = number of events; N = number of patients in each group on intention to treat basis. (Reprinted from Heys S et al. *Ann Surg* 1999;229:467–477. With permission.)

repeatedly been shown to convey clinical benefits to malnourished cancer patients if administered prior to major surgery. Clinical trials have shown improved outcomes in patients undergoing surgery for gastrointestinal malignancies, largely due to ~50% reductions in perioperative infections and as a result sizeable shortening in the duration of hospitalization.[136–139] Indeed, two meta-analyses, the larger of which incorporated 22 trials, concluded that the use of these formulas resulted in a 35%–50% reduction in perioperative infections in elective cancer surgery[140,141] (see Figure 7.4). The greatest benefit was seen in those who began formula feeds several days before surgery. The clinical benefits extended, in some trials, to patients who were not significantly malnourished.[142] Whether these special formulas will also benefit cancer patients in other settings, such as those receiving intensive chemotherapy has not yet been extensively studied.

7.2.6 VITAMIN AND MINERAL DEFICIENCIES ASSOCIATED WITH SPECIFIC CIRCUMSTANCES

In addition to anorexia and malnutrition, GI malignancy patients also face select vitamin deficiencies as a consequence of the tumor itself or the medical interventions required for treatment. This section will highlight a few representative examples of these deficiencies that an astute clinician should bear in mind.

Malabsorption of fat-soluble nutrients and divalent cations with hepatobiliary disease or ileal dysfunction. Biliary obstruction due to malignancy, biliary diversion, or extensive loss of ileal function due to resection or radiation leads to fat malabsorption. In biliary disease, for instance, enough bile does not reach the small intestine preventing fat emulsification. With ileal dysfunction, insufficient bile acids are recycled by the ileum. The liver is unable to upregulate bile acid synthesis to overcome this loss leading to malabsorption. Indeed, ileal disease or resection exceeding 100 cm is usually associated with steatorrhea. This limitation in fat malabsorption leads to weight loss but also loss of fat-soluble vitamins and divalent cationic minerals like calcium, magnesium, zinc, and copper. The likelihood of this occurring is proportional to the elevation in bilirubin.[143] A chronic total bilirubin above 5 mg/dL should raise suspicion for these deficiencies. Patients with these deficiencies may only show subtle clinical signs so the clinician must have a high index of suspicion and test and treat appropriately to prevent overt symptoms.

B$_{12}$ deficiency due to ileal or gastric insults: Vitamin B$_{12}$ deficiency, like cancer diagnoses, becomes more common with age. As a consequence of atrophic gastritis (with a prevalence of 40% in individuals in the eighth decade of life) vitamin B$_{12}$ levels are often low at baseline in the elderly. Subtle deficiency of B$_{12}$ occasionally can occur when plasma levels are at the low end of the normative range, in which case it can be confirmed by a sensitive indicator of cellular depletion such as the presence of elevated serum methylmalonic acid. With this background in mind, it is not surprising that GI cancer patients, many of whom are elderly, often incur B$_{12}$ deficiency. The reductions in absorption from gastric acid suppression (by proton pump inhibitors (PPI's)), radiation damage, and surgical resection (especially when more than 90 cm of the ileum is affected) compound the risk.[144,145] Therefore, the clinician needs to remain vigilant for both the neurologic and hematologic manifestations of B$_{12}$ deficiency and not attribute these changes to the myriad of other effects of cancer and its therapy.

7.2.7   PRACTICAL CONCLUSIONS

1. Wasting is common in gastrointestinal cancers and carries with it negative consequences in regard to morbid events, ability to withstand therapy, and survival. An unintentional weight loss of 10% or more of usual body weight is a convenient and surprisingly accurate means of identifying patients with moderate-to-severe malnutrition.

2. Routine identification of those cancer patients with moderate-to-severe malnutrition is important because these patients benefit most from aggressive nutritional support. This support has the greatest impact in the preoperative setting and during chemotherapy and radiation.

3. In those about to undergo major surgery, immunomodulatory enteral formulas reduce perioperative infections and hospitalization length versus conventional tube feeds. This benefit may extend even to those not substantially malnourished.

4. Agents to treat anorexia including progestational agents, dronabinol, and prokinetics have modest benefits, with the progestational agents showing the most benefit.

5. GI cancer patients are at risk for specific vitamin deficiencies and clinicians need to be diligent in these situations to avert the morbidity associated with these deficiencies.

ACKNOWLEDGMENT

Supported in part by a grant from the Prevent Cancer Foundation (JBM) and the USDA Agricultural Research Service (Agreement No. 1950–5100-074-01S [JBM]). Any opinions, findings, conclusions or recommendations expressed in this publication are those of the author(s) and do not necessarily reflect the view of the U.S. Department of Agriculture.

REFERENCES

1. *Global Cancer Facts and Figures*, 2nd Edition. 2011. American Cancer Society. Published online: cancer.org.
2. Gonzalez CA, Riboli E. Diet and cancer prevention: Contributions from the European Prospective Investigation into Cancer and Nutrition (EPIC) study. *EJC* 2010;46:2555–2562.
3. World Cancer Research Fund/ American Institute for Cancer Research. *Food, Nutrition, Physical Activity, and the Prevention of Cancer: A Global Perspective*. Washington, DC: AICR, 2007.
4. Flegal KM, Carroll MD, Kit BK et al. Prevalence of obesity and trends in the distribution of body mass index among US adults. 1999–2010. *JAMA* 2012;307:491–497.
5. Bardou M, Barkun AN, Martel M. Obesity and colorectal cancer. *Gut* 2013, 12 March;62(6):933–947.
6. Harriss DJ, Atkinson G, George K et al. Lifestyle factors and colorectal cancer risk: Systematic review and meta-analysis of associations with body mass index. *Colorectal Dis* 2009;11:547–563.
7. Dai Z, Xu YC, Niu L. Obesity and colorectal cancer risk: A meta-analysis of cohort studies. *World J Gastroenterol* 2007;13:4199–4206.
8. Moghaddam AA, Woodward M, Huxley R. Obesity and risk of colorectal cancer: A meta-analysis of 31 studies with 70,000 events. *CEBP* 2007;16:2533–2547.
9. Okabayashi K, Ashrafian H, Hasegawa H et al. Body mass index category as a risk factor for colorectal adenomas: A systematic review and meta-analysis. *Am J Gastroentrol* 2012;107:1175–1185.
10. Kim BC, Shin A, Hong CW et al. Association of colorectal adenoma with components of metabolic syndrome. *Cancer Causes Control* 2012;23:727–736.
11. Rapp K, Klenk J, Ulmer H et al. Weight change and cancer risk in a cohort of more than 65,000 adults in Austria. *Ann Oncol* 2008;19:641–648.
12. Campbell PT, Newton CC, Dehal AN et al. Impact of body mass index on survival after colorectal cancer diagnosis: The cancer prevention study II Nutrition Cohort. *J Clin Oncol* 2012;30:42–52.
13. Dignam JJ, Polite BN, Yothers G et al. Body mass index and outcomes in patients who receive adjuvant chemotherapy for colon cancer. *J Natl Cancer Inst* 2006;98:1647–1654.
14. Matthews CE, Sui X, LaMonte MJ et al. Metabolic syndrome and risk of death from cancers of the digestive system. *Metabolism* 2010;59:1231–1239.
15. Guiu B, Petit JM, Bonnetain F et al. Visceral fat area is an independent predictive biomarker of outcome after first line bevacizumab-based treatment in metastatic colorectal cancer. *Gut* 2010;59:341–347.
16. Ghiringhelli F, Vincent J, Guiu B et al. Bevacizumab plus FOLFIRI-3 in chemotherapy-refractory patients with metastatic colorectal cancer in the era of biotherapies. *Invest New Drugs* 2012;30:758–764.
17. Ryan AM, Duong M, Healy L et al. Obesity, metabolic syndrome and esophageal adenocarcinoma: Epidemiology, etiology and new targets. *Cancer Epidemiol Biomarkers Prevent* 2011;35:309–319.

18. Kubo A, Corley DA. Body mass index and adenocarcinomas of the esophagus or gastric cardia: A systematic review and meta-analysis. *Cancer Epidemiol Biomarkers Prev* 2006;15:872–878.
19. Veugelers PJ, Porter GA, Guernsey DL, Casson AG. Obesity and lifestyle risk factors for gastroesophageal reflux disease, Barrett esophagus and esophageal adenocarcinoma. *Dis Esophagus* 2006;19:321–328.
20. Corley DA, Kubo A, Zhao W. Abdominal obesity and the risk of esophageal and gastric cardia carcinomas. *Cancer Epidemiol Biomarkers Prev* 2008;17:352–358.
21. Abnet CC, Freedman ND, Hollenbeck AR, Fraumeni Jr JF, Leitzmann M, Schatzkin A. A prospective study of BMI and risk of oesophageal and gastric adenocarcinoma. *Eur J Cancer* 2008;44:465–471.
22. Figueroa JD, Terry MB, Gammon MD et al. Cigarette smoking, body mass index, gastro-esophageal reflux disease, and non-steroidal anti-inflammatory drug use and risk of subtypes of esophageal and gastric cancers by P53 overexpression. *Cancer Causes Control* 2009;20:361–368.
23. Reeves GK, Pirie K, Beral V, Green J, Spencer E, Bull D. Cancer incidence and mortality in relation to body mass index in the Million Women Study: Cohort study. *BMJ* 2007;335:1134.
24. Ryan AM, Rowley SP, Fitzgerald AP, Ravi N, Reynolds JV. Adenocarcinoma of the oesophagus and gastric cardia: Male preponderance in association with obesity. *Eur J Cancer* 2006;42:1151–1158.
25. Anderson LA, Watson RG, Murphy SJ et al. Risk factors for Barrett's oesophagus and oesophageal adenocarcinoma: Results from the FINBAR study. *World J Gastroenterol* 2007;13:1585–1594.
26. Samanic C, Chow WH, Gridley G, Jarvholm B, Fraumeni Jr JF. Relation of body mass index to cancer risk in 362,552 Swedish men. *Cancer Causes Control* 2006;17:901–909.
27. Merry AH, Schouten LJ, Goldbohm RA, van den Brandt PA. Body mass index, height and risk of adenocarcinoma of the oesophagus and gastric cardia: A prospective cohort study. *Gut* 2007;56:1503–1511.
28. Steffen A, Schulze MB, Pischon T et al. Anthropometry and esophageal cancer risk in the European prospective investigation into cancer and nutrition. *Cancer Epidemiol Biomarkers Prev* 2009;18:2079–2089.
29. MacInnis RJ, English DR, Hopper JL, Giles GG. Body size and composition and the risk of gastric and oesophageal adenocarcinoma. *Int J Cancer* 2006;118:2628–2631.
30. Whiteman DC, Sadeghi S, Pandeya N et al. Combined effects of obesity, acid reflux and smoking on the risk of adenocarcinomas of the oesophagus. *Gut* 2008;57:173–180.
31. Coggon D, Barker DJ, Cole RB, Nelson M. Stomach cancer and food storage. *J Natl Cancer Inst* 1989;81(15):1178–1182.
32. Anonymous Live flukes and *Helicobacter pylori*. IARC Working Group on the Evaluation of Carcinogenic Risks to Humans, Lyon, June 7–14, 1994. *IARC Monogr Eval Carcinog Risks Hum* 1994;61:1–241.
33. Leek RM, Jr., Crabtree JE. Helicobacter infection and gastric neoplasia. *J Pathol* 2006;208:233–248.
34. Mera R, Fontham ET, Bravo LE, Bravo JC, Piazuelo MB, Camargo MC, Correa P. Long term follow up of patients treated for *Helicobacter pylori* infection. *Gut* 2005;54:1536–1540.
35. Shikata K, Kiyohara Y, Kubo M et al. A prospective study of dietary salt intake and gastric cancer incidence in a defined Japanese population: The Hisayama study. *Int J Cancer* 2006;119:196–201.
36. Lee SA, Kang D, Shim KN, Choe JW, Hong WS, Choi H. Effect of diet and *Helicobacter pylori* infection to the risk of early gastric cancer. *J Epidemiol* 2003;13:162–168.

37. D'Elia L, Rossi G, Ippolito R et al. Habitual salt intake and risk of gastric cancer: A meta-analysis of prospective studies. *Clin Nutr* 2012;31:489–498.
38. Takahashi M, Hasegawa R. Enhancing effects of dietary salt on both initiation and promotion stages of rat gastric carcinogenesis. *Princess Takamatsu Symp* 1985;16:169–182.
39. Correa P. The biological model of gastric carcinogenesis. *IARC SciPubl* 2004;157: 301–310.
40. Ferlay J, Bray F, Parkin DM, Pisani P, Editors. *Gobocan 2000: Cancer Incidence and Mortality Worldwide (IARC Cancer Bases No. 5)*. Lyon: IARC Press; 2001.
41. Gancz H, Jones KR, Merrell DS. Sodium chloride affects *Helicobacter pylori* growth and gene expression. *J Bacteriol* 2008;190:4100–4105.
42. Loh JT, Torres VJ, Cover TL. Regulation of *Helicobacter pylori* cagA expression in response to salt. *Cancer Res* 2007;67:4709–4715.
43. Jenab M, Riboli E, Ferrari P et al. Plasma and dietary carotenoid, retinol, and tocopherol levels and risk of gastric adenocarcinomas in EPIC. *Br J Cancer* 2006;95:406–415.
44. Graham DY, Anderson SY, Lang T. Garlic or jalapeno peppers for treatment of *Helicobacter pylori* infection. *Am J Gastroenterol* 1999;94:1200–1202.
45. Iimuro M, Shibata H, Kawamori T et al. Suppressive effects of garlic extract on *Helicobacter pylori* induced gastritis in Mongolian Gerbils. *Cancer Lett* 2002;187:61–68.
46. You WC, Brown LM, Zhang L et al. Randomized double-blind factorial trial of three treatments to reduce the prevalence of precancerous gastric lesions. *J Natl Cancer Inst* 2006;98:974–983.
47. Dorant E, Van den Brandt PA, Goldbohm RA, Sturmans F. Consumption of onions and a reduced risk of stomach carcinoma. *Gastroenterology* 1996;110:12–20.
48. Hansson LE, Nyren O, Bergstrom R et al. Diet and risk of gastric cancer: A population-based case-control study in Sweden. *Int J Cancer* 1993;55:181–189.
49. Kim HJ, Chang WK, Kim MK, Lee SS, Choi BY. Dietary factors and gastric cancer in Korea: A case-control study. *Int J Cancer* 2002;97:531–535.
50. Ma J, Zhang L, Brown L et al. Fifteen year effect of H. pylori, garlic, and vitamin treatments on gastric cancer incidence and mortality. *J Natl Cancer Inst* 2012;104: 488–492.
51. Kim YJ, Kwon O. Garlic intake and cancer risk: An analysis using the food and drug administration's evidence-based review system for the scientific evaluation of health claims. *Am J Clin Nutr* 2009;89:257–264.
52. Ko I, Park S, Park B et al. Isoflavones from phytoestrogens and gastric cancer risk: A nested case-control study with the Korean Multicenter Cancer Cohort. *Cancer Epidemiol Biomarkers Prevent* 2010;19:1292–1300.
53. Gonzalez CA, Jakszyn P, Pera G et al. Meat intake and risk of stomach and esophageal adenocarcinoma within the European prospective investigation into cancer and nutrition (EPIC). *J Natl Cancer Inst* 2006;98:345–354.
54. Zhu H, Yang X, Zhang C et al. Red and processed meat intake is associated with higher gastric cancer risk: A meta-analysis of epidemiological observational studies. *PLoS One* 2013;8:e70955.
55. Halliwell B. Vitamin C and genomic stability. *Mutat Res* 2001;475:29–35.
56. Jarosz M, Dzieniszewski J, Dabrowska-Ufniarz E, Wartanowicz M, Ziemlanski S, Reed PI. Effects of high dose vitamin C treatment on *Helicobacter pylori* infection and total vitamin C concentration in gastric juice. *Eur J Cancer Prev* 1998;7:449–454.
57. Zhang ZW, Farthing MJ. The roles of vitamin C in *Helicobacter pylori* associated gastric carcinogenesis. *Chin J Dig Dis* 2005;6:53–58.
58. Drake IM, Davies MJ, Mapstone NP, Dixon MF, Schorah CJ, White KL, Chalmers DM, Axon AT. Ascorbic acid may protect against human gastric cancer by scavenging mucosal oxygen radicals. *Carcinogenesis* 1996;17:559–562.

59. Khanzode SS, Khanzode SD, Dakhale GN. Serum and plasma concentration of oxidant and antioxidants in patients of *Helicobacter pylori* gastritis and its correlation with gastric cancer. *Cancer Lett* 2003;195:27–31.
60. Correa P, Fontham ET, Bravo JC et al. Chemoprevention of gastric dysplasia: Randomized trial of antioxidant supplements and anti-*Helicobacter pylori* therapy. *J Natl Cancer Inst* 2000;92:1881–1888.
61. Correa P, Fontham ET, Bravo JC et al. Re: Chemoprevention of gastric dysplasia: Randomized trial of antioxidant supplements and anti-*Helicobacter pylori* therapy (letter). *J Natl Cancer Inst* 2001;93:559.
62. Mera R, Fontham ET, Bravo LE et al. Long term follow up of patients treated for *Helicobacter pylori* infection. *Gut* 2005;54:1536–1540.
63. Buckland G. Adherence to Mediterranean diet and risk of gastric adenocarcinoma within EPIC. *Am J Clin Nutr* 2010;91:381–390.
64. Samieri C, Sun Q, Townsend MK et al. The association between dietary patterns at midlife and health in ageing, on observational study. *Ann Intern Med* 2013;159(9):584–591.
65. Byers T. Diet, colorectal adenomas and colorectal cancer. Editorial. *NEJM* 2000;342:1206–1207.
66. Fuchs CS, Giovannucci E, Colditz, GA et al. Dietary fiber and the risk of colorectal cancer and adenoma in women. *N Engl J Med* 1999;340:169–176.
67. Terry P, Giovannucci E, Michels KB et al. Fruit, vegetables, dietary fiber, and risk of colorectal cancer. *J Natl Cancer Inst* 2001;93:525–533.
68. Park Y, Hunter DJ, Spiegelman D et al. Dietary fiber intake and risk of colorectal cancer: A pooled analysis of prospective cohort studies. *JAMA* 2005;294(22):2849–2857.
69. Pietinen P, Malila N, Virtanen M et al. Diet and the risk of colorectal cancer in a cohort of Finnish men. *Cancer Causes Control* 1999;10:387–396.
70. Schatzkin A, Lanza E, Corle D et al. Lack of effect of low fat high fiber diet on the recurrence of colorectal adenomas. *N Engl J Med* 2000;342:1149–1155.
71. Alberts DS, Martinez ME, Roe DJ et al. Lack of effect of a high fiber cereal supplement on the recurrence of colorectal adenomas. *N Engl J Med* 2000;342:1156–1162.
72. Bingham SA, Day NE, Luben R et al. Dietary fibre in food and protection against colorectal cancer in the EPIC: An observational study. *Lancet* 2003;361:1496–1501.
73. Bingham S, Norat T, Moskal A et al. Is the association with fiber from foods in colorectal cancer confounded by folate intake? *CEBP* 2005;14:1552–1556.
74. Murphy N, Norat T, Ferrari P et al. Dietary fibre intake and risks of cancers of the colon and rectum in the European Prospective Investigation into Cancer and Nutrition (EPIC). *PLoS ONE* 2012;7(6):e39361.
75. Voorrips, I, Goldbohm R, Van Poppel G et al. Vegetable and fruit consumption and risks of colon and rectal cancer in a prospective, cohort study. *Am J Epidemiol* 2000;152:1081–1092.
76. Michels K, Giovannucci E, Joshipura K et al. Prospective study of fruit and vegetable consumption and incidence of colon and rectal cancers. *J Natl Cancer Inst* 2000;92:1740–1752.
77. Matsuura N, Miyamae Y, Yamane K et al. Aged garlic extract inhibits angiogenesis and proliferation of colorectal carcinoma cells. *J Nutr* 2006;136:S842–S846.
78. Katsuki T, Hirata K, Ishikawa H, Matsuura N, Sumi SI, Itoh H. Aged garlic extract has chemopreventative effects on 1,2-dimethylhydrazine-induced colon tumors in rats. *J Nutr* 2006;136:S847–S851.
79. Tanaka S, Haruma K, Yoshihara M et al. Aged garlic extract has potential suppressive effect on colorectal adenomas in humans. *J Nutr* 2006;136:S821–S826.
80. Fleischauer AT, Poole C, Arab L. Garlic consumption and cancer prevention: Meta-analyses of colorectal and stomach cancers. *Am J Clin Nutr* 2000;72:1047–1052.

81. Deeb KK, Termp DL, Johnson CS. Vitamin D signaling pathways in cancer: Potential for anticancer therapeutics. *Nat Rev Cancer* 2007;7:684–700.
82. Huncharek M, Muscat J, Kupelnick B et al. Colorectal cancer risk and dietary intake of calcium, Vitamin D, and dairy products. A meta-analysis of 26,335 cases from 60 observational studies. *Nutr Cancer* 2009;61:47–69.
83. Jenab M, Bueno-de-Mesquita HB, Ferrari P et al. Association between pre-diagnostic circulating vitamin D concentration and risk of colorectal cancer in European populations; a nested case-control study. *BMJ* 2010;340:b5500.
84. Cho E, Smith-Warner S, Spiegelman D et al. Dairy foods, calcium, and colorectal cancer: A pooled analysis of 10 cohort studies. *J Natl Cancer Inst* 2004;96:1015–1022.
85. Baron J, Beach M, Mandel J et al. Calcium supplements for the prevention of colorectal adenomas. *NEJM* 1999;340:101–107.
86. Grau MV, Baron J, Sandler RS et al. Prolonged effect of calcium supplementation on risk of colorectal adenomas in a randomized trial. *J Natl Cancer Inst* 2007;99(2): 129–136.
87. Norat T, Bingham S, Ferrari P et al. Meat, fish, and colorectal cancer risk: The European Prospective Investigation into cancer and nutrition. *J Natl Cancer Inst* 2005;97:906–916.
88. Giovannucci E, Rimm E, Stampfer M, Colditz G, Ascherio A, Willett W. Intake of fat, meat, and fiber in relations to risk of colon cancer. *Cancer Res* 1994;54:2390–2397.
89. Xu B, Sun J, Huang L et al. No evidence of decreased risk of colorectal adenomas with white meat, poultry, and fish intake: A meta-analysis of observational studies. *Ann Epidemiol* 2013;April 23(4):215–222.
90. Ferrari P, Jenab M, Norat T et al. Lifetime and baseline alcohol intake and risk of colon and rectal cancers in the European prospective investigation into cancer and nutrition (EPIC). *Int J Cancer* 2007;121(9):2065–2072.
91. Gibson TM, Weinstein SJ, Pfeiffer RM et al. Pre- and postfortification intake of folate and risk of colorectal cancer in a large prospective cohort study in the United States. *Am J Clin Nutr* 2011;94:1053–1062.
92. Kim YI. Role of folate in colon cancer development and progression. *J Nutr* 2003;133(Suppl 1):3731S–3739S.
93. Vollset S, Clarke R, Lewington S et al. Effects of folic acid supplementation on overall and site-specific cancer incidence during the randomized trials: Meta-analyses. *Lancet* 2013;381:1029–1036.
94. Mason JB. Folate consumption and cancer risk: A confirmation and some reassurance but we're not out of the woods quite yet. *Am J Clin Nutr* 2011;94:965–966.
95. Clark L, Combs G, Turnbull B et al. Effects of delenium supplementation for cancer prevention in patients with carcinoma of the skin. A randomized controlled trial. *JAMA* 1996;276:1957–1963.
96. Duffield-Lillico A, Reid M, Turnbull B et al. Baseline characteristics and the effect of selenium supplementation on cancer incidence in a randomized clinical trial. *Cancer Epidemiol Biomarkers Prevent* 2002;11:630–639.
97. Marshall J, Tangen C, Sakr W et al. Phase III trial of selenium to prevent prostate cancer in men with high grade PIN: SWOG S9917. *Cancer Prev Res* 2011;4:1761–1769.
98. Vinceti M, Dennert G, Crespi CM, Zwahlen M, Brinkman M, Zeegers MPA, Horneber M, D'Amico R, Del Giovane C. Selenium for preventing cancer. *Cochrane Database Syst Rev* 2014;(3): Article No: CD005195. DOI: 10.1002/14651858.CD005195. pub3.
99. Mayne S, Ferrucci L, Cartmel B. Lessons learned from randomized clinical trials of micronutrient supplementation for cancer prevention. *Ann Rev Nutr* 2012;32:369–390.
100. Dewys WD, Begg C, Lavin P et al. Prognostic effect of weight loss prior to chemotherapy in cancer patients. *Am J Med* 1980;69:491–497.

101. Mick R, Vokes E, Weichselbaum RR et al. Prognostic factors in advanced head and neck cancer patient undergoing multimodality therapy. *Otolaryngol Head Neck Surg* 1991;105:62–73.

102. Nixon DW, Heymsfield SB, Cohen AE et al. Protein-calorie undernutrition in hospitalized cancer patients. *Am J Med* 1980;68:683–690.

103. Andreyev H, Norman A, Oates J et al. Why do patients with weight loss have a worse outcome when undergoing chemotherapy for gastrointestinal malignancies? *Eur J Cancer* 1998;34:503–509.

104. Patil PK, Patel SG, Mistry RC et al. Cancer of the esophagus:esophagogastric anastomotic leak—A retrospective study of predisposing factors. *J Surg Oncol* 1992;49:163–167.

105. Van Bokhorst-de van der Schuer MA, Van Leeuwan PA, Kuik D et al. The impact of nutritional status on the prognosis of patients with advanced head and neck cancer. *Cancer* 1999;86:519–527.

106. Lanzotti VJ, Thomas DR, Boyle LE et al. Survival with inoperable lung cancer. *Cancer* 1977;39:303–313.

107. Kama NA, Coskun T, Yuksek YN et al. Factors affecting post-operative mortality in malignant biliary tract obstruction. *Hepatogastroenterology* 1999;46:103–107.

108. Feron KCH, Preston T. Body composition in cancer cachexia. *Infusions-therapie* 1990;17(Suppl 3):63–66.

109. Strovfroff M, Fraker D, Swedenborg J et al. Cachetin/tumor necrosis factor, a possible mediator of cancer anorexia in the rat. *Cancer Res* 1988;48:920–925.

110. Opara E, Laviano A, Meguid M et al. Correlation between food intake and CSF IL1 in anorectic tumor bearing rats. *Neuro Report* 1995;6:750–752.

111. Langstein H, Doherty G, Fraker D et al. The roles of gamma-interferon and tumor necrosis factor alpha in an experimental rat model of cancer cachexia. *Cancer Res* 1991;51:2302–2306.

112. Lundholm K, Bylund A, Holm J et al. Skeletal muscle metabolism in patients with malignant tumor. *Eur J Cancer* 1976;12:465–473.

113. Cabal-Manzano R, Bhargava P, Torres-Duarte A et al. Proteolysis-inducing factor is expressed in tumors of patients with gastrointestinal cancers and correlates with weight loss. *Br J Cancer* 2001;84:1599–1601.

114. Zhang L, Tang H, Kou Y et al. MG132-mediated inhibition of the ubiquitin-proteasome pathway ameliorates cancer cachexia. *J Cancer Res Clin Oncol* 2013;139:1105–1115.

115. Rofe A, Bourgeois C, Coyle P et al. Altered insulin response to glucose in weight losing cancer patients. *Anticancer Res* 1994;14:647–650.

116. Islam-Ali B, Khan S, Prince SA, Tisdale MJ. Modulation of adipocyte G-protein expression in cancer cachexia by a lipid-mobilizing factor (LMF). *Br J Cancer* 2001;85(5):758.

117. Holyrode C, Babuzda T, Putnam R et al. Altered glucose metabolism in metastatic carcinoma. *Cancer Res* 1975;35:3710–3714.

118. Hill G. Body composition research: Implications for the practice of clinical nutrition. *JPEN J Parenter Enteral Nutr* 1992;16:197–218.

119. Prijatmoko D, Strauss B, Lambert J et al. Early detection of protein depletion in alcoholic cirrhosis: Role of body composition analysis. *Gastroenterology* 1993;105:1839–1845.

120. Buzby GP, Page CP, Reinhardt G et al. The veterans administration TPN cooperative study group. Perioperative total parenteral nutrition in surgical patient. *NEJM* 1991;325:525–532.

121. Bozzetti F, Bavazzi C, Miceli R et al. Perioperative TPN in malnourished, GI cancer patients: A randomized, clinical trial. *JPEN J Parenter Enteral Nutr* 2000;24:7–14.

122. Shirabe K, Matsumata T, Shimada M et al. A comparison of parenteral hyperalimentation and early enteral feeding regarding systemic immunity after major hepatic resection—A randomized, prospective study. *Hepatogastroenterology* 1997;44:205–209.

123. Flynn M, Leightty F. Preoperative outpatient nutritional support of patient with squamous cancer of the upper aerodigestive tract. *Am J Surg* 1987;154:359–362.
124. Senft M, Fietkau R, Iro H et al. The influence of supportive nutritional therapy via percutaneous endoscopically guided gastrostomy on the quality of life of cancer patients. *Support Care Cancer* 1993;1:272–275.
125. Paccagnella A, Morello M, Da Mosto M et al. Early nutritional intervention improves treatment tolerance and outcomes in head and neck cancer patients undergoing chemoradiotherapy. *Support Care Cancer* 2010;18:837–845.
126. Atasoy B, Yonal O, Demirel B et al. The impact of early PEG placement on treatment completeness and nutritional status in locally advanced head and neck cancer patients receiving chemoradiotherapy. *Eur Arch Otorhinolaryngol* 2012;269:275–282.
127. Cappell M. Risk factors and risk reduction of malignant seeding of the PEG track from pharyngoesophageal malignancy: A review of all 44 known reported cases. *Am J Gastro* 2007;102:1307–1311.
128. Jin D, Phillips M, Byles J. Effects of parenteral nutrition support and chemotherapy on the phasic composition of tumor cells in gastrointestinal cancer. *JPEN J Parenter Enteral Nutr* 1999;23:237–241.
129. Von Roenn J, Armstrong D, Kotler D et al. Megestrol acetate in patients with AIDS related cachexia. *Ann Intern Med* 1994;121:393–399.
130. Bruera E, Macmillan K, Kuehn N et al. A controlled trial of megestrol acetate on appetite, caloric intake, nutritional status, and other symptoms in patients with advanced cancer. *Cancer* 1990;66:1279–1282.
131. Jatoi A, Windschitl H, Loprinzi C et al. Dronabinol versus megestrol acetate vs combination therapy for cancer-associated anorexia: A North Central Cancer Treatment Group Study. *J Clin Oncol* 2002;20:567–573.
132. Bruera E, Roca E, Cedaro L, Carraro S, Chacon R. Action of oral methylprednisolone in terminal cancer patients: A prospective randomized double-blind study. *Cancer Treat Rep* 1985;69(7–8):751.
133. Loprinzi CL, Kugler JW, Sloan JA et al. Randomized comparison of megestrol acetate versus dexamethasone versus fluoxymesterone for the treatment of cancer anorexia/cachexia. *J Clin Oncol* 1999;17(10):3299.
134. Itariu B, Zeyda M, Hochbrugger E et al. Long-chain n-3 PUFAs reduce adipose tissue and systemic inflammation in severely obese nondiabetic patients: A randomized controlled trial. *Am J Clin Nutr* 2012;96:1137–1149.
135. Price SA, Tisdale MJ. Mechanism of inhibition of a tumor lipid-mobilizing factor by eicosapentaenoic acid. *Cancer Res* 1998;58(21):4827.
136. Saito H, Trocki O, Wang S et al. Metabolic and immune effects of dietary arginine supplementation after burn. *Arch Surg* 1987;122:784–789.
137. Fanslow W, Kulkarni A, Van Buren C et al. Effect of nucleotide restriction and supplementation on resistance to experimental murine candidiasis. *JPEN* 1988;12:49–52.
138. Fox A, Kripke S, DePaula J et al. Effect of glutamine-supplemental enteral diet on methotrexate induced enterocolitis. *JPEN* 1988;12:325–331.
139. Ziegler T, Young L, Benfell K et al. Clinical and metabolic efficacy of glutamine-supplemented parenteral nutrition after bone marrow transplantation. *Ann Intern Med* 1992;116:82–88.
140. Schloerb P, Amare M. Total parenteral nutrition with glutamine in bone marrow transplantation and other clinical applications. *JPEN* 1993;17:407–413.
141. Gianotti L, Braga M, Vignali A et al. Effect of route of delivery and formulation of postoperative nutrition support in patients undergoing major operations for malignant neoplasms. *Arch Surg* 1997;132:1222–1230.

142. Braga M, Gianotti L, Radeelli G et al. Perioperative immunonutrition in patients under-going cancer surgery: Results of a randomized double blind phase 3 trial. *Arch Surg* 1999;134:428–433.
143. Senkal M, Zumtobel V, Vauer K-H et al. Outcome and cost-effectiveness of perioperative enteral immunonutrition in patient undergoing elective upper gastrointestinal tract surgery: A prospective, randomized trial. *Arch Surg* 1999;134:1309–1316.
144. Daly J, Weintraub F, Shou J et al. Enteral nutrition during multimodality therapy in upper gastrointestinal cancer patients. *Ann Surg* 1995;221:327–338.
145. Heys S, Walker L, Smith I et al. Enteral nutritional supplementation with key nutrients in patients with critical illness and cancer: A meta-analysis of randomized controlled clinical trials. *Ann Surg* 1999;229:467–477.

8 Nutritional Considerations in Gastroesophageal Reflux Disease and Eosinophilic Esophagitis

Bethany Doerfler and Nirmala Gonsalves

CONTENTS

8.1 INTRODUCTION

Gastroesophageal reflux disease (GERD) and Eosinophilic esophagitis (EoE) are common gastrointestinal disorders seen by both primary care physicians and gastroenterologists. GERD is estimated to affect 13%–29% of the U.S. population and recent estimates suggest the prevalence of EoE in adults to be 1 in 10,000.[1,2] Both medical and dietary therapies are effective treatments for these conditions.[3-8] This chapter will highlight the dietary approach to treating these disorders.

8.2 GASTROESOPHAGEAL REFLUX DISEASE

GERD occurs when refluxed gastric acid and pepsin cause necrosis and inflammation of the esophageal mucosa. One of the mechanisms that results in excessive gastric acid reflux includes esophagogastric junction incompetence. Three main mechanisms of esophagogastric junction incompetence are identified: (1) transient lower esophageal sphincter (LES) relaxations which are a vagovagal reflux in which LES relaxation is brought on by gastric distension, (2) LES hypotension, or (3) anatomic distortion of the esophagogastric junction inclusive of hiatus hernia.[3,5] The most common mechanism thought to cause reflux is excessive transient LES relaxation, which occurs in 90% of cases. Other factors that predispose to reflux include obesity, disruption of esophageal peristalsis which affects the clearance of esophageal acid, pregnancy, gastric hypersecretory states, delayed gastric emptying, and excessive eating.

Proton pump inhibitor (PPI) therapy remains the most widely used and efficacious medical treatment for GERD. Despite its efficacy and popularity, only 40% of GERD patients experience complete relief and report breakthrough symptoms despite medical therapy.[4] Additionally, many patients express concerns over using these medications long term due to possible decreased micronutrient digestion and absorption.[9-11] Recent concerns over increased hip fracture risk with long-term PPI use suggest careful medical and nutritional monitoring for patients with GERD who need to use PPI therapy long term.[9,11]

Lifestyle and dietary modifications for GERD have long been recognized as important factors in effective GERD management yet no formal "anti-reflux" diet exists.[12,13] Traditional dietary advice includes limiting "refluxegenic foods" such as highly acidic, fatty, or spicy foods. However, there is limited evidence that global avoidance of these foods improves GERD symptoms.[14] Current consensus guidelines suggest lifestyle modifications including weight loss and head of bed positioning as more effective strategies to manage symptoms than limiting highly acidic or spicy foods.[14] Section 8.3 focuses on effective lifestyle strategies for treating GERD and will explore the nutritional impact of PPI therapy.

8.3 LIFESTYLE AND DIETARY THERAPY FOR GERD

Most GERD symptoms are reported in the postprandial period, and thus the role of diet in driving GERD symptoms has been suggested.[12,15] Patients with GERD have historically been directed to avoid aggravating foods such as orange juice, caffeine, chocolate, peppermint, carbonation, and fatty foods. This type of dietary therapy has been based on symptom reporting as well as evidence suggesting certain foods can weaken LES pressures and allow for more reflux. Although alcohol, chocolate, and high fat foods decrease LES pressure; esophageal pressures do not appear to improve with avoidance.[13] While global elimination of foods thought to trigger reflux such as coffee, caffeine, chocolate, and acidic foods are no longer recommended, individualized limitations are recommended.[14,15] Patients should be encouraged to keep a food and symptom diary examining types of foods and amounts of foods that appear to trigger symptoms. Eliminating suspected triggers and experiencing subsequent symptom relief is one technique to advise dietary avoidance of offending foods. Recumbent positioning after eating does impact GERD symptoms. Studies have demonstrated an improvement in both GERD symptoms and esophageal pH monitoring when the head of the bed is raised using foam blocks.[16–18] Using pillows does not appear to provide the same benefit as foam wedges.[18] Maintaining a healthy body weight could be one of the most important treatments for GERD as recent studies suggest weight loss can completely resolve symptoms in some patients. Ness-Jansen and colleagues assigned 332 overweight and obese adults (BMI 25–39.9 kg/m^2) to a structured weight loss program, which included decreasing calories, increased physical activity, and behavioral changes. After 6 months of intervention, 81% of the subjects had a reduction in GERD symptom scores, and 65% experienced complete resolution of symptoms. Weight loss in the study (an average of 28.5 lbs per subject) was related to improved GERD symptom scores and a dose–response was observed between weight and symptom decrease. In similar studies, weight loss improves treatment success when paired with anti-reflux medications such as PPIs. Studies have also shown that decreasing waist circumference and body mass index (BMI) may have curative impact on GERD symptoms and loss of LES integrity.[19,20]

The benefits of weight loss appear to positively impact GERD events and symptoms whether patients are slightly overweight or obese. Escalating BMI alone predicts increased reflux episodes and symptoms.[21,22] Normal weight women with a BMI increase of >3.5 units were almost three times more likely to develop GERD and associated symptoms (OR = 2.8, 95% CI 1.63–4.84).[21] The mechanism of weight gain and increased abdominal adiposity on GERD is thought to occur because of physical and hormonal changes that influence esophageal motility and acid clearance in overweight and obese subjects compared to healthy controls.[23,24] In the absence of GERD, the presence of overweight status and obesity alone predict increased episodes of transient lower esophageal sphincter relaxation (TLESR) and acid reflux in the postprandial period ($p < 0.001$).[24] Additionally, abdominal adiposity likely affects GERD due to increased intraabdominal pressure, which can influence LES function.

One of the most effective methods of weight loss reduction includes calorie reduction. In the past decade, the media has embraced many diet approaches ranging from low carbohydrate diets to gluten-free diets. Irrespective of the type of diet started, creating a calorie deficit is the most effective way to promote weight loss. Therefore, multiple weight loss strategies could be effective. Barriers to successful weight loss include easy access to highly palatable and unhealthy food, increased sedentary lifestyles, increased dining out, and larger portion sizes. Patients interested in weight loss should be referred to a registered dietitian to identify weight loss barriers and to develop a healthy weight loss plan. Common lifestyle driven weight loss strategies are listed in Table 8.1. When lifestyle and dietary changes alone are not effective in controlling GERD, patients are typically started on anti-reflux medications. Most commonly used anti-reflux medications are proton-pump inhibitors. While these medications can effectively control esophageal acid exposure, there are some recent concerns about their effects on micronutrient absorption and bone health.

TABLE 8.1
Dietary Strategies to Promote Weight Loss in Patients with GERD

Increase awareness: Keeping a food journal changes eating behaviors.

Shave calories: Reduce excess sugary drinks and high calorie condiments like cheese, mayonnaise, gravies, and sauces. Ask for dressings on the side of a salad to use less.

Trim portion sizes when dining out: Share entrees or order an appetizer portion to help trim calories.

Avoid multitasking when eating: Eating while watching TV or using the computer increases mindless eating of unwanted calories.

Make better choices: Eat more fruits and vegetables at meals to improve fullness and satiety. Extra fiber and water in these foods helps people eat less of other foods.

Practice eating less: Practice stopping eating when almost full. Eating until the point of fullness increases reflux and unwanted calorie consumption.

Long-term use of PPI therapy in adults could influence the absorption of several micronutrients such as calcium, B_{12}, vitamin C, vitamin D, and iron.[25] Modifying gastric pH can impact bioavailability of these nutrients, which translates to lower circulating serum values. Serum iron appears to be particularly impacted by lack of stomach acid. The odds of having a 1.0 g/dL drop in serum hemoglobin in adults using PPI therapy is five times greater than in adults not taking PPI therapy (OR = 5.03 [95% CI, 1.71–14.78, P = 0.01]). Similarly, a 3% drop in hematocrit is approximately five times more likely in patients taking PPIs compared with patients not taking medication (OR = 5.46 [95% CI, 1.67–17.85, P = 0.01]).[25] While this finding does not always translate into iron deficiency, the hematologic impact should be considered in patients at risk of iron deficiency and those needing treatment for existing anemia.

B_{12} absorption can also be impacted by gastric acid suppression. B_{12} exists in a protein matrix within animal products and fortified foods. Gastric acid is required to liberate this protein-bound nutrient for adherence to intrinsic factor and subsequent absorption in the terminal ileum.[26] Several studies support lower intestinal absorption and lower circulating serum values of B_{12} in individuals on long-term PPI therapy.[27,28] This may be most profound in the elderly and those with *H-pylori* infection. Outcome data on the consequence of this finding is lacking and, therefore, routine screening of serum B_{12} levels among patients on PPI therapy has not been recommended.

Although PPI use can alter the absorption of key nutrients, additional supplementation in patients taking PPI therapy has not yet been suggested. Routine screening in high risk patients is reasonable, however.

Emphasis on a healthy diet or supplementation required by life stage (i.e., pregnant or lactating women) should be driving supplementation recommendations. Approximately 10%–30% of adults 50 or older experience diminished absorption of B_{12} from foods. Therefore, foods supplementation from a multivitamin or from fortified foods is recommended in this age group. Medical monitoring of serum values of B_{12} and iron is recommended for adults receiving PPI therapy.

Because PPIs can alter the absorption of ionized calcium and vitamin D, they have been implicated in the increased risk of hip fracture. Impacting micronutrient

TABLE 8.2

Dietary Reference Intakes for Adult Men and Women for Calcium, Vitamin D, and B$_{12}$

Nutrient	Women < 50	Women > 50	Men < 50	Men > 50
Calcium	1000 mg	1200 mg	1000	1200
Vitamin D[a]	600–800 IU	600–800 IU	600–800 IU	600–800 IU
Vitamin B$_{12}$	2.4 µg	2.4 µg	2.4 µg	2.4 µg

[a] Some people may need additional or prescription levels of vitamin D if deficiency exists. The tolerable upper level of vitamin D intake is 4000 IU based on current USDA guidelines.

metabolism or directly affecting bone remodeling are possible mechanisms for increased risk of osteoporosis in adults.[25,29,30] Several observational studies demonstrate a modest increased risk of hip and vertebral fractures among adults using PPI therapy.[31,32] In 2010, the Food and Drug Administration (FDA) released new warnings associated with the use of PPI therapy for patients and health care professionals.[33] These warnings suggest an increased risk of hip, wrist, and vertebral fracture among adult users who are at high risk for fractures. However, the exact mechanisms for an increased risk of fractures with PPI therapy are unknown, and there are currently no randomized controlled trials evaluating the connection between PPI use and fractures. Conflicting observational evidence exists. Recent meta-analysis demonstrate no statistically significant increased risk of hip or vertebral fracture among individuals using PPI therapy >1 year compared with nonusers (OR = 1.30; 95% CI = 0.98–1.70).[29] Case control studies found no association (estimated RR = 0.9; 95% CI = 0.7–1.1) among adults ages 50–70 years old who were considered low fracture risk and were on PPI therapy >1 year. In the Manitoba Bone Mineral Density Database, the study with the longest follow-up to date, cases with osteoporosis at the hip or lumbar spine were matched to three controls with normal bone mineral density. PPI use over the previous 5 years was not associated with having osteoporosis in either the hip (OR = 0.84; 95% CI = 0.55–1.34) or the lumbar spine (OR = 0.79; 95% CI = 0.59–1.06).[34] Current guidelines suggest PPI use can continue in patients with osteoporosis or those at risk of developing osteoporosis with careful monitoring.[14] However, patients and providers need to increase surveillance parameters of bone health through bone density screenings and by optimizing serum markers of key nutrients involved in bone health including calcium and vitamin D. Based on current dietary reference intakes for adults, the following daily amounts of calcium and vitamins D and B$_{12}$ are listed in Table 8.2.[35]

8.4 EOSINOPHILIC ESOPHAGITIS

EoE is an inflammatory condition of the esophagus, which can result in dysphagia and food impaction in adults.[36–38] Consensus guidelines define EoE as a chronic, immune/antigen-mediated esophageal disease characterized clinically by symptoms related to esophageal dysfunction and histologically by eosinophil-predominant inflammation.[36–38] The role of food allergens in the development of EoE was first introduced by Kelly and Sampson in a landmark study.[39] They found that treatment with an elemental or amino acid-based formula resulted in symptom and histologic resolution in a cohort of pediatric patients who had symptoms of GERD and histologic features of esophageal eosinophilia.[39,40] Symptom recurrence occurred after open food challenges, further supporting this link between food allergens and EoE. Common food triggers found in pediatric EoE patients are cow's milk, soy, wheat, peanut, and egg.[39,40] The role of food allergens in EoE has been replicated in subsequent, larger pediatric series.[36,41–45]

Due to this link, dietary therapy has been one of the most effective treatments for EoE. Three approaches to dietary elimination in EoE patients have evolved. The first is total elimination of all food allergens by placing patients on an elemental or amino acid-based formula for at least 6 weeks.

While this is the most effective diet at controlling histologic eosinophilia, there are practical limitations to this approach.[41] The formulas can be costly, and children often require the use of feeding gastrostomy tubes to administer the formula, due to the palatability. Most adults, however, are able to take the nutrition orally. The need for repeated endoscopies during food reintroduction process and the length of time to complete food reintroduction is a concern with this approach.

Another approach to dietary therapy has been allergy-directed diets using the information gained from allergy testing to help guide the foods that are to be restricted. While this has been shown to be helpful in some pediatric cohorts, this has had limited utility in adult populations due to the lack of correlation with allergy testing and food triggers.[37,46,47] The third approach is an empiric elimination diet called the six food elimination diet (SFED) where patients empirically eliminate milk, wheat, soy, egg, nuts/peanuts, and fish/shellfish for a period of 6 weeks. Kagalwalla and colleagues in a retrospective study of pediatric patients described this first. They evaluated the outcomes of patients undergoing SFED as compared to those undergoing a traditional elemental diet (ED). These investigators found that 74% of patients who were treated with SFED had a histologic resolution as defined by <10 eos/hpf (eosinophils/high power field) after therapy compared with 88% in patients undergoing ED. Given this comparable response, they concluded that SFED offers advantages of better acceptance, cost, and compliance and, therefore, should be considered as an alternate initial dietary treatment option in EoE.[42,45]

8.4.1 EFFECTIVENESS OF EMPIRIC ELIMINATION DIETS IN ADULTS

Recently, empiric dietary elimination has also been shown to be effective in adults.[38,46] Gonsalves et al.[38] prospectively studied the efficacy of the SFED in 50 adults (25 M/25 F) with EoE. After 6 weeks of SFED, 70% of patients had histologic response of <10 eos/hpf, 94% had symptomatic improvement, and 74% had endoscopic improvement. In patients who responded, serial food reintroduction was undertaken and identified the common food allergens as wheat (60%), milk (50%), soy (10%), nuts (10%), and egg (5%). Allergy testing was undertaken prior to the elimination diet but was predictive of food triggers in only 13% of cases.[37,38] Another recent study from Spain demonstrated similar results in 67 adults with EoE after empiric elimination of wheat, rice, corn, legumes, peanuts, soy, egg, milk, fish, and shellfish resulting in histologic resolution of <15 eos/hpf in 73% of patients.[4] Food reintroduction identified the common triggers as milk (61%), wheat (28%), eggs (26%), and legumes (23%). A result of allergy testing in this cohort of patients was also not predictive of their food trigger.[46] In this study, continued elimination of these food triggers was effective in maintaining remission.

8.4.2 APPROACH TO DIETARY THERAPY IN ADULT EoE

Since dietary therapy is effective in adults, it can be used as an alternative to swallowed topical corticosteroids.[36] Dietary elimination with food reintroduction has the ability to identify the actual triggers of the disease. This allows patients to have more control in their ability to alter their allergen intake and, therefore, their esophageal inflammation. Avoidance of food allergens eliminates the need for chronic medication/corticosteroids to help control the disease and also has the advantage of getting to the root cause of the disease, that is, food allergen avoidance rather than symptom and histologic control. The decision to use medical or dietary therapy should be individualized based on patient preference as well as available resources. Implementing diet therapy appropriately is essential and is discussed in Section 8.4.4.

8.4.3 IMPLEMENTING SFED IN CLINICAL PRACTICE: THE CHICAGO EXPERIENCE

Dietary elimination is an alternative to topical corticosteroids for patients who meet criteria for EoE.[36,47] After 6 weeks of the elimination diet, an upper endoscopy with biopsy is undertaken to assess treatment response and the same biopsy protocol as used for diagnosis is completed. If the treatment is successful, systematic food reintroduction is pursued. Once the food trigger(s) has/have been identified, patients are counseled on avoidance of the trigger food/s. Long-term food allergen avoidance has been effective in controlling EoE in both children and adults. Avoiding whole food groups requires specific nutritional counseling to ensure both allergen avoidance as well as nutritional balance. Detailed nutritional protocols demonstrating food reintroduction protocols and healthy allergy-free meal plans have been published.[47]

8.4.3.1 Wheat Avoidance

Wheat is a major dietary trigger in two adult dietary studies.[37,38,47] Areas of potential wheat consumption and cross contamination of wheat can include the grain itself as well as breading, gravies, sauces, marinades, and fried foods.[46]

Products labeled as gluten and wheat free are increasingly popular and have grown by 28% since 2004.[48,49] Despite their popularity, wheat-free products are largely refined and are not fortified with iron or B vitamins such as folic acid, as are conventional grains.[49] Nutritional balance of key nutrients can be accomplished by the addition of whole, gluten-free grains such as quinoa, oats, brown rice, and millet. These whole grains are rich sources of B vitamins, iron, and trace minerals including magnesium.[50,51]

8.4.3.2　Milk Avoidance

Among children and adults, cow's milk protein is one of the most common allergens, accounting for more than 50% of the food triggers in patients with EoE.[46,52] Nutritionally, dairy products are rich in protein and are fortified with vitamins A and D as well as thiamin, riboflavin, B_{12}, and calcium. Milk avoidance can result in a low dietary intake of these key nutrients. Fortified rice milk, fortified hemp, and flax milk are acceptable fortified milk substitutes to augment dietary quality. Consumers should be aware of hidden dairy derivatives including added butter, casein and whey proteins powders, chocolate, and marinades. Occasionally, products such as deli meats, sausages, hot dogs, chicken nuggets, and other processed meats can contain cheese flavorings, which serve as a source of contamination.

8.4.4　Egg Avoidance

Eggs are rich in protein, choline, and B-vitamins. However, these nutrients can be obtained by the addition of legumes, seeds, quinoa, and lean animal proteins. Hidden sources of egg protein include mayonnaise, meringues, foams, marzipan, pastas, nougat, and baked goods. The prevalence of egg allergies among adults participating in the SFED ranges from 5% to 26.2%.[38,47]

8.4.4.1　Soy Avoidance

Soy beans and soy products are vegan proteins with a complete amino acid profile similar to animal proteins. Additionally, they are rich in nutrients such as calcium, folic acid, fiber, iron, and essential fatty acids.[53]

Highly refined soybean oil and soy lecithin are exempt from being labeled as an allergen by the FDA. Soybean oils and soy lecithin can be consumed during the SFED unless an IgE-mediated allergic response to soy is known. Soybean oils labeled as cold pressed, expeller pressed, or extruded oils should still be avoided as they still contain soy protein.[53] Common sources of soy protein include soy sauce, Asian foods, snack products, veggie burgers, protein shakes, margarine, and nondairy creamer.

8.4.4.2　Peanut and Tree Nut Avoidance

Peanut and tree nut allergies are less common than wheat and cow's milk protein in adults with EoE.[38] The most common sources of peanut and tree nut contamination include baked goods, cereals, snack foods, and whole grain breads. Consumers should be aware that fried foods, breaded dishes, breads, desserts, condiments, salads, and food prep surfaces are all potential sources of nut contamination when dining out.[54,55]

8.4.4.3　Avoiding Fish and Shellfish

Among adults with EoE, fish and shellfish allergies are rare compared with other foods.[38] Hidden sources of fish and shellfish proteins can often include ethnic cuisine, Worcestershire sauce, fish oil or omega-3 fortified products, soups containing fish stock, risotto, and stews. Fish is a rich source of protein and omega-3 fatty acids and this can be achieved by incorporation of lean poultry and seeds such as flax seeds and chia seeds.

8.4.4.4   Label Reading and Avoiding Cross Contamination

In 2006, the U.S. Congress passed the Food Allergen Labeling and Consumer Protection Act which mandated that companies list foods containing major allergens including milk, eggs, fish, shellfish, peanuts, tree nuts, wheat, and soy in plain language.[56] Unlike celiac disease and IgE-mediated food allergies, no clear agreement exists on the amount of allergens necessary to elicit an allergic reaction in EoE. Therefore, a SFED should emphasize avoiding the allergen directly and avoiding hidden sources of contamination. When at home or dining out, common sources of cross contamination can include shared cooking equipment, shared cooktop surfaces, sponges, salad bars, and condiments.

8.4.4.5   Managing Nutritional Limitations of SFED

Any restricted diet can pose significant nutritional risks and set the stage for both micronutrient and macronutrient deficiencies. Dietary intake of key nutrients including zinc, B-vitamins, calcium, vitamin D, magnesium, selenium, as well as fiber, calories, and protein can be jeopardized if alternative sources of these vitamins are not incorporated. Current dietary guidelines for adults include a nutrient intake emphasizing a balance of fruits, vegetables, whole grains, lean proteins, and heart healthy fats.[57,58] These requirements can be achieved while on SFED with proper nutritional preplanning and the expertise of a registered dietitian skilled in food allergies, and restricted diets. Utilizing food logs can help provide accountability and insight to optimize the response to SFED.

Assessing response to dietary therapy is confirmed typically 6 weeks after the SFED is begun with an EGD. Patients achieving histologic improvement (<5 eos/hpf) begin systematically adding back food groups for 2 weeks with symptom monitoring. After two food groups have been reintroduced, a repeat EGD is suggested to verify inactive disease status prior to continuing on with the food reintroduction trial. If a food is found to be a trigger, then a 6-week wash out period of avoidance of that trigger food is needed before moving on to the next food group. Although fish and shellfish are tested within the same time period, patients can separately test fin fish for 1 week and shellfish for another week to better evaluate symptoms and potential reactions. This reintroduction process is continued until all six food groups are completed.[37,38,47] Ultimately, the process and timeline of elimination diets and food reintroduction can differ between centers. This process of food elimination and reintroduction is illustrated in Figure 8.1.

8.5   CONCLUSION

GERD and EoE are common gastrointestinal disorders seen by both primary care physicians and gastroenterologists. In addition to medical management of these esophageal disorders, lifestyle, and dietary modifications are important adjunctive therapy. In GERD, an emphasis on weight loss, head of bed positioning, and meal volume reduction enhance PPI therapy. In EoE, removal of food allergens allows for a balanced, allergy-free dietary treatment plan that significantly improves histopathologic features, symptoms, and endoscopic findings in EoE. A multidisciplinary approach to these disorders involving gastroenterologists, allergists, and dietitians is important in optimal treatment and management of these conditions.

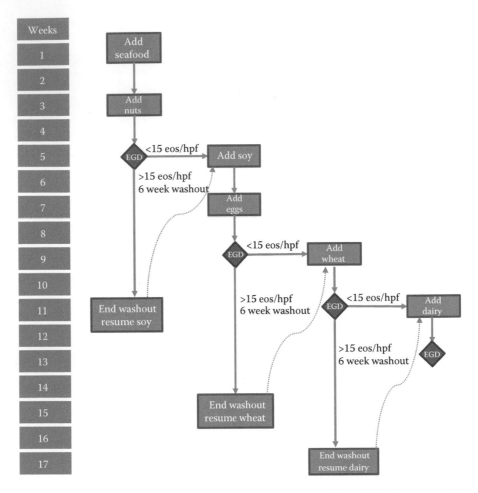

FIGURE 8.1 SFED dietary therapy: food reintroduction algorithm following successful response to SFED.

8.6 CASE STUDY

TF is a 58-year-old female who was referred to GI for management of dysphagia which had been occurring weekly for past few years. She had a history of allergic rhinitis but was otherwise healthy and denied any previous surgery. She began altering her eating pattern by taking smaller bites of food, having drinks with meals and eating moist foods. She was managing well but recently noted increased episodes of feeling food stuck. This seemed to resolve with ample fluids. Overall, she denied heartburn or chest pain on a regular basis. She presented to GI with food impaction that lasted for approximately 18 h after eating chicken. An emergent EGD was performed with subsequent food disimpaction. Visual changes of the esophagus consistent with EoE were noted including ringed esophagus, longitudinal furrows, small caliber esophagus, and white plaques. Initial biopsy revealed EoE with micro abscesses of up to 80 eos/hpf. She was started on omeprazole 40 mg daily for 6 weeks and repeat EGD was performed, which revealed mildly increased number of intraepithelial eosinophils, 13 eos/hpf in the proximal esophagus, and 17 eos/hpf in the distal esophagus. Although, the patient was PPI responsive, she had persistent mild eosinophilia. A clinical office visit was scheduled to discuss treatment options for EoE including diet or medication and the risk and benefits of each therapy. The patient chose to begin the SFED as a primary treatment for EoE.

Baseline Physical Assessment:
Neck: no adenopathy or thyromegaly
Cardiac: regular rate and rhythm
Lungs: clear to auscultation and percussion
Abdomen: soft nondistended nontender; bowel sounds active
Extremities: no edema, sclerodactyly
Skin: no telangiectasia
Labs: unremarkable
Weight/height: 5′9″, 179#, BMI = 26

TF met with the registered dietitian for assessment and education of SFED in which the top six allergic foods are avoided including wheat, dairy, nuts/tree nuts, fish/shellfish, eggs, and soy. She was counseled on how to avoid allergens in both obvious and hidden forms. She was given extensive materials that included allergy-free sample menus that were nutritionally balanced, and label reading and dining out guides. She was also instructed to add in an allergy-free multivitamin and 1000 mg calcium as well as 800 IU vitamin D daily.

After following the SFED for approximately 6 weeks, she reported feeling well and noted less dysphagia. Interim food diary review indicated good dietary adherence and good dietary balance. Repeat EGD demonstrated inactive EoE. She was allowed to begin with the food reintroduction protocol. At this time, her weight decreased to 160 lbs, which was consistent with a healthy weight and the patient reported being happy with her weight loss. Dietary recall revealed that the weight loss was largely due to avoidance of high sugar foods and fast foods that she would previously consume and was currently limiting. Her diet quality was excellent, and she was happy with her weight loss at this point. She reintroduced fish/shellfish for 2 weeks and then nuts/tree nuts for 2 weeks and underwent a follow-up EGD. Biopsies revealed inactive disease. She continued with the protocol, adding in soy for 2 weeks and eggs for 2 weeks on top of her baseline diet. Symptomatically, TF continued to report feeling well.

Follow-up EGD revealed inactive disease. This process was repeated until she reintroduced dairy. After approximately 3 days of food reintroduction, she noted increased throat pain and increased mucous production. After 1 week of increased symptoms, EGD was repeated which revealed anatomical signs of active disease including edema, linear furrows, and white exudates. Biopsies revealed 40 eos/hpf. Both the combination of acid reflux and cow's milk protein allergy were dual agents in driving her EoE activity.

TF was encouraged to stay on her omeprazole and a milk-free diet to maintain remission of her EoE, and to return to see her GI every year for surveillance EGD.

REFERENCES

1. Dent J, El-Serag HB, Wallander M-A, Johansson S. Epidemiology of gastro-oesophageal reflux disease: A systematic review. *Gut* 2005;54(5):710–717.
2. Straumann A, Simon HU. Eosinophilic oesophagitis: Escalating epidemiology? *J Allergy Clin Immunol* 2005;115:418–419.
3. Kahrilas P, Shaheen N, Vaezi M. American Gastroenterological Association Medical Position Statement on the management of gastroesophageal reflux disease. *Gastroenterology* 2008;135:1383–1391.
4. Kahrilas PJ, Boeckxstaens G. Republished: Failure of reflux inhibitors in clinical trials: Bad drugs or wrong patients? *Postgrad Med J* 2013;89(1048):111–119.
5. Longo D, Fauci A, Kasper D, Hauser S, Jameson J, Loscalzo J. *Harrison's Principles of Internal Medicine*, Vol. 1 and 2. USA: McGraw Hill; 2011.
6. Liacouras CA, Furuta GT, Hirano I et al. Eosinophilic esophagitis: Updated consensus recommendations for children and adults. *J Allergy Clin Immunol* 2011;128(1):3–20.
7. Kern E, Hirano I. Emerging drugs for eosinophilic esophagitis. *Expert Opin Emerging Drugs* 2013;18(3):353–364.
8. Delon ES, Gonsalves N, Hirano I et al. ACG clinical guideline: Evidence based approach to the diagnosis and management of esophageal eosinophilia and eosinophilic esophagitis (EoE). *Am J Gastroenterol* 2013;108(5):679–692.
9. Heidelbaugh JJ. Proton pump inhibitors and risk of vitamin and mineral deficiency: Evidence and clinical implications. *Ther Adv Drug Saf* Jun 2013;4(3):125–133.
10. Insogna KL. The effect of proton pump inhibiting drugs on mineral metabolism. *Am J Gastroenterol* 2009;104:S2–S4.
11. Koop H. Review article: Metabolic consequences of long-term inhibition of acid secretion by omeprazole. *Aliment Pharmacol Ther* 1992;6:399–406.
12. Festi D, Eleonora Scaioli E, Baldi F et al. Body weight, lifestyle, dietary habits and gastroesophageal reflux disease. *World J Gastroenterol* 2009;15(14);1690–1701.
13. Kaltenbach T, Crockett S, Gerson LB. Are lifestyle measures effective in patients with gastroesophageal reflux disease? An evidence-based approach. *Arch Intern Med* 2006;166:965–971.
14. Katz PO, Gerson LB, Vela MF. Guidelines for the diagnosis and management of gastroesophageal reflux disease. *Am J Gastroenterol* 2013;108(3):308–328.
15. DeVault KR, Castell DO. Updated guidelines for the diagnosis and treatment of gastroesophageal reflux disease. *Am J Gastroenterol* 2005;100:190–200.
16. Stanciu C, Bennett JR. Effects of posture on gastro-oesophageal reflux. *Digestion* 1977;15:104–109.
17. Hamilton JW, Boisen RJ, Yamamoto DT et al. Sleeping on a wedge diminishes exposure of the esophagus to refluxed acid. *Dig Dis Sci* 1988;33:518–522.
18. Pollmann H, Zillessen E, Pohl J et al. Effect of elevated head position in bed in therapy of gastroesophageal reflux. *Z Gastroenterol* 1996;34(suppl 2): 93–99.
19. Ness-Jensen E, Lindam A, Lagergren J, Hveem K. Weight loss and reduction in gastroesophageal reflux. A prospective population-based cohort study: The HUNT study. *Am J Gastroenterol* 2013;108(3):376–382.
20. Singh M, Lee J, Gupta N et al. Weight loss can lead to resolution of gastroesophageal reflux disease symptoms: A prospective intervention trial. *Obesity* 2012;2:284–290.
21. Jacobson BC, Somers SC, Fuchs CS et al. Body-mass index and symptoms of gastroesophageal reflux in women. *N Engl J Med* 2006;354:2340–2348.

22. El-Serag HB, Hashmi A, Garcia J et al. Visceral abdominal obesitymeasured by CT scan is associated with an increased risk of Barrett's oesophagus: A case control study. *Gut* 2014;63(2):220–229.
23. Penagini R, Carmagnola S, Cantu P, Allocca M, Bianchi PA. Mechanoreceptors of the proximal stomach: Role in triggering transient lower esophageal sphincter relaxation. *Gastroenterology* 2004;126:49–56.
24. Wu JC, Mui LM, Cheung CM, Chan Y, Sung JJ. Obesity is associated with increased transient lower esophageal sphincter relaxation. *Gastroenterology* 2007;132:883–889.
25. McColl K. Effect of proton pump inhibitors on vitamins and iron. *Am J Gastroenterol* 2009;104(suppl 2):S5–S9.
26. Allen RH, Seetharam B, Podell E et al. Effect of proteolytic enzymes on the binding of cobalamin to R protein and intrinsic factor. *J Clin Invest* 1978;61:47–54.
27. Marcuard SP, Albernaz L, Khazanie PG. Omeprazole therapy causes malabsorption of cyanocobalamin (Vitamin B12). *Ann Intern Med* 1994;120:211–215.
28. Steinberg WM, King CE, Toskes PP. Malabsorption of protein-bound cobalamin but not unbound cobalamin during cimetidine administration. *Dig Dis Sci* 1980;25:188–191.
29. Ngamruengphong S, Leontiadis G, Radhi S, Dentino A, Nugent K. Proton pump inhibitors and risk of hip fractures: A systematic review and meta-analysis of observational studies. *Am J Gastroenterol* 2011;106:1209–1218.
30. Yang YX, Lewis JD, Epstein S, Metz DC. Long-term proton pump inhibitor therapy and risk of hip fracture. *JAMA* 2006;296:2947–2953.
31. Kaye JA, Jick H. Proton pump inhibitor use and risk of hip fractures in patients without major risk factors. *Pharmacotherapy* 2008;28:951–59.
32. Gray SL, LaCroix AZ, Larson J et al. Proton pump inhibitor use, hip fracture, and change in bone mineral density in postmenopausal women: Results from the women's health initiative. *Arch Intern Med* 2010;170:765–771.
33. FDA Drug Safety Communication: Possible increased risk of fractures of the hip, wrist, and spine with the use of proton pump inhibitors. Available at: http://www.fda.gov/drugs/drugsafety/postmarketdrugsafetyinformationforpatientsandproviders/ucm213206.htm. Accessed November 22, 2013.
34. Targownik LE, Lix LM, Leung S et al. Proton pump inhibitor use is not associated with osteoporosis or accelerated bone mineral density loss. *Gastroenterology* 2010;138:896–904.
35. Food and Nutrition Board. Institute of Medicine Dietary Reference Intakes for Vitamins and Minerals. Available at http://www.iom.edu/Activities/Nutrition/SummaryDRIs/~/media/Files/Activity%20Files/Nutrition/DRIs/5_Summary%20Table%20Tables%201–4.pdf. Accessed September 2, 2014.
36. Liacouras CA, Furuta GT, Hirano I, Atkins D, Attwood SE et al. Eosinophilic esophagitis: Updated consensus recommendations for children and adults. *J Allergy Clinc Immunol* 2011;128(1):3–20.
37. Gonsalves N, Ritz S, Yang GY, Ditto A, Hirano I. A prospective clinical trial of allergy testing and food elimination diets in adults with eosinophilic esophagitis. *Gastroenterology* 2008;132.
38. Gonsalves N, Yang GY, Doerfler B et al. Elimination diet effectively treats eosinophilic esophagitis in adults; food reintroduction identifies causative factos. *Gastroenterology* 2012;142(7):1451–1459.
39. Kelly KJ, Lazenby AJ, Rowe PC, Yardley JH, Perman JA, Sampson HA. Eosinophilic esophagitis attributed to gastroesophageal reflux: Improvement with an amino acid based forumula. *Gastroenterology* 1995;109(5):1503–1512.
40. Markowitz JE, Spergel JM, Ruchelli E, Liacouras CA. Elemental diet is an effective treatment for esoinophilic esophagitis in children and adolescents. *Am J Gastroenterol* 2003;98:777–782.

41. Liacouras CA, Spergel JM, Ruchelli E et al. Eosinophilic esophagitis: A 10-year experience in 381 children. *Clin Gastroenterol Hepatol* 2005;3:1198–1206.
42. Kagalwalla AF, Sentongo TA, Ritz et al. Effect of six food elimination diet on clinical and histologic outcomes in esoinophilic esophagitis. *Clin Gastroenterol Hepatol* 2006;4:1097–1102.
43. Orenstein SR, Shalaby TI, Di Lorenzo C et al. The spectrum of pediatric eosinophilic esophagitis beyond infancy: A clinical case series of 30 children. *Am J Gastroenterol* 2009;95:1422–1430.
44. Spergel JM, Brown-Whitehorn TF, Cianferoni A, Shuker M, Wang ML, Verma R, Liacouras CA. Identification of causative foods in children with eosinophilic esophatitis treated with an elimination diet. *J Allergy Clin Immunol* 2012;130(2):461–467.
45. Kagalwalla AF, Shah A, Li UK et al. Identification of specific foods responsible for inflammation in children with eosinophilic esophagitis successfully treated with empiric elimination diet. *JPGN* 2011;53(2):145–149.
46. Lucendo AJ, Arias A, Gonzalez-Cervera J, Compadres Y, Angueira T et al. Emperic 6-food elimination diet induced and maintained prolonged remission in patients with adult eosinophilic esophagitis: A prospective study on the food cause of the disease. *J Allergy Clin Immunol* 2013;131(3):797–804.
47. Doerfler B, Bryce P, Hirano I, Gonsalves N. Practical approach to implementing dietary therapy in adults with eosinophilic esophagitis: The Chicago experience. *Dis Esophagus* 2014;(1):42–58.
48. Gaesser GA, Angadi SS. Gluten free diet: Imprudent dietary advice for the general population? *J Acad Nutr Diet* 2012;112(9):1330–1333.
49. Pagano AE. Whole grains and the gluten free diet. *Pract Gastroenterol* 2006;29: 66–78. http://www.practical gastro.com/pdf/October06/PaganoArticle.pdf. Accessed September 1, 2014.
50. Case S, Fenster C. Gluten free whole grains. Available at: http://www.glutenfreediet.ca/img/WholeGrainHandoutFinal2012.pdf. Accessed April 12, 2013.
51. Lee AR, Ng DL, Dave EJ, Ciaccio EH, Green PH. The effect of substituting alternative grains in the diet on the nutritional profile of the gluten free diet. *J Hum Nutr Diet* 2009;22:359–363.
52. Kagalwalla AF, Amsden K, Shah A, Ritz S, Manuel-rubio M, Dunne K, Nelson SP et al. Cow's milk protein elimination: A novel dietary approach to treat eosinophilic esophagitis. *J Pediatr Gastroenterol Nutr* 2012;55(6):711–716.
53. National Soybean Research Laboratory Illinois: Basic Soybean Facts. Available at: http://www.nsrl.uiuc.edu/aboutsoy/soynutrition.html. Accessed April 24, 2014.
54. Ahuja R, Sicherer SH. Food allergy management from the perspective of restaurant and food establishment personnel. *Ann Allergy Asthma Immunol* 2007;98(4):344–348.
55. Furlong TJ. DeSimone J, Sicherer SH. Peanut and tree nut allergic reactions in restaurants and other food establishments. *J Allergy Clin Immunol* 2001;108:867–870.
56. United States Food and Drug Administration: Food Allergen Labeling and Consumer Protection Act 2004: Public Law 108–282 Title II. Available at: http://www.fda.gov/Food/GuidanceRegulation/GuidanceDocumentsRegulatoryInformation/Allergens/ucm106187.ht. Accessed June 6, 2014.
57. Food and Nutrition Board Institute of Medicine Dietary Reference Intakes for Energy, Carbohydrate, Fiber, Fat, Fatty Acids, Cholesterol, Protein, and Amino Acids. Available at: http://iom.edu/Reports/2002/Dietary-Reference-Intakes-for-Energy-Carbohydrate-Fiber-Fat-Fatty-Acids-Cholesterol-Protein-and-Amino-Acids.aspx. Accessed September 1, 2014.
58. Dietary Guidelines for Americans, 2010. Available at: http://www.health.gov/dietary guidelines/2010.asp. Accessed August 21, 2014.

9 Nutrition and Celiac Disease

Jacalyn A. See and Joseph A. Murray

CONTENTS

9.1   DIAGNOSIS OF CELIAC DISEASE

Celiac disease (CD) is the culmination of an aberrant inflammatory response to "gluten" that refers to the storage proteins gliadins and glutenins from wheat, secalins from rye, and hordeins from barley. This reaction results in inflammation of and damage to the structures and function of the small intestine. The inflammatory response not only produces tissue injury in the small intestine, which is largely dependent on a cellular-based, but also a humoral response that results in antibodies present in the circulation. These antibodies are most often IgA-based antibodies directed against both gluten components as well as the autoantigen tissue transglutaminase (tTG) and the covalent complexes formed by both.

The symptoms occur largely because of the damage to the small intestine. This damage can lead to symptoms due to local inflammation as well as maldigestion and malabsorption of nutrients. Increases in secretion and decreases in absorption of liquid result in diarrhea. There may also be changes in motility and perhaps even sensory inputs can result in altered gut sensations. While CD in the past has been considered a solely classic malabsorptive disorder, which results in substantial malnutrition, weight loss, or failure to thrive in children, hence steatorrhea, the majority of patients no longer present with those symptoms. Indeed, even diarrhea is not universal in patients with CD. There is a tremendous reserve capacity of the small intestine for making up for some of the perturbations caused by CD. This can allow for scavenging of excess calories and reduction of fluid to prevent diarrhea occurring. Many patients present with monosymptomatic symptoms, such as diarrhea, anemia, particularly iron deficiency anemia, and occasionally other gastrointestinal symptoms such as nausea, vomiting, and abdominal distention postprandially, as well as subtle symptoms as excess flatulence. Some patients may not complain of symptoms at all because their symptoms are so insidious the patient comes to regard them as normal. Patients may present primarily with deficiency states—deficiencies of iron, vitamin D, vitamin B_{12}, and other fat-soluble vitamins are relatively common, at least in adults though perhaps less common in children.

Secondary manifestations of CD outside of the gastrointestinal tract may be due to consequences that may or may not be nutritional—for example, infertility. Neurologic disorders, including peripheral neuropathy, cognitive impairment, and balance disorders such as ataxia may be the first presentation of CD. Neuropsychiatric disorders, including chronic fatigue, are common symptoms, but lack specificity for CD. There is some overlap in the symptom complex associated with CD and irritable bowel syndrome (IBS), though the data on the actual overlap between these is somewhat controversial, as population-based studies do not demonstrate a significant association between IBS-like symptoms and hidden CD. The data on testing patients with overt IBS symptoms are variable and certainly consideration for testing for CD is important in this setting.

Children may present with delayed development, failure to thrive, and growth retardation. Most often, presentation in children now occurs in somewhat older children 7–12 years of age as opposed to the past when it was often much younger, shortly after introduction of gluten into the diet.

Individuals who have symptoms or syndromes associated with CD should be considered for testing for CD. In addition, those who have a family history of CD or who have other conditions that put them at substantially increased risk of CD should also be considered for testing. This includes patients with Down syndrome, type 1 diabetes, and other autoimmune diseases.

There are some circumstances where CD is a rare cause of their syndrome, but where it would be a particularly treatable cause. For example, pulmonary hemosiderosis is a very rare complication of CD, but when CD is detected in this setting and treated, the hemosiderosis usually resolves. In addition, several studies suggest that patients with chronic dyspepsia are not particularly enriched with CD but, when it is discovered, the dyspepsia can be readily treated with treatment of CD. Another circumstance would be recent-onset ataxia for which CD would be a rare cause, but with early intervention the ataxia may be reversible. CD is also far more common among non-Hispanic whites compared to others.

9.2   DETECTION OF CD

Most often, CD is first detected by the use of celiac-specific serology. Serologic tests for CD have been available for many decades. They started first with anti-gluten antibodies, were subsequently replaced with anti-gliadin antibodies, and more recently it is the auto-antibodies directed against tTG that have supplanted these earlier tests. The endomysial antibody (EMA) introduced first in 1987 is directed against the connective tissue fibers surrounding smooth muscle bundles in the monkey esophagus and has subsequently been shown to reflect an antibody response directed against tTG as it is extruded extracellularly in its activated form. The antibodies in CD are predominately IgA based, though IgG antibodies can be seen. Furthermore, the antibodies are quite sensitive to the removal of gluten from the diet. A newer adaptation of the gliadin antibodies are the so-called deamidated gliadin peptide antibodies. This test takes advantage of the fact that tTG deamidates particular glutamine residues in the gliadin molecule, making them into glutamic acids. This change in charge structure changes the affinity of the antigen to the major histocompatibility complex (MHC) molecule that presents these epitopes of gliadin to the gluten response of T cells. This deamidation step increases the affinity dramatically and greatly enhances the infective response to gluten or to these gliadin peptides by T cells. In addition, this deamidation state of gliadin leads to the development of antibodies directed against deamidated gliadin, which is far more specific for CD than antibodies directed against native gliadin antibody. The use of the deamidated gliadin antibodies is actually to supplement that of the tTG IgA. In addition, tTG can transamidate gliadin leading to stable neo-compounds that could be potent immunogens. Antibodies to this neo-epitope may be useful in detecting early-stage disease.

Endomysial antibodies, being an old test and requiring increased resources and expertise being subject to interpretation error, utilizes monkey esophagus for indirect immunofluorescence. The EMA, however, has the benefit of very high specificity and, when used sequentially with a positive tTG, greatly enhances the positive likelihood ratio of CD. The use of deamidated gliadin antibodies is supplemental to that of tTG IgA and might increase the sensitivity moderately. The primary use of deamidated gliadin antibodies is in patients with known IgA deficiency. In these patients, tTG IgA is unreliable and, when CD is suspected, tTG IgG and/or deamidated gliadin IgG antibodies can be performed.

Serological testing for CD has dramatically improved in specificity and sensitivity and indeed awareness of how these tests should be combined is important. For example, tTG IgA is the best single test and, in patients who are known not to be IgA deficient, is generally very effective. However, in some patients, especially those with lessor degree of injury, deamidated gliadin antibodies may provide additional sensitivity. In addition, if someone is double positive, it may increase the likelihood that they actually have CD. It is also important to know that false positives occur, especially when the positive results are close to the negative threshold. The more positive the tTG IgA, the greater likelihood of CD. The European Society for Pediatric Gastroenterology and Nutrition has recommended that a diagnosis of CD can be made in children who have symptoms of CD with a tTG that is >10 times the upper limit of normal if a subsequent separate blood sample is shown to be EMA positive and the patient carries the appropriate HLA risk genes for CD.[1] Selective IgA deficiency is rare in the community, maybe 1 in 600, but it is relatively common in patients with CD, and approximately 10% of people with IgA deficiency will subsequently develop CD. Hence, most strategies for the serologic diagnosis of CD incorporate the measurement of IgA. An alternative is to routinely measure IgG isotypes of the antibodies, but these tend to lack specificity, further detracting from the overall strategy.[2]

Confirmation of CD is done by undertaking small bowel biopsies. These typically are biopsies taken endoscopically in a sedated patient from the first and second part of the duodenum. Biopsies, while long considered the gold standard for the diagnosis of CD, have lately come under pressure, especially as it is realized that the biopsies are much more difficult to interpret than thought before.[3] Biopsies often show a spectrum of change from patients with total villous atrophy, an increased intraepithelial lymphocytosis, and crypt hyperplasia all the way down to partial villous atrophy with similar changes as above, to patients without any atrophy at all but increased intraepithelial lymphocytes. This latter state of what is called lymphocytic duodenosis is just increased intraepithelial lymphocytosis without villous atrophy or crypt hyperplasia. Patients with lymphocytic duodenosis most often (80%) do not have CD, and those few who do are often sero-positive and/or carry the HLA type associated with CD. In patients with lymphocytic duodenosis who are on a normal gluten-containing diet, it is especially important to consider other causes such as helicobacter, use of medications including nonsteroidal anti-inflammatory drugs (NSAIDs), presence of inflammatory bowel disease further downstream, or bacterial overgrowth, before concluding CD is the cause.[4]

In patients whose first diagnostic test is a biopsy showing villous atrophy, an assumption for CD should not be made without confirmation by serology as approximately 10% of patients who have villous atrophy in developed countries identified on biopsies will not have CD. The differential is very broad and includes conditions such as tropical sprue (can be identified by travel history), drug-associated enteropathy (including olmesartan, mycophenolate mofetil also known as CellCept, etc.), as well as other rare disorders such as common variable immunodeficiency, autoimmune enteropathy, and diffuse lymphoproliferative disorders of the intestine.

9.2.1 Nonceliac Gluten Sensitivity

Nonceliac gluten sensitivity has become recently recognized as a clinical entity of patients who often have gastrointestinal symptoms similar to IBS which respond to gluten exclusion. This is despite the absence of markers for CD, which are typically sero-negative. They may or may not carry the HLA type associated with CD, and this is a diagnosis of exclusion and requires a durable and specific response to the patient's symptoms to gluten exclusion. It is not even clear this is related to gluten; it may be in part due to other components of the wheat such as amylase trypsin inhibitors (ATI).[5]

9.2.2 Dermatitis Herpetiformis

Dermatitis herpetiformis is an extremely itchy vesiculating rash that affects primarily the extensor surfaces of the body, though excoriations often remove the blisters very quickly. It can occur in other parts of the body. It occurs more typically in adults than in children and is the skin manifestation of the enteric gluten-sensitive enteropathy. It shares the same genetic basis and indeed can occur within the same family or even in the same individual as a manifestation of gluten-sensitive enteropathy.[6] Patients who present with a skin manifestation typically have very little or no gastrointestinal symptoms. Approximately 75% of them will have enteropathy on biopsy, though 25% may have no or little enteropathy detectable. The severity of dermatitis herpetiformis may be independent of the severity of the intestinal disease and does not necessarily reflect the likelihood of gastrointestinal symptoms. The skin will exacerbate with gluten ingestion, though there may be a substantial delay between gluten ingestion and subsequent symptom exacerbation. The cause of the disorder beyond the gluten-sensitive enteropathy is not entirely known; however, it is thought that molecular mimicry between tTG, which is recognized by the autoantibodies in CD, overlaps with epidermal tTG, which is present in the skin. These IgA antibodies may become deposited at the site of epidermal tTG, especially in the papillae at the dermoepidermal junction. A neutrophil-based response to these IgA deposits may ensue and can cause blistering and substantial itching. The itching may be so severe that the patients will rapidly scratch off the top of the vesicles, leaving small sores that heal with scarring. These can occur and recur over months or years before diagnosis or can come on abruptly.

The diagnosis of dermatitis herpetiformis is typically made by appreciation of the appearance, pattern and pruritic nature of the rash, and biopsies. Biopsies taken from a lesion identify blistering and separation of the dermoepidermal junction with a neutrophilic infiltration, and a perilesional biopsy stained for IgA identifies the granular deposits of IgA immunofluorescence along the papillae. The presence of tTG antibodies and more recently epidermal tTG antibodies also support the diagnosis of dermatitis herpetiformis.[7]

The treatment of dermatitis herpetiformis is twofold. One is the removal of gluten from the diet as removal of the root cause, and the second can include the use of dapsone as a suppressive therapy, which suppresses the rash. The dapsone has no effect on the gastrointestinal effects of the disease. Typically, the gluten-free diet (GFD) works slowly and often incompletely in terms of relief of the rash, and dapsone is necessary at least on an interim basis to suppress the rash. About 70% of patients will be able to get off dapsone once they have been on a GFD at least 18 months. Often, a gradual reduction of dapsone is undertaken the longer the patient has been on a GFD. In some patients, very small amounts of gluten ingestion do not seem to stimulate the rash, but once the inflammatory process is initiated due to repeated dietary indiscretions, it can take months of a GFD for it to resolve. Rarely, in patients who are resistant, institution of an iodine-restricted diet may be necessary. There is anecdotal evidence that an elemental diet may be helpful in patients with severe rash and itching despite a GFD and dapsone. Skin application of gluten through skin contact is usually not an issue, as it requires enteric administration of gluten to produce a response. The use of dapsone needs to be monitored, in particular because of its effects on hemolysis and rarely causing agranulocytosis, which can be very serious and often acute in onset. Usually this occurs early after institution of treatment, and monitoring of blood counts is suggested. Fatigue and headaches are common side effects, which are dose related, as is methemoglobinemia, which can interfere with the carriage of oxygen. The need for duodenal biopsy is not needed to make a diagnosis of dermatitis herpetiformis, but rather to identify whether there is substantial enteropathy. Most of the nonskin manifestations are complications related to the enteropathy, not to the skin disease.

9.3   MANAGEMENT OF CD

The only available treatment for CD at this time is the strict avoidance of gluten, the protein found in wheat, rye, and barley.[8] The GFD should not begin until a diagnosis of CD has been confirmed. The purpose of a GFD is to control symptoms, improve quality of life (QOL), and prevent complications. Most people with CD will experience complete resolution of symptoms, normalization of serologies, and improvement of histology, although complete healing may take several years and is less certain in adults than in children.[9] A strict GFD also appears to prevent many of the potential complications of CD including, but not limited to, osteoporosis, intestinal malignancies, and neurologic complications. It may also slow or prevent the progression of other autoimmune diseases associated with CD but the data are conflicting.

It is important to have a team approach for the management of CD, including a physician, a celiac-competent registered dietitian, and others as needed, for example, an endocrinologist, oncologist, psychologist, and neurologist may also be needed depending on complications. Engagement with a support group can also be a valuable part of the team.

Because the diet is the core tenet of management, early referral to an expert celiac dietitian is recommended soon after diagnosis.[8,10] Insufficient education about the disease and diet is likely to lead to poor compliance, nonresponsive CD, frustration and anxiety for the patient and increased healthcare costs in the long run. Indeed, a GFD has been shown to reduce healthcare costs as well as long-term complications of CD.[11–13] Unfortunately, referral to a registered dietitian is often delayed sometimes for years after initial diagnosis.

9.3.1 NUTRITIONAL ASSESSMENT

An initial consultation should include a thorough nutrition assessment including weight status, medical history, biochemical data, and social situation.[10] The assessment should include a review of typical intake, food preferences, food intolerances or allergies and adequacy of nutrient intake, who prepares meals, where meals are eaten, the patient's food preparation skills, work travel and workplace exposure to airborne gluten. Other important data for planning and implementing a successful transition to a gluten-free lifestyle include accessibility to gluten-free foods, budget constraints, time constraints, social support, comorbidities (including psychiatric), educational level, and patient readiness. Does the patient accept the diagnosis, and what the treatment entails?

9.3.2 NUTRITIONAL DEFICIENCIES

Nutritional deficiencies are common in patients at the time of diagnosis of CD.[14,15] The severity and type of deficiencies depend in part on the duration of time the patient has had untreated CD as well as the extent and site of damage of the intestine. The actual deficiencies in CD are the result of the pathophysiologic changes that CD brings about. Of course, there is a substantial degree of fat malabsorption frequently seen in CD, and this can be associated with failure of absorption and therefore deficiencies of the fat soluble vitamins D, E, A, and K. In addition, the predilection for damage to the proximal small intestine, which is the site of absorption of iron, often leads to iron deficiency. Folic acid and B_{12} deficiencies may also occur for a variety of reasons, including inadequate opportunity for the effective transport of vitamin B_{12} along with its R factor and intrinsic factor and effective folic acid assimilation. In addition, zinc, calcium, magnesium and, occasionally, copper deficiencies may occur. It is estimated that at least half of the patients diagnosed with CD will have iron deficiency often with, but not always accompanied by, anemia. Iron deficiency is more common in patients during periods of rapid growth, such as early childhood, adolescence, pregnancy and during the active reproductive years with menstruation. Patients who have diarrhea with steatorrhea are most at risk for fat-soluble vitamin deficiencies. Serum calcium may also be depressed, and there may be a secondary hyperparathyroidism that can occur because of the vitamin D and calcium deficiency secondary to malabsorption. Often this metabolic bone disease can be quite subtle, with slight elevation of alkaline phosphatase evident. Substantial bone disease can occur in the absence of gastrointestinal symptoms. Some of the syndromes that can occur in response to deficiency states are outlined in Table 9.1. Rarely, scurvy from vitamin C, or other vitamin deficiencies, including B_1 and B_2 can be seen. Rarely, protein calorie malnutrition occurs and usually only in the most severe cases of CD.[16]

Deficiencies can be corrected by appropriate supplementation as seen in Table 9.1 and follow-up to assess response to treatment (Table 9.2). For severe bone disease, malabsorption doses of vitamin D, such as 50,000 units weekly, may be necessary to overcome the malabsorption. The continued use of malabsorption doses of

TABLE 9.1

Nutritional Deficiencies in CD and Their Treatment

Nutritional Deficiency	Clinical Manifestation	Treatment
Iron	Microcytic anemia, fatigue, restless legs	Iron replacement with either oral iron combined with vitamin C or parenteral iron if patient is unable to absorb oral iron
B_{12}	Macrocytic anemia, neurologic symptoms (peripheral neuropathy, ataxia, cognitive impairment)	In patients without any symptoms of B_{12} deficiency, oral B_{12} may be started and retested in 1 month. If the patient has symptoms of macrocytic anemia or neurologic syndromes, then parenteral B_{12} should be started promptly
Folic acid	Macrocytic anemia, fatigue, increased vascular disease	PO folic acid can be started at 1 mg/day though this should be delayed until any B_{12} deficiency is treated
Vitamin D	Osteomalacia, osteoporosis, proximal muscle weakness, increased somatic pain	50,000 units weekly for 12 weeks plus calcium
Zinc	Skin rash, oral ulceration, hair loss	25–50 mg zinc acetate/day
Vitamin E	Neurologic symptoms	Fat-soluble vitamin supplement
Vitamin A	Dark adaptation, vision impairment	
Vitamin K	Bleeding	
Calcium and magnesium	Tetany, muscle weakness, muscle spasm	Calcium: 1200 mg daily in divided dose Magnesium: 400 mg twice daily
Copper	Anemia, neurologic syndromes	2 mg bid; avoid dosing with zinc
Vitamin B_6	Peripheral neuropathy, fatigue	50 mg daily until replete, then 5 mg daily for maintenance

vitamin D requires monitoring of calcium excretion to avoid neophrocalcinosis due to hypercalciuria.

9.3.3   How Nutritious is a GFD

Vitamin and mineral deficiencies are not only a concern at the time of diagnosis of CD; several studies have suggested that a GFD is lacking in specific nutrients, and additional measures may be needed to address this issue. A number of studies show that people on a GFD do not meet the recommended intake for calcium, vitamin D, iron, B vitamins, whole grains, and fiber, and have higher intakes of fat.[17–20] In some ways, the GFD can be healthier than the standard North American diet if it contains more fruits and vegetables as, by default, these foods are naturally gluten free, and less processed foods and additives. On the downside, it also may contain

TABLE 9.2

Follow-Up of Celiac Disease

- Baseline
  - Cataloguing of frequency and severity of symptoms to detection of deficiency states
    - Iron stores (hemoglobin, mean corpuscular volume, ferritin)
    - 25-hydroxy vitamin D
    - B_{12}
    - Folic acid
    - Zinc
    - Copper[a]
    - Vitamin E[a]
    - Vitamin K (INR)
    - Vitamin A[a]
- 3–6 months
  - Symptom improvement
  - Dietary adjustment
  - Serology (tTG IgA)
  - TSH if patient on thyroid replacement
- 12 months
  - Symptom resolution
  - Serology negative or near negative
  - Retest for persistent deficiencies
  - Dietary adherence achieved
  - Rechallenge with lactose if lactose intolerant at beginning
  - Assess additional dietary issues, such as nutritional completeness, undesirable weight gain
- 2 years
  - Symptoms resolved
  - Continued adherence to a gluten-free diet
  - Serology negative
  - Repeat biopsy showing histologic improvement
  - Consider TSH

[a] Measure if symptoms of deficiency.

more meat, cheese, and eggs, which are generally gluten free but may not be heart healthy. Patients should be encouraged to choose lean meats, poultry, fish, and lower fat dairy products.

Lack of calcium and vitamin D in the diet is likely related to lactose intolerance, especially those who have persistent lactose intolerance, and these patients may need supplementation.

The majority of gluten-free flours and starches used for cereals and grain products are refined and lack B vitamins, minerals, and fiber. Most gluten-free cereals, pastas, bread, and other grain products are not fortified or enriched like their wheat-based counterparts. With increasing awareness of the lack of fortification and enrichment of processed gluten-free foods, more manufacturers are starting to enrich their gluten-free products with B vitamins and iron, and patients should be advised to choose these foods over brands that are not fortified/enriched. Patients should also be encouraged to use more gluten-free whole grains, such as amaranth, buckwheat, quinoa, millet, brown rice, flax, gluten-free oats, and others. Legumes, nuts, and seeds are also good sources of B vitamins, minerals, and fiber and are usually gluten free in their natural state.

There are no known adverse nutritional outcomes associated with a carefully planned GFD, however, the nutritional adequacy of a GFD varies substantially with the individual's food choices, and sometimes patients become so focused on gluten free that they forget about choosing foods that are nutritious, as well. A multivitamin mineral supplement may be considered if the intake of nutrients is marginal or low, especially in those patients who depend on commercially produced gluten-free processed foods.

9.3.4 Education

Everyone deals with the diagnosis of CD in their own way. A brief grieving process may be normal, however, this grieving process is highly individualized and the time it takes to move past this stage varies greatly. Patients who have been symptomatic for a long time may experience relief and welcome the diagnosis, which will likely improve their QOL through reduction of symptoms. These patients may be ready to tackle the GFD head on. Others may get into a state of denial, anger, or even depression over the diagnosis. Often these are patients who are relatively asymptomatic and/or were found by screening, particularly as part of a family, or were discovered by accident. These patients may find the GFD more burdensome and may need more time and support to accept the gluten-free lifestyle.[21] Indeed, there are various significant stages of readiness and abilities of patients; hence, the approach to education will need to be individualized (Table 9.3). For any patient, the complex nature of the diet, higher cost of gluten-free food, and impact on social activities can be challenging. If possible, information should be introduced in stages (Table 9.4).

The first stage is to provide basic survival skills. Patients should be counseled that not only will they learn about what they cannot eat, but also what they can eat (Table 9.5). Many are pleasantly surprised that they can still eat many 'normal' foods as well as the variety of gluten-free substitutes available. At this stage, patients can be encouraged to shop on the periphery of the supermarket where they will find primarily fresh produce, meat, poultry, fish, eggs, and dairy, which are naturally gluten free. There are also many packaged foods labeled gluten free, often conveniently arranged in gluten-free sections, which can take the stress out of decision making until the patient learns safe label reading skills. This approach helps relieve some of the stress patients may experience as they begin to feel the significant impact of the restrictions of a GFD.

Once the patient is able to identify the primary sources of gluten, the diet and skills can be refined. At this point, teach the patient to avoid sources of gluten by deciphering ingredients on labels and also to identify potential sources of cross contact in food preparation or processing. Cross contact can occur anywhere foods come together—in the home, in restaurants, food manufacturing plants, or in fields. Some patients prefer establishing a gluten-free kitchen; others develop a system for keeping

TABLE 9.3
CD Education Checklist

What is gluten and where is it found?
Rationale for strict GFD
Foods allowed, foods to avoid
Label reading
Cross contamination
- At home
- In restaurants
- In stores
- Environmental

Eating out
Travel, going visiting
School
Resources
- Where to shop
- Support groups
- Social media
- Shopper's guides

Nonfood sources of gluten
- Medications
- Supplements
- Communion wafers
- Play dough[a]

Calcium/vitamin D needs
Other deficiencies
Comorbidities—diabetes, weight issues, psychological, other
Potential barriers
- Educational
- Emotional
- Social
- Financial
- Lack of family support
- Attitude

[a] Only products that enter the mouth can cause harm. Gluten does not pass through the skin. However, hands need to be properly washed after handling play dough and prior to eating to avoid cross-contamination.

their gluten-free foods separate from other household members' gluten-containing foods. Most people find it easiest if most of the food prepared for the entire family is gluten free, but this is a personal and family choice. However, family members should not go on a strict GFD until after they have been tested for CD. Because of the higher cost of gluten-free items, some people prefer to reserve gluten-free products, such as bread, crackers, and cereals, for those with CD and for special occasions. Patients are best supported by families who work together to set up a system that works for all.

TABLE 9.4

Stepwise Approach to GFD

Basic survival skills
- Eliminate fundamental sources of gluten
- Gather knowledge
- Begin healing and acceptance

Branching out
- Evaluating choices
- Eating away from home
- Label reading
- Adapting socially

Life-long maintenance
- Make healthy food choices
- Prevent long-term complications
- Maintain a healthy weight
- Live a normal life
- Preserve social activities
- Keep current
- Prevent other chronic illnesses

Additionally, social isolation can have an effect on the patient's QOL. Exploring ways to eat safely outside the home is reasonable and part of the expectation of modern living on a GFD. Patients should be encouraged to participate in all the social activities they did before diagnosis, but with more preplanning necessary. Although several restaurants offer gluten-free menus, patients with CD still need to be vigilant for possible cross contact of their foods with gluten-containing foods that might result in substantial contamination and exposure (see Section 9.3.7 for more information).

The goals of long-term nutrition therapy for patients with CD include maintaining healthy eating patterns with emphasis on a variety of nutrient-dense foods to improve and, indeed, to maintain overall health. It is no longer enough to be simply gluten free but one must be healthy and gluten free as should the gluten-free foods that patients eat. Following the United States Department of Agriculture (USDA) Dietary Guidelines for Americans may help to reduce risk of heart disease, diabetes, osteoporosis, and other chronic illnesses.

9.3.5 CHALLENGES LIVING GLUTEN FREE

Because a GFD is the only current treatment for CD, this places the major burden of treatment on the patient. The ultimate goal, of course, is patient adherence to a GFD, achieved by being prudent but not becoming paranoid. Fortunately, the GFD has become easier due to the increased availability of gluten-free foods, although these products may not be available in smaller communities or to people who do not use the Internet. The quality has also improved, although the palatability may not meet the patient's expectations of what the product should taste like; for example, we

TABLE 9.5
Gluten-Free Diet

Allowed Grains

Amaranth	Job's tears	Sorghum[a]
Arrowroot	Millet[a]	Soy flour[a]
Bean flours	Nut flours	Tapioca
Buckwheat, 100% (Soba)[a]	Oats, gluten free[a]	Teff
Cassava	Potato starch or flour	Wild Rice
Corn flour, cornmeal	Quinoa	Yucca
Flax	Rice	
Indian rice grass	Sago	

Grains to Avoid

Wheat in any form:

Einkorn	Matzo	Barley, malt
Emmer	Semolina	Rye
Spelt	Orzo	
Kamut	Farro	
Bulgur	Graham	
Durum	Couscous	
Panko	Udon	
Farina	Wheat bran	
Wheat germ		

Overlooked Sources of Gluten[b]

Beer/ale	French fries	Sauces
Bouillon/broth	Gravy	Self-basting turkey
Brown rice syrup	Luncheon meats, hotdogs	Snack chips
Candy	Marinade	Soups
Communion wafers	Rice mixes	Soy sauce

[a] Even though these grains are gluten free as grown, they may be cross-contaminated during harvesting or processing. Use only products that a manufacturer guarantees are gluten free. Oats are the most likely to be cross-contaminated, but risk also exists for buckwheat, millet, sorghum, and soy.[61] Gluten-free oats may be tolerated by some patients, but should not be attempted until after healing occurs. Oats contain avenin, which some patients are sensitive to.

[b] Many of these foods can be found gluten free. When in doubt, check with the food manufacturer.

often advise patients to avoid gluten-free bread for the first month or two after being diagnosed to allow taste memory to fade.

The extra cost of gluten-free foods can also be a burden to the patient with CD. Indeed, most gluten-free specialty products cost 2–3 times more than their gluten-containing counterparts. Patients can downplay costs by relying more on naturally gluten-free whole foods, saving costly gluten-free products for special occasions, buying gluten-free foods in quantity, and baking from scratch versus buying prepared, ready-to-eat foods. Taxpayers can deduct expenses for medical care of the taxpayers' spouse, or dependents, if expenses exceed a certain proportion of adjusted gross income (see current tax code) (http://celiac.org/celiac-disease/resources/tax-deductions/). Flexible spending accounts may be an efficient way to capture some of the tax deductibility of the excess costs associated with gluten-free foods as long as they are required for medical therapy (http://celiacdisease.about.com/od/theglutenfreediet) and (https://www.wageworks.com/employers/benefits/healthcare-flexible-spending-account-fsa.aspx). Medical care includes, in the case of CD, the cost of gluten-free foods in the amount that exceeds the cost of regular food. A diagnosis and prescription from a physician are necessary for the documentation of eligibility.

9.3.6 LABEL READING

Grains, especially wheat, are so prevalent in the American food supply that it is difficult to avoid them. Derivatives of gluten-containing grains are also used in nongrain-based foods, which makes avoidance even more difficult. Label reading to identify less obvious sources of gluten is a critical feature of the patient's education.

Although label reading for gluten has improved considerably in the past decade, labeling foods as containing gluten is still not required. Label reading in the United States has undergone a significant change, both due to a change in the law as well as increased market desirability for foods marked gluten free. The FDA's "Food Allergen Labeling and Consumer Protection Act" (FALCPA) passed in 2004 requires companies to identify in plain language if the food contains any of the eight most prevalent food allergens—eggs, fish, milk, peanuts, shellfish, soybeans, tree nuts, and wheat (www.FDA.gov/food/guidanceregulation/guidancedocumentsregul atoryinformation/allergens/ucm106890). If wheat protein or anything derived from wheat is used as an ingredient, even in the tiniest amount (e.g., incorporated into flavoring or seasoning), it must be clearly stated in the ingredient list or in the allergy statement on the label. The labeling requirements under the FALCPA, however, do not address gluten as something that must be labeled, so, for example, something made from barley or rye would not be covered. If the food ingredient label does not indicate wheat, the patient must still carefully scrutinize the list of ingredients for these other gluten-containing grains. The FALCPA also laid out a requirement that the FDA formulate regulations to define what the term "gluten free" would mean on labels. Finally, in 2013, these guidelines were promulgated and went into effect in 2014 (www.FDA.gov/food/guidanceregulation/guidancedocumentsregulatoryinfor-mation/allergens/ucm362510). Basically, these guidelines require that if a manufacturer wishes to use the term gluten free, the content of gluten in the food must be <20 ppm (parts per million) in a finished product. It is not known what the threshold amount required to produce a problem in any individual is, but careful toxicological considerations suggested to the FDA that <20 ppm should be considered safe for most people with CD. Another reason 20 ppm was selected is that this is the lowest level that can be consistently detected in foods using valid scientific analytic tools and has also been adopted worldwide under the Codex Alimentarius. Some independent gluten-free certification programs have more stringent guidelines and require foods that bear their seal to have <5 ppm of gluten. However, thus far the reliability of the methods used to detect gluten at such low limits has not been demonstrated. Twenty ppm remains the level of gluten that can reliably and consistently be detected in a variety of food matrices.

The food labeling regulations for wheat and gluten free do not extend to USDA-regulated foods—meat, poultry, and eggs (http://www.fsis.usda.gov/OPPDE/larc/Ingredients/Allergens.htm). However, it is expected that most USDA manufacturers follow the FALCPA guidelines. In USDA-regulated foods, labeled meat, poultry and egg products, dextrin, starch, and modified food starch may be derived from wheat and the source would not need to be identified.

9.3.7 Eating Away from Home

As now the majority of all food consumed in the United States is prepared and/or eaten outside the home, eating out is no longer an occasional treat but has rather become the dominant way of life for many people. Dining away from home is one of the more challenging features of a GFD, especially for the newly diagnosed patient. This can include travel, eating at people's homes, and special events, as well as eating in restaurants.

With CD becoming more common and the GFD becoming more fashionable though unproven for a variety of reasons (weight control, athletic performance, energy), it is in the restaurateurs' best interest to offer gluten-free options, and there are a growing number of chain and independently owned restaurants that offer gluten-free menus or at least accommodate GFD requests. However, it is important that both patients and restaurant personnel realize that it is not just the ingredients but how the food is handled that makes or keeps products gluten free. For example, cross contact can occur by cooking gluten-free foods on a grill or in a fryer that was used for gluten-containing foods, or using same serving utensils for both gluten-free and gluten-containing foods. It is also worth noting that the employee turnover is very high in the restaurant business and, for the most reliable service, it is best to talk to the manager.

Planning is key when traveling, going to peoples' homes, or attending special events. There are many travel websites and mobile apps with information identifying gluten-free friendly restaurants, hotels, and grocers near one's travel destination. Gluten-free dining cards in various languages are handy for those who like to travel abroad and some airlines will provide gluten-free meals during intercontinental flights.

Eating in other peoples' homes can be more of a challenge due to the risk of cross-contamination in foods prepared by celiac-naive hosts/hostesses. Calling ahead to find out what is being served at a dinner party or banquet can help take the guesswork out of those experiences. Another solution would be to take along a gluten-free dish to share. Directly contacting caterers for larger events may also be effective to insure that they can safely provide gluten-free options for participants. Schools and institutions may provide special challenges. For example, students in colleges may need to seek accommodations or be excused from compulsory participation in the standard foodservice accommodations at school; similarly, nursing homes may need to undertake special accommodations for residents who require a GFD, and this can require significant education of all personnel involved in food provision as well as their suppliers.

9.3.8 Gluten in Drugs

A potential source of gluten is both prescription and over-the-counter (OTC) drugs and supplements. OTC drugs are required to list both active and inactive ingredients on the label, but the FDA does not require labels to note when wheat or gluten are used. Prescription drugs are not required to list inactive ingredients on their labels. Inactive ingredients, so-called excipients, often make up the bulk of most medications and this is where gluten is most likely to occur. Potential sources of gluten in excipients include starch (which could be wheat starch), dextrates, dextrin, dextrimaltose, or caramel coloring. Although the risk that a medication which may contain gluten is low, it does exist. If a patient takes a medication on a regular basis, it should be verified gluten free; however, the risk is small enough that in an emergent situation the gluten-free status of a drug should not interfere with using it.

The best way to determine if a medication or supplement is gluten free is to contact the manufacturer or perhaps a pharmacist. Websites that list gluten-free drugs may not be entirely reliable if the information is not current. Indeed, even pharmacists are challenged by the ability to obtain reliable information on excipient ingredients, especially as the suppliers of generic medications may rapidly change. There are groups petitioning to get the FDA to require gluten-free labeling on all prescription and OTC drugs, or even banning gluten in drugs.

9.3.9 Children

A strict GFD is critical for children with CD to insure appropriate nutritional growth and development and to prevent long-term complications. At the time of diagnosis, some children may have iron deficiency anemia, vitamin deficiencies, low bone density, and dental enamel defects. Except for the dental defects, these usually reverse quickly once the child is on a strict GFD.[22] Once fully recovered and maintaining a GFD, children with CD are at no higher risk for nutritional deficiencies than those who do not have CD.[23] Once fully recovered, the intestine will remain healed as long as a strict GFD is maintained.

Children who remain on a strict GFD generally do very well and appear to recover more quickly and more completely than adults. This is also true of loss of or failure to obtain optimal bone mass. However, it is also quite common for adherence problems to occur in teenagers who may have subtle physical or emotional consequences that they do not connect to gluten contamination.

Adjusting to the gluten-free lifestyle is difficult for an adult, but it can be even more difficult for children, especially teenagers. Most young children adapt quite easily, but older children and teens often have a difficult time coping with social situations of feeling "different," as well as with sound decision-making. Children who do not have bothersome symptoms may find it more difficult to follow a strict GFD.

It is important that children and their families encounter a smooth transition to a gluten-free lifestyle. This translates to fewer stressors at home, a safe school environment, and maintaining an active social life, leading to an overall improved QOL. As early as possible, parents should have their children participate in their own care, learning how to identify safe foods, prepare foods, read labels, eat out safely, and speak up when needed. These are lifelong skills a child will need to best insure adherence and to safely navigate the outside world when the child leaves home.

Communication is key in controlling your child's diet when someone else is in charge. Educating teachers, relatives, and other parents about the importance of gluten consequences and how to assure a gluten-free experience must include steps to prevent cross contact with gluten-containing foods. Many well-meaning relatives, friends, and other caregivers often overlook this aspect of the GFD.

Under the Americans with Disabilities Act, children with CD are entitled to be provided a gluten-free school lunch (www.celiaccentral.org/kids/parents/guides/Kids-Youth/Navigating-The-School-System/209).

One concern often overlooked is the child's mental health and the psychological impact of living with CD. Psychopathology, especially anxiety or even depression, has been shown to correlate with psychosocial stressors commonly associated with CD. These social stressors include social alienation, low self-esteem, and feelings of worthlessness and worry. Children should be allowed and encouraged to participate in all the school and social activities other children do, but with extra precautions regarding food.

Peer support groups can serve a beneficial role in promoting adjustment to a gluten-free lifestyle, not only for children but for anyone diagnosed with CD. Support groups or workshops focusing on handling social events and peer influence in particular can also improve adherence in adolescents. It is equally important that it not be viewed by the teenager that the diet is imposed upon them and, where possible, the teenager should be involved in all relevant decision making.

A local support group is an invaluable way for newly diagnosed patients with CD to learn from others. It is a place to gain empathy and compassion, learn coping skills, share product and restaurant information, and stay current with news related to CD. Many people find great comfort in knowing other people are dealing with the same issues. Just having someone to talk and relate to can make a big difference. If there is not a support group accessible to the patient or if the patient does not feel comfortable in a group setting, there are many other forms of social media to help connect the patient with the celiac community, including Facebook, Twitter, MySpace, and blogs. Advise the patient that much of the information on these sites is opinion rather than fact, and to find reputable organizations for the most reliable information (Table 9.6).

9.3.10 INFANT FEEDING

Studies have suggested that timing of gluten exposure in genetically susceptible infants may affect their chance of developing CD.[24] It appears the best time for introduction of gluten is between 4 and 6 months of age, and it should be introduced gradually.[25] In some studies, longer breastfeeding or breastfeeding during the time of introduction of gluten has been shown to be protective, but this is not a consistent finding.[25,26] Certainly, excessively early or delayed introduction of gluten seems to be associated with an increased risk of developing CD in childhood. It is not clear whether these feeding regimens provide permanent protection or simply delay the onset. It is reasonable to avoid introducing gluten to infants <4 months old or not to

TABLE 9.6

Resources

American Celiac Disease Alliance	www.americanceliac.org
Canadian Celiac Association	www.celiac.ca
Celiac Disease Foundation	www.celiac.org
Celiac Support Association CSA/USA	www.csaceliacs.org
Children's Digestive Health and Nutrition Foundation	www.celiachealth.org
Gluten Intolerance Group (GIG)	www.gluten.net
National Foundation for Celiac Awareness	www.celiaccentral.org
National Institutes of Health	http://digestive.niddk.nih.gov/ddiseases/pubs/celiac/
North American Society for Pediatric Gastroenterology, Hepatology, and Nutrition (NASPGHAN)	www.naspghan.org/sub/celiac_disease.asp
ROCK (Raising Our Celiac Kids)	www.celiackids.com

delay it to after 7 months of age, and also to try to encourage breastfeeding to continue during the time of initial gluten introduction.[27]

While the reason for the benefit of specifically timed gluten exposures is unknown, it may be related to an immature microbiological environment in the infant gut as well as a maturing immune system. In addition, breastfeeding may increase immunity and disease resistance in the infant. Ongoing research hopes to elicit more on this topic and, indeed, work relating to prevent CD is eagerly awaited.

9.3.11 BONE HEALTH

Approximately one-third of adult patients with CD have osteoporosis, one-third of patients have diminished or low bone mass, and another third have normal bone density at diagnosis. Unlike the general population in which women are at greater risk, men with CD have about the same risk as women and the disease tends to be more severe. The longer CD goes undetected and untreated, the greater the bone loss. The sooner CD is diagnosed and treated, the greater the opportunity to lessen the debilitating effects of osteoporosis, the most serious of which is hip fracture. Equally disabling can be compression fractures of the spine. The data on prevention of fractures in patients diagnosed with CD is mixed with some showing no short-term improvement in those diagnosed as adults. Measurement of bone mineral density at or close to the time of diagnosis of CD is advised.

Since the bone loss in CD is primarily due to malabsorption, a strict GFD is the most important treatment for bone loss. A strict GFD cannot cure osteoporosis, but it can slow or stop bone loss. Other factors contributing to bone loss in patients with CD include low calcium and vitamin D intake due to lactose avoidance, steroid use in patients with poorly responsive CD or comorbid autoimmune diseases, and low body weight. Inflammatory factors may also play a role in the bone disease.

Weight bearing and resistance exercise should be encouraged for bone strengthening. Patients at high risk for fracture would benefit from professional advice before starting an exercise program, particularly to avoid falls as well as compression fractures. Regular exercise is also part of any healthy lifestyle. Additional benefits for people with CD include empowerment, weight management, mood stabilization, stress management, anddiabetes management.

There are several prescription medications available for treating osteoporosis, however, in many cases these should not be considered, especially the anti-resorptive agents, for about 1 year after diagnosis in order to allow for maximum correction of the bone loss on a GFD alone as well as because of limitations of absorption of these agents in the context of a damaged intestine.

All patients with CD, regardless of their bone density, should try to meet the daily calcium goals in the FDA Recommended Daily Intake (RDI) from either food or supplements. Patients with low bone mineral density may need additional calcium and vitamin D and, if vitamin D deficient, a large malabsorption dose of vitamin D, 50,000 IU weekly until replete. Oral bisphosphonates are of limited value in CD and anecdotally ineffective, especially in untreated or unhealed CD. Other agents require adding calcium or vitamin D in order to be successful in improving bone density. Hence, attention to and management of CD is most crucial for the management of severe bone mineral loss in patients with CD.

Lactose intolerance is common due to intestinal damage and loss of lactase activity, but often improves with healing. Patients who experience gastrointestinal symptoms following the ingestion of milk may benefit from limiting lactose intake until healing occurs. In some patients, the lactose intolerance may be permanent, but most will recover.

9.3.12 Weight Concerns

While weight loss is traditionally regarded as one of the classic symptoms of CD, recent studies suggest that people with CD, including children, are far more likely to be obese or overweight at the time of diagnosis than what was once thought.[28-30]

Patients who have lost weight prior to diagnosis should spontaneously be able to gain weight once they start the GFD and the intestine starts to heal. Failure to gain weight in an underweight patient may be due to ongoing deliberate or accidental gluten ingestion, reduced caloric intake due to over restriction of food, or perhaps could be due to another pathology—for example, pancreatic insufficiency. Treatment should begin with a thorough dietary assessment to make sure the patient is on a strict GFD and consuming adequate calories and other nutrients. Strategies to increase calories in underweight patients can include choosing more energy-dense gluten-free foods and beverages, eating frequent meals and snacks, and supplementing with a nutritional drink. Most of the leading nutritional drinks, including Boost™, Ensure™, and Scandishakes™, are gluten free.

An excessive gain of weight can occur in those patients who have been able to eat more without gaining weight due to inefficient absorption prior to diagnosis.[31] These patients generally gain weight because their absorption improves along with their continued high calorie intake. In addition, gluten-free foods may be higher in fat and calories than their gluten-containing counterparts and further contribute to unwanted weight gain. On the other hand, some overweight patients lose weight on a

GFD because they are eating healthier and are more discriminate in their eating.[29,32] Patients who present with weight loss before diagnosis are more likely to gain weight and should be advised of the possibility of excess weight gain.

Prevention and treatment of excessive weight gain is similar to other weight management programs—reduce calories and increase exercise. Patients should be instructed not to cheat on their GFD for the purpose of controlling weight, as excess weight gain can be associated with poor adherence to a GFD.

9.3.13   DIABETES

The prevalence of CD in type 1 diabetes is estimated to be between 5% and 10% and is more common in type 1 diabetics who are Caucasian. CD in diabetes is often silent, exhibiting little or no symptoms, and may only be found serendipitously upon testing or screening. Still, there is controversy about whether or not to screen all patients with type 1 diabetes mainly because of some concerns about the double disease burden effect on individuals. Thus, a careful consideration of the appropriate timing to test for CD in a diabetic patient is important.[33–35] Clinicians caring for patients with type 1 diabetes need to be especially vigilant for CD that can present with gastrointestinal symptoms. Clinical manifestations of CD, such as abdominal pain, gas, bloating, diarrhea, and weight loss, may be present but are often mistaken for poor control of diabetes, gastroparesis, or diabetic neuropathy. Blood sugar control may or may not be affected by CD. Untreated CD may result in erratic blood sugars, hypoglycemia, or reduced insulin requirements due to malabsorption or may have no effect on diabetic control.[28,36] Once a GFD is started, an increase in insulin requirements may occur as the intestine heals and absorption improves. Patients should monitor their blood sugars more frequently and adjust their insulin dose as needed.

CD is generally diagnosed after the diagnosis of type 1 diabetes. Adding a GFD to an already restricted diet can be overwhelming for some patients, and it may be easier for the patient to maintain the usual diabetic eating plan and make adjustments for gluten over a period of time. The dietitian who counsels the patient should have expertise in both CD and type 1 diabetes. Regular follow-up with a dietitian and the diabetes nurse educator is strongly encouraged. The key to success in these patients is the support needed to help patients cope with the double burden. Young children with type 1 diabetes often transition better to a GFD as this is managed largely by parents, though this may increase the burden on parents.

Because some gluten-free products are higher in carbohydrates and calories than standard starch exchanges, carb counting is recommended over the exchange system for diabetes management. In addition, patients may find it easier to count grams of carbs rather than convert gluten-free products to carb choices. Label reading is crucial, not only for carb content, but also for gluten-containing ingredients.

Many of the gluten-free grain products are highly refined and have a higher glycemic index, which can also affect blood sugar control. These include rice flour and potato, corn, and tapioca starches. Encouraging the patient to use higher fiber grains, such as brown rice, quinoa, and others may help with diabetes management and also help reduce the risk of cardiovascular complications often associated with diabetes.

It should also be noted that some diabetic foods may have nonabsorbable sugars (sugar alcohols) that may have diarrheogenic effects unrelated to CD.

9.3.14 CONSTIPATION

Due to the refined nature of many gluten-free grain products, constipation can become a problem. Patients should be advised to increase their fiber from fruits, vegetables, legumes, and gluten-free whole grains. Many fiber supplements such as Citrucel and Metamucil are gluten free.

9.3.15 FOLLOW-UP

After initial diagnosis, patients should return for periodic follow-up visits ideally with both the registered dietitian and physician.[8] This practice improves adherence to the GFD, minimizes complications, and can result in an improved QOL. This practice has also been shown to be highly valued by patients.[37,38] In children, follow-up should include assessment of growth, development, and socialization.

Nonadherence to a GFD, both intentional or inadvertent, is common due to the restrictive and complex nature of the diet. Indeed, nonadherence has been estimated to be anywhere between 36% and 96% and the most common cause of persistent symptoms in patients with CD.[39–41] Inadvertent gluten ingestion occurs more often than deliberate or intentional ingestion.[40]

Repeat serologic testing can be used to assess response to the treatment, but is not particularly sensitive in that it does not always correlate with histology. Persistently elevated serologies, however, do indicate a high likelihood of ongoing gluten ingestion, often in substantial quantities. A small bowel biopsy should be repeated after 2 years to assess for healing in patients diagnosed as adults. This could be considered optional, but is certainly our practice. Failure to heal the intestine may be associated with long-term complications, such as increased risk of malignancy and in some studies a potential increase in mortality, though in the largest study from Sweden, failure to have a follow-up biopsy was associated with an increase in mortality, but not failure to heal.

9.3.16 NONRESPONSIVE CD

Adherence to the GFD improves symptoms in most patients; however, some patients continue to have symptoms, persistently elevated serologies, and intestinal damage. Symptoms may fail to improve initially or may recur years later. These patients often need a full reevaluation using a systematic approach (Figure 9.1). In most patients, continued gluten ingestion is the cause of persistent symptoms[39–41]; however, other causes must be ruled out, including lactose intolerance, which may be apparent early when a patient's symptoms do not completely respond to a GFD; microscopic colitis; small intestinal bacterial overgrowth; pancreatic insufficiency, especially if continued steatorrhea is occurring; functional gastrointestinal disease or, less commonly, refractory celiac disease (RCD).

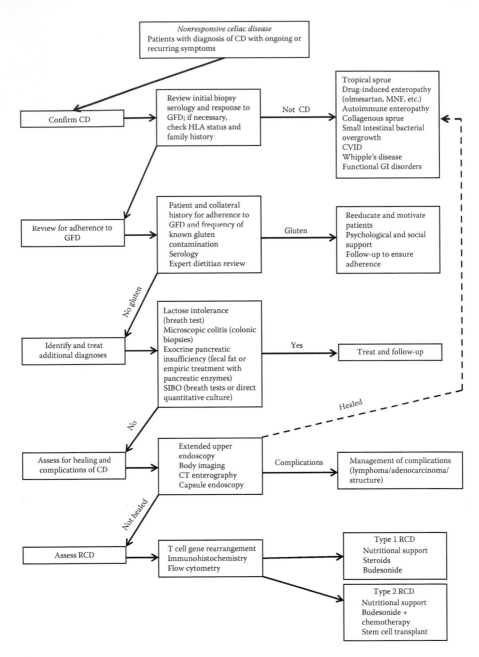

FIGURE 9.1 The systematic approach to the patient who presents with persistent or recurring symptoms of celiac disease. Abbreviations: CD = celiac disease; CVID = common variable immunodeficiency; GFD = gluten-free diet; SIBO = small intestinal bacterial overgrowth; RCD = refractory celiac disease.

Consultation with a dietitian skilled in the GFD is crucial to help identify sources of inadvertent (or intentional) gluten ingestion. Ongoing gluten ingestion is often due to inadequate education about CD and the GFD. However, even the most knowledgeable patients can experience inadvertent gluten exposure due to the ubiquitous nature of gluten in our environment. And, even patients who are convinced they are on a strict GFD may be surprised when the dietitian identifies some gluten they were not aware of in their diet. Thus, all patients who do not get better should have a thorough review by the dietitian. Assessment for nonresponsive CD should include a review of all food and beverage consumed at home and away from home (school, restaurants, others' homes), including brand names of products and who prepared the food (Table 9.7). A detailed food diary kept by the patient is helpful in identifying inadvertent sources of gluten. The diary should be kept for 4–7 days and include weekends as well as weekdays. It is important to review the patient's label-reading practices, skills at eating in places outside the home and what precautions they take to prevent cross-contamination in their own home. Frequent causes of inadvertent gluten exposure include shared condiments and spreads, shared toasters, communion wafers, commercially processed or packaged foods, unclear labels, regular oats, and restaurant foods. Other sources of potential gluten exposure should also be considered including medications, vitamins, dietary supplements, and environmental exposures, for example, working in a bakery.

There is a small subset of extra sensitive patients whose CD does not improve despite a strict GFD. These patients may benefit by a diet that reduces risk of contamination by largely avoiding processed foods, including GF processed foods, or at least those not made in a gluten-free dedicated facility.

If the gluten ingestion is intentional, the reasons should be explored and dealt with, whether it be denial/acceptance, lack of social support, attitude, financial or other psychosocial circumstances.

Up to 25% of adult patients suffer from persistent gastrointestinal symptoms despite apparently strict adherence to a GFD and complete intestinal healing. A common reason for ongoing gastrointestinal symptoms is IBS.[42–44] According to a recent meta-analysis, patients with IBS are 4 times more likely to have CD than the general population, though these data vary depending on the source of patients.[45,46]

Many patients who report ongoing symptoms, particularly pain and diarrhea, despite a GFD and complete healing, experience psychological distress and poor coping.[47–51] Psychosocial factors may have a stronger effect on health-related QOL than CD.[47,48] Patients with CD, especially women, seem to suffer from a higher rate of anxiety and depression than the general population.[52–54] There also may be greater catastrophizing, history of abuse, and substantial life stressors. These patients are more likely to utilize healthcare resources than patients without psychological distress. Management should include psychological support to reduce psychological distress, improve coping skills, manage functional gastrointestinal disorders, and thus improve overall health and reduce healthcare costs.

9.3.17 QUALITY OF LIFE

In recent years, health-related QOL has been the subject of much interest. Studies have suggested that people with CD have a poor quality life, especially in the social

TABLE 9.7

Checklist for Assessing Patients with Nonresponsive CD

Intentional ingestion
- Reason
- Frequency

Inadvertent ingestion
- Hidden ingredients
  - Cereals with malt
  - Regular oats
  - Medication
  - Supplements
  - Play dough
  - Others due to vague labeling
- Cross-contamination
  - Shared toaster
  - Shared condiments/spreads
  - Shared utensils
    - Grill/fryer
    - Colander
    - Strainer
    - Cutting board
    - Rolling pin
  - Open bins
  - Restaurants
  - School
  - Others' homes
  - Environmental exposure (work environment, such as a bakery)

Patient knowledge
- Label reading
- Eating out
- Contamination
- Resources

Barriers
- Educational
- Emotional
- Social
- Financial
- Family support
- Attitude

Educational media
- Support groups
- Internet
- Newsletters/magazines
- Mobile apps

Previous diet instruction
- No registered dietitian
- General registered dietitian
- Celiac registered dietitian
- Other health care provider (HCP)

realm, including eating out, traveling, and social events,[55,56] and this is often associated with noncompliance.[47,50,57] Patients with persistent symptoms are also more likely to have reduced QOL.[58,59]

The strict nature of the GFD necessary for CD can impact the patient's QOL, especially considering that it is the only treatment available for CD and that management is completely in the hands of the patient. This places considerable burden of responsibility on the patient to manage his/her condition. Studies suggest that QOL is lower, particularly in women than in men, patients who are symptomatic or who had severe symptoms of long duration before diagnosis, and patients with psychiatric, gastrointestinal, and neurologic comorbidities.[50,55,58,59] Poor QOL also may be more likely in patients diagnosed during working age.[59] Early diagnosis and management of comorbidities may have an impact on QOL in these patients.

Patients are frequently diagnosed because they are in high-risk groups. Many of these patients may lack symptoms; hence, the level of health-related anxiety may be increased following detection of CD. The GFD often enhances QOL in patients with symptomatic CD but also may be a burden to those without symptoms.[21,49,50,58,60] For some patients, QOL improves with the length of time since diagnosis and treatment[55] and in patients who follow a strict GFD.[57]

Patient education may have a significant impact on QOL.[37,38] Healthcare providers should provide information about living with CD, including the social aspects, as well as being sensitive to the potential for a grief reaction and the need for family and social support for the patient. Support groups can offer a sense of empathy and support that may be useful and appreciated by many patients.

9.3.18 ALTERNATIVE OR ADDITIONAL THERAPIES

The mainstay of treatment for CD is a GFD. There are no approved alternative treatments. Adjunctive therapies are largely focused on compensating for associated disorders, such as pancreatic exocrine insufficiency, small intestinal bacterial overgrowth, microscopic colitis, motility disorders of the stomach or small intestine, or secondary complications such as osteoporosis. There are, however, several agents that are in development for treatment of CD, and these have been elucidated to the pathogenesis of CD. These changes can involve enzyme degradation of the deleterious peptides from gliadin in the stomach and small intestine before they access the immune system. Such agents are in clinical trials. In addition, an agent that alters intestinal permeability, larazotide acetate, shows promise in clinical trials. Budesonide, a topically active, potent corticosteroid that has a high rate of inactivation by first pass metabolism in the liver, may suppress symptoms, accelerate healing in newly diagnosed patients according to one study, and also may be useful for patients with RCD, suppressing inflammation and providing symptomatic improvement. Additional targets, including T cell regulation, interleukin 15, the binding of gliadin molecules within the lumen, and blocking the interaction between the gliadin peptide and the binding groove of the HLA DQ molecule are all in preclinical development. One completed clinical trial using a chemokine inhibitor had never been reported despite having been completed over 5 years ago. It is expected that one or more of these therapies will successfully make it to market within the next 5–6 years.

9.3.19 COMPLICATIONS OF UNTREATED CD

Many organ systems can be affected by CD and particularly difficult, but not so common, are the nervous system associations. The most common is a peripheral symmetric predominately sensory neuropathy thus may recover once the patient has been treated, though recovery may be delayed for 1–2 years. Central nervous disorders, including ataxia often associated with cerebellar atrophy, cognitive decline and even premature dementia, movement disorders, and epilepsy or seizure disorders particularly associated with calcification of the occipital lobe may be particularly difficult to manage and not especially obvious. Many patients presenting with neurologic syndromes lack classic gastrointestinal symptoms. The mechanism by which these neurologic disorders occur could be immunological, nutritional, or idiopathic. The malignancies, particularly lymphoma or adenocarcinoma of the small intestine and also esophageal carcinoma, other visceral cancers and disseminated lymphoma may be seen more commonly in patients with CD than the general population. Most commonly, these occur in patients with severe symptoms whose diagnosis of CD was delayed until late adulthood. Disorders of reproduction have been described, in particular both male and female infertility, premature birth, and recurring spontaneous miscarriage, though the association is probably quite low and the attributable risk of CD toward infertility is also quite low. The reproductive capacity of patients with CD may be modestly impaired prior to diagnosis, but catching up usually occurs following diagnosis and treatment.

Other circumstances bear mention. Thyroid disease, one of the most frequent autoimmune diseases seen in patients with CD, may also present management problems due to relative malabsorption of the thyroid medication necessitating higher-than-usual doses. In addition, medications in general may be malabsorbed, leading to a lack of effectiveness.

9.3.20 REFRACTORY CELIAC DISEASE

RCD is a clinical syndrome which consists of symptomatic malabsorption allied with severe enteropathy confirmed by biopsy despite being on a GFD for at least 1 year. Typically these patients are sero-negative as serology sero-positivity is dependent on ongoing gluten ingestion. RCD does not include those patients who are ingesting significant amounts of gluten, either based on an expert dietary review or on persistently positive celiac-specific serology. RCD is a particularly serious disorder and often patients are anemic, hypoproteinemic with a low serum albumin, have significant weight loss, and often other nutrient deficiencies and particularly advanced bone disease. It is a rare condition in children or young adults. It can be a primary abnormality that occurs with first symptomatic presentation of CD or more commonly occurs later with a relapse in symptoms some months or years after diagnosis. RCD can be divided into two types.

9.3.20.1 Type 1 RCD

Type 1 is largely an autoimmune type where there is self-perpetuating inflammation in the intestine. The inflammatory cells in the lining of the intestine are characterized by an oligo- or polyclonal T cell response. Whilst this disorder can result in significant or even severe malnutrition, it typically responds well to immunosuppression and corticosteroids. Most centers now use topically active steroids of the first line, namely budesonide. It is important when utilizing budesonide that the intent is to deliver the budesonide to the area of the intestine most affected. Most commercial versions of budesonide are designed for delivery in the distal small bowel or colon and these preparations must be disrupted in some way to allow for earlier distribution of the medication in the upper small intestine. There are no approved medications for the treatment of RCD. Additional work has suggested that perhaps 5ASA compounds, which also act topically, may have some benefit when used in concert with budesonide. Systemic corticosteroids or steroid-sparing regimens, such as azathioprine, may also be used though concerns about absorption of systemically active drugs may be in question in patients with severe enteropathy.

9.3.20.2   Type 2 RCD

Type 2 RCD is one in which there is a monoclonal expansion of T cells arising from the intraepithelial lymphocyte layer. These T cells, in addition to being monoclonal, are aberrant in that they often no longer express the classic CD8 T cell markers on their surface and may instead express NK receptors. These monoclonal aberrant T cells are often responding to IL-15 in an unregulated fashion and become cytotoxic. In most cases of enteropathy-associated lymphoma occurring in the context of CD is a rise from these aberrant cells. These cells may spread laterally into stomach and colon compartments, surface compartments may spread systemically. Type 2 RCD may be detected by a number of methods of varying accuracy. Immunohistochemistry of the surface epithelium of the intestine utilizing stains of CD3, CD8, and CD4 may readily identify a population of cells that still express CD3 on immunohisto-chemistry, which is in the cytoplasm, and no longer express the usual CD8 or CD4 markers. A general rule of thumb is followed that, if <50% of the intraepithelial lymphocytes seen express CD8, this indicates an aberrant population as present. T cell gene rearrangement may also identify clonal expansion of T cell receptors and this tends to be a sensitive but not necessarily specific test as individuals with uncomplicated CD or even normal individuals may have clonal expansion detected. Flow cytometry of biopsies from the intestine has also been used as a sensitive way of identifying a percentage of intraepithelial lymphocytes that lack the surface CD3, CD8, and CD4 markers. This requires a dedicated research laboratory to undertake accurately. Cytogenetics do not usually identify abnormalities in RCD; however, in established enteropathy-associated lymphoma, trisomy of chromosome 1 may occur. Histologically, other than inflammation and the architectural change, there is little to distinguish these cells from type 2 RCD or even enteropathy-associated lymphoma from normal. Treatment of type 2 RCD is difficult and, in addition to the measures instituted for type 1 RCD, predominately steroids, experimental measures or approaches such as near myloablative chemotherapy followed by autologous stem cell support has been used with some success. Single agent acute chemotherapeutics like cladabrine or other agents have anecdotally been shown to have effectiveness for reduction of inflammation but not necessarily prevention of progression of the disease to lymphoma.

The prognosis for RCD is dependent on the type, with type 2 RCD having a much more guarded prognosis than type 1. Many patients with type 1 RCD who successfully respond to steroid therapy are able to get off the steroid therapy and continue on a GFD successfully. Type 2 RCD is more questionable. Some patients will respond quite well to steroid therapy and the authors continue these patients, if successful, on budesonide long term. Careful follow-up of all patients with RCD is necessary, particularly those with type 2 RCD, in order to identify complications. Endoscopic changes, such as extensive ulcerative jejunitis, may be a marker for type 2 RCD or even evolving enteropathy-associated T cell lymphoma.

Patients with persistent or ongoing symptoms with CD need to be evaluated for malignant complications. The two most common malignancies are enteropathy-associated T cell lymphoma and adenocarcinoma of the small intestine. The lymphoma can present with systemic lymphoma symptoms or with local complications. Adenocarcinoma typically presents with local complications with perforation, anemia, bleeding, or obstruction.

9.3.21 CASE STUDY

A 55-year-old woman presents with microcytic anemia associated with a low ferritin. The patient had a negative colonoscopy and negative occult blood testing. The patient has a history of postprandial bloating, excess flatulence, and abdominal discomfort. Patient avoids lactose-containing foods and has done so for 20 years. On evaluation, the patient reports a sibling who has had a diagnosis of CD some 10 years before. Based on this, a blood test is sent for serologic testing, including total IgA (which is normal) and tTG IgA (which is >100, normal range <4). The patient underwent upper endoscopy; the endoscopist identified changes compatible with villous atrophy in the duodenal mucosa and biopsies confirm the findings with partial villous atrophy, increased epithelial lymphocytes, and crypt hyperplasia. On further evaluation, the patient was found to have 25-hydroxy vitamin D that is very low (equals 6) and vitamin B_{12} of 102 (normal range >180).

The assessment is that the patient has CD presenting primarily with anemia in the context of family history of CD that has been confirmed by histology and positive serology. In addition, the patient has suffered likely consequences of CD, including iron deficiency anemia, vitamin D deficiency, diminished bone density, and osteoporosis ± osteomalacia, as well as thus far asymptomatic vitamin B_{12} deficiency. The patient is referred to an expert dietitian and commenced on a GFD and supplementation with iron, oral B_{12}, and vitamin D. After 30 days, the patient's vitamin B_{12} has risen to 350, indicating adequate oral absorption and vitamin B_{12} orally is continued. At 3 months, the patient reported an excellent response of her symptoms and at 6 months her deficiencies have corrected. Her hemoglobin is normal, though ferritin remained low at 9 (normal range: 12). When she is seen at 1 year, she has developed watery diarrhea. Biopsies of her small intestine showed healed small intestine with restoration of villous architecture; biopsies of the colon reveal lymphocytic colitis. Secondary diagnosis is lymphocytic colitis commonly seen in association with CD, and the patient is treated with budesonide with an excellent response.

This case illustrates the common presentation of CD with iron deficiency anemia, the elucidation of the family history of CD being what triggered testing. It should be noted that patients will not necessarily volunteer this information unless they are asked. The patient has significant deficiencies associated with her disease. The lymphocytic colitis is an unfortunate association of CD and, in this case, responded to budesonide.

9.4 CONCLUSION

In the past decade, the diagnosis and management of CD have improved vastly due to better detection methods, earlier screening/detection, and greater awareness by professionals and industry. Ongoing research will further this process and, indeed, these are exciting times. With timely diagnosis, intervention, and routine follow-up, many of the devastating complications observed in the past can be minimized or prevented. As the number of patients being diagnosed with CD increases, heightened awareness of CD by physicians, dietitians, and other health care providers is imperative. Finally, to maximize successful treatment, improve outcomes and reduce the burden of illness in patients diagnosed with CD, management needs to include awareness of their psychosocial needs and health-related QOL as well as their physiological needs. Novel strategies provide the promise of alternative, adjunctive treatment options which may help reduce complications and improve QOL.

REFERENCES

1. Husby S, Koletzko S, Korponay-Szabo IR et al. European Society for Pediatric Gastroenterology, Hepatology, and Nutrition guidelines for the diagnosis of coeliac disease. *J Pediatr Gastroenterol Nutr* 2012;54:136–160.
2. Rashtak S, Ettore MW, Homburger HA, Murray JA. Combination testing for antibodies in the diagnosis of coeliac disease: Comparison of multiplex immunoassay and ELISA methods. *Aliment Pharmacol Ther* 2008;28:805–813.
3. Husby S, Murray JA. New aspects of the diagnosis of celiac disease in children, adolescents, and adults. *Mayo Clin Proc* 2013;88:540–543.
4. Vande Voort JL, Murray JA, Lahr BD et al. Lymphocytic duodenosis and the spectrum of celiac disease. *Am J Gastroenterol* 2009;104:142–148.
5. Junker Y, Zeissig S, Kim SJ et al. Wheat amylase trypsin inhibitors drive intestinal inflammation via activation of toll-like receptor 4. *J Exp Med* 2012;209:2395–2408.
6. Oxentenko AS, Murray JA. Celiac disease and dermatitis herpetiformis: The spectrum of gluten-sensitive enteropathy. *Int J Dermatol* 2003;42:585–587.
7. Jakes AD, Bradley S, Donlevy L. Dermatitis herpetiformis. *BMJ* 2014;348:g2557.
8. Rubio-Tapia A, Hill ID, Kelly CP, Calderwood AH, Murray JA. ACG clinical guidelines: Diagnosis and management of celiac disease. *Am J Gastroenterol* 2013;108:656–676; quiz 677.
9. Rubio-Tapia A, Rahim MW, See JA, Lahr BD, Wu TT, Murray JA. Mucosal recovery and mortality in adults with celiac disease after treatment with a gluten-free diet. *Am J Gastroenterol* 2010;105:1412–1420.
10. Dietetics AoNa. Academy of nutrition and dietetics evidence analysis library celiac disease evidence-based nutrition practice guideline. 2012. http://www.adaevidencelibrary.com/default.cfm?auth=.

11. Ukkola A, Kurppa K, Collin P, Huhtala H, Forma L, Kekkonen L, Maki M, Kaukinen K. Use of health care services and pharmaceutical agents in coeliac disease: A prospective nationwide study. *BMC Gastroenterol* 2012;12:136–145.
12. Heymann AD, Leshno M, Endevelt R, Shamir R. The high cost of celiac disease in an Israeli Health Maintenance Organization. *Health Econ Rev* 2013;3:23–28.
13. Green PH, Neugut AI, Naiyer AJ, Edwards ZC, Gabinelle S, Chinburapa V. Economic benefits of increased diagnosis of celiac disease in a national managed care population in the United States. *J Insur Med* 2008;40:218–228.
14. Caruso R, Pallone F, Stasi E, Romeo S, Monteleone G. Appropriate nutrient supplementation in celiac disease. *Ann Med* 2013;45:522–531.
15. Theethira TG, Dennis M, Leffler DA. Nutritional consequences of celiac disease and the gluten-free diet. *Expert Rev Gastroenterol Hepatol* 2014;8:123–129.
16. Jamma S, Rubio-Tapia A, Kelly CP, Murray J, Najarian R, Sheth S, Schuppan D, Dennis M, Leffler DA. Celiac crisis is a rare but serious complication of celiac disease in adults. *Clin Gastroenterol Hepatol* 2010;8:587–590.
17. Ohlund K, Olsson C, Hernell O, Ohlund I. Dietary shortcomings in children on a gluten-free diet. *J Hum Nutr Diet* 2010;23:294–300.
18. Ferrara P, Cicala M, Tiberi E, Spadaccio C, Marcella L, Gatto A, Calzolari P, Castellucci G. High fat consumption in children with celiac disease. *Acta Gastro-Enterol Belg* 2009;72:296–300.
19. Niewinski MM. Advances in celiac disease and the gluten-free diet. *J Am Diet Assoc* 2008;108:661–672.
20. Wild D, Robins GG, Burley VJ, Howdle PD. Evidence of high sugar intake, and low fibre and mineral intake, in the gluten-free diet. *Aliment Pharmacol Ther* 2010;32:573–581.
21. Aggarwal S, Lebwohl B, Green PH. Screening for celiac disease in average-risk and high-risk populations. *Ther Adv Gastroenterol* 2012;5:37–47.
22. Cheng J, Malahias T, Brar P, Minaya MT, Green PH. The association between celiac disease, dental enamel defects, and aphthous ulcers in a United States cohort. *J Clin Gastroenterol* 2010;44:191–194.
23. Lily H. Children with celiac disease: Effect of gluten-free diet on growth and body composition (review). *Top Clin Nutr* 2013;28:93–98.
24. Ludvigsson JF, Fasano A. Timing of introduction of gluten and celiac disease risk. *Ann Nutr Metab* 2012;60(suppl 2):22–29.
25. Stordal K, White RA, Eggesbo M. Early feeding and risk of celiac disease in a prospective birth cohort. *Pediatrics* 2013;132:e1202–1209.
26. Akobeng AK, Ramanan AV, Buchan I, Heller RF. Effect of breast feeding on risk of coeliac disease: A systematic review and meta-analysis of observational studies. *Arch Dis Child* 2006;91:39–43.
27. Ivarsson A, Myleus A, Norstrom F, et al. Prevalence of childhood celiac disease and changes in infant feeding. *Pediatrics* 2013;131:e687–694.
28. Rizkalla Reilly N, Dixit R, Simpson S, Green PH. Celiac disease in children: An old disease with new features. *Minerva Pediatr* 2012;64:71–81.
29. Reilly NR, Aguilar K, Hassid BG, Cheng J, Defelice AR, Kazlow P, Bhagat G, Green PH. Celiac disease in normal-weight and overweight children: Clinical features and growth outcomes following a gluten-free diet. *J Pediatr Gastroenterol Nutr* 2011;53:528–531.
30. Tucker E, Rostami K, Prabhakaran S, Al Dulaimi D. Patients with coeliac disease are increasingly overweight or obese on presentation. *J Gastrointestin Liver Dis* 2012;21:11–15.
31. Kabbani TA, Goldberg A, Kelly CP, Pallav K, Tariq S, Peer A, Hansen J, Dennis M, Leffler DA. Body mass index and the risk of obesity in coeliac disease treated with the gluten-free diet. *Aliment Pharmacol Ther* 2012;35:723–729.

32. Cheng J, Brar PS, Lee AR, Green PH. Body mass index in celiac disease: Beneficial effect of a gluten-free diet. *J Clin Gastroenterol* 2010;44:267–271.
33. Hill ID, Dirks MH, Liptak GS et al. Guideline for the diagnosis and treatment of celiac disease in children: Recommendations of the North American Society for Pediatric Gastroenterology, Hepatology and Nutrition. *J Pediatr Gastroenterol Nutr* 2005;40:1–19.
34. Sud S, Marcon M, Assor E, Palmert MR, Daneman D, Mahmud FH. Celiac disease and pediatric type 1 diabetes: Diagnostic and treatment dilemmas. *Int J Pediatr Endocrinol* 2010;2010:161285–161300.
35. Simpson SM, Ciaccio EJ, Case S, Jaffe N, Mahadov S, Lebwohl B, Green PH. Celiac disease in patients with type 1 diabetes: Screening and diagnostic practices. *Diabetes Educ* 2013;39:532–540.
36. Abid N, McGlone O, Cardwell C, McCallion W, Carson D. Clinical and metabolic effects of gluten free diet in children with type 1 diabetes and coeliac disease. *Pediatr Diabetes* 2011;12(pt 1):322–325.
37. Jacobsson LR, Friedrichsen M, Goransson A, Hallert C. Impact of an active patient education program on gastrointestinal symptoms in women with celiac disease following a gluten-free diet: A randomized controlled trial. *Gastroenterol Nurs* 2012;35:200–206.
38. Rajani S, Sawyer-Bennett J, Shirton L, DeHaan G, Kluthe C, Persad R, Huynh HQ, Turner J. Patient and parent satisfaction with a dietitian- and nurse-led celiac disease clinic for children at the Stollery Children's Hospital, Edmonton, Alberta. *Can J Gastroenterol* 2013;27:463–466.
39. Abdulkarim AS, Burgart LJ, See J, Murray JA. Etiology of nonresponsive celiac disease: Results of a systematic approach. *Am J Gastroenterol* 2002;97:2016–2021.
40. Hall NJ, Rubin GP, Charnock A. Intentional and inadvertent non-adherence in adult coeliac disease. A cross-sectional survey. *Appetite* 2013;68.56–62.
41. Dewar DH, Donnelly SC, McLaughlin SD, Johnson MW, Ellis HJ, Ciclitira PJ. Celiac disease: Management of persistent symptoms in patients on a gluten-free diet. *World J Gastroenterol* 2012;18:1348–1356.
42. Aziz I, Sanders DS. The irritable bowel syndrome-celiac disease connection. *Gastrointest Endosc Clin N Am* 2012;22:623–637.
43. Kurien M, Barratt SM, Sanders DS. Functional gastrointestinal disorders and coeliac disease in adults—Negative impact on quality of life. *Aliment Pharmacol Ther* 2011;34:1044–1045; author reply 1045–1046.
44. Usai P, Manca R, Cuomo R, Lai MA, Boi MF. Effect of gluten-free diet and co-morbidity of irritable bowel syndrome-type symptoms on health-related quality of life in adult coeliac patients. *Dig Liver Dis* 2007;39:824–828.
45. Ford AC, Chey WD, Talley NJ, Malhotra A, Spiegel BM, Moayyedi P. Yield of diagnostic tests for celiac disease in individuals with symptoms suggestive of irritable bowel syndrome: Systematic review and meta-analysis. *Arch Intern Med* 2009;169:651–658.
46. Sainsbury A, Sanders DS, Ford AC. Prevalence of irritable bowel syndrome-type symptoms in patients with celiac disease: A meta-analysis. *Clin Gastroenterol Hepatol* 2013;11:359–365 e351.
47. Dorn SD, Hernandez L, Minaya MT, Morris CB, Hu Y, Lewis S, Leserman J, Bangdiwala SI, Green PH, Drossman DA. Psychosocial factors are more important than disease activity in determining gastrointestinal symptoms and health status in adults at a celiac disease referral center. *Dig Dis Sci* 2010;55:3154–3163.
48. Sainsbury K, Mullan B, Sharpe L. Reduced quality of life in coeliac disease is more strongly associated with depression than gastrointestinal symptoms. *J Psychosom Res* 2013;75:135–141.

49. Ukkola A, Maki M, Kurppa K, Collin P, Huhtala H, Kekkonen L, Kaukinen K. Diet improves perception of health and well-being in symptomatic, but not asymptomatic, patients with celiac disease. *Clin Gastroenterol Hepatol* 2011;9:118–123.

50. Hauser W, Stallmach A, Caspary WF, Stein J. Predictors of reduced health-related quality of life in adults with coeliac disease. *Aliment Pharmacol Ther* 2007;25:569–578.

51. Addolorato G, Leggio L, D'Angelo C et al. Affective and psychiatric disorders in celiac disease. *Dig Dis* 2008;26:140–148.

52. Arigo D, Anskis AM, Smyth JM. Psychiatric comorbidities in women with celiac disease. *Chronic Illn* 2012;8:45–55.

53. Hauser W, Janke KH, Klump B, Gregor M, Hinz A. Anxiety and depression in adult patients with celiac disease on a gluten-free diet. *World J Gastroenterol* 2010;16:2780–2787.

54. van Hees NJ, Van der Does W, Giltay EJ. Coeliac disease, diet adherence and depressive symptoms. *J Psychosom Res* 2013;74:155–160.

55. Lee AR, Ng DL, Diamond B, Ciaccio EJ, Green PH. Living with coeliac disease: Survey results from the USA. *J Hum Nutr Diet* 2012;25:233–238.

56. Rose C, Howard R. Living with coeliac disease: A grounded theory study. *J Hum Nutr Diet* 2014;27:30–40.

57. Nachman F, del Campo MP, Gonzalez A et al. Long-term deterioration of quality of life in adult patients with celiac disease is associated with treatment noncompliance. *Dig Liver Dis* 2010;42:685–691.

58. Gray AM, Papanicolas IN. Impact of symptoms on quality of life before and after diagnosis of coeliac disease: Results from a UK population survey. *BMC Health Serv Res* 2010;10:105–111.

59. Paarlahti P, Kurppa K, Ukkola A, Collin P, Huhtala H, Maki M, Kaukinen K. Predictors of persistent symptoms and reduced quality of life in treated coeliac disease patients: A large cross-sectional study. *BMC Gastroenterol* 2013;13:75–83.

60. Leffler DA, Dennis M, Hyett B, Kelly E, Schuppan D, Kelly CP. Etiologies and predictors of diagnosis in nonresponsive celiac disease. *Clin Gastroenterol Hepatol* 2007;5:445–450.

61. Thompson T, Lee AR, Grace T. Gluten contamination of grains, seeds, and flours in the United States: A pilot study. *J Am Diet Assoc* 2010;110:937–940.

10 Nutrition in IBS

Anil K. Asthana, Jane G. Muir, and Peter R. Gibson

CONTENTS

10.1 INTRODUCTION

Irritable bowel syndrome (IBS) is a chronic functional gastrointestinal disorder with prominent features including bloating, abdominal pain, and altered bowel frequency. As per the Rome III criteria,[1] the diagnosis is based on symptom duration of at least 12 consecutive weeks of the preceding 12 months; these include abdominal pain or discomfort as well as the following features: relief with defecation; and/or onset associated with a change in frequency of stool; and/or onset associated with a change in form (appearance) of stool. About one in seven of the population suffers from IBS. There are multiple pathophysiological abnormalities described ranging from dysbiosis of gut microbiota, abnormal visceral perception, gastrointestinal dysmotility to psychological morbidity, and perception issues. The brain–gut axis (BGA) is at the center of IBS symptom generation with dysregulation of the autonomic, enteric, and central nervous systems (CNSs).[2]

In conservative medicine, dietary approaches have only recently become a central strategy in management of the symptoms of IBS, rather than a peripheral issue or the domain of complementary and alternative medicine. A major reason for the slow uptake has been the difficulty in providing widely acceptable levels of evidence for dietary approaches due to the complexity of food itself and of interventional trial design. This chapter will address the eating behavior of patients with IBS and the approaches that have been taken by health professionals, but will concentrate on the perspectives of understanding the physiology of individual food components and of how they potentially affect the gut to impact symptoms.

10.2 PATIENT PERCEPTIONS OF FOOD AS A TRIGGER FOR IBS SYMPTOMS

Multiple studies have observed that a high proportion (60%–84%) of patients with IBS report ingestion of food as a trigger to their IBS symptoms and express intense interest in food choice.[3–5] Patients also act upon such perceptions. For example, in a Norwegian study, food items were limited or excluded from diets in 62% of IBS patients whilst 12% of them had instigated significant dietary changes.[4] In a survey of 1242 patients aimed at determining patient perceptions and desires, 52% felt that a lack of digestive enzymes and 38% malnutrition caused IBS and 62% were interested to learn more about foods to avoid.[6] Indeed a qualitative study of women with IBS indicated that modifying dietary intake was the major way used to control symptoms.[7]

Understanding how patients with IBS eat may provide clues to the pathogenesis of the condition and/or of symptom induction, and lead to therapeutic strategies. Firstly, what specific foods that are avoided might be instructive. Some of the culprit ingredients included hot spices, alcohol, and fatty food in the Swiss Norwegian study mentioned above. In a Swedish study, 84% of 197 patients with IBS reported ingestion of at least one of a list of food items were associated with their gut symptoms.[3] The number of food items identified correlated with the severity of the IBS and its impact on quality of life, but not with anxiety or depression. There was a wide range of culprit foods that included food rich in incompletely absorbed carbohydrates in more than two-thirds, dairy products, foods rich in biogenic amines, histamine-releasing foods, and fried and fatty foods. IBS patients also perceive lactose to be a culprit trigger, often reducing the consumption of milk products and increasing the consumption of alternate milk products.[8] The interpretative limitation is that what a patient blames as the specific inducing symptom might be an innocent bystander.

Secondly, evaluating actual intake in patients with IBS compared with those unaffected might provide insight, although there are few studies reported. In a Romanian population study,[9] patients with IBS consumed more frequently canned food ($p < 0.01$), processed meat ($p < 0.01$), legumes ($p < 0.01$), whole cereals ($p < 0.01$), confectionary ($p < 0.01$), and herbal teas ($p < 0.001$). The limitation of this approach is that it cannot be ascertained whether the differences might represent cause, effect, or neither.

With the association between specific food ingestion and induction of symptoms and consequent dietary modification made by the patient, the nutritional adequacy of the diet might suffer. The few studies performed that have examined the general nutritional adequacy of the diet of cohorts of patients with IBS from Spain and Poland[10,11] have revealed few abnormalities overall, whether performed by food frequency questionnaire or prospective food diaries. However, a Norwegian study has shown that 12% of IBS patients may have a nutritionally inadequate diet as a result of exclusions.[4] The avoidance of dairy foods in response to perceptions that lactose in the culprit may result in a lower intake of vitamin B_2, phosphorus, and calcium.[8]

Thus, studies of the dietary habits and perceptions of patients have shown an intense interest in diet and a belief that food choice matters. However, the broad spectrum of culprit foods provides limited clues to what dietary approaches might be used. The complexity of food and the strong influence of overriding belief patterns limit the value of this type of interrogation. This is best illustrated by the poor predictive value of perceived lactose intolerance for actual lactose malabsorption.[12]

10.3 DIETARY APPROACHES TO MANAGEMENT OF IBS

Multiple broad changes to the diet guided by theories based upon concepts steeped in pseudoscience have been proposed and propagated largely via the internet to help reduce the symptoms of IBS. These have included the paleolithic, specific carbohydrate, anti-candida, low food-chemical, and gluten-free diets (GFDs), amongst others.[13] All have anecdotes for efficacy and have gained a strong lay, celebrity, and sometimes medical support-base, despite lack of any quality evidence. In some ways, it is not surprising that sweeping changes to dietary intake have short-term benefits, but the restrictions and changes are often so great that adherence is difficult and, more worryingly, the impact across multiple nutrient groups raise serious questions about nutritional adequacy.

Alternatives to the more philosophical "one-diet-fits-all" approach have also been applied. One method is to identify the specific foods that cause problems using biomarkers. The most infamous of these has been the use of circulating food-specific IgG.[14] The presence of an immune response would then indicate that that food should be avoided. This approach has been highly criticized as healthy people without IBS also raise such antibodies to some foods as exposure of the immune system to food-associated antigens is normal. In a similar way, skin prick or patch testing with various foods has been applied in order to identify food allergies. This approach has a poor positive predictive value,[15] not surprising since the systemic not the gut-associated immune system is being challenged. Colonoscopic injection of foods into the cecal mucosa, looking for rapid wheal formation has been applied with apparent success, but this is not practised widely and has clear practical difficulties.[16] The likelihood of patients continuing with such restrictions and whether they have durable symptomatic benefits are not known.

A second approach is to accept that there are no guiding biomarkers and to apply an exclusion diet-rechallenge technique. If the symptoms resolve on a very bland exclusion diet, then a series of rechallenges with whole foods are given. While double-blind placebo-controlled rechallenges are the gold standard, the recent experience where gluten was challenged, has questioned the reliability of such an approach.[17] Nocebo response rates can be very high, although one group has described no nocebo response in their population.[18] Such exclusion diet techniques can have impressive efficacy in short-term studies, but the durability of the benefits achieved and the ongoing adherence of patients to such changes in the diets have not been reported. These approaches are time consuming and require highly levels of motivation for both patient and health professional, and have few reports of more than short-term results.

The third approach is to accept that food is complex and to take a "reductionist" approach by examining the specific components of food that might induce pathophysiological changes and symptoms. Symptoms induced by eating food where wheat flour is a major component provide a salient example of this approach. Wheat contains protein, carbohydrates, lipids, and lectins. If one component, such as gluten or fructans, can be proven to be the inducer of symptoms, then other foods that contain gluten or fructans can be sought and subsequently reduced in the diet. A GFD will then extend to other grains, whereas a fructan-reduced diet will include onions and other vegetables. The key is in proving that the individual component is the inducer of symptoms. Examples of such approaches include the low FODMAP (fermentable oligosaccharides, disaccharides, monosaccharides, and polyols) diet, the GFD and the low food chemical diets. Hence, it is preferable to understand the components of food that might be pathogenically involved with symptom genesis. To do that, a framework of the pathophysiology of IBS upon which potential interaction of those food components can be more rationally defined will be addressed.

10.4   PATHOPHYSIOLOGICAL MECHANISMS IN IBS

The pathophysiological mechanisms that underlie the symptoms of IBS are complex. Conceptually, IBS can be considered a disorder of the BGA and a pathogenic framework as illustrated in Figure 10.1. The key components are

- *The components of the BGA:* These comprise the gut wall, enteric nervous system (ENS), autonomic nervous system (ANS), CNS, and the hypothalamo–pituitary–adrenal (HTPA) axis. Its complexities and pathways involved have been recently extensively reviewed.[19]

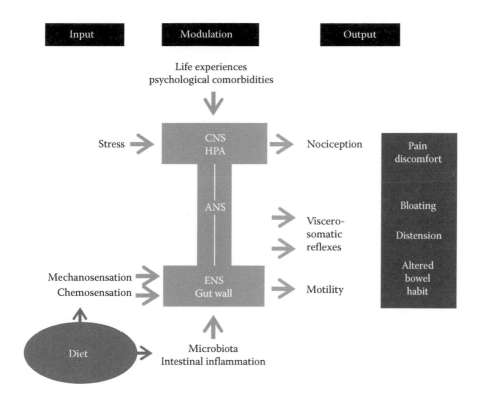

FIGURE 10.1 A pathogenic framework for IBS. The brain–gut axis (BGA, denoted as "CNS," "ANS," and "ENS", in light gray) is the core component and is considered for this diagram a "black box." "Input" refers to rapidly changing stimuli for the BGA, "Modulation" refers to factors that modulate the BGA on a longer term basis. "Output" refers to how the BGA leads to the symptoms of IBS. Dietary intake will affect the sensory input at the gut level and the modulation that microbiota and inflammation may cause.

- *The input into the BGA:* This comprises stimulation of mechano- and chemosensory receptors in the gut wall, and cerebral input from life experiences.
- *The output of the BGA (i.e., the manifestation of IBS):* This comprises central responses (such as pain and sensation of bloating), motility responses (altered bowel habit), and viscerosomatic reflexes (such as abnormal abdominal distension).
- *Modulating factors:* There are many factors that can modulate or even dictate the function of the BGA (see discussion below).

The major physiological manifestations of the disordered BGA are visceral hypersensitivity, ANS dysfunction, gut dysmotility, abnormal viscera-somatic reflexes, and abnormal perception. Such abnormalities are intimately interrelated and not independent of each other. Any individual patient will have a unique combination of any number of these key abnormalities. Hence, it is not unexpected that a heterogeneity of responses to therapies directed specifically at any one of the abnormalities or of the modulating factors will be observed, and that multiple and diverse therapeutic options are utilized in managing patients with IBS. In order to understand where food intake and dietary interventions might fit in this pathophysiological model, each component will be described including factors that potentially modulate them.

10.4.1 VISCERAL HYPERSENSITIVITY

One of the key mechanisms inducing abdominal pain is visceral hypersensitivity. The gut is bombarded by sensory stimuli from mechano- and chemosensory receptors in the gut wall. Most of these stimuli do not lead to the induction of pain/discomfort or change in motility unless of great intensity. In the presence of visceral hypersensitivity, such low level stimuli will tend to result in an output from the BGS (i.e., symptoms). This is thought to be a combination of peripheral and central mechanisms including increased expression or sensitivity of gut wall receptors leading to greater neuronal transmission from the gut wall, and central mechanisms generally referred to as "central sensitization" that involve altered neuronal transmission in the spinal cord and brain.[20]

Centrally, IBS patients may demonstrate heightened activation of the anterior cingulated cortex (ACC) to painful visceral stimuli.[21] This was ascertained by distension of different colonic regions. The central component of visceral hypersensitivity is due to increased afferent signaling to the brain in IBS rather than altered processing of signals at the level of the brain. Structural white matter changes occur as well as functional gray matter changes in IBS patients; this consists of changes in areas of the brain involved with pain and hemostasis.[22] Thus, the role of structural and functional abnormalities in the CNS in IBS patients is important to consider.

Injury at the enteric mucosa level triggers a reaction cascade manifesting as visceral hypersensitivity. Injury results in the release of chemical and inflammatory mediators such as prostaglandin; this then triggers the afferent neurons as well as mast cells and associated chemicals leading to visceral pain.[23] Serotonin can stimulate primary efferent neurons secondary to distension of the gut resulting in abdominal pain and visceral hypersensitivity.[2] Bradykinin, additionally, has been shown to regulate visceral hypersensitivity during the processes of intestinal injury and inflammation.

10.4.2 ANS DYSFUNCTION

Regulation of intestinal secretions occurs via input from the peripheral ANS, hypothalamus and ENS. It is now becoming evident that the ANS has a crucial role in the gut inflammatory process; in particular, in IBS patients, there is overactivity of the sympathetic nervous system and underactivity of the peripheral ANS.[24] This is particularly relevant for altered intestinal secretions in IBS patients, particularly in relation to the efferent neurons. IBS patients may also have other associated conditions related to ANS dysfunction such as migraines, back pain, and heartburn.[2]

10.4.3 GUT DYSMOTILITY

Abnormal motility patterns per se with IBS have not been consistently reported, with some exceptions such as increased frequency of colonic high amplitude propagated contractions IBS with diarrhea.[25] However, evidence is stronger that the motility response to sensory input is abnormal in many patients with IBS. For example, stress-induced colonic motility is increased in IBS-D with hyper-responsiveness to corticotrophin releasing factor (CRF).[26] In the fasting state, gas insufflation of the jejunum (representing a distending stimulus) leads to inappropriate motility responses with gas retention in a proportion of patients with IBS.[27,28] Furthermore, intestinal infusion of lipids impairs intestinal gas clearance in healthy patients, an effect that was exaggerated in patients with IBS.

Identification of the pathways and neurochemicals involved is important in defining new therapies. The main components involved are the ANS and ENS. In particular, serotonin has been implicated in gut dysmotility,[29] in particular by stimulation of its receptors (5-HT$_3$ and 5-HT$_4$) resulting in increased gut motility.[30] There is also evidence that gut motility, driven by the above physiological changes, is affected by psychological, other somatic and immune processes.[31]

10.4.4 ABNORMAL VISCERO-SOMATIC REFLEXES

Somatic reflex responses to intestinal stimuli, such as luminal distension, have more recently provided insight into mechanisms of gross abdominal distension that occurs in some patients, without apparent marked distension of the intestine. The intraabdominal volume is controlled in part by the tone of the diaphragmatic and anterior abdominal wall musculature. Intestinal distension leads to relaxation of the diaphragm and increased tone of the anterior abdominal wall muscles. Paradoxical responses have been observed to occur in patients who have major problems with abdominal distension in association with bloating.[32] Such abnormal reflexes are similar to the pelvic floor dyssynergia that occurs in some patients with constipation and is associated with abdominal bloating and distension.[33]

10.4.5 PSYCHOLOGICAL COMORBIDITIES

Psychological comorbidities are reported to be present in about one-half of patients with functional gastrointestinal disorders.[34] These include anxiety disorders, depression, somatoform disorders, and phobic disorders. Such a background psychological state may influence the clinical expression of the condition, such as lowering pain thresholds, increased health-seeking behavior, and a tendency to catastrophization.[35,36] Coping strategies tend to be passive and may be considered dysfunctional for a patient with chronic illness. Childhood and life experiences are likely to contribute to the background psychological state; for example, a high frequency of a history of sexual and physical abuse has been reported.[34]

10.4.6 MODULATING FACTORS

There is ample evidence that several factors modulate these pathophysiological mechanisms. At the level of the gut, these include the gut microbiota and neuro-inflammatory changes in the gut wall. There is great interest in the controversial concept of small intestinal bacterial overgrowth and its role in symptom induction, especially with the high level evidence now showing modest efficacy of antibiotics in patients with diarrhea-predominant IBS, the demonstration of dysbiosis of intestinal microbiota in patients with IBS,[37] and the influence of the gut microbiota on brain function.[38] Mild inflammatory changes in the intestinal mucosa of patients with postinfectious IBS, the putative role of mast cell activation in IBS and centrally, and the effect of intestinal inflammation on nociceptive receptors in the gut have focused attention on neuroinflammatory events and their role in inducing, for example, visceral hypersensitivity.[39] At a central level, evidence for a role of psychological factors such as stress, anxiety, and depression in modulating the central responses to input from the gut is strong.

10.5 INTERACTION OF FOOD WITH PATHOPHYSIOLOGICAL MECHANISMS

Ingestion of food can potentially interact with the BGS and its modulating factors in many ways that might include the following:

- *Major source of sensory input into the gut wall and ENS:* This can occur via luminal distension and stimulation of chemosensory receptors. Indeed, food ingestion per se is an important stimulus to the motility of the gut via, for example, the gastrocolic reflex. However, specific food components can stimulate mechanoreceptors via inducing luminal distension (such as poorly absorbed short-chain carbohydrates), or stimulate taste receptors (such as glutamate stimulating glutamate receptors and capsaicin stimulating TRP-V1 receptors).[40]
- *Alteration of the gut microbiota:* Food, particularly carbohydrates can modulate the structure and function of the gut microbiota, which is now recognized to have key interactions with the body's immune system, metabolism, and possibly cognition.[31]
- *Induction of inflammation in the gut wall:* This can range from the obvious (e.g., T-cell-mediated responses to gluten in celiac disease) to food allergies, to the putative activation of mast cells by food chemicals such as salicylates.
- *Altering receptor expression and/or function is the gut wall:* Food chemicals influence chemoreceptor expression,[41] but studies have been largely limited to experimental animals. The exception is capsaicin, for which chronic exposure leads to a downregulation of its receptor.
- *Modulation of mental health:* This can potentially occur by altering HPTA activity,[42] or by changing mood, such as gluten inducing current feeling of depression in patients who believe they have nonceliac gluten sensitivity (NCGS).[43]

Thus, there are multiple entry points to the abnormal BGA that food might be pathogenic and, more importantly, where food choice might be able to be used as a therapy to alleviate symptoms or even reverse underlying pathophysiological abnormalities.

10.5.1   Food

As outlined above, there is little doubt that ingestion of food has a temporal relationship to the induction of symptoms in patients with IBS. This can be nonspecific; the so-called gastrocolic reflex has been well described. Abnormal colonic motor responses to food ingestion have been demonstrated in patients with IBS, with faster transit in those with predominantly diarrhea and slower transit in those with predominantly constipation.[44] With such a background, it can be hazardous attributing the triggering of symptoms to specific foods, and such cause–effect relationships have been notoriously inaccurate. Furthermore, food is complex and attribution of symptoms to one known component can override other potential triggers. This has been most evident with gluten; wheat has many potential inducers of symptoms, yet gluten is often blamed, and often unfairly. For these reasons, identification of specific dietary triggers of symptoms has been difficult and inaccurate. A recent report of dietary triggers identified multiple food types that induced symptoms in patients, including vegetables and fatty foods.[45]

Hence identification of specific dietary triggers of symptoms requires a different approach. Food is a complex of substances comprising macronutrients, micronutrients, food chemicals, and inert substances.[46] If individual components of food that may trigger IBS symptoms by any or all of the mechanisms discussed above can be identified then more pathogenically related dietary changes may be more rationally designed. Some of the evidence in this line of enquiry is outlined in the following.

10.5.2   Carbohydrates

Traditionally, specific carbohydrates have been isolated as causative for symptoms of IBS, in particular lactose and fructose. Carbohydrates are the most abundant organic molecules found in nature and classified according to their chain length or degree of polymerization (DP). The nomenclature is, therefore, based on the number of carbon atoms present—monosaccharides and polyols (sugar alcohols) with a single DP, disaccharides for DP 2, oligosaccharides for DP 3–10, and polysaccharides for DP greater than 10. Examples of monosaccharides include glucose and fructose, disaccharides include sucrose and lactose, oligosaccharides include galacto-oligosaccharides (GOS) and fructo-oligosaccharides (FOS), polysaccharides include starches, pectin and cellulose, and polyols include sorbitol and mannitol. The structure of these molecules is affected by presence of either α or β bonds within them.

The carbohydrates that cause problems associated with IBS are those that are indigestible and/or poorly absorbed in the small intestine. This relates to their propensity to be water retaining and/or fermentable by intestinal bacteria. Only these will be considered. While the indigestible carbohydrates can be classified by structure and size, a new, functional classification into three groups—fiber (laxation), FODMAPs (IBS symptom induction), and prebiotics (selective growth of favorable bacteria)—has recently been proposed.[47] While these groups are highly overlapping, it provides the basis of a better understanding of the complexities of altering carbohydrate intake.

10.5.3 Dietary Fiber

The definition of fiber is at best controversial. It is generally defined as those carbohydrates of a DP more than two that are not hydrolyzed or absorbed in the upper part of the gastrointestinal tract.[48] An alternative definition is nonstarch carbohydrates derived from plant foods and poorly digested by human body enzymes, but this excludes resistant starch.[48] Specifically, ingestion of total fiber consists of the sum of dietary fiber plus any added fiber, which usually comprises of nondigestible carbohydrates providing good physiological benefits.[49] The recommended average daily requirement of dietary fiber in adults is 20–35 g/day.

10.5.3.1 Laxation

The principle function of fiber from the gastrointestinal point of view is laxation. Once in the colon, fibers may remain unfermented, be partially fermented or be totally fermented.[50] Fiber has a key role in laxation via two mechanisms. The first is a bulking effect related to retention of water and the increase in the bacterial biomass as a consequence of fermentation.[51] Secondly, it decreases colonic transit time related to the increased bulk and the pro-motility effects of short-chain fatty acids (SCFA) as a by-product produced of fermentation. Gas (methane, hydrogen, and carbon dioxide) is also released during fermentation, which may be associated with the release of excessive flatus and sensations of bloating.

10.5.3.2 Types of Fiber

Dietary fibers are heterogeneous in their effects on the basis of varying solubility, fermentability, and, to a lesser extent, chain length. There are multiple systems of fiber classification but a recently proposed system of five types based upon those variables is preferable since it takes a more functional approach.[51] *Solubility* dictates the ability to hold water, *fermentability* dictates where fermentation is likely to occur in the large bowel and to some extent the effect on colonic transit (e.g., the more rapid the fermentation in the proximal colon, the less effect it will have on transit), and regarding *chain length*, those of very short-chain length, particularly oligosaccharides, will have more rapid fermentation and proximal gas production is greater without a laxative effect. Thus, dietary fiber should not be viewed as a single entity but as a heterogeneous group of indigestible carbohydrates that have heterogeneous effects.

10.5.3.3 Fiber Use in IBS

As outlined above, studies of fiber supplementation in patients with IBS have reported heterogeneous outcomes, as outlined in Table 10.1. Ispaghula (or psyllium), a fiber of intermediate solubility and fermentability, improves global symptoms with a pooled relative risk of symptom relief being 1.55 (95% CI, 1.35–1.78). In a double-blind randomized placebo-controlled trial in 80 IBS patients, constipation significantly improved with psyllium ($p = 0.026$), transit time decreased in the fiber group ($p = 0.001$) but there was no significant difference in the improvement of abdominal pain or bloating.[52] In contrast, wheat bran, the fiber content of which is insoluble and slowly fermented,[53] is similar to placebo in improving global IBS symptoms (relative

TABLE 10.1

Summary of Studies Addressing the Efficacy of Fiber Supplements for Symptoms of Irritable Bowel Syndrome (IBS)

Type of Study	Fibers Studied	No. of Studies	Numbers Studied	Response	Reference
Meta-analysis	Bran, ispaghula/psyllium, one unspecified	12	591	Fiber more effective than placebo	111
	Corn fiber, ispaghula, psyllium, bran	13	607	Inconsistent results; OR 1.9	112
Systematic reviews	Psyllium, ispaghula, calcium polycarbophil Corn, wheat bran	17	1363	Benefits for global IBS symptoms were marginal; soluble fiber OR 1.55, insoluble fiber OR 0.89	54
	Insoluble and soluble fibers	12	621	No benefit of bulking agents	113
	Psyllium, coarse bran, concentrated fiber, polycarbophil, ispaghula	13	341	Efficacy not clearly established. All three high-quality studies showed significant improvement in nonspecific outcomes, for example, ease of stool passage, constipation	114
	Corn fiber, ispaghula, bran fiber, polycarbophil, plantago ovate	7	288	Effective for treating constipation but little evidence for improving entire IBS symptom complex	115

risk 0.89; 95% CI, 0.72–1.11) in a systematic review.[54] Some individual studies have suggested wheat bran to be beneficial[55] or detrimental to the symptoms of IBS,[56] but generally they have been underpowered. It is clear, however, that, as in patients with simple constipation, wheat bran can improve constipation by reducing colonic transit and increasing daily stool weight, but at the cost of greater pain and bloating.

In summary, the use of commercial fiber supplements carries the risks of worsening pain, bloating, and gas production, presumably by distending the sensitive colon due to gas production and increased bulk of the contents. Another hidden hazard is the fact that wheat bran that contains nonstarch polysaccharides that are very slowly fermented also has a moderate content of oligosaccharides.[57] The use of nonfermentable fiber such as sterculia or methylcellulose in constipated patients in whom gas and bloating are major issues is logical, but there is a paucity of evidence for or against this approach. On the positive side, ispaghula (and wheat bran) do have positive effects on constipation. Hence, contrary to previous anecdotal recommendations when fiber intake was universally advised for IBS symptoms, current literature illustrates that this may not always be an optimal strategy. When deciding upon the use of fiber for the treatment of IBS patients, the characteristics of each agent, such as its fermentability and subsequent impact on symptoms, should be considered.

10.5.4   FODMAPs

In the 1980s and 1990s, lactose and fructose were identified as inducers of IBS symptoms.[58,40] Breath-hydrogen testing was used to look for evidence of fructose malabsorption in IBS patients compared to controls. However, when fructose malabsorption was found to be of similar frequency in patients with IBS as in controls, it was not thought to play an important role in the etiology of IBS. Likewise, lactose restriction in those with lactose intolerance was found to be an ineffective strategy for symptoms of IBS.[59] Not to be deterred, the suggestion that fructose and fructans in the diet were common triggers of IBS symptoms was made in a retrospective evaluation of patients with fructose malabsorption on breath hydrogen testing who had been educated on a diet that restricted both fructose in excess of glucose and fructans.[60] This was strongly supported by a subsequent randomized blinded rechallenge cross-over study in such patients, in which fructose and fructans both induced symptoms while glucose did not.

On the basis of shared putative effects on the intestine and by observations of additive effects on symptoms of individual sugars (e.g., fructose and fructans, fructose and sorbitol), a hypothesis was published that suggested *all* dietary poorly absorbed fermentable short-chain carbohydrates should be grouped together and restricted in the diet to gain optimal benefit of gut symptoms.[61] These short-chain carbohydrates were collectively termed "FODMAPs" (*F*ermentable *O*ligosaccharides, *D*isaccharides, *M*onosaccharides, *A*nd *P*olyols), and the FODMAP concept was born. Characteristics, common sources, and physiological consequences of the ingestion of FODMAPs are shown in Table 10.2.

10.5.4.1   Small Intestinal Absorption of FODMAPs

Before delving deeper into specific evidence-based diets, it is important to understand the physiology of carbohydrate absorption in the small intestine. Monosaccharides are the basic component of carbohydrates; all other complex molecules, such as disaccharides and polysaccharides, need to be hydrolyzed by hydrolases, found in the intestinal brush border. The major monosaccharides consist of glucose, galactose, and fructose, each with different methods of absorption. Glucose and galactose are absorbed by SGLT1, a high affinity transporter in the small intestine. This transporter is responsible for transport of luminal glucose when luminal concentrations are low and tends to be absent in patients with glucose–galactose malabsorption.[62] Fructose has two major transporters—GLUT2 and GLUT5—although other transporters of uncertain functional significance have recently been described.[63] The GLUT2 transporter is present on the basolateral membrane where it transports hexoses out of the cell down the concentration gradient.[64] It carries glucose, galactose, and fructose. Importantly, this is a high-capacity glucose-dependent fructose cotransporter. This system, therefore, allows lower luminal concentrations of glucose to be taken up by the cells which in turn activates a system which can take up

TABLE 10.2
Characteristics, Common Sources, and Physiological Consequences of FODMAPs

		Main Constituents	Common Food Sources	Physiological Effects
F	Fermentable			Increased osmotic effect
O	Oligosaccharides	Fructo-oligosaccharides	Onion, wheat, barley, garlic, beetroot, artichoke, leek, rye, peach, watermelon	Rapid bacterial fermentation resulting in gas production. Favors hydrogen over methane production
		Galacto-oligosaccharides	Lentils, legumes	↑ Gastroesophageal reflux and small bowel motility
D	Disaccharides	Lactose	Milk, yoghurt, ice cream	Fatigue
M	Monosaccharides	"Free fructose"	Honey, pears, apples, watermelon, asparagus, high-fructose corn syrup	Prebiotic effects
A	And			
P	Polyols	Mannitol, sorbitol, xylitol	Cherries, nectarines, plums, peaches, mushrooms, cauliflower, avocado, prune, confectionery	Possible effects via binding to taste receptors

all hexoses more efficiently. On the other hand, GLUT5 is a facultative transporter (glucose independent) requiring a concentration gradient for movement and is specific for fructose. This dual absorption system for fructose means that the efficiency of fructose absorption is dependent upon the luminal concentrations of glucose. If there are at least equal concentrations of glucose and fructose, fructose tends to be absorbed rapidly in the proximal small intestine; fructose is absorbed slowly along the length of the small intestine if its concentration exceeds that of luminal glucose. Thus, coingestion of glucose enhances fructose absorption via the GLUT2 mechanism. "Fructose malabsorption" is defined by its fermentation by intestinal bacteria before its absorption can occur. Thus, fructose malabsorption will occur if the GLUT5 transporter expression is low, if there is rapid small intestinal transit, if the load of fructose in excess of glucose in the lumen is very high, or in the presence of small intestinal bacterial overgrowth.[47]

Polyols (sugar alcohols) appear to be absorbed by passive diffusion and is slow, occurring right along the small intestine. A proportion of people will not fully absorb a load of polyols and they will be fermented by intestinal bacteria. Like fructose, they will be malabsorbed if the load is high, if transit is fast, or if the absorptive rate is altered. The current concept is that their diffusion across the epithelium is via epithelial pores.[65] The size of these pores may indeed be altered by mucosal disease;[66] sorbitol absorption is increased in celiac disease and mannitol absorption is greater in patients with IBS than that in healthy controls.[67]

Oligosaccharides are not hydrolyzed in the small intestine since mammalian small intestine does not possess the hydrolases needed. More than 90% of oligosaccharides are delivered to the colonic lumen.[68]

10.5.4.2 Pathophysiology of Symptom Generation

The putative mechanism by which FODMAPs trigger symptoms is via luminal distension with subsequent stimulation of mechanoreceptors. The evidence that this occurs is substantial and occurs via two main mechanisms:

- *Increasing luminal water content*: This increases due to the osmotic effect of the FODMAPs, since they are poorly absorbed and the luminal osmolality is equivalent to that in the tissues. This effect has been confirmed by showing an increase in ileostomy water output with a modest increase in dietary FODMAP intake.[68] The luminal distension probably does predominantly occur in the small intestine as demonstrated by calculation of the small intestinal luminal water volume using magnetic resonance imaging.[69,70] This effect will be greater the smaller the molecule. Thus, fructose and polyols will exert the greatest osmotic effect. It does not require them to malabsorbed since mannitol markedly increased small intestinal water despite its complete absorption in most patients with IBS and fructose malabsorption (on breath hydrogen testing) was not needed to increase small intestinal water.[79] Indeed, symptoms induced by both mannitol and fructose were independent of its malabsorption, suggesting that a major cause of the symptoms was distension of the small intestine.[67]
- *Increased intestinal gas production:* The ready fermentation of FODMAPs leads to increased production of hydrogen, carbon dioxide, and methane, presumably mainly in the colon. This occurred throughout the day when the patterns of breath methane and hydrogen production with consumption of a high compared to low-FODMAP diet in healthy controls and patients with IBS were examined.[71] Furthermore, there was preferential production of hydrogen over methane in healthy subjects although no significant difference was observed in IBS patients. This suggests that there is increased volume of gas produced per molecule of carbohydrate when FODMAPs are consumed in high amounts.

There are other potential mechanisms by which FODMAPs might trigger symptoms. SCFAs are also one of the main by-products of carbohydrate fermentation, and these increase water and sodium absorption as well as promote motility.[13] High luminal production can also increase visceral sensitivity, at least in rats.[72] Their effects on FFA receptors are poorly understood. Ingestion of FODMAPs can also change gastro-esophageal motility causing increased reflux. Mechanisms for this effect are not known. The effect of FODMAPs on taste receptors in the gut are also an unexplored area of research. Acute exposure of patients with IBS to FODMAPs in food was associated with the induction of tiredness, but this effect was not seen in healthy controls. Mechanisms for such effects are unclear, but it is possible that stimulation of taste or other receptors may be involved or indeed other metabolic products of their fermentation have been postulated.[73]

10.5.4.3 Low-FODMAP Diet

The overriding concept behind the low-FODMAP diet is that if FODMAPs trigger gut symptoms from distending the lumen, then reducing their intake in the diet will lead to reduce sensory input from mechanosensors and lead to a marked reduction of symptoms in those with visceral hypersensitivity. Indeed, evidence is accumulating for the efficacy of the diet in about three out of four patients with IBS. However, whether the presence of visceral hypersensitivity predicts response has yet to be studied. Details of the evidence base for efficacy of the low-FODMAP diet in patients with IBS are shown in Table 10.3. The most recently reported study used gold-standard techniques in a randomized single-blinded cross-over study comparing a diet of usual FODMAP content with that of reduced FODMAPs by feeding the subjects all their food.[74] Overall abdominal symptoms were approximately halved across the 30 patients studied by reducing FODMAPs. In addition, eight healthy subjects were also studied and no differences in symptoms were seen between the diets, supporting the notion that the low-FODMAP diet is one for alleviating symptoms in patients with IBS,[117] not one for good health in general.

The structure of the diet follows the simple principles that foods with a high content of FODMAPs be avoided and be replaced with those low in FODMAPs. Adjunct techniques such as the use of glucose coingestion with foods high in free fructose (as discussed above) can be used and lactase can be taken with lactose-containing food in those with lactose malabsorption. This plan depends upon accurate and comprehensive knowledge of the FODMAP content of food. Since such information was only presented in a patchy manner when the diet was initially set up, a program of food analysis is needed which uses validated enzymatic assay techniques and high pressure liquid chromatography.[75–77] As the database thus created continues to grow, published information on food content needs frequent updating. Published literature often contains errors as the knowledge grows. In order to permit ready access of patients to accurate food lists, the Monash University Low-FODMAP Diet App was launched (http://www.med.monash.edu/cecs/gastro/fodmap/iphone-app.html). This has provided a vehicle that can be updated regularly. There are still limitations in the database. It has predominantly tested Australian foods, but a program of testing international foods is underway and, in the near future, filters in the app will permit country-specific information to be accessed.

All published data on the diet has involved education of patients by dietitians trained in delivering the diet. It is recommended that the diet be followed strictly for 4 weeks to assess its efficacy. In controlled trials, response is seen within 1 week, but it may take longer than this for the patients to adjust to the new dietary plan. If there has been an excellent response after 4 weeks, a cautious food-reintroduction plan should be followed to determine the individual's tolerance to specific FODMAPs. It is not envisaged that this is a strict diet for life in all but those more severely

TABLE 10.3

Published Studies Addressing the Efficacy of the Low-FODMAP Diet on Gastrointestinal Symptoms

Type of Study	Diets Studied	Number Studied	Patient Group(s)	Responses	Reference
Observational	Fructose/fructan restriction	62	IBS[a] with fructose malabsorption	74% with durable response	63
	Low FODMAP	90	Unselected IBS	72% satisfied with response	81
	Low FODMAP	15	IBD[b] with ileorectal anastomosis or ileo-anal pouch anastomosis	67% improved; no improvement in those with pouchitis	116
	Low FODMAP	72	Quiescent IBD with IBS-like symptoms	>50% responded	83
Nonrandomized comparative	Low FODMAP versus standard dietary advice	72	Unselected IBS	76% versus 54% for comparator satisfied with response ($p = 0.038$)	117
Randomized controlled	Rechallenge cross-over: fructose versus fructans versus fructose and fructans versus glucose	25	IBS with fructose malabsorption who had responded to fructose/fructan restriction	Symptoms not adequately controlled in 70% fructose, 77% fructans, 79% combination, 14% glucose ($p < 0.002$)	60
	Low versus high FODMAP cross-over—all food provided	30	Unselected IBS (15), healthy (15)	Gut symptoms and lethargy worse with high-FODMAP diet; only flatus worse in healthy subjects	74
	Low FODMAP versus habitual	41	Unselected IBS	Adequately controlled symptoms: 68% versus 23% ($p = 0.005$)	88
	Low versus typical Australian FODMAP cross-over—all food provided	38	Unselected IBS (30), healthy (8)	Overall symptoms less on low-FODMAP diet ($p < 0.001$); 70% response; no difference in healthy subjects	74

[a] IBS = irritable bowel syndrome.

[b] IBD = inflammatory bowel disease.

affected by IBS. Rather it is anticipated that the majority of those responding would be able to follow less strict restriction with continuing efficacy.

10.5.4.4 Role for Breath Hydrogen Testing

Hydrogen breath testing is the most common method of assessing for carbohydrate malabsorption. The test is based on the principle that hydrogen gas production, in humans, only occurs as a result of bacterial metabolism of carbohydrates.[78] It has been an important research tool, but whether its application has a role beyond detection of lactose malabsorption has recently been questioned.[47] The basis for its use was to assess an individual's ability to absorb FODMAPs which are variably absorbed in order to better design the dietary approach. However, recent data showing that symptom induction by fructose and polyols is independent of their malabsorption and issues about the intra-individual reproducibility of tests for fructose malabsorption indicate that the results will not influence dietary approaches. However, in a prospective observational series, having breath tests seem to prepare patients better for dietary intervention and the presence of fructose malabsorption predicted response to subsequent dietary change.[79]

10.5.4.5 Adherence to a Low-FODMAP Diet

The low-FODMAP diet requires considerable effort by the patient to follow and adherence to the low-FODMAP diet has been shown to be a strong predictor of response to it. Somewhat surprisingly, the adherence rate to a precursor diet (fructose malabsorption diet) was 77% (always or frequently adherent)[80] and subsequent retrospective studies have observed similar high rates. Predictors of adherence have been evaluated in two studies. The first in patients with IBS-like symptoms and IBD, response was clearly related to adherence and this was better in those who had reached a higher education level, worked less than 35 h/week and had access to appropriate cookbooks. In the second study in patients with IBS, 60% stated that the diet was easy to follow and 44% were able to incorporate the diet easily into their life.[79] Adherence was associated with a dietitian consultation, receiving written information, having support from family and friends, and accessing low-FODMAP cookbooks and online information. Furthermore, adherence rates were higher in those patients who liked the overall taste of the diet and found it easy to follow. Interestingly, the patients who had breath hydrogen testing felt that it helped them to understand the role of the diet. Thus, the diet is not as difficult to follow as some imagine, and the method of delivery of the diet—by a dietitian and with access to quality written or electronic information—is an important part of optimizing adherence to the diet.

10.5.4.6 Clinical Applications Other Than IBS

Reduction of FODMAP intake has been shown to provide an effective therapy in patients with stable IBD but with the presence of functional symptoms. A wide array of symptoms, such as abdominal pain, bloating, wind, and diarrhea improve with dietary intervention ($p < 0.02$ for all).[81] Reduction of functional symptoms in Crohn's disease patients were associated with adherence to the diet ($p = 0.033$) and inefficacy with nonadherence ($p = 0.013$). A low-FODMAP diet has also been shown to reduce stool frequency in patients who have undergone a colectomy with pouch formation but without pouchitis.[82] The median stool frequency in this study fell from 8 to 4 ($p = 0.001$) in the seven patients without pouchitis. None of the eight patients who had pouchitis improved but these patients did have a tendency to be associated with a low baseline FODMAP diet.

Other functional gastrointestinal disorders might benefit from a low-FODMAP diet. Functional dyspepsia has not been evaluated. However, intake of FODMAPs increases physiologically-assessed gastroesophageal reflux as well as heartburn in patients with gastroesophageal reflux disease,[83] but whether reducing FODMAP intake will improve symptoms of reflux has not been addressed. Observations that the volume output from an ileostomy will fall with reduction of FODMAPs[68] suggests this approach might have application in ieostomates with a high output. This has not been formally studied. It has been hypothesized that FODMAPs in enteral nutrition formulas might be one factor responsible for enteral nutrition-associated diarrhea. A retrospective study of factors associated with diarrhea in such a population did suggest an association with formulas with higher FODMAP content,[84] but recent data has indicated that the measurement of FODMAP content of enteral formulas is problematic and a study *in vivo* indicated that they are not likely to have high content of FODMAPs.[85]

10.5.4.7   Potential Hazards Associated with the Low-FODMAP Diet

A critical issue when making large changes to diet is to ensure maintenance of nutritional adequacy. The nutritional adequacy of a low-FODMAP diet has been assessed in a randomized controlled trial; patients were randomized to the interventional low-FODMAP diet or the habitual diet for 4 weeks. As expected, the dietary intake of starch, carbohydrates, and total sugars were lower following the 4 weeks of this interventional diet.[86] Calcium intake was also lower but protein, fat, total energy, and nonstarch polysaccharides were not different between the two groups. It was surprising that fiber intake was not reduced, since FODMAPs and nonstarch polysaccharides coexist. It is thus important, when advising patients to follow a low-FODMAP diet, to ensure adequacy of carbohydrate in general and dietary fiber specifically, and that calcium substitution is achieved. This is another major advantage of patients being taught the diet by dietitians who pay specific attention to nutritional adequacy.

As outlined below, many FODMAPs, particularly the oligosaccharides, exhibit prebiotic activity. In other words, a low-FODMAP diet reduces natural prebiotic intake. Indeed, changes occur to the fecal microbiota while following the diet. For example, following a low-FODMAP diet for 4 weeks led to lower absolute and relative abundances of fecal *Bifidobacteria* compared with those on habitual diet.[86] In a cross-over study in which the effects of 3 weeks' diets differing in their FODMAP content (with similar overall fiber levels) on fecal microbiota were examined and compared with that on their habitual diet, absolute abundance of putatively beneficial bacteria, especially strongly butyrate-producing *Clostridia* groups and *Bifidobacteria*, were reduced in the low FODMAP arm, as might be expected with the reduction of fermentable substrates.[87] Large differences in the relative abundance of the *Clostridia* groups and the putatively health-promoting mucus-associated bacterium, *Akkermansia muciniphila*, were also observed as might also be anticipated if prebiotics are markedly restricted. However, most of the differences related to an apparent prebiotic effect associated with the dietary arm with the highest oligosaccharide intake (where gut symptoms were the greatest), rather than an "anti-prebiotic" effect of the low FODMAP arm. Such effects might have implications in the long term, although this is purely theoretical. However, it does underline the concept that the low-FODMAP diet should only be followed strictly in the short term and the level of tolerance to FODMAPs needs to be determined.

10.6   PREBIOTICS

Prebiotics are nondigestible dietary components that result in specific changes in the composition and/or activity of the gastrointestinal microbiota. They are substances which tend to be resistant to digestion, are usually fermentable and promote the growth of beneficial bacteria.[88] In other words, the ingestion of prebiotics may be a tool to favorably change the gut microbiota.

Such an effect has potential benefit for patients with IBS, based upon the apparent dysbiosis in the fecal microbiota that has been reported in populations of patients with IBS and the belief that such dysbiosis is causally related to IBS. Inconsistencies in abnormalities documented, the small and poorly phenotyped patient groups studied and small apparently healthy controls for comparison have left the issue of dysbiosis inconclusive.[89] However, more recent studies have shown consistent microbiota patterns in subgroups that might permit stratification of patients into a postinfectious/diarrhea-predominant IBS[90] or into subgroups in which gut or CNS abnormalities appear to predominate.[91] Furthermore, in a recent study in gnotobiotic rats, visceral hypersensitivity could be transferred via fecal microbiota from patients,[92] offering evidence that the microbiota might be a driving force at least in some patients.

Nearly all work on prebiotics has been done using dietary additives such as inulin, fructo-oligosaccharides (FOS, oligofructose), or synthetic GOS. Only a few studies have been performed in patients with functional gut symptoms. Of three that have used FOS, one using 20 g/day made patients worse than in controls,[93] one had not apparent effect at a dose of 6 g/day,[94] and third using 5 g/day found significant improvement in IBS symptoms compared with placebo-treated patients.[95] An additional study examined the effect of 3.5 g/day of a synthetic GOS in patients with IBS. A prebiotic effect was observed with increased fecal *Bifidobacteria* and symptoms improved.[96]

There are a few reasons why heterogeneity of effects might be observed in studies of prebiotic supplements. The first is the dose used. High doses like 20 g FOS per day is likely to exceed the maximal dose at which a prebiotic effect will be observed, the excess oligosaccharide will be nonspecifically fermented, and, as it is FODMAP, will induce symptoms. Secondly, in no study was the dietary intake of prebiotics (such as FOS and GOS) assessed. This is likened to studying the effect of drug on a clinical end point when all subjects currently use that drug, but the dose is not known. There has been little attention paid to natural prebiotics in the diet in health promotion.

The dilemma is that FODMAPs are being restricted to control IBS symptoms, yet FODMAPs with prebiotic actions are being tested as therapy for IBS. This apparent paradox is compounded by the loss of prebiotic effect when FODMAPs are markedly restricted (as outlined above). Resolution of this conflict, if possible, will involve both the judicious selection of prebiotics to use (a longer chain molecule like inulin will have less osmotic effect and may be less rapidly fermented) and the application of a dose that exerts a prebiotic effect and minimizes nonspecific fermentation. It is also evident that it is not known whether the specific prebiotic effects of oligosaccharides do indeed correct the dysbiosis found in some patients with IBS.

10.7 PROTEIN

The role of dietary proteins in IBS is a lot less established and more controversial than that of carbohydrates. Proteins might act in the pathogenesis of IBS or its symptoms in several ways.

10.7.1 FOOD ALLERGY

Food allergy is not uncommon, but seldom masquerades as IBS. Such reactions may be IgE- or non-IgE mediated. Attempts to implicate proteins from various sources in the genesis of IBS by skin testing (prick or patch) or by detecting specific IgE or IgG to food antigens have not met with success as the sensitivity and specificity of positive tests have been generally very poor.[15] For example, the use of food-specific IgG to direct dietary changes has been highly criticized and not recommended because the presence of such antibodies is a normal phenomenon and the supporting data for efficacy was unconvincing.[97] The use of colonoscopically performed prick tests in the proximal colon, with the read-out being wheal formation has promise, but has only been reported by one group and has not been widely applied.[16]

Another type of food allergy to proteins has been described mainly in the setting of wheat sensitivity. The condition has many immune-mediated phenomena associated with it, including atopic phenotype, eosinophilic infiltration of the small and large intestinal mucosa and, interestingly, the intraepithelial compartment in about one-third of patients, the presence of anti-gliadin antibodies in about 40%, and the presence of eosinophilic cationic protein in feces and a positive basophil activation test in the majority of patients.[98] It is recognized initially by a double-blind, placebo-controlled challenge of capsules containing wheat. Two groups of patients have been defined—those only with wheat sensitivity and those with multiple food sensitivity. Surprisingly, it comprised about one-third of a large population of patients presenting with IBS and all of those had at least short-term resolution of symptoms on appropriate dietary restrictions. This condition has yet to be described in other centers and needs independent confirmation.

10.7.2 GLUTEN

Celiac disease can present with typical symptoms of IBS. Given the importance of making that diagnosis and initiating a GFD to improve not only symptoms but outcome, it is essential that all patients with IBS be screened for celiac disease and that GFD is not instituted until such an assessment has been made because of the difficulty excluding celiac disease after gluten has been withdrawn. However, there are increasing numbers of patients with IBS who are taking a GFD on the advice of medical practitioners and naturopaths, or from books, celebrities, and the internet. Those who have improved on a GFD, and have had celiac disease and wheat allergy excluded, fulfill the criteria for NCGS.

That wheat is a major trigger for symptoms of IBS has been known for years. Many authors had assumed that this represented the effect of withdrawal of gluten and many rechallenge studies have used wheat products. Unfortunately, FODMAPs commonly coexist with gluten.[57] The other issue in the NCGS story has been the blurring between NCGS and celiac disease; several studies have included many patients with intraepithelial lymphocytosis and some with celiac-specific serology suggesting that the NCGS populations described were contaminated by patients with celiac disease and minimal intestinal lesions. This aspect is fully reviewed elsewhere.[99] Two publications from the one investigating group describing three randomized controlled trials in patients who fulfilled the criteria for NCGS have further muddied the waters.[17,100] Both utilized FODMAP-deplete gluten, the only studies to do this, and studied only patients with normal celiac-specific serology and duodenal histology while consuming adequate gluten or who were HLA-DQ2 and DQ8 negative. The first pilot study was a parallel group design in which the patient groups consumed muffins and bread spiked or not with gluten.[100] It involved only 35 patients and overall symptoms significantly worsened with gluten ($p = 0.047$). This was also true for individual symptoms. Contrary to previous studies, there were no differences in any end point between individuals who were positive or negative for HLA-DQ2/8.

This study prompted a second, well-powered study in 37 subjects which utilized a cross-over design where all food was provided in an attempt to avoid potential confounders such as variations in the intake of FODMAPs.[17] In addition, all patients were educated in lowering FODMAPs in a run-in period during which time all patients improved their gut symptoms (despite remain gluten-free throughout). The intervention was for 7 days and comprised high gluten (16 g/day), low gluten (2 g/day) and no gluten, with whey protein making up the control. Symptoms worsened to a similar degree in all three arms and only three patients had gluten-specific effects. A second controlled trial was then performed in 22 of these patients. Again no differences were observed between gluten, placebo and whey protein arms and the three patients with gluten-specific induction of symptoms in the prior trial did not reproduce this effect. In all three trials, no evidence of immune activation, change in intestinal permeability, and systemic or intestinal inflammation were noted. Since this publication represented the gold standard from rechallenge dietary experiments (repeated double-blinded, placebo-control where all food was provided), it is likely that it represents strong evidence that at least this group of patients did not have NCGS on the basis of gut symptoms.

However, the plot thickens. Many of the patients continued a GFD after the results were revealed as they felt better. This was addressed in a preliminary study in which the effect of 3 days' gluten on current feelings of anxiety and depression using the State Trait Personality Inventory.[43] Indeed, current feelings of depression were observed in the gluten-treated arm but not the placebo or whey protein arms. This can only be regarded as a preliminary pilot study and interpretation of the findings must be guarded until a more definitive study is performed.

Thus, recent high-quality evidence places serious doubts on the prescription of a GFD for IBS symptoms, at least as a first-line dietary therapy. Further research is needed from other centers for its true role to be defined.

10.8   FAT

The belief that fat is a dietary trigger for symptoms is common amongst IBS patients when there is no evidence confirming this. An important pathophysiological feature of IBS is of visceral hypersensitivity; lipids have been found to increase colonic hypersensitivity. A colonic distension trial was carried out on IBS patients and healthy controls[101]; a barostat was used to measure distension pressures before and after a duodenal lipid infusion.[118] IBS patients were found to have an altered viscerosomatic referral pattern and increased colonic sensitivity post lipid infusion. Based on this, it would be reasonable to suggest avoidance of high-fat content intake in IBS patients. Caldarella et al. confirmed a similar principal using graded rectal distensions pre- and postintraduodenal lipid infusions. IBS patients had increased visceral sensitivities compared to healthy controls ($p < 0.05$).[102] Fats can also worsen abnormalities in gastric accommodation and functional dyspeptic symptoms.[103] Interestingly, polyunsaturated fatty acids have been shown to induce beneficial effects on intestinal inflammation[104] but there is not sufficient evidence to advocate its use clinically. Thus, fat intake is a credible factor in worsening visceral hypersensitivity and this aspect can be considered as part of the patient's IBS management plan.

10.9   FOOD CHEMICALS

Food chemicals are substances which are found widespread in food and have been implicated in systemic syndromes (e.g., salicylates). The main chemicals are salicylates, glutamates, and amines. These have important functional roles in plants, for example, enhancing pollination through colors and odors, bad taste for protection and antimicrobial actions.[46] It is thought that these food chemicals may have a particularly important interaction with the nervous system and the process of neuroinflammation rather than the immune system.[46,105] A low food chemical diet has been described in the past but there is no high-quality evidence to support this.[106] An alternative use for food chemicals is as a therapeutic strategy. Capsaicin in red pepper has been used for receptor desensitization and this was significant in reducing the intensity of abdominal pain and bloating compared to placebo.[107] Hence, food chemicals comprise an important area to study and to further our understanding of functional symptoms; well-designed trials are required to explore this.

10.10   CONCLUSIONS

Gastroenterology has come a long way in the past two decades with respect to management of IBS. Initially being a diagnosis of exclusion, IBS is now correctly acknowledged as a complex pathophysiological condition with contributions from the BGA, dysbiosis, inflammation, visceral hypersensitivity, and dysmotility. Diet, as outlined in this chapter, has a pivotal role in shifting the equilibrium in most, if not all of these pathophysiological processes. The advent of the low-FODMAP diet has revolutionized how we utilize diet as a therapeutic strategy to improve symptoms in an evidence-based manner. It is imperative to continue expanding this evidence-based platform as there persists excessive, nonevidence-based restrictive diets that are followed by the general public under the guidance of self-proclaimed dietary gurus and the media. This is indeed a dangerous situation as restrictive diets may be accompanied by nutritional inadequacy, which can harm the patient. Thus, following evidence-based dietary recommendations will be in the best interests of the patients. In the future, there is potential to explore predictive patient factors to the low-FODMAP diet, using diet as a therapeutic drug and the role of food chemicals in the management of IBS, in addition to further study of gluten as a dietary villain in the absence of celiac disease.

10.11   CASE STUDY

A 36-year-old female executive attorney visits the gastroenterology clinic for your expert opinion on her self-diagnosed IBS; the main troublesome symptoms consist of bloating, abdominal pain, and constipation. These can worsen with stress at work and home. She admits having lost weight but has put this down to stress in her life. She has been advised to follow the paleolithic diet, which has not improved her symptoms. She also takes a marketed highly soluble fiber product after reading about its benefits in her weekly magazine. She has been strictly gluten free for 2 years because she was convinced that gluten had worsened her symptoms in the past and feels certain that she has undiagnosed celiac disease. She admits to drinking 2–3 standard glasses of wine each evening. She lives at home with a family of three children and her husband, who, like herself, works in a high-pressure environment. She is otherwise healthy with no significant past medical history and currently consumes no regular medications or over-the-counter products. How would you approach this diagnostic problem?

This women has several issues to tease out and they need to be addressed in a systematic manner.

1. *Define the correct diagnosis:* Her symptoms do sound consistent with IBS but her past response to a GFD (one that is apparently not continuing in the longer term) is important to note and further explore. After eliciting a detailed history and performing a physical gastrointestinal examination, some basic blood tests would be helpful. The aims would be to exclude celiac disease with celiac-specific serology comprising tissue transglutaminase and deamidated gliadin peptide antibodies or endomysial antibody levels depending upon availability and a serum concentration measurement IgA, screen for inflammatory disease with C-reactive protein, serum albumin, and blood hematology, assess for nutritional deficiencies in light of her restrictive diets and weight loss with, for example, iron studies and vitamin D and zinc levels, and check her thyroid status with estimation of thyroid-stimulating hormone levels. Celiac serology was negative, but in view of her prolonged adherence to a GFD, celiac

disease cannot be confidently excluded. HLA testing for DQ2 and DQ8 is then indicated. She was negative and thus, celiac disease can be excluded. If she were positive, gluten challenge would be necessary with subsequent duodenal biopsy and serology. The result indicated no "red flags" and normal nutritional indices; a confident diagnosis of IBS was made. She cannot be labeled as having "NCGS" without careful consideration to gluten rechallenge.

2. *Referral to a specialist dietitian:* The patient has an intense interest in diet, but her current combination of gluten-free and paleolithic diet seems nutritionally challenging. It is also noted that she continues on both despite their lack of impact on her gastrointestinal symptoms. This is a common finding.[108] She ought to be referred to a specialized gastrointestinal dietitian who has experience of managing IBS patients. The purpose is threefold—to evaluate the nutritional adequacy of her diet, to advise regarding nonspecific measures for improving dietary habits (such as eating regularly including breakfast, modulating fiber intake including avoiding the fiber supplement, reducing fat intake, and reducing alcohol intake), and for specific advice that would include instruction on the low-FODMAP diet. A longer-term desire would be to divert her away from the GFD, but this would be inappropriate as an initial approach and would depend upon success in achieving other changes and in relieving her symptoms.

3. *Treating her constipation:* Effective treatment of constipation preferably—avoiding bulk-creating strategies such as osmotic laxatives and fiber, with a preference for pro-kinetic agents and/or bowel retraining with biofeedback if pelvic floor dyssynergy is suspected—is associated with improved bloating and should be attempted.[109]

4. *Attention to psychological issues:* The BGA has a crucial role in the pathophysiology of IBS; this woman would benefit from management of her stress by nonpharmacological and pharmacological strategies.[110] The possibility of active depression would need to be explored and addressed; a multidisciplinary approach would be highly advisable with the possibility of cognitive behavior therapy or hypnotherapy entertained (according to local availability and patient preference). Such an approach should be followed for most complex IBS patients to achieve optimal outcomes. An empathetic physician would benefit her greatly in this situation and regular follow-up with the physician and dietitian would ensure optimal care is delivered.

The outcome of this approach was excellent. She accepted dietary advice and had six 1-h sessions of gut-directed hypnotherapy. The hypnotherapy provided better strategies for stress alleviation and helped her undertake dietary change, in addition to the possible benefits on her underlying gut visceral hypersensitivity. The low FODMAP approach achieved considerable symptomatic improvement in association with liberalization from her previous restrictions. She even gained sufficient confidence to abandon the GFD. The constipation improved with this dietary approach and the aggressive treatment planned was not needed.

The learnings from this case are several. Firstly, appropriate diagnostic work-up is important to enable confident delivery of a diagnosis and institution of specific therapies. Secondly, dietary change carries risks of worsening behavioral and psychological health if not delivered appropriately. Given the strong nocebo effect that food ingestion has when the individual believes that specific foods induce symptoms, it raises the importance of avoiding unsubstantiated food restrictions in patients with IBS. Furthermore, many patients seem to accumulate dietary restriction even when ineffective, rather than replace one with another. At the extreme end, the patients can become "dietary cripples"—and without symptomatic benefit. Thirdly, dietary manipulation in more complex situations is not stand-alone therapy. Attention to psychological issues, for instance, is an important adjunct. In this case, hypnotherapy may have increased her willingness to lift long-standing dietary restrictions. Finally, time and multidisciplinary involvement are keys to gaining optimal outcomes.

REFERENCES

1. Longstreth, G.F., W.G. Thompson, W.D. Chey, L.A. Houghton, F. Mearin, and R.C. Spiller. Functional bowel disorders. *Gastroenterology* 2006;130:1480–1491.
2. Karantanos, T., T. Markoutsaki, M. Gazouli, N.P. Anagnou, and D.G. Karamanolis. Current insights in to the pathophysiology of irritable bowel syndrome. *Gut Pathog* 2010;2:3.
3. Simren, M., A. Mansson, A.M. Langkilde et al. Food-related gastrointestinal symptoms in the irritable bowel syndrome. *Digestion* 2001;63:108–115.
4. Monsbakken, K.W., P.O. Vandvik, and P.G. Farup. Perceived food intolerance in subjects with irritable bowel syndrome—Etiology, prevalence and consequences. *Eur J Clin Nutr* 2006;60:667–672.
5. Bohn, L., S. Storsrud, H. Tornblom, U. Bengtsson, and M. Simren. Self-reported food-related gastrointestinal symptoms in IBS are common and associated with more severe symptoms and reduced quality of life. *Am J Gastroenterol* 2013;108:634–641.
6. Halpert, A., C.B. Dalto, O. Palsson et al. What patients know about irritable bowel syndrome (IBS) and what they would like to know. National survey on patient educational needs in IBS and development and validation of the patient educational needs questionnaire (PEQ). *Am J Gastroenterol* 2007;102:1972–1982.
7. Jamieson, A.E., P.C. Fletcher, and M.A. Schneider. Seeking control through the determination of diet: A qualitative investigation of women with irritable bowel syndrome and inflammatory bowel disease. *Clin Nurse Spec* 2007;21:152–160.
8. Ostgaard, H., T. Hausken, D. Gundersen, and M. El-Salhy. Diet and effects of diet management on quality of life and symptoms in patients with irritable bowel syndrome. *Mol Med Rep* 2012;5:1382–1390.
9. Chirila, I., E.D. Petrariu, I. Ciortescu, C. Mihai, and V.L. Drug. Diet and irritable bowel syndrome. *J Gastroenterol Liver Dis* 2012;21:357–362.
10. Cabre, E. Irritable bowel syndrome: Can nutrient manipulation help? *Curr Opin Clin Nutr Metab Care* 2010;13:581–587.
11. Prescha, A., J. Pieczynska, R. Ilow et al. Assessment of dietary intake of patients with irritable bowel syndrome. *Rocz Panstw Zakl Hig* 2009;60:185–189.
12. Vernia, P., V. Marinaro, F. Argnani, M. Di Camillo, and R. Caprilli. Self-reported milk intolerance in irritable bowel syndrome: What should we believe? *Clin Nutr* 2004;23:996–1000.
13. Shepherd, S.J., M.C. Lomer, and P.R. Gibson. Short-chain carbohydrates and functional gastrointestinal disorders. *Am J Gastroenterol* 2013;108:707–717.

14. Atkinson, W., T.A. Sheldon, N. Shaath, and P.J. Whorwell. Food elimination based on IgG antibodies in irritable bowel syndrome: A randomised controlled trial. *Gut* 2004;53:1459–1464.
15. Niec, A.M., B. Frankum, and N.J. Talley. Are adverse food reactions linked to irritable bowel syndrome? *Am J Gastroenterol* 1998;93:2184–2190.
16. Bischoff, S.C., J. Mayer, J. Wedemeyer et al. Colonoscopic allergen provocation (COLAP): A new diagnostic approach for gastrointestinal food allergy. *Gut* 2007;40:745–753.
17. Biesiekierski, J.R., S.L. Peters, E.D. Newnham, O. Rosella, J.G. Muir, and P.R. Gibson. No effects of gluten in patients with self-reported non-celiac gluten sensitivity after dietary reduction of fermentable, poorly absorbed, short-chain carbohydrates. *Gastroenterology* 2013;145:320–328.
18. Carroccio, A., P. Mansueto, G. Iacono et al. Non-celiac wheat sensitivity diagnosed by double-blind placebo-controlled challenge: Exploring a new clinical entity. *Aliment Pharmacol Ther* 2012;107:1898–1906.
19. Camilleri, M. Physiological underpinnings of irritable bowel syndrome: Neurohormonal mechanisms. *J Physiol* 2014;592(Pt 14):2967–2980.
20. Fichna, J. and M.A. Storr. Brain-gut interactions in IBS. *Front Pharmacol* 2012;3:127.
21. Hall, G.B., M.V. Kamath, S. Collins et al. Heightened central affective response to visceral sensations of pain and discomfort in IBS. *Neurogastroenterol Motil* 2010;22:276–280.
22. Chen, J.Y., U. Blankstein, N.E. Diamant, and K.D. Davis. White matter abnormalities in irritable bowel syndrome and relation to individual factors. *Brain Res* 2011;1392:121–131.
23. Tracey, D.J. and J.S. Walker. Pain due to nerve damage: Are inflammatory mediators involved? *Inflammation Res* 1995;44:407–411.
24. Adeyemi, E.O., K.D. Desai, M. Towsey, and D. Ghista. Characterization of autonomic dysfunction in patients with irritable bowel syndrome by means of heart rate variability studies. *Am J Gastroenterol* 1999;94:816–823.
25. Chey, W.Y., H.O. Jin, M.H. Lee, S.W. Sun, and K.Y. Lee. Colonic motility abnormality in patients with irritable bowel syndrome exhibiting abdominal pain and diarrhea. *Am J Gastroenterol* 2001;96:1499–1506.
26. Fukudo, S., T. Nomura, and M. Hongo. 1998. Impact of corticotropin-releasing hormone on gastrointestinal motility and adrenocorticotropic hormone in normal controls and patients with irritable bowel syndrome. *Gut* 1998;42:845–849.
27. Salvioli, B., J. Serra, F. Azpiroz et al. Origin of gas retention and symptoms in patients with bloating. *Gastroenterology* 2005;128:574–579.
28. Maxton, D.G., D.F. Martin, P.J. Whorwell, and M. Godfrey. Abdominal distension in female patients with irritable bowel syndrome: Exploration of possible mechanisms. *Gut* 1991;32:662–664.
29. Gershon, M.D. The enteric nervous system: A second brain. *Hosp Pract* 1999;34:31–2, 5–8, 41–42 passim.
30. Talley, N.J., S.F. Phillips, A. Haddad et al. GR 38032F (ondansetron), a selective 5HT3 receptor antagonist, slows colonic transit in healthy man. *Dig Dis Sci* 1990;35:477–480.
31. Cooke, H.J. Neurotransmitters in neuronal reflexes regulating intestinal secretion. *Ann NY Acad Sci* 2000;915:77–80.
32. Villoria, A., F. Azpiroz, E. Burri, D. Cisternas, A. Soldevilla, and J.R. Malagelada. Abdomino-phrenic dyssynergia in patients with abdominal bloating and distension. *Am J Gastroenterol* 2011;106:815–819.
33. Shim, L., G. Prott, R.D. Hansen, L.E. Simmons, J.E. Kellow, and A. Malcolm. Prolonged balloon expulsion is predictive of abdominal distension in bloating. *Am J Gastroenterol* 2010;105:883–887.

34. Drossman, D.A., F.H. Creed, K.W. Olden, J. Svedlund, B.B. Toner, and W.E. Whitehead. Psychosocial aspects of the functional gastrointestinal disorders. *Gut* 1999;45(suppl 2):II25–II30.

35. Seres, G., Z. Kovacs, A. Kovacs et al. Different associations of health related quality of life with pain, psychological distress and coping strategies in patients with irritable bowel syndrome and inflammatory bowel disorder. *J Clin Psychol Med Settings* 2008;15:287–295.

36. van Tilburg, M.A., O.S. Palsson, and W.E. Whitehead. Which psychological factors exacerbate irritable bowel syndrome? Development of a comprehensive model. *J Psychosom Res* 2013;74:486–492.

37. Cremon, C., G. Carini, R. De Giorgio, V. Stanghellini, R. Corinaldesi, and G. Barbara. 2010. Intestinal dysbiosis in irritable bowel syndrome: Etiological factor or epiphenomenon? Expert review of molecular diagnostics. *World J Gastroenterol* 2010;10(4):389–393.

38. Collins, S.M. and P. Bercik. Gut microbiota: Intestinal bacteria influence brain activity in healthy humans. *Nature Rev Gastroenterol Hepatol* 2013;10:326–327.

39. Feng, B., J.H. La, E.S. Schwartz, and G.F. Gebhart. Irritable bowel syndrome: Methods, mechanisms, and pathophysiology. Neural and neuro-immune mechanisms of visceral hypersensitivity in irritable bowel syndrome. *Am J Physiol Gastrointest Liver Physiol* 2012;302:G1085–G1098.

40. Nelis, G.F., M.A. Vermeeren, and W. Jansen. Role of fructose-sorbitol malabsorption in the irritable bowel syndrome. *Gastroenterology* 1990;99:1016–1020.

41. Gibson, P.R. and S.J. Shepherd. Food choice as a key management strategy for functional gastrointestinal symptoms. *Am J Gastroenterol* 2012;107:657–666.

42. Belvederi Murri, M., C. Pariante, V. Modelli et al. HPA axis and aging in depression: Systematic review and meta-analysis. *Psychoneuroendocrinology* 2014;41:46–62.

43. Peters, S.L., J.R. Biesiekierski, G.W. Yelland, J.G. Muir, and P.R. Gibson. Randomised clinical trial: Gluten may cause depression in subjects with non-coeliac gluten sensitivity—An exploratory clinical study. *Aliment Pharmacol Ther* 2014;39:1104–1112.

44. Deiteren, A., M. Camilleri, D. Burton, S. McKinzie, A. Rao, and A.R. Zinsmeister. Effect of meal ingestion on ileocolonic and colonic transit in health and irritable bowel syndrome. *Dig Dis Sci* 2010;55:384–391.

45. Hayes, P., C. Corish, E. O'Mahony, and E.M. Quigley. A dietary survey of patients with irritable bowel syndrome. *J Hum Nutr Diet* 2014;27(suppl 2):36–47.

46. Gibson, P.R., J.S. Barrett, and J.G. Muir. Functional bowel symptoms and diet. *Intern Med J* 2013;43:1067–1074.

47. Tuck, C.J., J.G. Muir, J.S. Barrett, and P.R. Gibson. Fermentable oligosaccharides, disaccharides, monosaccharides and polyols: Role in irritable bowel syndrome. *Expert Rev Gastroenterol Hepatol* 2014;15:1–16.

48. Floch, M.H. and R. Narayan. Diet in the irritable bowel syndrome. *J Clin Gastroenterol* 2002;35(suppl 1):S45–S52.

49. Zuckerman, M.J. The role of fiber in the treatment of irritable bowel syndrome: Therapeutic recommendations. *J Clin Gastroenterol* 2006;40:104–108.

50. Flamm, G., W. Glinsmann, D. Kritchevsky, L. Prosky, and M. Roberfroid. Inulin and oligofructose as dietary fiber: A review of the evidence. *Crit Rev Food Sci Nutr* 2001;41:353–362.

51. Eswaran, S., J. Muir, and W.D. Chey. Fiber and functional gastrointestinal disorders. *Am J Gastroenterol* 2013;108:718–727.

52. Prior, A. and P.J. Whorwell. Double blind study of ispaghula in irritable bowel syndrome. *Gut* 1987;28:1510–1513.

53. Ritchie, J.A. and S.C. Truelove. Treatment of irritable bowel syndrome with lorazepam, hyoscine butylbromide, and ispaghula husk. *Br Med J* 1979;1(6160):376–378.

54. Bijkerk, C.J., J.W. Muris, J.A. Knottnerus, A.W. Hoes, and N.J. de Wit. Systematic review: The role of different types of fiber in the treatment of irritable bowel syndrome. *Aliment Pharmacol Ther* 2004;19:245–251.

55. Manning, A.P., K.W. Heaton, and R.F. Harvey. Wheat fiber and irritable bowel syndrome. A controlled trial. *Lancet* 1977;2(8035):417–418.

56. Cann, P.A., N.W. Read and C.D. Holdsworth. What is the benefit of coarse wheat bran in patients with irritable bowel syndrome? *Gut* 1984;25:168–173.

57. Gibson, P.R. and J.G. Muir. Not all effects of a gluten-free diet are due to removal of gluten. *Gastroenterology* 2013;145:693.

58. Ravich, W.J., T.M. Bayless, and M. Thomas. Fructose: Incomplete intestinal absorption in humans. *Gastroenterology* 1983;84:26–29.

59. Parker, T.J., J.T. Woolner, A.T. Prevost, Q. Tuffnell, M. Shorthouse, and J.O. Hunter. Irritable bowel syndrome: Is the search for lactose intolerance justified? *Eur J Gastroenterol Hepatol* 2001;13:219–225.

60. Shepherd, S.J., F.C. Parker, J.G. Muir, and P.R. Gibson. Dietary triggers of abdominal symptoms in patients with irritable bowel syndrome: Randomized placebo-controlled evidence. *Clin Gastroenterol Hepatol* 2008;6:765–771.

61. Gibson, P.R. and S.J. Shepherd. Personal view: Food for thought—Western lifestyle and susceptibility to Crohn's disease. The FODMAP hypothesis. *Aliment Pharmacol Ther* 2005;21:1399–1409.

62. Ferraris, R.P. Dietary and developmental regulation of intestinal sugar transport. *Biochem J* 2001;360(Pt 2):265–276.

63. Putkonen, L., C.K. Yao, and P.R. Gibson. Fructose malabsorption syndrome. *Curr Opin Clin Nutr Metab Care* 2013;16:473–477.

64. Gibson, P.R., E. Newnham, J.S. Barrett, S.J. Shepherd, and J.G. Muir. Review article: Fructose malabsorption and the bigger picture. *Aliment Pharmacol Ther* 2007;25:349–363.

65. Langkilde, A.M., H. Andersson, T.F. Schweizer, and P. Wursch. Digestion and absorption of sorbitol, maltitol and isomalt from the small bowel. A study in ileostomy subjects. *Eur J Clin Nutr* 1994;48:768–775.

66. Fordtran, J.S., F.C. Rector, T.W. Locklear, and M.F. Ewton. Water and solute movement in the small intestine of patients with sprue. *J Clin Invest* 1967;46:287–298.

67. Yao, C.K., H.L. Tan, D.R. van Langenberg et al. Dietary sorbitol and mannitol: Food content and distinct absorption patterns between healthy individuals and patients with irritable bowel syndrome. *J Hum Nutr Diet* 2014;27(suppl 2):263–275.

68. Barrett, J.S., R.B. Gearry, J.G. Muir et al. Dietary poorly absorbed, short-chain carbohydrates increase delivery of water and fermentable substrates to the proximal colon. *Aliment Pharmacol Ther* 2010;31:874–882.

69. Marciani, L., E.F. Cox, C.L. Hoad et al. Postprandial changes in small bowel water content in healthy subjects and patients with irritable bowel syndrome. *Gastroenterology* 2010;138:469–477.

70. Murray, K., V. Wilkinson-Smith, C. Hoad et al. Differential effects of FODMAPs (fermentable oligo-, di-, mono-saccharides and polyols) on small and large intestinal contents in healthy subjects shown by MRI. *Am J Gastroenterol* 2013;109:110–119.

71. Ong, D.K., S.B. Mitchell, J.S. Barrett et al. Manipulation of dietary short chain carbohydrates alters the pattern of gas production and genesis of symptoms in irritable bowel syndrome. *J Gastroenterol Hepatol* 2010;25:1366–1373.

72. Xu, D., X. Wu, G. Grabauskas, and C. Owyang. Butyrate-induced colonic hypersensitivity is mediated by mitogen-activated protein kinase activation in rat dorsal root ganglia. *Gut* 2013;62:1466–1474.

73. Depoortere, I. Taste receptors of the gut: Emerging roles in health and disease. *Gut* 2014;63:179–190.

74. Halmos, E.P., V.A. Power, S.J. Shepherd, P.R. Gibson, and J.G. Muir. 2014. A diet low in FODMAPs reduces symptoms of irritable bowel syndrome. *Gastroenterology* 2014;146:67–75.
75. Muir, J.G., S.J. Shepherd, O. Rosella, R. Rose, J.S. Barrett, and P.R. Gibson. Fructan and free fructose content of common Australian vegetables and fruit. *J Agr Food Chem* 2007;55:6619–6627.
76. Muir, J.G., R. Rose, O. Rosella et al. Measurement of short-chain carbohydrates in common Australian vegetables and fruits by high-performance liquid chromatography (HPLC). *J Agric Food Chem* 2009;57:554–565.
77. Biesiekierski, J.R., O. Rosella, R. Rose et al. Quantification of fructans, galacto-oligo-sacharides and other short-chain carbohydrates in processed grains and cereals. *J Hum Nutr Diet* 2011;24:154–176.
78. Simren, M. and P.O. Stotzer. Use and abuse of hydrogen breath tests. *Gut* 2006;55:297–303.
79. de Roest, R.H., B.R. Dobbs, B.A. Chapman et al. The low FODMAP diet improves gastrointestinal symptoms in patients with irritable bowel syndrome: A prospective study. *Int J Clin Pract* 2013;67(9):895–903.
80. Shepherd, S.J. and P.R. Gibson. Fructose malabsorption and symptoms of irritable bowel syndrome: Guidelines for effective dietary management. *J Am Diet Assoc* 2006;106:1631–1639.
81. Gearry, R.B., P.M. Irving, J.S. Barrett, D.M. Nathan, S.J. Shepherd, and P.R. Gibson. Reduction of dietary poorly absorbed short-chain carbohydrates (FODMAPs) improves abdominal symptoms in patients with inflammatory bowel disease-a pilot study. *J Crohns Colitis* 2009;3:8–14.
82. Croagh, C., S.J. Shepherd, M. Berryman, J.G. Muir, and P.R. Gibson. Pilot study on the effect of reducing dietary FODMAP intake on bowel function in patients without a colon. *Inflammatory Bowel Dis* 2007;13:1522–1528.
83. Piche, T., S.B. des Varannes, S. Sacher-Huvelin, J.J. Holst, J.C. Cuber, and J.P. Galmiche. Colonic fermentation influences lower esophageal sphincter function in gastroesophageal reflux disease. *Gastroenterology* 2003;124:894–902.
84. Halmos, E.P., J.G. Muir, J.S. Barrett, M. Deng, S.J Shepherd, and P.R. Gibson. Diarrhoea during enteral nutrition is predicted by the poorly absorbed short-chain carbohydrate (FODMAP) content of the formula. *Aliment Pharmacol Ther* 2010;32:925–933.
85. Halmos, E.P. Role of FODMAP content in enteral nutrition-associated diarrhea. *J Gastroenterol Hepatol* 2013;28(suppl 4):25–28.
86. Staudacher, H.M., M.C. Lomer, J.L. Anderson et al. Fermentable carbohydrate restriction reduces luminal bifidobacteria and gastrointestinal symptoms in patients with irritable bowel syndrome. *J Nutr* 2012;142:1510–1518.
87. Halmos, E.P., C.T. Christophersen, A.T. Bird, S.J. Shepherd, P.R. Gibson, and J.G. Muir. Submitted. Diets that differ in their FODMAP content alter the colonic luminal micro-environment. *Gut* (in re-review).
88. Whelan, K. Mechanisms and effectiveness of prebiotics in modifying the gastrointestinal microbiota for the management of digestive disorders. *Proc Nutr Soc* 2013;72:288–298.
89. Simren, M., G. Barbara, H.J. Flint et al. Intestinal microbiota in functional bowel disorders: A Rome foundation report. *Gut* 2013;62:159–176.
90. Jalanka-Tuovinen, J., J. Salojärvi, A. Salonen et al. Faecal microbiota composition and host-microbe cross-talk following gastroenteritis and in postinfectious irritable bowel syndrome. *Gut* 2013; in press.
91. Jeffery, I.B., P.W. O'Toole, L. Ohman et al. An irritable bowel syndrome subtype defined by species-specific alterations in faecal microbiota. *Gut* 2012;61:997–1006.

92. Crouzet, L., E. Gaultier, C. Del'Homme et al. The hypersensitivity to colonic distension of IBS patients can be transferred to rats through their fecal microbiota. *Neurogastroenterol Motil* 2013;25:e272–e282.
93. Olesen, M. and E. Gudmand-Hoyer. Efficacy, safety, and tolerability of fructooligosaccharides in the treatment of irritable bowel syndrome. *Am J Clin Nutr* 2000;72:1570–1575.
94. Hunter, J.O., Q. Tuffnell, and A.J. Lee. Controlled trial of oligofructose in the management of irritable bowel syndrome. *J Nutr* 1999;129(suppl 7):1451S–1453S.
95. Paineau, D., F. Payen, S. Panserieu et al. The effects of regular consumption of short-chain fructo-oligosaccharides on digestive comfort of subjects with minor functional bowel disorders. *Br J Nutr* 2008;99:311–318.
96. Silk, D.B., A. Davis, J. Vulevic, G. Tzortzis, and G.R. Gibson. Clinical trial: The effects of a trans-galactooligosaccharide prebiotic on faecal microbiota and symptoms in irritable bowel syndrome. *Aliment Pharmacol Ther* 2009;29:508–518.
97. Ligaarden, S.C., S. Lydersen, and P.G. Farup. IgG and IgG4 antibodies in subjects with irritable bowel syndrome: A case control study in the general population. *BMC Gastroenterol* 2012;12:166.
98. Carroccio, A., P. Mansueto, A. D'Alcamo, and G. Iacono. Non-celiac wheat sensitivity as an allergic condition: Personal experience and narrative review. *Am J Gastroenterol* 2013;108:1845–1852.
99. Gibson, P.R. and J.G. Muir. Not all effects of a gluten-free diet are due to removal of gluten. *Gastroenterology* 2013;145:693.
100. Biesiekierski, J.R., J.G. Muir, and P.R. Gibson. Is gluten a cause of gastrointestinal symptoms in people without celiac disease? *Curr Allergy Asthma Rep* 2013;13:631–638.
101. Biesiekierski, J.R., E.D. Newnham, P.M. Irving et al. Gluten causes gastrointestinal symptoms in subjects without celiac disease: A double-blind randomized placebo-controlled trial. *Am J Gastroenterol* 2011;106:508–514.
102. Simren, M., H. Abrahamsson, and E.S. Bjornsson. Lipid-induced colonic hypersensitivity in the irritable bowel syndrome: The role of bowel habit, sex, and psychologic factors. *Clin Gastroenterol Hepatol* 2007;5:201–208.
103. Caldarella, M.P., A. Milano, F. Laterza et al. Visceral sensitivity and symptoms in patients with constipation- or diarrhea-predominant irritable bowel syndrome (IBS): Effect of a low-fat intraduodenal infusion. *Am J Gastroenterol* 2005;100:383–389.
104. Feinle-Bisset, C. and F. Azpiroz. Dietary and lifestyle factors in functional dyspepsia. *Nat Rev Gastroenterol Hepatol* 2013;10:150–157.
105. Marion-Letellier, R., P. Dechelotte, M. Iacucci, and S. Ghosh. Dietary modulation of peroxisome proliferator-activated receptor gamma. *Gut* 2009;58:586–593.
106. Raithel, M., H.W. Baenkler, A. Naegel et al. Significance of salicylate intolerance in diseases of the lower gastrointestinal tract. *J Physiol Pharmacol* 2005;56(suppl 5):89–102.
107. Allen, D.H., S. Van Nunen, R. Loblay, L. Clarke, and A. Swain. Adverse reactions to foods. *Med J Aust* 1984;141(suppl 5):S37–S42.
108. Bortolotti, M. and S. Porta. Effect of red pepper on symptoms of irritable bowel syndrome: Preliminary study. *Dig Dis Sci* 2011;56:3288–3295.
109. Biesiekierski, J.R., E.D. Newnham, S.J. Shepherd, J.G. Muir, and P.R. Gibson. Characterisation of adults with a self-diagnosis of nonceliac gluten sensitivity. *Nutr Clin Pract* 2014; in press.
110. Yang, L.S., A. Khera, and M.A. Kamm. Outcome of behavioural treatment for idiopathic chronic constipation. *Intern Med J* 2014; in press.
111. Asthana, A.K. and P.R. Gibson. IBS in IBD and psychological implications. In: A. Micocka-Walus and S. Knowles, Eds. *Psychological Aspects of Inflammatory Bowel Disease: A Biopsychosocial Approach*, 2014; Great Britain: Barnes & Noble.

112. Ford, A.C., N.J. Talley, B.M. Spiegel et al. Effect of fiber, antispasmodics, and peppermint oil in the treatment of irritable bowel syndrome: Systematic review and meta-analysis. *Br Med J* 2008;337:a2313.
113. Lesbros-Pantoflickova, D., P. Michetti, M. Fried, C. Beglinger, and A.L. Blum. Meta-analysis: The treatment of irritable bowel syndrome. *Aliment Pharmacol Ther* 2004;20:1253–1269.
114. Ruepert, L., A.O. Quartero, N.J. de Wit, G.J. van der Heijden, G. Rubin, and J.W. Muris. Bulking agents, antispasmodics and antidepressants for the treatment of irritable bowel syndrome. *Cochrane Database Syst Rev* 2011;(8):CD003460.
115. Jailwala, J., T.F. Imperiale, and K. Kroenke. Pharmacologic treatment of the irritable bowel syndrome: A systematic review of randomized, controlled trials. *Ann Intern Med* 2000;133:136–147.
116. Akehurst, R. and E. Kaltenthaler. Treatment of irritable bowel syndrome: A review of randomised controlled trials. *Gut* 2001;48;272–282.
117. Staudacher, H.M., K. Whelan, P.M. Irving, and M.C. Lomer. Comparison of symptom response following advice for a diet low in fermentable carbohydrates (FODMAPs) versus standard dietary advice in patients with irritable bowel syndrome. *J Hum Nutr Diet* 2011;24:487–495.
118. Salvioli, B., J. Serra, F. Azpiroz, and J.R. Malagelada. Impaired small bowel gas propulsion in patients with bloating during intestinal lipid infusion. *Am J Gastroenterol* 2006;101:1853–1857.

11 Nutrition in Inflammatory Bowel Disease

Robert Shulman and Seema Mehta Walsh

CONTENTS

Inflammatory bowel disease (IBD) is a chronic, immune-mediated gastrointestinal disorder comprised of two major phenotypes, Crohn's disease (CD) and ulcerative colitis (UC). The inflammatory process in CD can affect any part of the gastrointestinal tract and is transmural. In contrast, UC affects only the colon and inflammation is limited to the mucosa. Despite these differences, nutrition increasingly has been identified as an important consideration in IBD. As the location of nutrient absorption, the gastrointestinal tract is constantly exposed to dietary antigens. Diet also plays a key role influencing the composition and function of the gastrointestinal microbial population (microbiome). Thus, it is understandable that investigators have evaluated various dietary habits and their potential causative role in the development of IBD, the nutritional deficits resulting from IBD, and the potential therapeutic role of nutrition in treating IBD.[1] This chapter will review these intriguing relationships in further detail.

11.1 DIETARY CONSTITUENTS AS RISK FACTORS FOR IBD

The exact pathogenesis of IBD remains unknown; however, its complex nature supports the notion that the origin is multifactorial.[2] It is hypothesized that the interplay of a genetically susceptible host, an environmental trigger, the intestinal microbiota, and a dysregulated immune response result in the chronic gastrointestinal tract inflammation seen in IBD (see Figure 11.1).[2,3]

Given IBD is a disease of the gastrointestinal tract, dietary antigens have generated considerable interest as potential environmental triggers in the pathogenesis of

239

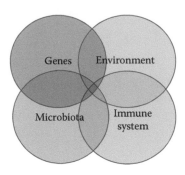

FIGURE 11.1   Key interactions involved in susceptibility to the development of inflammatory bowel diseases. A genetic predisposition leading to altered innate immune function, immunoregulation, and/or altered gut barrier function lead to changes in gut microbiota which is influenced by, among other factors, environment (e.g., hygiene, antibiotics). Diet may interact by affecting immune function, gut microbiome composition, among other pathways. (From Gentschew L, Ferguson LR. *Mol Nutr Food Res* 2012;56:524–535.)

IBD.[4–6] Dietary constituents that have been of interest include carbohydrates, fats, fruits and vegetables, fiber, and animal protein. A recent systematic review evaluated the risk of developing IBD based on preillness dietary consumption of these nutrients.[6] A greater risk was observed with increased consumption of polyunsaturated fats, omega-6 fatty acids, and animal protein. Diets high in fiber and fruit consumption were found to have a protective effect against CD. Data linking carbohydrates to IBD were inconsistent. The majority of the studies reviewed utilized a retrospective case-control design which is subject to recall bias.[6]

Four recent prospective studies corroborate some of these observations. The IBD in the European Prospective Investigation into Cancer and Nutrition (EPIC) study identified an association between high dietary intake of linoleic acid and the risk for UC in middle-aged and elderly individuals.[7] In addition, a decreased risk for UC was noted with high dietary consumption of docosahexaenoic acid. These results are in keeping with data from the prospective Nurses' Health Study cohort study in which high intake of n-3 polyunsaturated fatty acids was found to be associated with a trend for a lower risk of UC (HR 0.72, 95% CI 0.51–1.01).[8] The E3N study discovered that a diet high in animal protein intake is associated with a greater risk for IBD.[9] This study did not find a notable association between total lipid and carbohydrate intake and the risk for IBD. Similar to the IBD in EPIC study, the E3N study population consisted of only women ages 40–65 years.[9] Another study, using data from the Nurses' Health Study, identified that increased dietary fiber consumption is associated with a lower risk of CD but not UC.[10] The Nurses' Health Study population also consisted only of adult women.[10] A prospective, population based case-control study from New Zealand suggested that vegetable intake and breastfeeding an infant were protective against both CD and UC.[11]

Since the onset of IBD typically peaks between 15 and 35 years, the dietary consumption in children also has been investigated, but studies are limited and none is prospective. Results of a case-control multicenter study in children reviewing nutritional intake of the subjects in the previous year revealed that diets high in vegetables, fruits, fish, and nuts were associated with a lower risk of CD.[12] Similarly, increased intake of omega-3 fatty acids was associated with a lower risk of CD.[12] No significant association was noted between carbohydrate intake and the risk of CD although fiber intake was lower in CD patients.[12] These findings are similar to those noted in adult studies.[6] A further analysis of the pediatric study evaluated dietary patterns.[4] In girls, a western diet (meat, fried food, and fast food) was associated with CD. In contrast, in both girls and boys, a prudent diet (fruits, vegetables, olive oil, fish, and grains) was associated with decreased risk of CD.[4] A cheese snack (cheeses, snacks, and desserts) and beverage pattern (sodas, milkshakes) were not associated with CD.[4]

Recent studies highlighting the connection between diet and the composition of the gut microbiome have raised interest in the possibility of an indirect link between diet and the risk of developing IBD.[13] Diet is considered to be one of the main factors contributing to the diversity of the human gut microbiota.[13] Changes in gut microbiome composition can be seen within 24 h of altering diet composition.[14] However, long-term changes in dietary composition will have a greater impact on the gut microbiome. Individuals consuming primarily carbohydrates and simple sugars for long term have a predominance of *Prevotella* while those consuming protein and animal fat have a predominance of *Bacteroides*.[14] In a study comparing the gut microbiome of children from an underdeveloped village in Africa with children from developed countries in Europe, the children of Africa were found to have a predominance of *Prevotella*.[15] Interestingly, the prevalence of IBD in Africa and other underdeveloped parts of the world is low when compared to developed areas such as Europe and North America.[15] As a result of these and similar studies, it has been hypothesized that diet may influence the composition of the gut microbiota in a way that increases the risk for IBD.[13,15] However, to date, studies investigating the relationship between diet and IBD have not revealed a direct cause and effect relationship. That said, the ability of enteral nutrition to modify the course of CD lends credence to the connection between diet, gut microbiota, and CD (see Section 11.2).

11.2 ETIOLOGY OF NUTRITIONAL DEFICIENCIES IN IBD

Optimizing nutritional status is an essential priority in the management of children and adults with IBD. Both CD and UC can cause protein–calorie malnutrition and nutritional deficiencies that can result in increased morbidity and even mortality.[16] Nutritional considerations are even more critical for the pediatric population as onset of puberty, and linear growth can be significantly delayed in the setting of malnutrition.[17–19] These complications can subsequently have a negative impact on a child's psychosocial development and quality of life.

The etiology of nutritional deficiencies and malnutrition in IBD is thought to be multifactorial. The inflammatory process, clinical symptoms, and even medical therapy, all have an impact on nutritional status.[16,17,20] Contributors to malnutrition are shown in Table 11.1.[21]

Reduced dietary intake is one of the leading causes of malnutrition in IBD.[17,22] Patients may experience anorexia especially when their disease is active.[17,23] Symptoms

TABLE 11.1

Causes of Malnutrition in Inflammatory Bowel Disease

Decreased nutrient intake
   Anorexia
   Altered taste
   Intake-associated pain or discomfort
   Iatrogenic dietary restrictions
Malabsorption
   Mucosal abnormalities
   Diminished absorptive surface
      Surgery
      Extensive disease
   Bacterial overgrowth
Excessive losses
   Protein-losing enteropathy
   Bleeding
   Fistula outputs
Increased requirements
   Hypercatabolic states
      Fever
      Sepsis
   Growth in children
Iatrogenic
   Surgical complications
   Drugs
      Corticosteroids
      Sulfasalazine
      Cholestyramine
      5-Aminosalicylic acid
      Metronidazole

Source: Adapted from Graham TO, Kandil HM. *Gastroenterol Clin North Am* 2002;31:203–218.

of IBD, primarily abdominal pain, diarrhea, and nausea, may also dissuade them from eating. Their intake may be limited secondary to early satiety related to gastroparesis.[24] Restricted diets, whether prescribed by the physician or self-adopted by the patient, may result in inadequate dietary intake because the specific restrictions limit food options or make food taste unpleasant[17] and also may result in nutrient deficiencies. For example, patients following a lactose-free diet may need calcium and vitamin D supplementation because of avoidance of milk and cheese.

Malabsorption can occur in patients with active CD. It can result from inflammation of the small intestine, decreased small intestinal length secondary to surgical resection(s), fistulas, and strictures that can result in intestinal stasis and bacterial overgrowth. All of these conditions result in decreased intestinal mucosal surface area for nutrient digestion and absorption. Indeed, a small study ($n = 16$) in adults with CD in remission suggested that body mass index (BMI) is related to the degree of malabsorption and not to an increase in resting energy expenditure (REE) (see also below).[25]

Enteric protein loss may occur in a number of conditions in the setting of active mucosal inflammation.[26,27] Consequently, it is not surprising that fecal alpha-1-antitrypsin, a measure of enteric protein loss, is increased in children and adults with IBD.[28,29] However, intestinal protein loss has not been reported consistently to correlate with disease activity.[28,29] This may reflect the vagaries of clinical measures of disease activity (e.g., CD activity index) used in these older studies. It stands to reason that the greater the severity (degree of inflammation and length of bowel involved) of mucosal inflammation in IBD, the greater the likelihood of clinically significant enteric protein loss.[30]

Increased energy requirements associated with active inflammation or disease complications such as fever and sepsis also could contribute to protein–calorie malnutrition seen in patients with IBD. As recently reviewed, a number of studies suggest that REE increased in both adults and children with CD and UC.[31] However, REE may be expressed a number of ways (e.g., per body weight, fat-free mass, etc.). Studies using dual-energy x-ray absorptiometry, currently considered the gold standard for measuring body composition, suggest that many adults and children, even with quiescent CD and UC, have deficits in lean tissue (fat-free mass) that exceed those of BMI.[32] Expressing REE per fat-free mass would, by definition, result in an increased value, thus accounting for many reports of increased REE in IBD.[31] Consequently, changes in body composition must be accounted for when measuring REE. For example, it would be anticipated that weight loss would lead to decreased REE. Yet, an average weight loss of 9.4 ± 5.5 kg does not result in a significant change in REE if changes in fat and fat-free mass are taken into account.[33] When controlling for factors potentially influencing REE and body composition (e.g., clinical activity index, sedimentation rate, and C-reactive protein), current evidence questions whether changes in REE and body composition relate to disease activity.[31,32] Overall, interpretation of studies measuring REE and body composition in patients with IBD are limited by great variation in the methodologies used (many of which have been superseded by more accurate methods), the range of severity of clinical disease in the patients, and the measures used to assess disease activity.[31,32] Clearly, more rigorous studies are needed. This is underscored by a longitudinal study in children with CD that showed that although BMI normalized over 2 years, deficits in fat-free mass did not.[34] Thus, improvements in weight were accounted for by fat accretion, not lean body mass (muscle).[34]

Glucocorticoids, a therapy commonly used for the treatment of IBD, also can negatively impact growth in pubertal children with IBD.[35] Glucocorticoids can suppress growth in multiple ways including interfering with endogenous growth hormone production, insulin-like growth factor-1 (IGF-1), and metabolic processes critical for normal growth such as bone formation.[36,37] Although glucocorticoids can interfere with growth, a larger dose of glucocorticoids for a greater length of time is likely to be used in patients with severe disease. It may be difficult to separate the effect of steroid therapy from disease severity and other factors (e.g., serum cytokine levels) in assessing the etiology of growth failure in patients receiving glucocorticoids.[38]

11.3   NUTRITIONAL COMPLICATIONS OF IBD

Both macronutrient and micronutrient deficiencies have been described in children and adults with IBD, with varying degrees of clinical significance (Table 11.2).[21] Clinical complications resulting from macronutrient deficiencies classically associated with IBD include weight loss, protein–calorie malnutrition, and, specific to the pediatric population, growth failure/pubertal delay.[21] Malnutrition is common in patients with active IBD with 20%–75% of patients experiencing weight loss with exacerbations.[21] Patients with CD may have insidious weight loss accompanied by the development of multiple, sometimes severe, nutrient deficiencies.[21] In contrast, UC patients may appear to be well nourished but suffer from acute nutritional deficiencies with accompanying disease exacerbations.[21]

Micronutrient deficiencies also are commonly encountered, primarily in children and adults with small bowel CD, and can cause complications such as anemia, bone disease, thrombophilia, and poor healing.[39] A survey of adult Canadian patients with

TABLE 11.2
Prevalence of Nutritional Deficiencies Reported in Inflammatory Bowel Disease

Deficiency	Crohn's Disease		Ulcerative Colitis	
	Adult (%)	Pediatric (%)	Adult (%)	Pediatric (%)
Weight loss	65–75		18–62	33
Growth failure	31			10
Pubertal delay		30		20
Hypoalbuminemia	25–80	59	25–50	35
Intestinal protein loss	75		R	
Negative nitrogen balance	69		R	
Anemia	60–80	73	81	58
Iron	39	73	81	58
Folic acid	54	56	36	30
Vitamin B_{12}	48	38	5	5
Calcium deficiency	13		R	
Magnesium deficiency	14–33		R	
Potassium deficiency	5–29		R	
Vitamin A deficiency	11–21		NR	
Vitamin D deficiency	75		35	
Vitamin K deficiency	R		NR	
Vitamin C deficiency	12		NR	
Zinc deficiency	50		R	
Selenium deficiency	35–40		NR	
Metabolic bone disease	30–50			

Source: From Graham TO, Kandil HM. *Gastroenterol Clin North Am* 2002;31:203–218.

CD indicated that despite normal BMIs, inadequate micronutrient intake was more likely to be encountered than was inadequate macronutrient intake (e.g., protein and calories).[40] All micronutrient intakes except vitamin B_{12} were below those recommended with the most severe shortfalls being folate, calcium, and vitamins C and E[40] Deficiencies did not vary according to the CD activity index.[40] Although micronutrient deficiencies may present with overt clinical symptoms (e.g., anemia due to iron deficiency, glossitis due to B vitamin deficiencies), they also can present with nonspecific symptoms such as fatigue and depression.[41]

Anemia is the leading extraintestinal manifestation of IBD (Table 11.2).[21,42,43] It can result from deficiencies of iron, folic acid, or vitamin B_{12}. Other causes include chronic inflammation and medications such as thiopurines, methotrexate, or sulfasalazine.[43]

Iron deficiency anemia is the most common cause of anemia in IBD with a prevalence of 36%–88%.[41,42] Chronic blood loss, inadequate dietary intake, impaired absorption and utilization of iron, all contribute to anemia in IBD.[44] Iron is absorbed in the duodenum and proximal jejunum.[39] Active CD, especially in these regions of the small intestine can significantly compromise iron absorption. In addition, the use of acid blocking therapies, proton-pump inhibitors, H_2 blockers, or antacids, can also negatively impact iron absorption by limiting the conversion of iron into its most efficiently absorbed form, heme (Fe^{2+}).[39] Serum ferritin is a good measure of storage iron, and a low level is virtually diagnostic of iron deficiency.[43] However, as an acute phase reactant, ferritin may be normal in the face of iron deficiency.[43]

The clinical manifestations of iron deficiency anemia range from physical symptoms such as fatigue, headache, shortness of breath, and nausea to those that are less obvious and often go unrecognized such as diminished quality of life and cognitive function.[44,45] Iron deficiency anemia can be treated with either oral or intravenous supplementation. According to guidelines on the management of anemia in IBD, intravenous iron supplementation is the preferred route although it is recognized that many patients will respond to oral therapy.[44] It is deemed to be more effective, better tolerated, and improves quality of life to a greater degree than does oral therapy.[44] That said, experience from one report suggests that only 5% of patients ($n = 78$) with hemoglobin between 10 and 12 g/dL (women) and 10–13 g/dL (men) developed an intolerance to oral therapy and needed to be switched to the intravenous route.[46]

The guidelines suggest the following as absolute indications for intravenous iron supplementation: severe anemia (hemoglobin <10 g/dL), intolerance and/or inappropriate response to oral iron supplementation, severe intestinal disease activity, concomitant therapy with an erythropoietic agent, or patient preference.[44] Studies comparing oral versus intravenous supplementation have revealed a faster and longer lasting response to intravenous therapy.[44] Oral supplementation can be poorly tolerated causing nausea, abdominal pain, and diarrhea. In addition, animal as well as human studies have shown that oral supplementation with iron sulfate can be associated with increased intestinal inflammation and disease activity, likely, through inducing oxidative stress when nonabsorbed iron interacts with hydrogen peroxide to produce reactive oxygen species.[47,48] Indeed, 90% of an oral dose of iron is not absorbed and passes into the distal bowel equating to maximal absorption of 10–20 mg.[44,49] Oral supplementation still is widely used as the first-line therapy for iron deficiency anemia, and in the right setting, it can be effective. Disadvantages of intravenous iron supplementation with iron dextran include the inconveniences of an infusion and risk of an infusion reaction, including anaphylaxis.[44] Intravenous iron sucrose appears to be safer than iron dextran.[44,50]

Folate deficiency can result in macrocytic, megaloblastic anemia. While the prevalence of folate deficiency in IBD has decreased overall, children and adults with IBD are still at risk.[51–53] Older studies have described prevalence values of up to 28%.[53] More recent studies using modern laboratory techniques put this figure closer to 4%.[54] Inadequate dietary intake is the leading cause of folate deficiency in IBD.[52,55,56] Other risk factors include active small bowel CD and/or history of small bowel resections.[16,39] In addition, sulfasalazine and methotrexate inhibit the cellular update of folate.[16,39] Oral folate supplementation is recommended for children and adults being treated with sulfasalazine or methotrexate, for pregnant females with IBD and anyone identified to be deficient.[39]

Vitamin B_{12} deficiency is also associated with a macrocytic, megaloblastic anemia. Since vitamin B_{12} is absorbed in the terminal ileum, children and adults with Crohn's ileitis or ileocolitis are at the greatest risk of developing vitamin B_{12} deficiency. Active inflammation, ileal resections, and ileal stricture resulting in small bowel dilation causing stasis and bacterial overgrowth can compromise vitamin B_{12} absorption.[16,57] Even though UC only involves the colon, vitamin B_{12} deficiency has been identified in patients who have had a proctocolectomy with ileoanal pouch anastomosis. It has been suggested that the cause of vitamin B_{12} deficiency in these patients is resection of a portion of the ileum during pouch construction or bacterial overgrowth in the pouch.[58] Assessing vitamin B_{12} deficiency is indicated in patients with macrocytic, megaloblastic anemia but routine screening also should be completed for children and adults with CD, specifically with active ileal disease or history of ileal resection.[39] A loss of 60 cm of the terminal ileum in an adult will result in the need for vitamin B_{12} supplementation, without which, deficiency will occur.[59] However, resections as small as 10 cm or less can be associated with vitamin B_{12} malabsorption in 38% of patients; the degree of malabsorption does not necessarily correlate directly with the length of ileum removed.[59] Given that deficiency may take years to develop, monitoring is warranted in all patients who have had such surgery. Vitamin B_{12} malabsorption is unlikely to improve with time.[59]

Metabolic bone disease is another well described clinical complication of IBD. Risk factors are listed in Table 11.3.[60] Osteoporosis and osteopenia occur more commonly and at an earlier age in adults with IBD when compared to the general population.[39] Some studies suggest that the rates of osteoporosis and osteopenia are similar in adult CD versus UC patients while other studies suggest a greater prevalence in CD (for reviews see References[21,39,61]). Reduced bone mineral density also occurs in children and adolescents with IBD and may be of greater significance since peak bone mass is usually attained by the end of adolescence.[62] Inability to attain and maintain optimal bone mass may compromise the lifelong bone health of children with IBD.[63,64] A greater risk for fractures is not seen in children with IBD but in adults.[65] Risk factors for bone disease specific to IBD include daily use of glucocorticosteroid therapy, presence of active intestinal inflammation, and malabsorption resulting in nutrient deficiencies such as vitamins D and K, and calcium.[66–69]

TABLE 11.3
Risk Factors for Osteopenia/Osteoporosis in Inflammatory Bowel Disease

- Malnutrition
- Malabsorption of vitamin D, calcium, and vitamin K
- Low BMI
- Low bone mineral intensity peak in IBD patients with pediatric onset
- Chronic inflammatory state
- Type of IBD (CD versus UC; small intestinal involvement)
- Increasing age
- Female gender
- Immobilization
- Use of corticosteroids
- Previous fragility fracture
- Hypogonadism
- Smoking
- Family history of osteoporosis

Source: From Ghishan FK, Kiela PR. *Am J Physiol Gastrointest Liver Physiol* 2011;300:G191–G201.
Note: IBD, inflammatory bowel disease; CD, Crohn's disease; UC, ulcerative colitis.

Additional risk factors are shown in Table 11.4.[69] Glucocorticoids adversely affect bone mineralization in a number of ways including induction of apoptosis of osteocytes and decreasing IGF-1(for reviews, see References[69,70]). Use of glucocorticoids at a dose of <7.5 mg/d or on alternate days lowers the risk of steroid associated bone disease.[38,71] Despite the common perception that decreased bone mineralization is related solely to glucocorticoid use; it may be seen in newly diagnosed patients who are naïve to steroid administration.

TABLE 11.4
Risk Factors for Glucocorticoid-Induced Osteoporosis

Advanced Age	Patients Over 60 versus Younger than 32
Low BMI	<24 in adults
Underlying disease	Inflammatory bowel disease, rheumatoid arthritis, chronic pulmonary disease, transplantation
Smoking	
Prevalent fractures	
Family history of hip fracture	
Glucocorticoid receptor genotype	Glucocorticoid sensitivity may be regulated by polymorphisms in glucocorticoid receptor gene
High glucocorticoid dose	High current dose, cumulative dose, long duration
Low bone mineral density	Patients with very low bone density may be at higher risk

Source: From Weinstein RS. *N Engl J Med* 2011;365:62–70.

Recent studies have focused on the central role of inflammation and cytokines in impairing both bone mineralization and growth (Figure 11.2). Proinflammatory cytokines can have a direct adverse effect on the hypothalamic–pituitary-growth axis, including reductions in hepatic production of IGF-1 as a consequence of growth hormone secretion.[65,72] In addition, they can directly adversely affect bone formation (in part, via inhibition of IGF-1) and/or increased bone resorption.[60,72] These observations are supported by the fact that treatment with tumor necrosis blocking agents (e.g., infliximab) in adults has been shown to improve bone formation and bone mineral density and in children to improve bone formation biomarkers (for review see References[65,73]). Many questions remain regarding the pathogenesis of bone disease in IBD with evidence that both decreased bone mineralization and increased bone resorption play a role.[60] Bone health should be assessed using dual energy x-ray absorptiometry (DXA) although there are limitations to its usefulness as an assessment tool (for reviews see References[73,74]). In children, the results should be expressed as a Z score and in the case of patients with CD, normalized to bone age.[75] Vitamin D is a fat-soluble vitamin necessary for normal bone mineralization. Low vitamin D levels can contribute to increased bone resorption and reduced bone mineral density. Since Vitamin D is absorbed primarily in the jejunum, children and adults with small bowel CD are at the greatest risk of developing Vitamin D deficiency.[39] Active small bowel inflammation, extensive small bowel resections, malabsorption, and gastrointestinal losses can negatively impact vitamin D absorption.

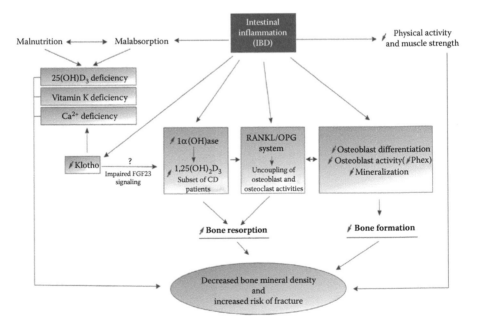

FIGURE 11.2 Factors and mechanisms associated with bone mass loss and increased risk of fractures in patients with inflammatory bowel diseases. IBD, inflammatory bowel disease; RANKL, receptor activator of NF-κB lifand; OPG, osteoprotegeria. (From Ghishan FK, Kiela PR. *Am J Physiol Gastrointest Liver Physiol* 2011;300:G191–G201.)

Vitamin D may play a much larger role than in just bone health. Vitamin D deficiency is common in patients with IBD. There is still much debate regarding whether this deficiency is a direct result of the disease process or a potential risk factor for development of IBD.[76]

Variations in CD prevalence and disease activity have been thought to be associated with geographic and seasonal changes in vitamin D levels.[77-79] Recent evidence also has shown that Vitamin D plays an important role in the regulation of the innate immune system and inflammatory response. Vitamin D promotes the antimicrobial response of macrophages and binds to dendritic cells, which also play a central role in antigen processing (for reviews see References[80,81]). Another recent study demonstrated a positive association between the plasma concentration of vitamin D and risk reduction for CD.[82] A randomized trial of vitamin D supplementation suggested that supplementation with 1200 U/day of vitamin D_3 may reduce the risk of relapse.[83] Further studies are warranted to delineate better, the relationship between Vitamin D deficiency and IBD.

Calcium absorption occurs in the duodenum and proximal jejunum.[39] Similar to vitamin D deficiency, calcium deficiency can occur in the setting of active small bowel inflammation, multiple small bowel resections, and malabsorption. Vitamin D deficiency contributes to poor calcium absorption because Vitamin D is a primary promoter of calcium absorption in the proximal intestine. Glucocorticoid therapy also can negatively impact calcium absorption by inhibiting absorption in the intestine and stimulating the excretion in the kidneys. Studies also have demonstrated that individuals with IBD have inadequate dietary intake of calcium secondary to avoidance of dairy products.[52]

Adequate intakes of vitamin D and calcium are essential to help maintain normal bone mineral status. However, as noted above, they alone may not be adequate because of the direct adverse effect of inflammation on bone mineralization. Recent recommendations for calcium and vitamin D intakes for healthy individuals are provided in Table 11.5. For patients with CD with low vitamin levels, vitamin D_3 appears superior to vitamin D_2, with a dose of 2000 IU/day superior to 400 IU/day based on a recent studies in children with CD.[84,85] Adults receiving glucocorticoids should receive 1200 mg of calcium per day in divided doses and 800–2000 IU/day of vitamin D.[69] Data are lacking the optimum serum vitamin D level (25-hydroxy vitamin D) for patients with IBD but the value probably should be maintained at ≥ 32 ng/mL.[73]

11.4   NUTRITIONAL ASSESSMENT

Nutritional assessment is a critical component of the medical care for patients with IBD. Early recognition of signs and symptoms indicative of poor nutritional status could prompt intervention to optimize nutrition and prevent nutritional complications such as bone disease, poor wound healing, and growth failure. This is particularly important for children with IBD.[86]

Nutritional assessment should be comprehensive and include a detailed history, physical examination, and laboratory evaluation.[16] Key historical points include fluctuations in weight, change in appetite, dietary history, current medications including

TABLE 11.5
Daily Recommended Allowances of Calcium and Vitamin D

Age	Calcium (mg)	Vitamin D (IU)
1–3 years old	700	600
4–8 years old	1000	600
9–13 years old	1300	600
14–18 years old	1300	600
19–30 years old	1000	600
31–50 years old	1000	600
51–70 years old males	1000	600
51–70 years old females	1200	600
71+years old	1200	800
14–18 years old, pregnant/lactating	1300	600
19–50 years old, pregnant/lactating	1000	600

Source: Adapted from Ross AC. *Public Health Nutr* 2011;14(5):938–939.

any nutritional supplements, new symptoms that might impact nutritional status such as vomiting or diarrhea, and socioeconomic factors that may impact access to food.[16,86]

Physical examination should include regular measurements of height and weight and calculation of BMI. For children, calculation of height velocity is also essential as it is the most sensitive indicator of impaired linear growth.[86] Linear growth impairment may be the earliest indication of disease in pediatric patients with CD. If additional information regarding a patient's body composition is needed, measurements such as the triceps skin fold thickness and mid-arm circumference, which assess body fat and lean body mass composition, respectively, may be useful.[16,86]

Tanner staging is another important component of the physical examination to monitor closely in children with IBD.[86] Other considerations include examining for signs of specific nutrient deficiencies such rashes, change in hair, and clubbing of nails.

Laboratory testing including serum albumin and those specific for nutrient deficiencies (i.e., 25-hydroxy vitamin D, iron/ferritin, and zinc) may offer additional information regarding the nutritional status of patients with IBD. Serum albumin level may by altered by factors other than nutritional status (e.g., enteric protein loss, urinary loss, etc.) but taken in context, does provide useful information such as being a predictor of clinical outcome during hospitalization or postsurgery.[87,88] Specific micronutrient deficiencies should be tested for in patients based on their diagnosis, location of the disease, disease activity, and nutritional status.[52] Once nutritional intervention is underway, the short half-life (24–48 h) of prealbumin allows it to be used to assess how effective enteral or parenteral nutritional support is in an undernourished patient in the context of assessing protein anabolism.[86]

11.5 THERAPEUTIC NUTRITION

11.5.1 ENTERAL NUTRITION

Exclusive enteral nutrition is the use of nutrition via the gastrointestinal tract (as opposed to parenteral) as the sole source of nutrition. In addition, it implies the use of a defined diet as opposed to an unrestricted, normal diet. Enteral nutrition diets generally can be subdivided into those in which the protein is intact (polymeric), partially hydrolyzed (semi-elemental), or completely broken down to amino acids (elemental). Semi-elemental and elemental enteral diets usually also have some proportion of their fat composition as medium chain triglycerides. All three types have been used in patients with IBD.[89–91]

Early interest in nutrition as a primary therapy for IBD was sparked in the 1970s when patients awaiting surgery for medically resistant CD went into remission while receiving enteral formula for preoperative nutritional support.[92] Although this study had several limitations, the idea that nutritional support could be used as primary therapy for IBD was appealing and prompted additional investigations. Since then, most studies have focused on the use of exclusive enteral nutrition as primary therapy for CD in children and adolescents. A number of recent meta-analyses and systematic reviews have been published regarding enteral nutrition in CD and UC, and the most recent are discussed below.[93–98] Enteral nutrition has not proven useful in the treatment of UC.[99]

The interpretation of the efficacy of enteral nutrition therapy in treating CD is complicated by differences among randomized, controlled trials. Studies have used different types of enteral nutrition diets (i.e., polymeric, semi-elemental, and elemental), tested efficacy as primary treatment for newly diagnosed disease or in established disease, or compared enteral nutrition to glucocorticoid treatment for inducing remission.

Polymeric, semi-elemental, and elemental diets all appear efficacious in inducing remission in active CD.[94,98] A Cochrane meta-analysis from 2008 and a more recent review reported that steroids were more effective than enteral nutrition in inducing remission in CD.[94,100] However, when only data for higher quality studies was used (based on blinding, randomization, etc.), there appeared to be no significant difference between the efficacy of steroids versus enteral nutrition.[41,94] Currently, the European Society for Parenteral and Enteral Nutrition recommends the use of enteral nutrition in adults with CD when use of glucocorticoids is not feasible.[101] Interestingly, a review and two pediatric meta-analyses concluded that exclusive enteral nutrition and corticosteroid therapy were equally effective suggesting that the pediatric population may have a more favorable response to enteral therapy when compared to adults.[93,98,102]

Fewer data are available that assess the utility of enteral nutrition in maintaining remission in CD. Uncontrolled trials have suggested that maintenance of remission can be prolonged by the addition of enteral nutrition to an unrestricted normal diet.[41] There are few randomized trials, but they also support the ability of enteral nutrition to maintain remission as reviewed by a Cochrane analysis and later systematic reviews.[96,97,100] The greater the proportion of enteral nutrition versus normal diet used, the greater the efficacy.[97] Several studies from Japan examine various potential benefits of enteral therapy including prevention of postoperative CD recurrence, improved response to infliximab therapy, and decreased hospitalization rate for CD patients. However, interpretation of these studies is complicated by their retrospective nature and the generally small number of patients.[103–106]

More data are needed to quantify the amount/proportion of enteral formula needed and the optimal duration of therapy.[107,108] Additionally, studies are required to identify what characteristics of CD patients (e.g., duration of disease, age; fistulizing, stenosing, or inflammatory) may influence the response to enteral nutrition. How and when to introduce a regular diet also remains a matter of debate.[100]

Exclusive enteral nutrition should be strongly considered as primary induction therapy for all children with CD. It should also be considered as primary therapy for children with CD with poor growth and nutritional status and those who are steroid dependent or suffering adverse effects of corticosteroids.[109]

Despite the observations of the efficacy of enteral nutrition, particularly in pediatrics, an international survey completed by physicians caring for children with CD identified that only 4% of pediatric gastroenterologists in the United States use exclusive enteral nutrition therapy, whereas 62% of European physicians use it regularly.[110] A survey of North American pediatric gastroenterologists revealed that experience with exclusive enteral nutrition, whether during training or current practice, correlated with regularity of use.[111]

The exact mechanism by which exclusive enteral nutrition treats CD is uncertain. Proposed mechanisms include suppression of proinflammatory mediators, decreased intestinal exposure to dietary antigens, modification of the intestinal microbiota, improvement of overall nutritional status, and bowel rest.[41,112–115] Interestingly, a recent study demonstrated that adults receiving enteral nutrition had less mesenteric adipose tissue hypertrophy, lower mesenteric adipose tissue levels of tumor necrosis factor alpha, a proinflammatory cytokine, and C-reactive protein with a corresponding increase in the anti-inflammatory cytokine adiponectin compared with patients who did not receive enteral nutrition.[116] These results are important because mesenteric fat is believed to play an important role in modulating the mucosal inflammation in CD.[117]

11.5.2 STANDARD DIETS

Several organizations and reviews focused on nutrition and gastrointestinal diseases have also outlined general nutritional guidelines for patients with IBD. Many of the dietary recommendations proposed are similar and focus on maintaining a well-balanced diet especially when patients are in remission.[100,118–120] Patients are encouraged to consume a variety of foods ensuring adequate intake of protein, carbohydrates, fats, and vitamins and minerals. This includes sufficient consumption of water to remain hydrated.

Supplementation with a multivitamin also is recommended.[118,119] Specific supplementation with vitamin D, vitamin B_{12}, and/or iron under the supervision of a physician should be used in specific clinical settings, as previously discussed.[118,120]

A number of diets have been explored that may promote maintenance of remission. Several eliminations diets, which involve the removal of foods that provoke symptoms, have been tried; however, no conclusive evidence exists to support promotion of these diets.[118,119,121]

The specific carbohydrate diet has gained a lot of attention over the years. This diet eliminates complex carbohydrates and refined sugars. This intervention purports to correct the imbalance of the gut microbiome caused by exposure to foods containing these products and thereby allow the intestine to heal. Two recent small studies, one retrospective, and the other a small, prospective, open label, nonrandomized pilot study, suggest that the specific carbohydrate diet may have some therapeutic benefit in patients with CD; however, larger prospective trials are needed to prove efficacy (http://breakingtheviciouscycle.info. Accessed June 25, 2014).[122,123]

Regardless, patients are often interested in trying dietary changes especially those who are aware of a "success story." These changes should be made under the supervision of the patient's medical team to ensure the patient is receiving a healthy, balanced diet.[118,119,121] Whether modifications to an enteral nutrition diet prescription can enhance efficacy remains to be proven. For example, the use of low fat enteral diets or those supplemented with fish oil has been suggested as being beneficial. However, the evidence to date is weak.[41,94]

Additional recommendations focus on periods of active disease. Certain dietary changes may be recommended in specific clinical situations. Lactose intolerance occurs frequently in patients with CD.[118] A lactose-restricted diet may provide these patients with some symptomatic relief, but this can be individualized according to the patient's tolerance.[119,120] However, caution should be taken to ensure that they receive adequate calcium and vitamin D.[124]

There are too few data upon which to recommend decreasing fiber intake in CD patients.[100,119,120] This diet has not shown any benefit in patients with nonstricturing CD.[112,125] Data are unclear regarding patients who have stricturing CD.[100,119,120] However, it stands to reason that a diet that promotes fermentation and gas production or contains a large amount of nondigestible starch may cause increased symptoms in patients with stricturing disease. Thus, a low fiber diet is recommended in patients with stenotic bowel segments and symptoms of obstruction.

Other dietary considerations during periods of active disease include limiting fat consumption to less than eight teaspoons per day, limiting consumption of dietary fermentable carbohydrates and sugar alcohols, avoiding beverages containing large amounts of sugar, caffeine, or alcohol. It is important to note that very limited evidence exists to support these dietary changes.

11.5.3 PARENTERAL NUTRITION

Nutritional therapy in the form of parenteral nutrition also has been used for IBD. Studies have compared parenteral to enteral nutrition in patients with active UC and CD. Parenteral nutrition was found to provide no benefit in the treatment of UC and to be equivalent to enteral nutrition in the treatment of adult patients with active CD.[126] In children, parenteral nutrition has been used for those with severe disease and growth failure.[127,128]

Enteral nutrition remains the preferred method of nutritional support secondary to the increased cost and risk of complications associated with parenteral nutrition.[112]

In settings where enteral nutrition is not tolerated or not effective, parenteral nutrition should be utilized.[86,112,128] It can be used in a short term for patients with bowel obstruction, perforation, or fistula and in the longer term for patients with short bowel secondary to multiple small intestine resections.[86,112] Complications related to parenteral nutrition are usually related to the use of a central venous catheter and include infection and thrombosis.[112]

11.6   CASE STUDY

Emily is a 16-year-old female with a new diagnosis of CD. She presented with a 1-year history of intermittent nonbloody diarrhea and abdominal pain. Her pediatrician also had noted that Emily's weight remained at the 3rd percentile despite her height being at the 15th percentile. On physical examination, she had fullness and mild tenderness in her right lower quadrant. The perianal area was normal, but the rectal exam revealed stool positive for occult blood.

Laboratory studies were done and revealed the following:

- Hemoglobin: 10.5 g/dL with a normal white blood cell and platelet count
- Serum ferritin: 8 ng/mL (normal 10–70)
- Serum 25-hydroxy vitamin D 15 ng/mL (normal ≥21)
- Serum vitamin B_{12} 300 pg/mL (normal 213–816)
- Normal liver panel
- Fecal calprotectin 1100 mg/g (normal <50)

Her upper gastrointestinal endoscopy was normal; however, her colonoscopy revealed severe inflammation in the terminal ileum. Magnetic resonance enterography was normal except for a 25 cm segment of the terminal ileum that was narrowed and inflamed.

The following treatment options were discussed with Emily and her family:

- Corticosteroids for induction and mercaptopurine as maintenance therapy
- Infliximab for induction and maintenance
- Exclusive enteral nutrition for induction and mercaptopurine as maintenance therapy
- Exclusive enteral nutrition for induction and as maintenance therapy

Emily's parents were very interested in exclusive enteral nutrition, but Emily initially refused because she did not like the idea of not being able to eat food. Eventually, Emily and her parents agreed to enteral nutrition therapy for induction of remission and mercaptopurine as maintenance therapy. They expressed concern regarding whether Emily would be unable to drink the required quantity of formula. The option of an indwelling nasogastric tube was presented. Emily refused because she thought that she would be teased at school and not be able to participate in gymnastics.

Emily was started on a daily multivitamin supplement. In addition, because of her iron deficiency anemia she was given oral ferrous sulfate at a dose of 325 mg thrice daily. Vitamin D_3 at a dose of 2000 U/day was also provided. A bone mineral density study was scheduled.

Emily, in the beginning, agreed to not eat and only drink various polymeric enteral diets. She met with a dietitian who recommended that she drink at least eight 8-oz cans of formula daily (equal to approximately 2000 kcal/day). After 2 weeks, she returned to the clinic and had a weight gain and a reduction in her abdominal pain and stooling frequency. She and her parents stated that she had been very conscious about only using the enteral diet.

Two weeks after her clinic visit, her mother called to report that Emily had been complaining of more abdominal pain, and they had noticed that she was again waking at night to complete bowel movement. On further questioning, it was revealed that her intake of the enteral diet had decreased substantially and, more often than not, was eating a regular diet. Emily stated that she had grown tired of the formulas and thought she could not drink more than 2–3 cans a day. She also wanted to eat food when she went out with her friends. It was suggested that she try night-time nasogastric tube feedings. Initially, Emily balked.

To inform Emily and her parents better about what was involved in tube feedings, they spoke with another child who had been using nasogastric feedings. He stated that at first, he did not want to use a nasogastric tube but had felt pressured by his parents to try tube feeding. However, he did have concerns about potential side effects of medicines and therefore had agreed to give tube feedings a try.

Emily was taught how to place the nasogastric tube each night and remove it in the morning. The overnight feeding provided approximately 1000 kcal. She initially complained of some early morning bloating and diarrhea; however, this improved after 1 week. She was also started on mercaptopurine. Over the next few weeks, her abdominal pain and stooling frequency diminished. A repeat fecal calprotectin was 450 mg/g.

At the time of her follow-up visit 6 weeks later, Emily's abdominal pain and diarrhea had resolved. Her weight was now appropriate for her height and her BMI had returned to its preillness percentile. She was passing one, semi-formed, stool daily. Her hemoglobin was 11.5, and her fecal calprotectin was 75 mg/g. Emily and her parents were very pleased with Emily's progress. However, she still wanted to have the overnight nasogastric tube feedings stopped. Agreement was made to discontinue the tube feeding with Emily committing to attempt to drink as enteral nutrition over a 24-h period, the same amount of calories she had been receiving overnight by nasogastric tube (i.e., 1000 kcal, equal to approximately 33 oz/day).

At follow-up, Emily continued to do well. Her intake of enteral nutrition varied between 500 and 750 kcal/day. She and her parents met again with the dietician to review food options that would help provide Emily with a healthy, balanced diet.

REFERENCES

1. Gassull MA, Cabre E. Nutrition in inflammatory bowel disease. *Curr Opin Clin Nutr Metab Care* 2001;4:561–569.
2. Sartor RB. Bacteria in Crohn's disease: Mechanisms of inflammation and therapeutic implications. *J Clin Gastroenterol* 2007;41(suppl 1):S37–S43.

3. Gentschew L, Ferguson LR. Role of nutrition and microbiota in susceptibility to inflammatory bowel diseases. *Mol Nutr Food Res* 2012;56:524–535.
4. D'Souza S, Levy E, Mack D et al. Dietary patterns and risk for Crohn's disease in children. *Inflammatory Bowel Dis* 2008;14:367–373.
5. Shoda R, Matsueda K, Yamato S et al. Epidemiologic analysis of Crohn disease in Japan: Increased dietary intake of n-6 polyunsaturated fatty acids and animal protein relates to the increased incidence of Crohn disease in Japan. *Am J Clin Nutr* 1996;63:741–745.
6. Hou JK, Abraham B, El-Serag H. Dietary intake and risk of developing inflammatory bowel disease: A systematic review of the literature. *Am J Gastroenterol* 2011;106:563–573.
7. Tjonneland A, Overvad K, Bergmann MM et al. Linoleic acid, a dietary n-6 polyunsaturated fatty acid, and the aetiology of ulcerative colitis: A nested case-control study within a European prospective cohort study. *Gut* 2009;58:1606–1611.
8. Ananthakrishnan AN, Khalili H, Konijeti GG et al. Long-term intake of dietary fat and risk of ulcerative colitis and Crohn's disease. *Gut* 2014;63:776–784.
9. Jantchou P, Morois S, Clavel-Chapelon F et al. Animal protein intake and risk of inflammatory bowel disease: The E3N prospective study. *Am J Gastroenterol* 2010;105:2195–2201.
10. Ananthakrishnan AN, Khalili H, Konijeti GG et al. A prospective study of long-term intake of dietary fiber and risk of Crohn's disease and ulcerative colitis. *Gastroenterology* 2013;145:970–977.
11. Gearry RB, Richardson AK, Frampton CM et al. Population-based cases control study of inflammatory bowel disease risk factors. *J Gastroenterol Hepatol* 2010;25:325–333.
12. Amre DK, D'Souza S, Morgan K et al. Imbalances in dietary consumption of fatty acids, vegetables, and fruits are associated with risk for Crohn's disease in children. *Am J Gastroenterol* 2007;102:2016–2025.
13. Albenberg LG, Lewis JD, Wu GD. Food and the gut microbiota in inflammatory bowel diseases: A critical connection. *Curr Opin Gastroenterol* 2012;28:314–320.
14. Wu GD, Chen J, Hoffmann C et al. Linking long-term dietary patterns with gut microbial enterotypes. *Science* 2011;334:105–108.
15. De Filippo C, Cavalieri D, Di Paola M et al. Impact of diet in shaping gut microbiota revealed by a comparative study in children from Europe and rural Africa. *Proc Natl Acad Sci U S A* 2010;107:14691–14696.
16. Massironi S, Rossi RE, Cavalcoli FA et al. Nutritional deficiencies in inflammatory bowel disease: Therapeutic approaches. *Clin Nutr* 2013;32:904–910.
17. Oliva MM, Lake AM. Nutritional considerations and management of the child with inflammatory bowel disease. *Nutrition* 1996;12:151–158.
18. Vasseur F, Gower-Rousseau C, Vernier-Massouille G et al. Nutritional status and growth in pediatric Crohn's disease: A population-based study. *Am J Gastroenterol* 2010;105:1893–1900.
19. Gupta N, Lustig RH, Kohn MA et al. Menarche in pediatric patients with Crohn's disease. *Dig Dis Sci* 2012;57:2975–2981.
20. Gerasimidis K, McGrogan P, Edwards CA. The aetiology and impact of malnutrition in paediatric inflammatory bowel disease. *J Hum Nutr Diet* 2011;24:313–326.
21. Graham TO, Kandil HM. Nutritional factors in inflammatory bowel disease. *Gastroenterol Clin North Am* 2002;31:203–218.
22. Thomas AG, Taylor F, Miller V. Dietary intake and nutritional treatment in childhood Crohn's disease. *J Pediatr Gastroenterol Nutr* 1993;17:75–81.
23. Murch SH, Lamkin VA, Savage MO et al. Serum concentrations of tumour necrosis factor alpha in childhood chronic inflammatory bowel disease. *Gut* 1991;32:913–917.

24. Grill BB, Lange R, Markowitz R et al. Delayed gastric emptying in children with Crohn's disease. *J Clin Gastroenterol* 1985;7:216–226.
25. Vaisman N, Dotan I, Halack A et al. Malabsorption is a major contributor to underweight in Crohn's disease patients in remission. *Nutrition* 2006;22:855–859.
26. Choudhary S, Gibson PR, Deacon MC et al. Measurement of faecal alpha 1-antitrypsin: Methodologies and clinical application. *J Gastroenterol Hepatol* 1996;11:311–318.
27. Shulman RJ, Buffone G, Wise L. Enteric protein loss in necrotizing enterocolitis as measured by fecal alpha 1-antitrypsin excretion. *J Pediatr* 1985;107:287–289.
28. Griffiths AM, Drobnies A, Soldin SJ et al. Enteric protein loss measured by fecal alpha 1-antitrypsin clearance in the assessment of Crohn's disease activity: A study of children and adolescents. *J Pediatr Gastroenterol Nutr* 1986;5:907–911.
29. Miura S, Yoshioka M, Tanaka S et al. Faecal clearance of alpha 1-antitrypsin reflects disease activity and correlates with rapid turnover proteins in chronic inflammatory bowel disease. *J Gastroenterol Hepatol* 1991;6:49–52.
30. Becker K, Frieling T, Haussinger D. Quantification of fecal alpha 1-antitrypsin excretion for assessment of inflammatory bowel diseases. *Eur J Med Res* 1998;3:65–70.
31. Wiskin AE, Wootton SA, Cornelius VR et al. No relation between disease activity measured by multiple methods and REE in childhood Crohn disease. *J Pediatr Gastroenterol Nutr* 2012;54:271–276.
32. Bryant RV, Trott MJ, Bartholomeusz FD et al. Systematic review: Body composition in adults with inflammatory bowel disease. *Aliment Pharmacol Ther* 2013;38:213–225.
33. Schwartz A, Kuk JL, Lamothe G et al. Greater than predicted decrease in resting energy expenditure and weight loss: Results from a systematic review. *Obesity (Silver Spring)* 2012;20:2307–2310.
34. Sylvester FA, Leopold S, Lincoln M et al. A two-year longitudinal study of persistent lean tissue deficits in children with Crohn's disease. *Clin Gastroenterol Hepatol* 2009;7:452–455.
35. Alemzadeh N, Rekers-Mombarg LT, Mearin ML et al. Adult height in patients with early onset of Crohn's disease. *Gut* 2002;51:26–29.
36. Allen DB. Growth suppression by glucocorticoid therapy. *Endocrinol Metab Clin North Am* 1996;25:699–717.
37. Kritsch KR, Murali S, Adamo ML et al. Dexamethasone decreases serum and liver IGF-I and maintains liver IGF-I mRNA in parenterally fed rats. *Am J Physiol Regul Integr Comp Physiol* 2002;282:R528–R536.
38. Gokhale R, Favus MJ, Karrison T et al. Bone mineral density assessment in children with inflammatory bowel disease. *Gastroenterology* 1998;114:902–911.
39. Hwang C, Ross V, Mahadevan U. Micronutrient deficiencies in inflammatory bowel disease: From A to zinc. *Inflammatory Bowel Dis* 2012;18:1961–1981.
40. Aghdassi E, Wendland BE, Stapleton M et al. Adequacy of nutritional intake in a Canadian population of patients with Crohn's disease. *J Am Diet Assoc* 2007;107:1575–1580.
41. Donnellan CF, Yann LH, Lal S. Nutritional management of Crohn's disease. *Ther Adv Gastroenterol* 2013;6:231–242.
42. Gasche C, Lomer MC, Cavill I et al. Iron, anaemia, and inflammatory bowel diseases. *Gut* 2004;53:1190–1197.
43. Cronin CC, Shanahan F. Anemia in patients with chronic inflammatory bowel disease. *Am J Gastroenterol* 2001;96:2296–2298.
44. Gasche C, Berstad A, Befrits R et al. Guidelines on the diagnosis and management of iron deficiency and anemia in inflammatory bowel diseases. *Inflammatory Bowel Dis* 2007;13:1545–1553.
45. Wells CW, Lewis S, Barton JR et al. Effects of changes in hemoglobin level on quality of life and cognitive function in inflammatory bowel disease patients. *Inflammatory Bowel Dis* 2006;12:123–130.

46. Gisbert JP, Bermejo F, Pajares R et al. Oral and intravenous iron treatment in inflammatory bowel disease: Hematological response and quality of life improvement. *Inflammatory Bowel Dis* 2009;15:1485–1491.
47. Werner T, Wagner SJ, Martinez I et al. Depletion of luminal iron alters the gut microbiota and prevents Crohn's disease-like ileitis. *Gut* 2011;60:325–333.
48. Erichsen K, Hausken T, Ulvik RJ et al. Ferrous fumarate deteriorated plasma antioxidant status in patients with Crohn disease. *Scand J Gastroenterol* 2003;38:543–548.
49. Rimon E, Kagansky N, Kagansky M et al. Are we giving too much iron? Low-dose iron therapy is effective in octogenarians. *Am J Med* 2005;118:1142–1147.
50. Coppol E, Shelly J, Cheng S et al. A comparative look at the safety profiles of intravenous iron products used in the hemodialysis population (February). *Ann Pharmacother* 2011. (Epub).
51. Kulnigg S, Gasche C. Systematic review: managing anaemia in Crohn's disease. *Aliment Pharmacol Ther* 2006;24:1507–1523.
52. Vagianos K, Bector S, McConnell J et al. Nutrition assessment of patients with inflammatory bowel disease. *JPEN J Parenter Enteral Nutr* 2007;31:311–319.
53. Hoffbrand AV, Stewart JS, Booth CC et al. Folate deficiency in Crohn's disease: Incidence, pathogenesis, and treatment. *Br Med J* 1968;2:71–75.
54. Oldenburg B, Fijnheer R, van der Griend R et al. Homocysteine in inflammatory bowel disease: A risk factor for thromboembolic complications? *Am J Gastroenterol* 2000;95:2825–2830.
55. Filippi J, Al-Jaouni R, Wiroth JB et al. Nutritional deficiencies in patients with Crohn's disease in remission. *Inflammatory Bowel Dis* 2006;12:185–191.
56. Wasko-Czopnik D, Paradowski L. The influence of deficiencies of essential trace elements and vitamins on the course of Crohn's disease. *Adv Clin Exp Med* 2012;21:5–11.
57. Headstrom PD, Rulyak SJ, Lee SD. Prevalence of and risk factors for vitamin B(12) deficiency in patients with Crohn's disease. *Inflammatory Bowel Dis* 2008;14:217–223.
58. Coull DB, Tait RC, Anderson JH et al. Vitamin B_{12} deficiency following restorative proctocolectomy. *Colorectal Dis* 2007;9:562–566.
59. Behrend C, Jeppesen PB, Mortensen PB. Vitamin B_{12} absorption after ileorectal anastomosis for Crohn's disease: Effect of ileal resection and time span after surgery. *Eur J Gastroenterol Hepatol* 1995;7:397–400.
60. Ghishan FK, Kiela PR. Advances in the understanding of mineral and bone metabolism in inflammatory bowel diseases. *Am J Physiol Gastrointest Liver Physiol* 2011;300:G191–G201.
61. Bjarnason I, Macpherson A, Mackintosh C et al. Reduced bone density in patients with inflammatory bowel disease. *Gut* 1997;40:228–233.
62. Sylvester FA, Wyzga N, Hyams JS et al. Natural history of bone metabolism and bone mineral density in children with inflammatory bowel disease. *Inflammatory Bowel Dis* 2007;13:42–50.
63. Pappa H, Thayu M, Sylvester F et al. Skeletal health of children and adolescents with inflammatory bowel disease. *J Pediatr Gastroenterol Nutr* 2011;53:11–25.
64. Panel NCD. Osteoporosis prevention, diagnosis, and therapy. *JAMA* 2001;285:785–795.
65. DeBoer MD, Denson LA. Delays in puberty, growth, and accrual of bone mineral density in pediatric Crohn's disease: Despite temporal changes in disease severity, the need for monitoring remains. *J Pediatr* 2013;163:17–22.
66. Lichtenstein GR, Sands BE, Pazianas M. Prevention and treatment of osteoporosis in inflammatory bowel disease. *Inflammatory Bowel Dis* 2006;12:797–813.
67. Bernstein CN. Inflammatory bowel diseases as secondary causes of osteoporosis. *Curr Osteoporosis Rep* 2006;4:116–123.

68. Bernstein CN, Blanchard JF, Leslie W et al. The incidence of fracture among patients with inflammatory bowel disease. A population-based cohort study. *Ann Intern Med* 2000;133:795–799.
69. Weinstein RS. Clinical practice. Glucocorticoid-induced bone disease. *N Engl J Med* 2011;365:62–70.
70. Ezri J, Marques-Vidal P, Nydegger A. Impact of disease and treatments on growth and puberty of pediatric patients with inflammatory bowel disease. *Digestion* 2012;85: 308–319.
71. Issenman RM, Atkinson SA, Radoja C et al. Longitudinal assessment of growth, mineral metabolism, and bone mass in pediatric Crohn's disease. *J Pediatr Gastroenterol Nutr* 1993;17:401–406.
72. Ahmed SF, Farquharson C, McGrogan P et al. Pathophysiology and management of abnormal growth in children with chronic inflammatory bowel disease. *World Rev Nutr Diet* 2013;106:142–148.
73. Mascarenhas MR, Thayu M. Pediatric inflammatory bowel disease and bone health. *Nutr Clin Pract* 2010;25:347–352.
74. Pappa HM, Gordon CM, Saslowsky TM et al. Vitamin D status in children and young adults with inflammatory bowel disease. *Pediatrics* 2006;118:1950–1961.
75. Hill RJ, Brookes DS, Lewindon PJ et al. Bone health in children with inflammatory bowel disease: Adjusting for bone age. *J Pediatr Gastroenterol Nutr* 2009;48:538–543.
76. Palmer MT, Weaver CT. Linking vitamin d deficiency to inflammatory bowel disease. *Inflammatory Bowel Dis* 2013;19:2245–2256.
77. Sonnenberg A, Jacobsen SJ, Wasserman IH. Periodicity of hospital admissions for inflammatory bowel disease. *Am J Gastroenterol* 1994;89:847–851.
78. Sonnenberg A, McCarty DJ, Jacobsen SJ. Geographic variation of inflammatory bowel disease within the United States. *Gastroenterology* 1991;100:143–149.
79. Lakatos PL. Environmental factors affecting inflammatory bowel disease: Have we made progress? *Dig Dis* 2009;27:215–225.
80. Chun RF, Liu PT, Modlin RL et al. Impact of vitamin D on immune function: Lessons learned from genome-wide analysis. *Front Physiol* 2014;5:151.
81. Yin K, Agrawal DK. Vitamin D and inflammatory diseases. *J Inflammation Res* 2014;7:69–87.
82. Ananthakrishnan AN, Khalili H, Higuchi LM et al. Higher predicted vitamin D status is associated with reduced risk of Crohn's disease. *Gastroenterology* 2012;142:482–489.
83. Jorgensen SP, Agnholt J, Glerup H et al. Clinical trial: Vitamin D3 treatment in Crohn's disease—A randomized double-blind placebo-controlled study. *Aliment Pharmacol Ther* 2010;32:377–383.
84. Pappa HM, Mitchell PD, Jiang H et al. Treatment of vitamin D insufficiency in children and adolescents with inflammatory bowel disease: A randomized clinical trial comparing three regimens. *J Clin Endocrinol Metab* 2012;97:2134–2142.
85. Wingate KE, Jacobson K, Issenman R et al. 25-Hydroxyvitamin D concentrations in children with Crohn's disease supplemented with either 2000 or 400 IU daily for 6 months: A randomized controlled study. *J Pediatr* 2014;164:860–865.
86. Kleinman RE, Baldassano RN, Caplan A et al. Nutrition support for pediatric patients with inflammatory bowel disease: A clinical report of the North American Society for Pediatric Gastroenterology, Hepatology and Nutrition. *J Pediatr Gastroenterol Nutr* 2004;39:15–27.
87. Windsor JA, Hill GL. Weight loss with physiologic impairment. A basic indicator of surgical risk. *Ann Surg* 1988;207:290–296.
88. Yamamoto T, Allan RN, Keighley MR. Risk factors for intra-abdominal sepsis after surgery in Crohn's disease. *Dis Colon Rectum* 2000;43:1141–1145.
89. Zachos M, Tondeur M, Griffiths AM. Enteral nutritional therapy for inducing remission of Crohn's disease. *Cochrane Database Syst Rev* 2001;3:CD000542.

90. Grogan JL, Casson DH, Terry A et al. Enteral feeding therapy for newly diagnosed pediatric Crohn's disease: A double-blind randomized controlled trial with two years follow-up. *Inflammatory Bowel Dis* 2012;18:246–253.
91. Verma S, Brown S, Kirkwood B et al. Polymeric versus elemental diet as primary treatment in active Crohn's disease: A randomized, double-blind trial. *Am J Gastroenterol* 2000;95:735–739.
92. Voitk AJ, Echave V, Feller JH et al. Experience with elemental diet in the treatment of inflammatory bowel disease. Is this primary therapy? *Arch Surg* 1973;107:329–333.
93. Day AS, Whitten KE, Sidler M et al. Systematic review: Nutritional therapy in paediatric Crohn's disease. *Aliment Pharmacol Ther* 2008;27:293–307.
94. Zachos M, Tondeur M, Griffiths AM. Enteral nutritional therapy for induction of remission in Crohn's disease. *Cochrane Database Syst Rev* 2007;1:CD000542.
95. Mills SC, von Roon AC, Tekkis PP et al. Crohn's disease. *Clin Evidence* (Online) 2011.
96. Akobeng AK, Thomas AG. Enteral nutrition for maintenance of remission in Crohn's disease. *Cochrane Database Syst Rev* 2007;3:CD005984.
97. Yamamoto T, Nakahigashi M, Umegae S et al. Enteral nutrition for the maintenance of remission in Crohn's disease: A systematic review. *Eur J Gastroenterol Hepatol* 2010;22:1–8.
98. Dziechciarz P, Horvath A, Shamir R et al. Meta-analysis: Enteral nutrition in active Crohn's disease in children. *Aliment Pharmacol Ther* 2007;26:795–806.
99. Rajendran N, Kumar D. Role of diet in the management of inflammatory bowel disease. *World J Gastroenterol* 2010;16:1442–1448.
100. Lee J, Allen R, Ashley S et al. British Dietetic Association evidence-based guidelines for the dietary management of Crohn's disease in adults. *J Hum Nutr Diet* 2014;27:207–218.
101. Lochs H, Dejong C, Hammarqvist F et al. ESPEN Guidelines on enteral nutrition: Gastroenterology. *Clin Nutr* 2006;25:260–274.
102. Heuschkel RB, Menache CC, Megerian JT et al. Enteral nutrition and corticosteroids in the treatment of acute Crohn's disease in children. *J Pediatr Gastroenterol Nutr* 2000;31:8–15.
103. Yamamoto T, Shiraki M, Nakahigashi M et al. Enteral nutrition to suppress postoperative Crohn's disease recurrence: A five-year prospective cohort study. *Int J Colorectal Dis* 2013;28:335–340.
104. Hirai F, Ishihara H, Yada S et al. Effectiveness of concomitant enteral nutrition therapy and infliximab for maintenance treatment of Crohn's disease in adults. *Dig Dis Sci* 2013;58:1329–1334.
105. Sazuka S, Katsuno T, Nakagawa T et al. Concomitant use of enteral nutrition therapy is associated with sustained response to infliximab in patients with Crohn's disease. *Eur J Clin Nutr* 2012;66:1219–1223.
106. Watanabe O, Ando T, Ishiguro K et al. Enteral nutrition decreases hospitalization rate in patients with Crohn's disease. *J Gastroenterol Hepatol* 2010;2025(suppl 1):S134–S137.
107. Wilschanski M, Sherman P, Pencharz P et al. Supplementary enteral nutrition maintains remission in paediatric Crohn's disease. *Gut* 1996;38:543–548.
108. Belli DC, Seidman E, Bouthillier L et al. Chronic intermittent elemental diet improves growth failure in children with Crohn's disease. *Gastroenterology* 1988;94:603–610.
109. Critch J, Day AS, Otley A et al. Use of enteral nutrition for the control of intestinal inflammation in pediatric Crohn disease. *J Pediatr Gastroenterol Nutr* 2012;54:298–305.
110. Levine A, Milo T, Buller H et al. Consensus and controversy in the management of pediatric Crohn disease: An international survey. *J Pediatr Gastroenterol Nutr* 2003;36:464–469.
111. Stewart M, Day AS, Otley A. Physician attitudes and practices of enteral nutrition as primary treatment of paediatric Crohn disease in North America. *J Pediatr Gastroenterol Nutr* 2011;52:38–42.

112. Goh J, O'Morain CA. Review article: Nutrition and adult inflammatory bowel disease. *Aliment Pharmacol Ther* 2003;17:307–320.
113. Fell JM, Paintin M, Arnaud-Battandier F et al. Mucosal healing and a fall in mucosal pro-inflammatory cytokine mRNA induced by a specific oral polymeric diet in paediatric Crohn's disease. *Aliment Pharmacol Ther* 2000;14:281–289.
114. Tjellstrom B, Hogberg L, Stenhammar L et al. Effect of exclusive enteral nutrition on gut microflora function in children with Crohn's disease. *Scand J Gastroenterol* 2012;47:1454–1459.
115. Alhagamhmad MH, Day AS, Lemberg DA et al. An update of the role of nutritional therapy in the management of Crohn's disease. *J Gastroenterol* 2012;47:872–882.
116. Feng Y, Li Y, Mei S et al. Exclusive enteral nutrition ameliorates mesenteric adipose tissue alterations in patients with active Crohn's disease. *Clin Nutr* 2013;33(5):850–858.
117. Kredel LI, Batra A, Stroh T et al. Adipokines from local fat cells shape the macrophage compartment of the creeping fat in Crohn's disease. *Gut* 2013;62:852–862.
118. Brown AC, Rampertab SD, Mullin GE. Existing dietary guidelines for Crohn's disease and ulcerative colitis. *Expert Rev Gastroenterol Hepatol* 2011;5:411–425.
119. Richman E, Rhodes JM. Review article: Evidence-based dietary advice for patients with inflammatory bowel disease. *Aliment Pharmacol Ther* 2013;38:1156–1171.
120. Bernstein CN, Fried M, Krabshuis JH et al. World gastroenterology organization practice guidelines for the diagnosis and management of IBD in 2010. *Inflammatory Bowel Dis* 2010;16:112–124.
121. Hou JK, Lee D, Lewis J. Diet and inflammatory bowel disease: Review of patient-targeted recommendations. *Clin Gastroenterol Hepatol* 2013;12(10):1592–1600.
122. Suskind DL, Wahbeh G, Gregory N et al. Nutritional therapy in pediatric Crohn disease: The specific carbohydrate diet. *J Pediatr Gastroenterol Nutr* 2014;58:87–91.
123. Cohen SA, Gold BD, Oliva S et al. Clinical and mucosal improvement with the specific carbohydrate diet in pediatric Crohn's disease: A prospective pilot study. *J Pediatr Gastroenterol Nutr* 2014;59(4):516–521.
124. Mishkin B, Yalovsky M, Mishkin S. Increased prevalence of lactose malabsorption in Crohn's disease patients at low risk for lactose malabsorption based on ethnic origin. *Am J Gastroenterol* 1997;92:1148–1153.
125. Levenstein S, Prantera C, Luzi C et al. Low residue or normal diet in Crohn's disease: A prospective controlled study in Italian patients. *Gut* 1985;26:989–993.
126. Koretz RL, Lipman TO, Klein S et al. AGA technical review on parenteral nutrition. *Gastroenterology* 2001;121:970–1001.
127. Heuschkel R, Salvestrini C, Beattie RM et al. Guidelines for the management of growth failure in childhood inflammatory bowel disease. *Inflammatory Bowel Dis* 2008;14:839–849.
128. Working Group of the Japanese Society for Pediatric Gastroenterology H, Nutrition, Konno M et al. Guidelines for the treatment of Crohn's disease in children. *Pediatr Int* 2006;48:349–352.
129. Ross AC. The 2011 report on dietary reference intakes for calcium and vitamin D. *Public Health Nutr* 2011;14(5):938–939.

12 Nutritional Management of Acute and Chronic Pancreatitis

Kishore Vipperla and S. J. O'Keefe

CONTENTS

12.1   ACUTE PANCREATITIS

Acute pancreatitis (AP) is the most common pancreatic disease. It is characterized by both local pancreatic and secondary system inflammatory responses resulting from the premature activation of the proteolytic proenzymes such as trypsinogen within the pancreatic acinar cells. Mild disease, contributing to >80% of hospital admissions, is confined to the pancreas and usually resolves within a few days of bowel rest and analgesia. The remaining 20% develop the severe disease (SAP) with cytokine-driven systemic complications associated with an overwhelming systemic inflammatory response syndrome and multiorgan failure (MOF). It is this group that contains all the morbidity and mortality, often resulting in prolonged intensive care unit (ICU) and hospital stay, and the need for surgery for pancreatic complications such as necrosis. SAP is one of the most catabolic of critical conditions encountered within the ICU, with high metabolic and nutritional requirements. Nutritional support is difficult because (a) enteral feeding may exacerbate the disease, (b) the inflamed swollen pancreas and associated fluid collections compress the upper gastrointestinal (GI) tract making feeding tube placement difficult, (c) total parenteral nutrition (TPN) rests the pancreas, but produces serious complications such as hyperglycemia and gut derived amplification of the inflammatory response.

12.1.1   Physiology of Pancreatic Secretion

The knowledge of physiological and pathological processes involved in pancreatic secretion and the adverse effects of dysregulated gut function on systemic inflammation helps us appreciate the challenges faced in providing nutritional support. The pancreatic acinar cells synthesizing powerful digestive juices are normally protected from "autodigestion" by secreting the proteolytic enzymes in their inactive forms (e.g., trypsinogen), which are subsequently activated within the intestinal lumen by the intestinal brush border peptidase, enterokinase. The pancreatic juices are secreted at a basal rate (~20%) associated with migrating motor complexes,[1] but are predominantly (~80%) secreted in response to ingested meals in three coordinated phases—cephalic, gastric, and intestinal phases that are mediated by complex neurohumoral pathways.[2] The mere sight of food, mastication, and swallowing stimulate pancreatic acinar cells directly via vagal cholinergic pathways during the "oral phase." The mechanical distention caused by the ingested food passing into the stomach activates the "gastric phase" of pancreatic secretion that is mediated by pancreatic vago-vagal reflex pathways. The passage of acidic gastric contents into the intestine through the pylorus causes the final and maximal pancreatic stimulation during the "intestinal phase" mediated by the coordinated cholinergic excitation of the entero-pancreatic reflex (neural) pathway and secretion of the enteroendocrine hormones, cholecystokinin (CCK) and secretin (humoral pathway). CCK is produced by the duodenal I-cells in response to peptides, amino acids, and fatty acids present in the chyme and stimulates the release of pancreatic juices rich in enzymes. On the other hand, secretin is released in response to the acidic chyme and stimulates the release of pancreatic juices rich in water and bicarbonate. Importantly, pancreatic secretion is inhibited via a negative feedback mechanism, known as the "ileal brake" that is mediated by enteroendocrine gut peptides such as glucagon-like peptide-1 (GLP-1) and peptide-YY (PYY) released in response to undigested food at the terminal ileum.[3] Therefore, the physicochemical characteristics (i.e., the proportion of fat, protein, and carbohydrates) of the gastric contents and their rate of delivery into the duodenum influence the composition and intensity of the pancreatic secretory response.

12.1.1.1   Pathophysiology of Pancreatic and Systemic Inflammation

Intracellular influx of calcium and premature activation of a variety of proenzymes within the pancreatic acinar cell results in proteolytic injury (autodigestion or "autophagia") that triggers a cascade of local as well as systemic inflammatory pathways.[4] Subsequently, signaling pathways such as nuclear factor-kappa B (NF-κB) and mitogen-activated protein (MAP) kinase pathways are activated to generate a flood of proinflammatory cytokines such as tumor necrosis factor-α (TNF-α), interleukins (IL)—IL-1b, IL-17, and IL-18.[5] In mild AP the inflammation is restricted to the pancreas but in SAP a plethora of these cytokines and other proinflammatory mediators are released into the systemic circulation triggering an intense systemic inflammation. Intestinal as well as pancreatic perfusion is compromised by the hypovolemia due to the fluid sequestration within the inflamed pancreatic bed and splanchnic vasoconstriction mediated by cytokines such as endothelin-A.[6] Intestinal ischemia from defective microcirculation disrupts the integrity of the mucosal defense barrier, and promotes bacterial and cytokine translocation. Bacterial translocation leads to local as well as systemic infections and promotes sepsis as is evidenced by frequent isolation of enteric organisms from pancreatic necrotic samples. The systemic proinflammatory cytokines aggravate the systemic inflammatory response syndrome (SIRS) and distant organ failure such as acute respiratory distress syndrome (ARDS) results.

12.1.2   Management of AP: Nutritional Support

Aggressive fluid resuscitation, symptomatic control of abdominal pain, nausea, and vomiting, and identification and treatment of the inciting etiological factor are the principal initial treatment strategies.[7] Nutritional support is a key component of the supportive therapeutic strategies in the management of AP (Figure 12.1).

12.1.2.1   Pancreatic Rest by *Nil per os*: Is It Good or Bad?

Nil per os (NPO), or bowel rest, has been the standard of care intended to prevent dietary stimulation of pancreatic enzyme secretion and potential aggravation of pancreatic injury and associated inflammation.[8] In addition, acute nausea and abdominal pain as a result of delayed gastric emptying and intestinal ileus, followed by extrinsic compression from the swollen pancreas, prevent the patients from being able to tolerate a diet. Bowel rest for 5–7 days does not significantly impact the nutritional status or clinical outcomes of patients with a milder disease and adequate baseline nutritional reserves. Their nutritional reserves can be replenished by gradually introducing an oral diet as the symptoms abate. However, prolonged fasting in severe or complicated AP can be detrimental by depriving these patients of essential nutrients. Lack of luminal nutrients for extended periods of time can weaken the gut mucosal

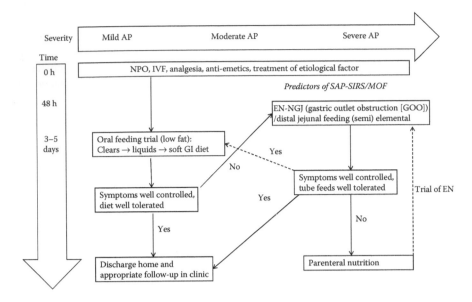

FIGURE 12.1 Nutritional support in acute pancreatitis. Nutritional support is a key supportive measure in the management of AP. Oral feeding trials can be initiated with resolution of symptoms after 3–5 days of bowel rest in mild to moderate AP cases. Enteral nutritional (EN) support, preferably in the form of NJ feeding, should be initiated at 48–72 h in SAP or predicted SAP patients. parenteral nutrition (PN) is reserved for SAP patients who fail enteral feeding trials.

integrity that allows bacteria, toxins, and cytokines to permeate into the systemic circulation and potentiate the SIRS. In fact enteric microbiota are frequently isolated from infected pancreatic necrosis and prophylactic antibiotics have not been shown to mitigate the infection risk suggesting the critical role of an intact mucosal defense barrier in preventing infection. Bacterial overgrowth and disturbed motility are other unwarranted consequences of prolonged fasting.

12.1.2.2 Why Is Nutritional Support Important in SAP?

Nutritional support is vital in providing the nutrients essential for the structural repair and healing of the inflamed pancreas as well as that of the other affected organs. Importantly, withholding nutrition in the event of a highly catabolic stressful state will quickly deplete the energy/protein reserves depending on the nutritional status of the patient at baseline and adversely affect the healing process. Besides providing the caloric and nitrogenous support essential to sustain the hypercatabolic stressful state, enteral nutrition (EN) offers the unique beneficial effects of promoting normal gut function by maintaining the gut defense barrier, blood flow, and motility. With a growing body of evidence suggesting the benefits of early feeding on improving infections, the need for surgical interventions, and mortality in SAP, the traditional practice of prolonged fasting in patients with moderate AP to SAP has been replaced by recommendations of initiating EN earlier to potentially modulate the disease course and improve clinical outcomes.[9]

12.1.2.3 How Can We Rest the Pancreas While Feeding?

The goals of nutrition support in SAP are ideally met when the protein and caloric needs to sustain the hypercatabolic state can be provided while causing the least stimulation of pancreatic secretion. Parenteral nutrition (PN) is the most effective way of circumventing feed-associated pancreatic stimulation, but is accompanied by risks of metabolic, thrombotic, and infectious complications that actually impair outcome, as outlined below. All oral or conventional forms of enteral feeding in humans have been shown to stimulate secretion of pancreatic juices rich in enzymes that can potentially aggravate pancreatic inflammation.[1] Importantly, the pancreatic secretory response and composition of digestive juices are influenced by the composition (i.e., proportion of fat, carbohydrate, and protein) and the site of delivery of the enteral feeding. Dietary fat and protein stimulate the release of CCK that causes enzyme-rich pancreatic secretion. Pancreatic secretion was shown to be reduced by ~50% by infusing an elemental diet (low fat and free amino acids) when compared to a polymeric diet that contained intact protein.[1] The site of nutrient delivery is another crucial factor that influences the degree of pancreatic stimulation (Figure 12.2). In a study evaluating the influence of the intestinal site of feeding on pancreatic stimulation, the rate of trypsin secretion was noted to be lower with increasing the distance of the tip of the feeding tube beyond the ligament of Trietz (LOT) associated with

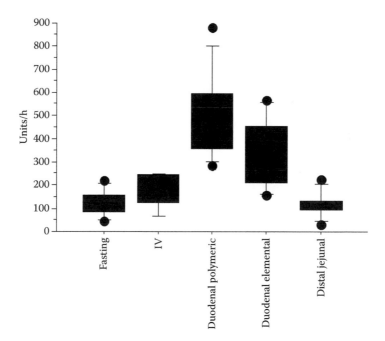

FIGURE 12.2 Influence of the form and site of feeding on pancreatic trypsin secretory response. DJ feeding is associated with the least pancreatic stimulation, evidenced by the least trypsin secretion, when compared with intravenous (IV) or either polymeric or elemental duodenal feeding. (With permission from O'Keefe, S. J. *Curr Opin Clin Nutr Metab Care* 2006;9(5):622–628. Copyright 2006; Lippincott Williams & Wilkins, Inc.)

increased stimulation of the ileal brake, highlighting the benefit of distal jejunal (DJ) feeding over gastric feeding in order to minimize stimulation of pancreatic secretion while at the same time bypassing the compression of the upper GI tract.[10] Infusion of enteral feeding into the proximal duodenum was shown to cause a 4-fold increase in basal trypsin secretion, whereas its infusion into mid-jejunum, ~60 cm from LOT, showed no stimulatory effect.[11] Based on these studies, we prefer to use transnasal endoscopic placement of DJ (>20 cm) feeding tubes, with double lumens so that gastric decompression can be performed simultaneously.[12,13]

12.1.3   ENTERAL FEEDING

The initial use of PN in the 1980s fell into disfavor following the recognition that complications outweighed potential nutritional benefits, exemplified by randomized control trials (RCT) that showed that patients randomized to no nutrition did better.[14] A better understanding of the crucial role of luminal nutrients in the preservation of the gut function and reduced concerns of pancreatic stimulation by distal intestinal feeding led to the performance of randomized comparative studies between postpyloric feeding and PN. The results of these studies and their meta-analysis showed clearly that EN was superior with regard to complications and patient outcome.[15,16] EN has now gained acceptance as the most important form of feeding in SAP. While NPO has its place in mild disease, proactive and earlier enteral feeding has to be considered when the AP course is anticipated to be severe and associated with complications. Clinical tools such as Ranson's criteria (score of ≥3), an acute physiology and chronic health evaluation (American Society for Parenteral and Enteral Nutrition [APACHE], score of ≥8), and CT findings (Balthazar score) often assist the clinician in objective assessment of the severity of disease and in ascertaining the need for initiation of EN.

The benefits of EN can be ascribed to two reasons. First, by preserving the gut function enteral feeding attenuates the inflammatory cascade of events. Second, by avoiding PN the risks of central line placement, line-related complications such as venous thrombosis, and blood stream infections could be avoided. Importantly, intravenous (IV) administration of glucose produces higher levels of hyperglycemia, and patients with SAP have impaired pancreatic endocrine function and insulin production making them at extreme risk of hyperglycemia. Finally, healthcare costs can be minimized by providing EN support at ~15% cost of PN.

12.1.3.1   What Is the Best Route for Delivery of EN?

Oral feeding is the best physiologic way of delivering nutrition, and patients with mild-to-moderate AP can have a diet rich in protein and carbohydrates and low in fat initiated once their symptoms resolve and then gradually advanced as tolerated. However, it is not feasible in patients with SAP who have severe symptoms (abdominal pain, nausea, or vomiting) and/or are heavily sedated for mechanical ventilation in the ICU. In such patients EN can be delivered through either nasogastric (NG) or nasojejunal (NJ) feeding. RCTs conducted by Eatock et al.[17] and Kumar et al.[18] comparing gastric and "jejunal" feeding started within 72 h of abdominal pain onset among SAP patients noted that they were well tolerated and, interestingly, mortality, length of hospital stay, number of patients requiring ICU, and infectious complications were not significantly different between these groups. Further, Eatock et al.[17] investigated the inflammatory responses and clinical course and did not find significant differences in the APACHE II scores, C-reactive protein levels, analgesic requirement, and mortality between the NG and NJ feeding groups of SAP. However, the position of the tip of the feeding tube was not radiographically confirmed in the NJ study arm in both these studies, raising the question of distinction between the NG and NJ feeding groups, as they both would have caused pancreatic stimulation, as discussed.[19] While reviews have suggested that NG should be first used as it is quicker and easier to place,[20] our experience is that patients with the most severe form of disease do not tolerate NG feeding because of failure of the stomach to empty.

While gastric feeding offers the simplicity of bedside administration, it is ineffective and/or even unsafe in patients with delayed gastric emptying and/or GOO from duodenal swelling or extrinsic compression by the pancreatic fluid collections. Gastric suctioning to mitigate the risk of aspiration of gastric contents precludes gastric feeding under these circumstances. Moreover, the risk of pancreatic stimulation remains with NG feeding. In this respect, DJ feeding offers the advantage of bypassing the gastric outlet obstruction and has been shown to be more effective than PN in providing nutrition while allowing the pancreas to rest.[21] A novel nasogastrojejunal (NGJ) tubing system comprising a double lumen tube designed to have a proximal port for gastric decompression and distal port for jejunal feeding beyond the obstruction eliminates the need for two separate tubes to serve those purposes.[12] The downside is that an experienced GI team is needed to place these tubes blindly (w/o fluoroscopy) at the bedside in the ICU. Patients who require surgical intervention for necrosis or fluid collections can be considered for surgical enterostomy tube (jejunostomy) placement when prolonged EN is anticipated.

12.1.3.2   When Is the Best Time to Start EN?

Emerging evidence now supports the beneficial effects of early enteral feeding on improved survival and lower complications in SAP. The ideal time of initiating enteral feeding has not been specifically addressed in prior studies, but fairly reasonable conclusions can be drawn from feeding studies in critically ill patients. Aggressive fluid resuscitation and symptom control measures take precedence in the treatment of SAP patients. Considering the severe net nitrogen losses that can be as high as 20–40 g/day it is not advised to delay nutritional support for more than 5–7 days in patients with optimal baseline nutritional status.[22] Marik et al. have noted that length of stay was shorter and infectious complications were delayed in non-AP ICU patients who had their EN initiated within 36 h when compared to those who received it after 36 h.[23] In a systematic review of RCTs comparing EN and PN in mild AP and SAP, the benefits of EN over PN in AP including the reduction in MOF, pancreatic infectious complications, and mortality were significantly different only when EN was administered within 48 h of admission.[24]

The idea of early feeding is intended to exploit the "window of opportunity" in the initial disease course when gut integrity can be reinforced by luminal nutrients in an effort to potentially attenuate the overwhelming inflammation.[25] It remains unclear, however, if trickle (slow) feeding (or hypocaloric feeding), and not neces-sarily full feeding, is sufficient enough to preserve the gut function, as a significant proportion of SAP patients are obese and fairly well nourished.[21]

12.1.3.3 Composition of EN

In addition to the average daily calorie requirement of 25–35 kcal/kg of energy and 0.8–1.5 g/kg of protein necessary for adults, patients with AP would require higher calorie and protein content to match the catabolic state. However, high levels of forced feeding in our experience should be avoided as most of our SAP patients are obese and body stores are sufficient to support hypocaloric feeding for at least 2 weeks. We feel that early trickle feeding (20 cc/h) is probably best to maintain intestinal function and prevent stasis, rather that improve nutritional status. Elemental formulas (composed of amino acids, simple sugars, and essential fatty acids) and semi-elemental formulas (containing peptides, glucose polymers, and medium-chain triglycerides) are preferred over the standard polymeric formulas (i.e., nonhydro-lyzed proteins, complex carbohydrates, and long-chain triglycerides) in AP patients as they are easily digestible, and cause less pancreatic stimulation, bearing in mind that we have measured pancreatic secretion during SAP and found it to be >80% reduced.[26] Isotonic solutions with high peptide and low fat (long-chain fatty acids/LCFA) formulae are considered to be ideal for AP patients when infused into the distal jejunum. However, in a recent meta-analysis, the risk of intolerance to feeding, infectious complications, and mortality were not significantly different between AP patients who received either polymeric or (semi) elemental formula.[27]

12.1.3.4 Administration of EN

Feeding must be initiated at a slow rate and then gradually advanced as tolerated. In either NG or NJ feeding, generally a liquid elemental nutrient formula can be initi-ated at 25 mL/h for the first 24 h, and then gradually advanced by 25 mL/h daily over the next 2–3 days to achieve the final goal rate calculated to provide 25 kcal energy/kg ideal body weight/day. Gastric residual volumes (GRV) need to be moni-tored every 4 h to detect intolerance to gastric feeding in order to minimize the risk of aspiration of stagnant gastric contents, which can be significant when GRV exceed 500 mL.[25] Keeping the head end of the bed elevated to ~30–45° helps minimize the risk of aspiration which is higher for NG than for NJ feeding. Having said that, lower rates of feeding throughout the acute episode may be optimal, as it might preserve gut function without significant intolerance. In the case of NGJ system, the gastric port (G-port) is connected to a low-pressure (50 mm Hg) intermittent suction while feeding is started until the GRVs drop below 500 mL/4 h, whence the G-port can be clamped and monitored as described above.

While diarrhea is commonly associated with EN, microbiotal dysbiosis (dys-regulated composition and function of intestinal microbiota and their metabolites) secondary to fasting, use of antibiotics and proton-pump-inhibitors, osmotic con-stituents of formula such as sorbitol, and/or fiber deficiency are the common culprits. Interestingly, fiber supplementation in critically ill patients with diarrhea was shown to improve the symptoms by modulating the colonic microbiota and their metabolic function.[28]

Enteral feeding is continued until the patient's clinical condition improves and appetite returns when oral feeding can be resumed gradually. Tolerance of <10% of the goal rate of feeding can be considered a failure of enteral feeding. Failure to tolerate EN requires consideration of PN for nutritional support in the second week.

12.1.3.5   Maintenance of Feeding Tube

Regular maintenance and monitoring is important for efficient functioning of feeding tubes.[12,29] The most common trouble-shooting issues encountered with the feeding tubes are clogging from congealed feed or powdered medications, migration or malpositioning, and dislodgement. Accidental dislodgement can be minimized by firmly securing the feeding tube, often using a "nasal bridle." Flushing the tubes regularly (e.g., ~30 mL of tap water can be used to flush once every 4–6 h using easily programmable infusion pumps) minimizes the risk of clogging. Importantly, the J-port of the NGJ feeding tube must be reserved for feeding and medications should be carefully administered as crushed or liquid preparations via the G-port or as intravenous preparations. GRV should be <500 mL for medication delivery through the G-port. Kinking of the enteral feeding tube within the intestinal lumen can be mistaken for "clogging" but does not respond to declogging maneuvers. Kinking can be usually identified on a plain abdominal radiograph that can be rectified by gently withdrawing the J-tube until flow is restored, but fluoroscopy guided maneuvering might be necessary.

Proximal recoil of the feeding tube tip can aggravate the AP symptoms by stimulating the pancreas[30] and may even cause devastating aspiration of feeding formula into the lungs. Suspected malpositioning of the feeding tube or presence of tube feeds in the tracheal aspirates in intubated patients should prompt immediate cessation of infusion of the feed and radiographic confirmation of the location of the tip of feeding tube for accuracy. The other common complications that can be caused by the feeding tube are nasopharyngeal discomfort, sinusitis, otitis media, esophageal erosions, and gastroesophageal acid reflux.

12.1.4   Parenteral Feeding

With our techniques of transnasal endoscopic DJ feeding tube placement we rarely use PN today. Theoretically, PN offers the unique advantage of providing the macro- and micronutrients necessary to sustain the metabolic stress of AP while allowing complete pancreatic rest, as it does not stimulate pancreatic secretion. However, the high-glucose concentration of hyper alimentation formulae promotes hyperinsulinemia and insulin resistance resulting in dysregulated glucose metabolism. Serum electrolytes have to be very closely monitored and any imbalance corrected promptly. Importantly, complete bowel rest deprives the intestines of luminal nutrient-driven regulation of the mucosal defense barrier and mucosa-associated lymphoid tissue (MALT); impairs the intestinal blood flow resulting in gut mucosal atrophy; facilitates endotoxemia from a compromised mucosal defense barrier; and small intestinal bacterial overgrowth from stagnation. These detrimental consequences of bowel rest further compound the inflammatory cascade of events triggered by AP that in combination aggravate sepsis. Experimental and clinical data suggest that PN is associated with stronger proinflammatory responses, impaired cellular and humoral immunity, compromised gut defense barrier, increased bacterial translocation, and risk of systemic infections. In addition, PN administration requires a central venous catheter that is associated with risks of bleeding during placement, central line associated blood stream infections and thromboses, which contribute to significant morbidity and mortality.

In light of the compelling evidence of its adverse effects, PN should be initiated in a carefully chosen subset of AP patients who have either failed a trial of enteral feeding or are at very high risk of nutritional compromise. With the advent of sophisticated NGJ feeding tubes and available expertise in managing them, PN support is rarely absolutely necessary nowadays.

12.1.5 IMMUNONUTRITION, PREBIOTICS, AND PROBIOTICS IN AP

Immunonutrition or usage of enteral feeding formulas enriched with the amino acids glutamine and/or arginine, omega-3 fatty acids, and/or antioxidants such as vitamins and micronutrients to boost the gut immune system in order to achieve better clinical outcomes has gained significant research attention in recent years. Experimental models of immunonutrition in AP revealed some tantalizing observations, but small-scale human studies yielded mixed results and a recent systematic review did not find immunonutrition to be beneficial in improving the incidence of MOF, length of hospitalization, or mortality in AP patients.[27] Studies on supplementation with prebiotics and probiotics aimed to modulate the gut immune system have revealed inconclusive results in AP patients, and moreover, the alarming finding of higher mortality (16% vs. 6%) in the group receiving prophylactic probiotics in a RCT is noteworthy.[31] Overall, the current available evidence is not strong enough to suggest immunonutrition in routine AP management and recommends against usage of probiotics in SAP.

12.1.6 SUMMARY

1. The majority of AP patients have a mild disease that resolves with supportive care, bowel rest, and an oral diet rich in carbohydrate and protein and low in fat that can be introduced within 3–4 days when symptoms abate.
2. SAP is the most catabolic disease encountered in the ICU, suggesting that nutritional requirements are higher than normal.
3. However, most SAP patients are obese and early feeding should be given more to maintain gut function and suppress systemic inflammatory responses.
4. NJ feeding tube offers the combined advantage of
   a. Maintaining the gut function
   b. Minimizing pancreatic stimulation and
   c. Bypassing the obstructed upper GI tract
5. PN is reserved for patients with complete intestinal obstruction, as it is associated with significant metabolic and infectious complications.

12.2 CHRONIC PANCREATITIS

Chronic pancreatitis (CP) refers to the progressive fibrosis and irreversible destruction of the glandular parenchyma as a result of persistent inflammation after an initial episode of AP, especially in patients who smoke, or have alcoholic, hereditary, or autoimmune pancreatitis.[32] CP is characterized by exocrine and endocrine insufficiencies that manifest as malnutrition from maldigestion and malabsorption due to impaired pancreatic digestive enzyme synthesis by the acinar cells and type-3 diabetes mellitus from loss of insulin secreting beta cells. CP is a disease spectrum manifesting as chronic nausea, bloating, and abdominal pain, steatorrhea, and/or failure to thrive depending on the degree of glandular destruction. Diagnosis of CP is established on the basis of tests for exocrine insufficiency and radiographic hallmark features such as pancreatic parenchymal calcifications, glandular atrophy, and pancreatic ductal dilatation in conjunction with the signs and symptoms suggestive of CP.[33] However, the typical clinical signs and symptoms of CP are evident only in advanced cases and it often takes 5–10 years or more for the diagnostic radiological findings to be prominent. Hence, diagnosis can be very challenging in the early stages when the symptoms are subtle or intermittent, pancreatic function tests are inconclusive, and characteristic radiographic changes are absent. While the progressive inflammatory glandular destruction cannot be significantly delayed, earlier detection and monitoring helps in identification of patients at risk for developing malnutrition, vitamin deficiencies, bone disease, and diabetes mellitus.

12.2.1 PATHOPHYSIOLOGY OF CP

The normal pancreatic glandular tissue is gradually replaced by fibrotic tissue in CP due to recurrent inflammation and healing. Irreversible morphological changes in the form of progressive fibrosis, acinar cell atrophy, and structuring of the pancreatic ducts and inspissation of secretions that may calcify within the ducts gradually diminish the pancreatic secretory function resulting in exocrine insufficiency. In general, digestion of lipids is more effected than that of the carbohydrates and proteins.[34] Salivary amylase and intestinal brush border oligosaccharidases compensate for the loss of pancreatic amylase delaying the manifestation of impaired carbohydrate digestion. Similarly, proteolytic activity of the gastric secretions and the enterocyte/intestinal brush border peptidases compensate for the trypsin deficiency. On the other hand, while salivary and gastric lipase can break the triglycerides to glycerol and free fatty acids, most of the lipid digestion takes place in the intestine and is driven by pancreatic lipase. Lipids need formation of micelles by bile acids that takes place only in the intestine, making pancreatic enzyme-mediated lipolysis very crucial for digestion and absorption of fat. Micronutrient deficiencies and fat-soluble vitamin deficiencies, particularly vitamins D and E, are commonly noted in CP.[35,36] In a recent systematic review osteoporosis was found to be prevalent in one quarter of CP patients and overall up to two-thirds of them possibly had osteopathy (osteoporosis or osteopenia).[37] Loss of islet cell function from fibrosis and possibly micro-ischemia from defective blood supply result in diminished insulin production resulting in endocrine insufficiency. Glucose intolerance from endocrine insufficiency is noted in 50%–90% of CP patients and insulin-dependent diabetes mellitus develops in ~30% of those with advanced CP.[38]

12.2.2 Malnutrition in CP

CP is characterized by progressive malnutrition that is mainly driven by maldigestion and malabsorption from exocrine pancreatic insufficiency (EPI). Importantly, malnutrition in CP is multifactorial resulting from poor dietary intake due to chronic abdominal pain with postprandial aggravation; often underlying alcoholism; and poor compliance with the modified diet recommended for fat malabsorption and/or diabetes mellitus, which contribute to the malnutrition.

12.2.2.1 Diagnosis of EPI

Diarrhea, steatorrhea, and weight loss/failure to thrive are the most common manifestations suggestive of EPI. Steatorrhea, characterized by large volume or bulky foul smelling, oily stools that float in water, is the classical symptom of fat malabsorption, but is not obvious until ~90% of the pancreatic function is impaired.[39] Conventional tests of pancreatic exocrine function depend upon stimulation of the pancreas with secretin and/or CCK for 2 h with the simultaneous collection of secretions into the duodenum. However, these tests are not widely available and performed only at a few institutions, chiefly for research purposes. In an endoscopic pancreatic function test based on the detection of trypsin in the periampullary juices collected after a test enteral feed, an activity of <5% of the average normal detected EPI (defined by loss of >90% pancreatic secretion) with a 96% specificity and 75% sensitivity.[40] In general, indirect testing of the pancreatic function is performed to measure fat malabsorption either by (a) a simple qualitative fecal fat test of microscopic identification of fecal fat droplets by Sudan III staining (>6 globules/hpf [high-power field]) or (b) the gold standard quantitative test of the measurement of 72-h fecal fat (>7 g of fat) whilst patients consume a normal diet containing 100 g fat. Because the latter is uncomfortable for the patient and investigator, alternatives continue to be searched for. Low fecal pancreatic elastase-1 levels (<200 μg/g stool), a pancreas-specific protein that is not degraded by the intestinal transit and enriched 5–7 fold in the feces, or low serum trypsin levels (<20 ng/mL) can be used instead to detect exocrine insufficiency.[41,42] Again, these tests have the highest sensitivity only in advanced cases of CP and neither test is specific for CP.

12.2.2.2 Nutritional Assessment

A comprehensive baseline nutritional status assessment should include anthropometric measurements including height, weight, and body mass index (BMI); biochemical/laboratory (complete blood count, liver function tests, albumin and prealbumin levels, vitamins D and A, and calcium levels); clinical (history and physical examination to identify nutritional deficiencies); and dietary evaluation (by 24-h dietary recall, food frequency questionnaires, and food diaries). Nutritional assessment needs to be undertaken at the initial evaluation of CP patients and then periodically as necessary at subsequent follow-up visits to monitor response to therapeutic interventions. BMI, calculated as weight/height^2 to measure body fat based on the weight and height, remains the most useful clinical measure of nutritional state despite its shortcomings in patients with edema or ascites. Anthropometric measurements such as mid-arm circumference and triceps skin fold thickness would give a better assessment of lean body mass and body fat stores when compared with age- and gender-specific centiles.

Osteopathy is an under-recognized problem that can contribute to significant morbidity by exposing CP patients to a high risk of fractures and patients should be screened regularly for osteoporosis and osteopenia using DEXA scans. Nutritional screening of CP patients using tools such as subjective global assessment (SGA) can help identify patients who are malnourished or at high risk for malnutrition.

12.2.3 MANAGEMENT OF CP

The management of CP is principally focused on adequate pain control, pancreatic enzyme supplementation for exocrine insufficiency, nutritional assessment and support, and lifestyle and dietary modifications.[43] A multidisciplinary team approach involving gastroenterologists, endocrinologists, dieticians, pain management specialists, surgeons, and patient support groups is vital for achieving the best clinical outcomes (Figure 12.3). The main objectives of optimizing nutritional status in patients with CP are dietary modification and supplementation with pancreatic enzymes.

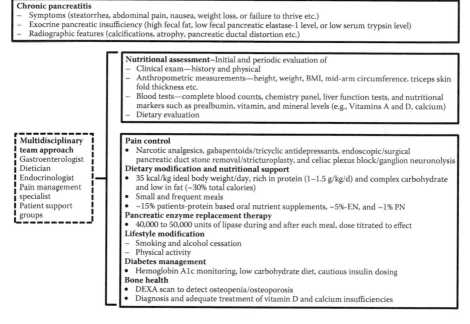

Chronic pancreatitis
- Symptoms (steatorrhea, abdominal pain, nausea, weight loss, or failure to thrive etc.)
- Exocrine pancreatic insufficiency (high fecal fat, low fecal pancreatic elastase-1 level, or low serum trypsin level)
- Radiographic features (calcifications, atrophy, pancreatic ductal distortion etc.)

Nutritional assessment–Initial and periodic evaluation of
- Clinical exam—history and physical
- Anthropometric measurements—height, weight, BMI, mid-arm circumference, triceps skin fold thickness etc.
- Blood tests—complete blood counts, chemistry panel, liver function tests, and nutritional markers such as prealbumin, vitamin, and mineral levels (e.g., Vitamins A and D, calcium)
- Dietary evaluation

Multidisciplinary team approach
Gastroenterologist
Dietician
Endocrinologist
Pain management specialist
Patient support groups

Pain control
- Narcotic analgesics, gabapentoids/tricyclic antidepressants, endoscopic/surgical pancreatic duct stone removal/stricturoplasty, and celiac plexus block/ganglion neuronolysis

Dietary modification and nutritional support
- 35 kcal/kg ideal body weight/day, rich in protein (1–1.5 g/kg/d) and complex carbohydrate and low in fat (~30% total calories)
- Small and frequent meals
- ~15% patients-protein based oral nutrient supplements, ~5%-EN, and ~1% PN

Pancreatic enzyme replacement therapy
- 40,000 to 50,000 units of lipase during and after each meal, dose titrated to effect

Lifestyle modification
- Smoking and alcohol cessation
- Physical activity

Diabetes management
- Hemoglobin A1c monitoring, low carbohydrate diet, cautious insulin dosing

Bone health
- DEXA scan to detect osteopenia/osteoporosis
- Diagnosis and adequate treatment of vitamin D and calcium insufficiencies

FIGURE 12.3 Nutritional management of chronic pancreatitis. A multidisciplinary team approach is paramount for evaluation and optimization of the nutritional status in CP patients. Nutritional support in CP involves a comprehensive nutritional assessment; pain management; counseling on dietary and lifestyle modification; identification of nutritional deficiencies; prescription of pancreatic enzymes, vitamin D, and calcium supplements; and monitoring therapeutic response.

12.2.3.1   Nutritional Management: Dietary Modification

Given the high resting energy expenditure in patients with CP, a normal-calorie diet of 35 kcal/kg ideal body weight/day is recommended. In general, a diet rich in protein (1–1.5 g/kg/day) and complex carbohydrate and low in fat (~30% total calories) is recommended for CP patients to be consumed in the form of small and frequent meals. However, severe fat restriction may sometimes worsen underlying nutritional deficiencies and high carbohydrate content can aggravate hyperglycemia in diabetic CP patients. Theoretically MCT can be used to improve fat absorption as they are directly absorbed without the need for lipase, colipase or bile acids (micelle formation) but compliance is low due to cramps, nausea, and diarrhea associated with its usage. Deficiency of fat-soluble vitamins (A, D, E, and K) and vitamin B_{12} are commonly observed in CP patients. Vitamin levels should be measured to confirm deficiency before prescribing supplements and monitored to ensure correction.

12.2.3.2   Pancreatic Enzyme Supplementation

A healthy human pancreas releases approximately 900,000 USP (United States Pharmacopeia) units of lipase with each meal, only 10% of which is necessary to achieve relatively normal absorption of fat and fat-soluble vitamins. Thus, 90,000 USP units of lipase per meal are theoretically needed to increase fat absorption. However, due to problems of insufficient mixing with the meals and motility, it is difficult to mimic what the exocrine pancreas physiologically performs and higher quantities will likely be needed to improve fat absorption. On the other hand, lipase production by the residual pancreatic tissue and the compensatory increase in gastric lipase secretion allows for even lower amounts of lipase for effective therapeutic use. Treatment is usually initiated with at least 40,000–50,000 USP units of lipase with each meal and half that amount with snacks, to be taken during and after the meal; splitting the doses between these times is commonly recommended. The dose can be titrated up or adjusted for clinical response in terms of reduction in diarrhea or steatorrhea, weight gain, or improvement in laboratory markers of nutrition.

Most pancreatic enzyme supplements are available in the form of enteric-coated microsphere capsules (e.g., Creon), while some formulations are not enteric coated (e.g., Viokase) with the latter requiring cotreatment with gastric acid-suppressing agents such as an H_2-blocker or proton-pump inhibitor if gastric acid secretion is high.[44] On the other hand, lowering gastric acidity allows the release of pH-sensitive enteric-coated more proximally in the duodenum where most normal fat and fat-soluble vitamin absorption takes place.

12.2.3.3   Nutritional Supplements, Enteral, and Parenteral Nutrition

In general, nutritional status can be improved and maintained in ~80% of patients with adequate pain control, dietary modification, and pancreatic enzyme supplementation. However, 10%–15% of CP patients require oral protein or peptide-based nutritional supplements when their nutrient intake remains low despite dietary intervention. A small percentage of patients may also require enteral feeding (~5%) or even PN (~1%) under special circumstances. NGJ feeding is required in patients with gastric outlet obstruction, acute inflammation, recurrent pancreatitis attacks, and before abdominal surgery when it improves postoperative morbidity and length of hospitalization.[12] A peptide based, low-fat enteral feeding formula is delivered via a NJ feeding tube. If the EN is well tolerated and needed for longer periods of time, a percutaneous jejunal feeding tube can be placed either by a surgeon laparoscopically, by interventional radiologists under fluoroscopic guidance, or endoscopically by gastroenterologists. In one study on 53 CP patients receiving jejunal enteral feeding via percutaneous endoscopic gastrostomy/jejunostomy (PEG/J) or percutaenous endoscopic jejunostomy (PEJ) tube, a significant improvement in percentage of patients with chronic abdominal pain (decrease from 96% to 23%) as well as nutritional status (~5 kg gain in weight) was noted during their 6 months of home enteral feeding support.[45] In our own experience, patients with CP complicated by weight loss, pain induced by eating, and gastric outlet obstruction have been successfully managed at home with NGJ feeding tubes to (a) bypass the outlet obstruction and (b) provide pancreatic rest for months allowing time for spontaneous resolution of symptoms without surgery.[12] Previously, all these patients were managed with home PN, but the metabolic (hyperglycemia due to coexistent impaired pancreatic endocrine function) and infective (catheter related sepsis) complications outweighed nutritional benefits, and we now avoid its use. PN is occasionally indicted for the management of complex internal and external pancreatic fistulae and, in the short term, to address severe malnutrition prior to surgery.

12.2.3.4 Life Style Modification

Alcohol abuse contributes to significant morbidity by being the major etiological factor of CP, compromising nutritional intake, and increasing the risk of osteoporosis. Smoking cessation, abstinence from alcohol, and weight-bearing physical activity are essential for preventing bone demineralization.

12.2.3.5 Pain Management

Chronic or intermittent abdominal pain can be debilitating and interfere with the patients' nutrition intake and quality of life. Adequate pain control could be achieved by using opioid analgesics and other adjunct pain modulators such as tricyclic antidepressants gabapentoids, and in some cases endoscopic or surgical relief of pancreatic ductal obstruction by stones or strictures.[43] Interestingly, exogenous supplementation of pancreatic enzymes decreases endogenous enzyme production by a negative feedback mechanism and potentially results in fewer and less severe painful episodes in the early stages of CP or recurrent AP.[46]

12.2.3.6 Management of Endocrine Insufficiency

The destruction of endocrine cells, the islets of Langerhans, as a consequence of chronic inflammation depletes the production of hormones such as insulin, glucagon, and somatostatin that are essential for the assimilation of nutrients that flow into the portal system following digestion. The endocrine insufficiency mainly manifests as type 3c diabetes mellitus and is characterized by hyperglycemia. Interestingly, the deficiency of counter-regulatory hormones such as glucagon, in the setting of frequently associated malnutrition and alcoholism in CP patients, renders this subset of diabetic patients more susceptible to hyper- and hypoglycemia and having "brittle diabetes."[47] An endocrinologist has to be involved in the care of these patients and as use of oral agents such as metformin might not be effective in controlling hyperglycemia, and given the higher risk of hypoglycemia when insulin is used and the patient stops eating for whatever reason.

12.2.4 SUMMARY

1. CP manifests as exocrine and endocrine insufficiencies from irreversible destruction of the pancreatic parenchyma.
2. Symptomatic EPI is not clinically evident until the disease has advanced with loss of significant pancreatic function that causes malnutrition, osteopathy, and micronutrient deficiencies.
3. CP diagnosis should be sought by radiographic and functional testing and comprehensive nutritional assessment has to be performed sooner rather than later in those at risk for malnutrition.
4. CP management involves a multidisciplinary team (involving gastroenterologist, endocrinologist, dietician, pain management specialist, surgeon, and patient support groups) approach with a focus on lifestyle and dietary modifications, adequate treatment of chronic pain, and mitigation of malabsorption by pancreatic enzyme supplementation.
5. Nutritional support in the form of supplements, EN, or rarely PN, is necessary in a select group of CP patients who fail to respond to dietary modification and enzyme supplementation.
6. Diagnosis and treatment of the endocrine insufficiency is warranted to mitigate the morbidity and mortality associated with diabetes mellitus.

REFERENCES

1. O'Keefe, S.J. et al. Physiological effects of enteral and parenteral feeding on pancreaticobiliary secretion in humans. *Am J Physiol Gastrointest Liver Physiol* 2003;284(1):G27–G36.
2. O'Keefe, S.J. Physiological response of the human pancreas to enteral and parenteral feeding. *Curr Opin Clin Nutr Metab Care* 2006;9(5):622–628.
3. Van Citters, G.W. and H.C. Lin. Ileal brake: Neuropeptidergic control of intestinal transit. *Curr Gastroenterol Rep* 2006;8(5):367–373.
4. Sah, R.P., P. Garg, and A.K. Saluja. Pathogenic mechanisms of acute pancreatitis. *Curr Opin Gastroenterol* 2012;28(5):507–515.
5. Norman, J. The role of cytokines in the pathogenesis of acute pancreatitis. *Am J Surg* 1998;175(1):76–83.
6. Inoue, K. et al. Further evidence for endothelin as an important mediator of pancreatic and intestinal ischemia in severe acute pancreatitis. *Pancreas* 2003;26(3):218–223.
7. Tenner, S. et al. American college of gastroenterology guideline: Management of acute pancreatitis. *Am J Gastroenterol* 2013;108(9):1400–1415.
8. Ragins, H. et al. Intrajejunal administration of an elemental diet at neutral pH avoids pancreatic stimulation. Studies in dog and man. *Am J Surg* 1973;126(5):606–614.
9. Hegazi, R. et al. Early jejunal feeding initiation and clinical outcomes in patients with severe acute pancreatitis. *JPEN J Parenter Enteral Nutr* 2011;35(1):91–96.
10. Kaushik, N. et al. Enteral feeding without pancreatic stimulation. *Pancreas* 2005;31(4):353–359.
11. Vu, M.K. et al. Does jejunal feeding activate exocrine pancreatic secretion? *Eur J Clin Invest* 1999;29(12):1053–1059.

12. O'Keefe, S. et al. Enteral feeding patients with gastric outlet obstruction. *Nutr Clin Pract* 2012;27(1):76–81.

13. O'Keefe, S.J., W. Foody, and S. Gill. Transnasal endoscopic placement of feeding tubes in the intensive care unit. *JPEN J Parenter Enteral Nutr* 2003;27(5):349–354.

14. Sax, H.C. et al. Early total parenteral nutrition in acute pancreatitis: Lack of beneficial effects. *Am J Surg* 1987;153(1):117–124.

15. Abou-Assi, S., K. Craig, and S.J.D. O'Keefe. Hypocaloric jejunal feeding is better than total parenteral nutrition in acute pancreatitis: Results of a randomized comparative study. *Am J Gastroenterol* 2002;97(9):2255–2262.

16. Marik, P.E. and G.P. Zaloga. Meta-analysis of parenteral nutrition versus enteral nutrition in patients with acute pancreatitis. *BMJ* 2004;328(7453):1407.

17. Eatock, F.C. et al. A randomized study of early nasogastric versus nasojejunal feeding in severe acute pancreatitis. *Am J Gastroenterol* 2005;100(2):432–439.

18. Kumar, A. et al. Early enteral nutrition in severe acute pancreatitis: A prospective randomized controlled trial comparing nasojejunal and nasogastric routes. *J Clin Gastroenterol* 2006;40(5):431–434.

19. O'Keefe, S.J. and S.A. McClave. Feeding the injured pancreas. *Gastroenterology* 2005;129(3):1129–1130.

20. Petrov, M.S., M.I. Correia, and J.A. Windsor. Nasogastric tube feeding in predicted severe acute pancreatitis. A systematic review of the literature to determine safety and tolerance. *JOP* 2008;9(4):440–448.

21. Abou-Assi, S., K. Craig, and S.J. O'Keefe. Hypocaloric jejunal feeding is better than total parenteral nutrition in acute pancreatitis: Results of a randomized comparative study. *Am J Gastroenterol* 2002;97(9):2255–2262.

22. Bouffard, Y.H. et al. Energy expenditure during severe acute pancreatitis. *JPEN J Parenter Enteral Nutr* 1989;13(1):26–29.

23. Marik, P.E. and G.P. Zaloga. Early enteral nutrition in acutely ill patients: A systematic review. *Crit Care Med* 2001;29(12):2264–2270.

24. Petrov, M.S., R.D. Pylypchuk, and A.F. Uchugina. A systematic review on the timing of artificial nutrition in acute pancreatitis. *Br J Nutr* 2009;101(6):787–793.

25. McClave, S.A. et al. Guidelines for the provision and assessment of nutrition support therapy in the adult critically ill patient: Society of Critical Care Medicine (SCCM) and American Society for Parenteral and Enteral Nutrition (A.S.P.E.N.). *JPEN J Parenter Enteral Nutr* 2009;33(3):277–316.

26. O'Keefe, S.J. et al. Trypsin secretion and turnover in patients with acute pancreatitis. *Am J Physiol Gastrointest Liver Physiol* 2005;289(2):10.

27. Petrov, M.S. et al. Systematic review and meta-analysis of enteral nutrition formulations in acute pancreatitis. *Br J Surg* 2009;96(11):1243–1252.

28. O'Keefe, S.J. et al. Effect of fiber supplementation on the microbiota in critically ill patients. *World J Gastrointest Pathophysiol* 2011;2(6):138–145.

29. O'Keefe, S.J. A guide to enteral access procedures and enteral nutrition. *Nat Rev Gastroenterol Hepatol* 2009;6(4):207–215.

30. O'Keefe, S.J. et al. Nutrition in the management of necrotizing pancreatitis. *Clin Gastroenterol Hepatol* 2003;1(4):315–321.

31. Besselink, M.G. et al. Probiotic prophylaxis in predicted severe acute pancreatitis: A randomised, double-blind, placebo-controlled trial. *Lancet* 2008;371(9613):651–659.

32. Yadav, D., M. O'Connell, and G.I. Papachristou. Natural history following the first attack of acute pancreatitis. *Am J Gastroenterol* 2012;107(7):1096–1103.

33. Forsmark, C.E. Management of chronic pancreatitis. *Gastroenterology* 2013;144(6): 1282–1291 e3.

34. Holtmann, G. et al. Survival of human pancreatic enzymes during small bowel transit: Effect of nutrients, bile acids, and enzymes. *Am J Physiol* 1997;273(2 Pt 1):G553–G558.

35. Quilliot, D. et al. Evidence that diabetes mellitus favors impaired metabolism of zinc, copper, and selenium in chronic pancreatitis. *Pancreas* 2001;22(3):299–306.
36. Van Gossum, A. et al. Deficiency in antioxidant factors in patients with alcohol-related chronic pancreatitis. *Dig Dis Sci* 1996;41(6):1225–1231.
37. Duggan, S.N. et al. High prevalence of osteoporosis in patients with chronic pancreatitis: A systematic review and meta-analysis. *Clin Gastroenterol Hepatol* 2014;12(2): 219–228.
38. Ewald, N. and P.D. Hardt. Diagnosis and treatment of diabetes mellitus in chronic pancreatitis. *World J Gastroenterol* 2013;19(42):7276–7281.
39. Lankisch, P.G. et al. Functional reserve capacity of the exocrine pancreas. *Digestion* 1986;35(3):175–181.
40. O'Keefe, S.J. et al. Physiological evaluation of the severity of pancreatic exocrine dysfunction during endoscopy. *Pancreas* 2007;35(1):30–36.
41. Naruse, S. et al. Fecal pancreatic elastase: A reproducible marker for severe exocrine pancreatic insufficiency. *J Gastroenterol* 2006;41(9):901–908.
42. Jacobson, D.G. et al. Trypsin-like immunoreactivity as a test for pancreatic insufficiency. *N Engl J Med* 1984;310(20):1307–1309.
43. Forsmark, C.E. Management of chronic pancreatitis. *Gastroenterology* 2013;144(6): 1282–1291.
44. Marotta, F. et al. Pancreatic enzyme replacement therapy. Importance of gastric acid secretion, H2-antagonists, and enteric coating. *Dig Dis Sci* 1989;34(3):456–461.
45. Stanga, Z. et al. Effect of jejunal long-term feeding in chronic pancreatitis. *JPEN J Parenter Enteral Nutr* 2005;29(1):12–20.
46. Gupta, V. and P.P. Toskes. Diagnosis and management of chronic pancreatitis. *Postgrad Med J* 2005;81(958):491–497.
47. O'Keefe, S.J., A.K. Cariem, and M. Levy; The exacerbation of pancreatic endocrine dysfunction by potent pancreatic exocrine supplements in patients with chronic pancreatitis. *J Clin Gastroenterol* 2001;32(4):319–323.

13 Enteral Access and Enteral Nutrition

Mark H. DeLegge and Mara Lee Beebe

CONTENTS

13.1 INTRODUCTION

Nutritional support for the malnourished, hospitalized patient is critical in order to improve patient outcomes. The past 50 years have shown tremendous improvement in our ability to deliver nutrition to at-risk patients. Parenteral nutrition (PN) was introduced in the 1960s and has continued to be an important tool for nutrition support for patients with inadequate gastrointestinal (GI) function. The development of specialized enteral nutrition (EN) feeding formulas creates another opportunity for nutrition-based disease management of unique patient populations.

The use of EN is usually preferred as compared to PN as it is less costly and has a reduced incidence of infectious and metabolic complications.[1] The use of early EN has also been shown to be important in stimulating the gut's immune system, an important tool in overall host defense.[2]

In a patient who can eat or drink, the provision of nutrition support is focused on the use of nutritional supplements, dietary counseling, and appetite stimulation. However, in those patients who cannot eat or drink due to some impairment of the GI system, the provision of enteral access becomes the foundation for delivering any EN.

The nurse, intensivist, gastroenterologist, radiologist, or surgeon usually is responsible for placing enteral access devices. These procedures are performed at the patient's bedside, in the endoscopy suite, radiology suite, or operating room depending on the specific device used and the expertise available at a given center. Medicare trends from 1992 to 2000 have shown a significant increase in percutaneous enteral access procedures performed amongst radiologists, closely followed by gastroenterologists,[3] while, the percentage of surgeons performing enteral access procedures had decreased.

13.2 NASOENTERIC TUBE ACCESS

Nasoenteric tube placement techniques include bedside passage or, the use of radiologic or endoscopic techniques. All of these placement techniques have their indications, benefits, and risks. The final position of an enteral access tube is either the stomach for gastric feeding or the jejunum for small bowel feeding. A patient who is intolerant of gastric feedings, such as a patient with gastroparesis, or a patient who has had his stomach surgically removed will require small bowel feeding. Nasoenteric tubes do have associated complications (Table 13.1).

TABLE 13.1

Complications of Nasoenteric Tubes

Nasal mucosal ulceration

Pharyngitis

Otitis media

Sinusitis

Aspiration pneumonia

Pneumothorax

Tracheoesophageal fistula

Tube migration

Tube obstruction

The use of small bowel feeding to prevent aspiration events is a contentious topic. Some studies have shown a reduction in aspiration episodes in patients who are fed into the small bowel as compared with the stomach.[4] Other studies have noted no difference in aspiration events between patients randomized to gastric versus small bowel feeding.[5] A consensus conference documented that small bowel feeding is recommended for the prevention of aspiration pneumonia in critically ill patients.[6]

Bedside nasoenteric tube placement is the most common enteral access technique used in hospitals and in long-term care environments. Either a nasogastric (NG) or a nasojejunal (NJ) may be placed. The decision on what tube to place is based on a patient's GI anatomy, tube feeding tolerance, and aspiration risk. There are many techniques available for blind, bedside nasoenteric tube placement. Typically, an 8–12 French (Fr) tube is lubricated and passed through the nose into the stomach or the small intestine. The patient can ingest sips of liquids and swallow to assist the tube being passed successfully. Many centers promote bedside auscultation for confirmation of an adequate position of the nasoenteric tube before use. However, this can be misleading as inappropriate tube locations (e.g., in the lung or coiled in the distal esophagus) may be misinterpreted as being in proper position by bedside ausculatory techniques. For this reason, every patient should have a radiograph to confirm proper position of an NG or NJ tube after blind bedside placement prior to initiating feeding.[7] It is not unusual for a clinician to be faced with a patient who is comatose and therefore, unable to swallow and assist with passage of a nasoenteric tube. In these instances, the patient should be monitored for coughing or wheezing consistent with a bronchial placement during tube passage.

A number of techniques have been described for passing an NJ tube with the goal of having the tube tip transverse through the pylorus and end in the jejunum. Filling the tube with a stylet(s) to stiffen it and using a corkscrew motion with forward passage of the tube has been described with success.[8] Another method placed the patient on their right side; the tube was tracked into a position in the small bowel by bedside auscultation, with a reported 83% success rate.[9] There have been reports of "self-propelled" tubes with a spiral tip that are "designed" to move from the stomach to the small bowel with GI motility.[10] In reality, most of these techniques have limited success when used widely in clinical practice.[12]

New technologies are available to allow bedside passage of a nasoenteric tube with the creation and utilization of an electromagnetic-generated image.[11] This bedside technique has been reported to result in a very high success rate of NJ tube passage to the proper location with minimal complications. Recent data have demonstrated that the use of this device can eliminate the need for radiographic confirmation of proper feeding tube tip position prior to feeding.[12]

There have been attempts to position an NJ tube beyond the pylorus with the use of pharmacologic agents which cause increased GI motility. The mixed results are: while one study reported no benefit of the use of metoclopramide in assisting the proper placement of NJ tubes, another study in contrast described success with the use of metoclopramide.[13,14] Both of these studies contained very small numbers of patients. In an overall literature review on the topic, it was reported that the propensity of data suggested that metoclopramide was beneficial in promoting placement of NJ tubes.[15]

Failure to pass an NJ tube blindly or with an electromagnetic guidance at the bedside requires the use of radiologic or endoscopic tube placement. The preference for either technique is center dependent. Those centers with available C-arm fluoroscopy and modified fluoroscopy beds, fluoroscopic passage of NJ tubes can be done at the patient's bedside. However, institutions without bedside fluoroscopic capabilities, transport of patients to the radiology suite, especially critically ill patients, can be time consuming, expensive, and hazardous.[16]

Endoscopic placement of NJ tubes can be done at the bedside. Table 13.2 lists the current most common endoscopic NJ tube placement techniques. The drag and pull method has the most history. In this procedure, a snare or a suture material is attached to the end of the NJ tube. The suture is grasped with a forceps. The NJ tube is pulled down into the jejunum with the snare or forceps. Difficulty usually occurs in attempting to release the suture from the grasping forceps or releasing the NJ tube from the snare without displacing the tube's position. A second common technique, over the guidewire technique, requires the placement of a guidewire through the biopsy channel of the endoscope into the small intestine. The endoscope may be passed orally or through the nasal cavity. The endoscope is removed, and an NJ tube is passed over the guidewire blindly or with fluoroscopy. A final technique requires filling the lumen of an NJ tube with a guidewire (0.052) to make it stiff. The endoscope is passed into the stomach. The NJ tube is pushed through the nare into the small bowel. The endoscope is used to visualize the NJ tube being pushed into

---

TABLE 13.2
Endoscopic Nasoenteric Tube Placement Methods

Methods	Technique
Drag-and-pull	Suture on end of the tube pulled with forceps into position
Over-the-guidewire	Tube pushed into position over a guidewire
Through-the-scope	Tube pushed through the biopsy channel of an endoscope (small diameter tube)
Stiffened "push" procedure	Guidewire filled, stiffened tube pushed into position under endoscopic visualization

the position. Occasionally, the tip of the endoscope is used to "nudge" the tip of the feeding tube toward the right direction.[17]

Nasoenteric tube placement is the most common method for enteral access. However, nasoenteric tubes may fail early, secondary to either tube occlusion or tube dislodgement and interrupt tube feeding and medication delivery regimens. The use of a commercial "bridle" may improve tube dislodgement without causing significant complications.[18] When using endoscopy to place a nasoenteric tube, the use of an endoscopic clip to attach the end of the feeding tube to the small bowel, mucosa, to prevent migration has been described. One prospective randomized trial noted a reduction in the need for repeat endoscopy for nasoenteric tube replacement by using the endoscopic clip.[19]

The decision to use a small diameter feeding tube, such as a J-tube, should also warrant some very specific instructions for the patient. In general, the lumen of a J-tube is much smaller than the lumen of a G-tube and, therefore, J-tubes are more prone to tube clogging and occlusion. J-tubes should never be used to check for gastric or small bowel residual content as this promotes tube occlusion. J-tubes should be flushed after every feed or medication instillation. Only liquid medications or completely dissolved medications should be placed through a J-tube to avoid tube clogging.

Because of their frequent tube failure over time, nasoenteric tubes should be relegated to patients requiring enteral feeding for <1 month. Patients requiring long-term enteral access or who experience repeated failure of nasoenteric enteral access should have a percutaneous feeding tube placed such as a gastrostomy, jejunostomy, or gastro/jejunostomy.

13.3   PERCUTANEOUS ENTERAL ACCESS

If a patient requires enteral access for >1 month, percutaneous procedures are preferred. These procedures can be performed by endoscopy, radiology, or by the surgeon dependent on the patient's need and the institutional expertise. Percutaneous procedures include gastrostomy, jejunostomy, and gastro/jejunostomy.

13.4   ENDOSCOPY

13.4.1   PERCUTANEOUS ENDOSCOPIC GASTROSTOMY

Percutaneous endoscopic gastrostomy (PEG) was developed by Ponsky and Gauderer in the early 1980s.[20] The procedure involves the placement of a percutaneous gastrostomy tube after endoscopic transillumination of the abdominal wall for an appropriate insertion site. The use of prophylactic antibiotics before the procedure is important for the prevention of postprocedure infections.[21] Recent information suggests that cephalosporins are no longer adequate preprocedure antibiotic coverage because of the prevalence of *Staphylococcus aureus* methicillin resistant bacteria and other resistant organisms.[22]

Placement of the PEG tube is most often accomplished by the Sachs-Vine (push) and the Ponsky (pull) technique. A decision to use one procedure or the other is simply a matter of patient's preference.[23] Prospective evaluations of PEG placement have shown these procedures to be associated with few major complications.

In patients where a push or a pull PEG placement may not be desired, such as in patients with head and neck cancer or esophageal cancer where tumor seeding of the gastrostomy site by cancer cells picked up by the PEG tube as it passes by the tumor, is a concern. In these instances, a "direct" method of PEG placement may be appropriate. In this technique, endoscopy is performed, and the abdominal wall is transilluminated. The anterior gastric wall is attached to the abdominal wall with 3–4 T-fasteners. An incision is made, and a gastrostomy site is created with a series of dilators passed over a guidewire. Ultimately, a PEG tube with its internal bumper in a peel away sheath is placed through the gastrostomy site into the stomach.[24] A meta-analysis comparing PEG placement by the pull technique to PEG placement by the direct method noted a reduction in peristomal infectious complications with the direct method.[25] However, this meta-analysis was hampered by the limited number of studies in this area and the high risk of biased interpretation of the data.

For patients who cannot open their mouth for endoscopy, transnasal endoscopy may be used for PEG placement with the direct method or a standard pull technique with a 20 Fr PEG tube which is pulled through the nare.[26]

PEG tube kits are available from multiple manufacturers. The most common sizes are 16–24 Fr. Most tubes are made of silicon or polyurethane. In general, these tubes start to degrade in 1–2 years with yeast implantation into the wall of the tube.[27]

Obstructed PEG tubes may be cleared with warm water and a syringe. In some cases, pancreatic enzymes mixed in a bicarbonate solution can be effective.[28] Data does not exist to support the use of juices, soft drinks, or meat tenderizer to clear a PEG tube. PEG tube brushes and an FDA approved mechanical action catheter and probe tip are also available for clearing obstructed PEG tubes.

Once a PEG tube malfunctions, degrades or is no longer needed, it can be removed at the bedside with a traction pull force of 7–10 lb. These tubes are labeled 'traction removable.[28] Some PEG tubes have a "stiff" internal bolster and can only be removed with an endoscope. These are labeled "endoscopic removable." These types of PEG tubes may be beneficial for patients who are combative and at risk for self-removal of their PEG tubes.

Replacement PEG tubes are broadly divided into two categories; replacement gastrostomy tubes and low profile devices. Replacement gastrostomy tubes usually have a balloon internal bolster. These tubes are inserted blindly through the gastrostomy site into the gastric lumen. The balloon is inflated to serve as the internal bolster. An external bolster is slid down the tube to rest against the abdominal wall to keep the tube from migrating. Replacement PEG tubes may also have a distensible internal bolster (Figure 13.1). The internal bolster is stretched with a stylet and pushed blindly through the gastrostomy site into the gastric lumen. The stylet is removed, and the internal bolster assumes its previous shape. Care must be taken to know the direction of the gastrostomy tract so that damage or rupture of the tract does not occur with the use of the stylet.

PEG tubes may be replaced with low-profile devices (Figure 13.2). These devices provide skin level access to the gastric lumen. The internal bolster may be an

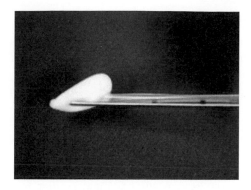

FIGURE 13.1   Internal bolster distended with stylet. (Photo from the Library of Dr. Mark DeLegge.)

inflatable balloon or a distensible internal bumper that requires a stylet for placement. The devices come in predetermined lengths. The gastrostomy tract length must be measured so the clinician can choose the correct length skin level device. To access these devices for feeding or medication delivery or for gastric decompression, an access tube must be used to engage a valve on the low profile device. Although, these devices are cosmetically appealing, the small internal diameter of the access tubing and valve make them more prone to valve and access tube occlusion and dysfunction.

After replacement of a PEG tube with a replacement gastrostomy device, appropriate placement of the tube within the gastric lumen must be confirmed. This can be done by a combination of auscultation of the stomach region of the abdominal wall for air rapidly infused through the PEG tube and visualization of gastric contents withdrawn from the PEG tube by a syringe. If there is a question about proper placement of the replacement gastrostomy tube, a contrast fluoroscopic study through the tube should be obtained. This is especially important when the original PEG tube has been in place for <1 month as the abdominal wall, and the anterior gastric wall may not have adhered together to create a viable fistula tract.

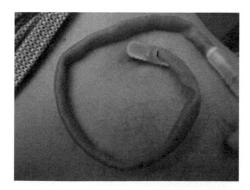

FIGURE 13.2   Low-profile device. (Photo from the Library of Dr. Mark DeLegge.)

13.4.2 PERCUTANEOUS ENDOSCOPIC GASTRO/JEJUNOSTOMY AND JEJUNOSTOMY

In patients for whom small bowel feedings are desired endoscopic, percutaneous small bowel access may be obtained by two methods. The first method, percutaneous gastro/jejunostomy (PEG/J) places a jejunal tube (J-tube) through an existing PEG tube using a variety of techniques. One of the most common techniques is the over-the-guidewire method. After PEG placement, a pediatric colonoscope is placed into the stomach. An alligator forceps is passed up through the PEG tube to the outside of the patient. A guidewire is grasped in the forceps and pulled into the gastric lumen. The guidewire, forceps, and pediatric colonoscope are advanced into the distal duodenum or proximal jejunum. A 9 or 12 Fr J-tube is passed over the guidewire through the existing PEG and into position in the small bowel. The colonoscope, forceps, and guidewire are removed. Very high success rates with this technique have been reported with no major complications.[29] The PEG/J tube system allows concurrent gastric decompression and small bowel feeding.

Other methods of endoscopic PEG/J placement have been described. An ultrathin endoscope may be passed directly through the PEG into the small bowel. A guidewire is passed through the endoscope into the small bowel, and the endoscope is removed. The J-tube is passed over the guidewire into proper position in the small intestine.[30] Another technique removes an existing PEG tube after it has been in place for at least 4 weeks. An endoscope is passed through the gastrostomy site into the small intestine. A guidewire is left in place in the small intestine, and the endoscope is removed. A combination G/J tube is passed over the guidewire into proper position.[31]

The second major method of percutaneous endoscopic jejunal tube placement is known as direct percutaneous endoscopic jejunostomy (DPEJ). A small bowel feeding tube is placed directly into the jejunum with an endoscope. This procedure requires the use of a pediatric colonoscope or an enteroscope to reach a point of entry beyond the ligament of Treitz. Good success with this technique has been described as far back as the early 1990s.[32,33] There were some reported minor complications with this procedure (including local site infection), but no cases of peritonitis or bowel infarction. One of the difficulties with the endoscopic DPEJ procedure was the frequent migration of the small bowel away from the introducer needle once an adequate entry site had been located by endoscopic transillumination. This was resolved by the use of a "2 needle stick" technique.[34] In this procedure, a smaller, sharper 19 gauge needle is first passed through the abdominal wall into the small intestine. This needle is grasped by a snare. The larger introducer needle is passed into the small bowel without pushing the small bowel away as it is now "trapped" in position. The snare is pulled off the smaller needle and placed around the introducer needle. The smaller needle is removed. A guidewire is passed through the introducer needle, grasped by the snare and pulled out of the oral cavity. A J-tube is attached to the guidewire and pulled into position using a standard PEG placement technique. Adequate positioning of the internal bumper in the small bowel is confirmed by repeat endoscopy.

Percutaneous endoscopic procedures are successful methods for obtaining enteral access. PEG should be performed in patients who can tolerate gastric feedings and who will require enteral access for >1 month. PEG/J allows both jejunal feeding and gastric decompression. It should be used in patients who require small bowel feedings for >1 month, but <6 months as the jejunal component of the tube system may fail secondary to tube occlusion or tube migration. DPEJ should be used by patients requiring jejunal feeding for >6 months.[35]

A retrospective study compared physician endoscopic reinterventions for J-tube dysfunction or complication in a group of patients who received DPEJ versus PEG/J for jejunal feeding. The DPEJ group had significantly fewer endoscopic reinterventions.[36]

13.4.3 Surgical Enteral Access

Surgical enteral access was the standard of care for many years. These procedures include gastrostomy, gastrojejunostomy and jejunostomy. These procedures may be performed with a standard open technique or with laparoscopic guidance. In recent years, the advent of endoscopic and radiologic percutaneous enteral access techniques has relegated surgical enteral access procedures to patients who are in the operating room for another procedure or in instances where endoscopic or radiologic enteral access is technically impossible to perform safely. Multiple studies have compared surgical gastrostomy to PEG. These studies have shown either operative time savings, cost savings or reduction in associated morbidity with PEG.[37,38]

In the standard open gastrostomy for feeding tube placement, an enterotomy is formed, and a feeding tube is placed into the gastric lumen. The anterior gastric wall is fixed to the abdominal wall. The open surgical gastrostomy was first described by Seidllot in 1849 and has not changed significantly in the following years.[39]

Surgical jejunostomy is a procedure where a feeding tube is placed into the proximal jejunal lumen. The first person to accomplish this procedure was Bush in 1858 in a patient with a nonoperable cancer.[40] In 1878, Surmay de Havre developed a technique in which a J-tube was introduced into the bowel through an enterostomy.[41] In 1891, Witzel first described the most well-known technique for the surgical jejunostomy which has subsequently undergone a number of modifications.[42]

The decision to place a surgical jejunostomy follows the same decision tree analysis as does the decision to place any jejunal feeding tube. Typically, patients who are intolerant to gastric feedings or in patients with a surgically absent or obstructed stomach will receive a surgical jejunostomy. Surgical jejunostomy is also common in trauma patients who have associated gastroparesis following trauma and surgical exploration and repair. In one study, patients received the surgical jejunostomy as an additional procedure during major abdominal trauma in 95% of cases and as a sole procedure in 5% of cases.[43]

Needle catheter jejunostomy (NCJ) involves the placement of a 5 or 7 Fr catheter into the jejunum through a submucosal tunnel. It was hypothesized that this technique would have fewer complications than a standard jejunostomy as the entrance to the jejunum was much smaller in comparison. Multiple studies have demonstrated a reduction in major complications when NCJ is compared to open jejunostomy.[44,45] However, because of the small tube size there are significantly more episodes of tube occlusion and dislodgement.

Laparoscopic placement of G- and J-tubes was developed in the early 1990s. Initially, it was believed these procedures would be associated with less morbidity and operative stress as compared to standard surgical gastrostomy and jejunostomy. However, these techniques were discovered to provide no significant advantage to the standard surgical gastrostomy and jejunostomy with relationship to operative time or morbidity.[46,47]

The use of early small bowel feeding in the intensive care unit (ICU) has been encouraged because of the beneficial effects of early enteral feeding. However, there is some concern amongst clinicians about the potential deleterious effects of enteral feeding on mesenteric blood flow and resultant ischemia that could develop in a hypotensive patient. One study reported a 4% incidence of bowel necrosis in 103 critically ill patients receiving tube feeding through a surgical jejunostomy.[48] The postmortem examination in these patients did not show any evidence of bowel torsion or mesenteric artery thrombosis suggesting that the jejunal feeding may have exacerbated a previous low flow state in the mesentery.[49] A more recent analysis of ventilated patients on vasopressors reported a reduction in overall mortality in patients receiving early EN as compared to late EN.[50]

13.4.4 RADIOLOGIC PERCUTANEOUS ENTERAL ACCESS

Placement of radiologic percutaneous gastrostomy, jejunostomy, and gastro/ jejunostomy has continued to blossom since their introduction in the 1980s.[51,52] These procedures are usually performed in the fluoroscopic or computed tomography (CAT/CT) scan suite. After topical anesthesia of the abdominal wall and occasional moderate sedation, the inferior margin of the liver is identified and marked on the patient's abdominal wall skin surface. A NG tube is passed into the stomach for insufflation. For those instances where a NG tube cannot be passed into the stomach, an access needle is passed into the stomach under ultrasound (US) or CT guidance. The stomach can be insufflated through this needle.[53] After gastric insufflation, the stomach is punctured with an introducer catheter. Most radiologists will attach the anterior gastric wall to the abdominal wall with T-fasteners. A guidewire is passed through the introducer into the stomach. The puncture site is serially dilated over a guidewire to a size of 10–14 Fr. A feeding tube is passed through the gastrostomy site into the stomach. If a gastrojejunostomy is desired, a tube can be passed through the gastrostomy site with the tip advanced to the jejunum.

The fluoroscopic approach to enteral access has excellent reported technical success.[54] CT-guided enteral access also has excellent technical success even in technically difficult patients, such as the obese patient.[55] The major criticism of these procedures focuses on associated complications. The majority of these complications involve either inadvertent puncture of contiguous organs or separation of the gastric and abdominal walls after tract dilation resulting in intraabdominal leakage and peritonitis. In addition, frequent occlusion of the radiologically placed feeding tubes may occur at a greater rate secondary to their small internal diameter. The placement of larger enteral access tubes by a radiologic technique may require modification of the standard placement procedure techniques.[56] When comparing endoscopic and radiologic gastrostomy tube placement, clinical outcomes, and associated complications are very similar.[57,58]

13.4.5 Indications and Contraindications for EN

Although most patients can be fed enterally, EN may be contraindicated in patients with a nonfunctional GI tract as noted in Table 13.3. EN is contraindicated in patients with a complete mechanical bowel obstruction. However, patients with a partial bowel obstruction or an ileus may tolerate EN with careful monitoring of tolerance.[59] Short bowel syndrome patients with <100 cm of small bowel remaining or patients with severe malabsorption may not be able to maintain adequate nutrition status with an oral diet or EN alone.[60] EN may not be possible in patients with GI fistulas that are too distal to bypass with a feeding tube or have increased fistula output with the initiation of EN. GI bleeds are not an absolute contraindication for EN. The feasibility of EN is affected by the cause, location, and severity of the bleed. Generally, most patients with lower GI bleeds can be fed enterally, but in patients with severe upper GI bleeds, such those from esophageal varices, EN should be held until the risk for bleeding has lessened.[61] Additionally, patients whose expected need for nutrition support is <5–7 days in the malnourished patient or 7–9 days in the adequately nourished patient may not benefit from the initiation of EN.[62] Withholding EN may be appropriate in end-of-life situations where aggressive medical care is being withdrawn.

13.4.6 Benefits of EN

EN provides many physiological benefits compared to PN. EN utilizes normal digestive and absorptive pathways. EN stimulates the release of cholecystokinin allowing normal gallbladder function to be maintained. Bowel rest can lead to loss of mucosal mass, absorptive function, and increase gut permeability whereas EN maintains gut mucosal integrity and gut-associated immune function and prevents bacterial translocation.[63,64] EN has been shown to decrease infectious complications such as sepsis, pneumonias and intraabdominal abscesses leading to decreased length of ICU and hospital stays.[65–69] EN is more economical than PN, not only in cost to provide nutrition support but also in cost savings related to decreased infection and hospital length of stay.[70,71] EN also allows for the delivery of nutrients not readily available in the parenteral form in the United States such as fiber, prebiotics, specialized fatty acids, glutamine, arginine, and nucleotides.

TABLE 13.3
Possible Contraindications to EN

Mechanical GI obstruction or paralytic ileus

Short-bowel syndrome (<100 cm small bowel)

Distal high output fistula

Severe GI bleed

Severe malabsorption

Unable to obtain enteral access

Short term need for nutrition support

Aggressive nutrition support is not warranted or desired

13.4.7   METHOD OF DELIVERY

EN formulas are available in ready-to-feed, ready-to-hang, and powder formulations. Ready-to-feed and ready-to-hang methods are most commonly used. Powdered formulas require reconstitution by mixing with water, which is time and labor intensive and requires a sanitary environment. This method is primarily used by institutions in the neonatal and pediatric populations. Institutions are moving away from the read-to-feed or "open-systems," which require the transfer of formula from a can, bottle, or brick pack to an enteral feeding bag for hanging. Ready-to-hang or closed systems come in sealed bags or rigid containers and have hang times of 24–48 h. Closed systems reduce the risk of contamination and nursing time required for administration.[72]

EN can be delivered a number of ways including bolus, intermittent, continuous, and cycled. The selection of the method of delivery is determined by the type of enteral access, current medical condition, and patient preference. Bolus feedings allow for the delivery of a large amount of enteral formula over a short period of time. Bolus feedings of 240 cc of formula are generally provided over 10–15 min every 3–6 h during the day through a large syringe as required to meet daily calorie, protein, and water needs. Bolus feedings can be initiated at one-half to one can (240 mL) per feeding and increased up to two cans per feeding. Bolus feeds are low cost and allow patients to have feeding schedules similar to normal meal patterns. However, bolus feeds may be poorly tolerated by patients with persistent nausea or delayed gastric emptying. Providing the feedings intermittently, by gravity drip over the course of 20–30 min can improve tolerance.

Continuous feedings provided by mechanical pump are commonly used in acutely ill hospitalized patients, patients with small bowel feeding tubes, or in patients who do not tolerate bolus/intermittent feeds. An enteral feeding pump is used to provide a controlled rate of formula. Continuous TFs are usually initiated at 20–30 mL/h and slowly advanced to the goal by 20–30 mL every 4–8 h. Some patients may tolerate a more aggressive advancement to goal. EN may be cycled using the enteral pump to infuse daily total nutrient needs over an 8–16 h time period, usually while the patient is sleeping. This method of delivery is often done in hospitalized patients who are transitioning to oral diets to encourage oral intake at meals during the day. Patients on home EN are also often transitioned to cycled feedings to allow free time away from the enteral pump and pole, which can promote improved quality of life and activity. Portable backpack pumps can be considered in these patients. Cycled feedings may not be tolerated in some patients due to increased infusion rates required to deliver the daily nutrient requirements over a shorter period of time.

13.4.8   ENTERAL FORMULATIONS

Numerous enteral formulas are commercially available and choosing the best formula for patients can be challenging, especially in patients with GI diseases (Table 13.4). Most formulas can be classified as polymeric or semi-elemental/elemental. Polymeric formulas contain intact nutrients, whereas semi-elemental or elemental formulas contain partially or completely hydrolyzed nutrients. Each category can be further classified into standard formulas with balanced amounts of macronutrients or

TABLE 13.4

Summary of Macronutrient Distribution and Fluid Content of Enteral Formulas

Product Name	Kcal/mL	% Calories from Protein	% Calories from Carbohydrate	% Calories from Fat	Fiber (g/L)	Osmolality (mOsm/kg H$_2$O)	% Free Water	Additional Ingredients per L
Standard polymeric								
Nutren 1.0[a]	1.0	16	51	33	0	315	85	
Nutren 1.0 Fiber[a]	1.0	16	51	33	14	315	85	
Replete[a]	1.0	25	45	30	0	300	85	
Replete Fiber[a]	1.0	25	45	30	14	300	85	
Promote[b]	1.0	25	52	23	0	340	84	
Promote Fiber[b]	1.0	25	52	23	14.4	340	83	
Jevity 1 Cal[b]	1.06	17	54	29	14.4	300	84	
Osmolite 1 Cal[b]	1.06	17	54	29	0	300	84	
Compleat[a]	1.07	18	48	34	6	340	85	
Fibersource HN[a]	1.2	18	53	29	10	490	81	
Jevity 1.2 Cal[b]	1.2	19	53	29	18	450	81	
Isosource HN[a]	1.2	18	53	29	0	490	85	
Osmolite 1.2[b]	1.2	19	53	29	0	360	82	
Isosource 1.5[a]	1.5	18	44	38	8	650	78	
Jevity 1.5[b]	1.5	17	54	29	22	525	76	
Osmolite 1.5[b]	1.5	17	54	29	0	525	76	
Nutren 2.0[a]	2.0	16	39	45	0	746	70	
TwoCal HN[b]	2.0	17	46	40	5	725	70	
Polymeric diabetic								
Glucerna 1.0 Cal[b]	1.0	17	34	49	14.4	355	85	
Nutren Glytrol[a]	1.0	18	40	42	15.2	280	84	
Diabetisource AC[a]	1.2	20	36	44	15	450	82	3.2 g arginine and 1 g EPA/DHA

(Continued)

TABLE 13.4 (*Continued*)
Summary of Macronutrient Distribution and Fluid Content of Enteral Formulas

Product Name	Kcal/mL	% Calories from Protein	% Calories from Carbohydrate	% Calories from Fat	Fiber (g/L)	Osmolality (mOsm/kg H$_2$O)	% Free Water	Additional Ingredients per L
Glucerna 1.2[b]	1.2	20	35	45	17	720	81	3 g ALA, 1 g EPA/DHA and
Glucerna 1.5[b]	1.5	22	33	48	17	875	76	3 g ALA and
Polymeric pulmonary								
Nutren Pulmonary[a]	1.5	18	27	55	0	330	78	
Pulmocare[b]	1.5	17	28	55	0	475	79	
Polymeric renal								
Nepro with Carb Steady[b]	1.8	18	34	48	15.6	585	72.5	
Suplena with Carb Steady[b]	1.8	10	42	48	16	600	71	
Novasource Renal[a]	2.0	18	37	45	0	800	72	
Renalcal[a]	2.0	7	58	35	0	600	70	
Polymeric hepatic								
Nutrihep[a]	1.5	11	77	12	0	790	76	
Polymeric immune enhancing								
Impact[a]	1.0	22	53	25	0	375	85	1.7 g EPA/DHA, 12.5 g arginine, 1.2 g nucleotides
Impact with Fiber[a]	1.0	22	53	25	10	375	87	1.7 g EPA/DHA, 12.5 g arginine, 1.2 g nucleotide
Oxepa[b]	1.5	17	28	55	0	535	79	4.6 g EPA, 4 g GLA
Pivot[b]	1.5	25	45	30	7.5	595	80	2.6 g EPA, 1.3 g DHA, 13 g arginine, 6.5 g glutamine
Elemental								
Tolerex[a]	1.0	8	90	2	0	550	84	2.4 g arginine, 3.5 g glutamine
Vital HN[b]	1.0	16.7	73.8	9.8	0	500	85	
Vivonex Plus[a]	1.0	18	76	6	0	650	83	6.3 g arginine, 9.5 g glutamine

TABLE 13.4 (Continued)
Summary of Macronutrient Distribution and Fluid Content of Enteral Formulas

Product Name	Kcal/mL	% Calories from Protein	% Calories from Carbohydrate	% Calories from Fat	Fiber (g/L)	Osmolality (mOsm/kg H₂O)	% Free Water	Additional Ingredients per L
Vivonex RTF[a]	1.0	20	70	10	0	630	85	5.9 g arginine
Vivonex TEN[a]	1.0	15	82	3	0	630	83	3.9 g arginine, 4.8 g glutamine
Semi-elemental								
Peptamen[a]	1.0	16	51	33	0	270	85	
Peptamen with Prebio[a]	1.0	16	51	33	0	300	85	
Peptamen AF[a]	1.2	25	36	39	5.2	390	81	2.4 g EPA/DHA
Peptamen 1.5[a]	1.5	18	49	33	0	550	77	
Peptamen 1.5 with Prebio[a]	1.5	18	49	33	0	550	77	
Vital 1.0 Cal[b]	1.0	16	51	33	4.2	390	84	
Vital 1.5[b]	1.5	18	49	33	6	610	76	
Semi-elemental immune-enhancing								
Peptamen Bariatric[a]	1.0	37	31	32	4.4	345	84	2 g EPA/DHA
Vital AF 1.2 Cal[b]	1.2	25	36	39	5.1	425	81	2.7 g EPA, 1.1g DHA,
Perative[b]	1.3	20.5	54.5	25	6.5	460	79	8 g arginine
Impact Glutamine[a]	1.3	24	46	30	10	630	81	2.7 g EPA/DHA, 15 g arginine, 15 g glutamine, 1.5 g nucleotides
Impact Peptide 1.5[a]	1.5	25	37	38	0	510	77	4.8 g EPA/DHA,18.7 g arginine, 1.8 g nucleotides

[a] Nestlé Nutrition.
[b] Abbott Nutrition.

specialty formulas with a modified nutrient profile designed for patients with specific diseases or clinical states. Multiple factors should be considered when determining the appropriate formula. Figure 13.3 illustrates an example pathway for enteral formula selection.[73]

13.4.9 POLYMERIC STANDARD FORMULA

Polymeric standard formulas are most often used for patients requiring EN. The nutrient composition of these formulas is designed to match the diet of a healthy individual and meet general dietary recommendations. Standard formulas can meet the nutrient needs of most patients and are significantly less expensive than specialty formulas.

Standard formulas are available in a range of nutrient concentrations (1.0–2.0 kcal/mL) to meet the fluid needs or restrictions of different patient populations. Patients with congestive heart failure, fluid overload, renal failure, ascites, syndrome of inappropriate antidiuretic hormone (SIADH), or hypervolemic hyponatremia may benefit from the concentrated 2 kcal/mL formulas. Concentrated formulas may also be beneficial for bolus or cyclic feedings as they allow for calorie requirements to be met with a smaller volume. However, clinicians must consider the fluid needs of patients and ensure the balance of fluid needs is being provided through oral intake, periodic free water flushes, or intravenous fluids.

Standard formulas also contain varying amounts of protein (16%–25%). Higher protein formulas (25%) may be beneficial in patients with acute pancreatitis (AP), ulcerative colitis, Crohn's disease, short bowel syndrome, or other GI diseases with increased protein requirements. It should be noted that most standard high protein formulas provide 1 kcal/mL and may not be appropriate for patients requiring fluid restriction.

Less commonly used blenderized formulas may be a substituted for standard formulas in patients who do not tolerate semisynthetic formulas or have a strong desire for a more natural formula. Blenderized formulas are made from table foods with added vitamins and minerals. Homemade blenderized formulas should be used with

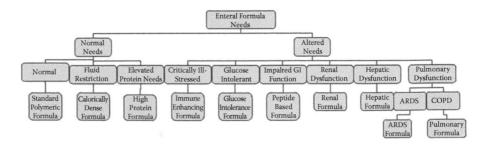

FIGURE 13.3 Guide to formula selection. (Reprinted from Enteral Formula Selection and Preparation. In: Boullata J., Nieman Carney L., and Guenter P., Eds. *A.S.P.E.N. Enteral Nutrition Handbook*. Silver Spring, MD: American Society for Parenteral and Enteral Nutrition; 2010. p. 95 with permission from the American Society for Parenteral and Enteral Nutrition (ASPEN). ASPEN does not endorse the use of this material in any form other than its entirety.)

caution due to possible risk of foodborne illness, potential to clog feeding tubes if not adequately blenderized, and difficultly confirming adequate calorie, protein, vitamin, and mineral provision. Currently, there is one commercially available blenderized formula made from chicken, peas, carrots, tomatoes, and cranberry juice.

13.4.10 FIBER

Fiber is often added to the standard and some specialty formulas. Fiber formulas are designed to promote bowel regularity. Most formulas contain a combination of soluble and insoluble fiber. Soluble fiber may be beneficial in patients with diarrhea by increasing water and sodium absorption.[74] On the other hand, insoluble fiber has been shown to increase fecal weight and peristalsis and may be beneficial for patients with constipation and for patients on long-term EN.

Fiber may provide other benefits including promoting healthy gut microflora.[75] Since humans are unable to digest fiber; it is fermented by bacteria in the colon to produce short-chain fatty acids (SCFAs). SCFA can be used as a fuel source for colonocytes and beneficial bacteria. Some formulas may also contain fructooligosaccharides (FOS) that are also fermented in the colon to produce SCFA. There is some evidence to suggest that fiber containing formulas may improve glycemic control.[76]

The use of fiber containing formulas should be monitored closely, and adequate fluids should be provided to avoid constipation or impaction in patients on long-term EN. Fiber containing formulas should be used with caution in the critically ill patients and should be avoided in hypotensive patients or patients at risk for developing ischemic bowel.[77]

13.5 DISEASE SPECIFIC

13.5.1 DIABETES/GLUCOSE INTOLERANCE

There are multiple enteral formulas promoted for patients with diabetes or glucose intolerance that contain less carbohydrate (31%–40%), higher amounts of fat (42%–49%), and a mixture of soluble and insoluble fiber (14–21 g/L). The fat content may be modified to provide increased amounts of monounsaturated fatty acid (MUFA) and less polyunsaturated and saturated fatty acids. Research on the efficacy of using a diabetic formula is conflicting with some studies showing a benefit and others showing no difference.[78–80] The recent *A.S.P.E.N. Clinical Guidelines: Nutrition Support of Adult Patients With Hyperglycemia* did not provide any recommendation for the use of diabetes formulas in hyperglycemic hospitalized patients stating that the research on glycemic and lipid control was inconclusive.[81] Routine use of diabetes formulas is not currently recommended but may be considered in patients who have uncontrolled blood glucose on a standard formula.

Additionally, diabetes formulas may not be appropriate for all patients with diabetes. Patients with gastroparesis may not tolerate the additional fiber if being fed into the stomach as fiber can slow gastric emptying. Additionally, the fat content of diabetes formulas (42%–49%) is significantly more than the 20%–35% of calorie from fat recommended for adults in the *2010 Dietary Guidelines for Americans.*[82] Despite higher amounts of MUFA, it is unclear what the long-term effect the diabetes formulas may have on cardiovascular health.

13.5.2 RENAL FAILURE

Enteral formulas for specific for patients with renal dysfunction are calorically dense and provide lower amounts of electrolytes (sodium, potassium, phosphorus, magnesium). The protein content of renal formulas varies (7%–18%). Formulas with lower amounts of protein should only be used in patients who have renal dysfunction but are not yet on renal replacement therapy (RRT). Patients on RRT have higher protein (1.1–1.3 g/kg)[83] and energy needs and may tolerate a fluid restricted standard formula. The use of a renal formula with more moderate levels of protein may be appropriate in patients on RRT with chronic hyperkalemia or hyperphosphatemia. Critically ill patients on continuous renal replacement therapy (CRRT) have even higher protein (2–2.5 g/kg)[84] and energy needs which cannot be met by renal formulas without the use of protein modulars. Since patients on CRRT may not require fluid or electrolyte restrictions, a standard high-protein formula may be most appropriate for these patients. There are no clinical trials comparing renal formulas to standard formulas in this population.

13.5.3 HEPATIC FAILURE

Hepatic formulas have increased amounts of branch-chain amino acids (BCAAs) and lower amounts of aromatic amino acids (AAAs) compared to standard formulas. The uptake of AAA across the blood–brain barrier leads to the synthesis of false neurotransmitters resulting in hepatic encephalopathy. The provision of BCAAs is thought to offset the imbalance of BCAA:AAA found in hepatic disease.[85] However, a 2003 Cochrane Review did not find any difference in the development of hepatic encephalopathy or mortality when using a hepatic formula.[86] Additionally, hepatic formulas are lower in protein and may not meet the increased protein needs of most end-stage liver disease patients. Hepatic formulas are more expensive than standard formulas.

13.5.4 IMMUNE ENHANCING

Immune-enhancing (IE) enteral formulas contain supplemental amounts of at least one of the following ingredients: arginine, glutamine, ω-3 fatty acids, nucleotides, and/or antioxidants. IE formulas are designed to improve immune cell function, attenuate inflammation, and decrease infections. Arginine and glutamine are considered nonessential amino acids but become conditionally essential during times of acute stress or illness.[87] Arginine is involved in cell growth and proliferation, collagen synthesis, wound healing, and is a precursor of nitric acid.[87] Glutamine is involved in many metabolic pathways during critical illness and is thought to protect against oxidative injury, enhance heat-shock protein expression, reduce cytokine release, and decrease apoptosis.[88] Additionally, glutamine is a fuel source for small intestine enterocytes and immune cells.[89] The ω-3 fatty acids eicosapentaenoic acid (EPA) and docosahexaenoic acid (DHA) modulate inflammation by limiting the production of arachidonic acid (AA), which is proinflammatory and immunosuppressive.[89] Nucleotide is essential for DNA and RNA production and antioxidants act on different oxidative processes of critical illness.[89]

IE formulas have been studied more than any other type of enteral formula, but use of IE formulas remains controversial. Multiple studies have shown a reduction of infectious complications (abdominal abscess, wound infection, and pneumonia), decreased complications associated with anastomotic leak, and reduced LOS in elective GI surgery patients.[90] Perioperative nutrition using IE is recommended for moderately and severely malnourished patients undergoing extensive head and neck surgery, GI surgery (esophagus, stomach, pancreas, and small/large intestine), and in patients with blunt and penetrating torso trauma.[91] Consumption of IE orally or via feeding tube is recommended for 5–7 days prior to surgery[90] and for 5 days after surgery when possible.[92] The use of IE in critical illness is less clear. The 2009 critical care guidelines published by the Society of Critical Care Medicine and American Society for Parenteral and Enteral Nutrition (ASPEN) recommend the use of IE in surgical ICU patients (grade A) and medical ICU patients (grade B) with caution in patients with severe sepsis.[93] The European Society for Parenteral and Enteral Nutrition (E.S.P.E.N.) also recommends the use of IE in critically ill patients without severe sepsis.[94] However, the Canadian Clinical Practice Guidelines do not recommend the use of arginine supplemented formulas in critically ill patients.[95]

13.5.5 PULMONARY FAILURE/ACUTE RESPIRATORY DISTRESS SYNDROME

Originally, pulmonary formulas were formulated with increased fat content and decreased carbohydrate content in an effort to decrease carbon dioxide production and improve vent weaning. However, evidence from clinical research showed that higher fat formulas did not improve clinical outcomes.[96–98] Additionally, an important study by Talpers et al.[99] demonstrated that overfeeding total calories had a more significant impact on carbon dioxide production than overall carbohydrate content.

Since then, IE pulmonary formulas have been developed with similar carbohydrate and fat content of the original pulmonary formulas but with higher amounts of EPA from fish oil and gamma-linolenic acid (GLA) from borage oil and antioxidants designed for patients with acute respiratory distress syndrome (ARDS) and acute lung injury (ALI). Studies have shown decreased pulmonary inflammation, ventilator days, ICU days and new organ failure with these pulmonary formulations in specific patient populations.[100–102] Multiple international critical care guidelines recommend the consideration of an enteral formula with added fish oils, borage oils, and antioxidants in patients with ARDS and ALI.[93–95]

13.5.6 WOUND HEALING

Adequate nutrition is imperative for wound healing, and multiple enteral formulas have been designed for patients with wounds or pressure ulcers to take orally or via a feeding tube. These formulas often contain increased amounts of protein and vitamin A, C, and E, zinc, and arginine, which all have been shown to be involved in the wound healing process. Consumption of a high protein oral supplement has been shown to reduce the development of pressure ulcers in high risk patients,[103] and high protein enteral feedings have been shown to accelerate healing of pressure ulcers compared with a standard formula.[104] It is important to remember that wound healing is multifaceted and impacted by hydration status, glucose control, incontinence, and mobility. Additionally, long-term use of formulas with supplemental amounts of vitamin A, C, and E and zinc should be avoided.[105]

13.5.7   Semi-Elemental/Elemental

Elemental and semi-elemental formulas are designed for patients with compromised GI function such as those with malabsorption, pancreatic insufficiency, and short bowel syndrome. Semi-elemental formulas contain protein hydrolyzed into dipeptides and tripeptides, whereas elemental formulas contain free amino acids. These formulas also contain an increased ratio of medium-chain triglycerides (MCT) to long-chain triglycerides (LCT). MCT are absorbed into the portal circulation and do not require chylomicron formation, bile salts, or lipase for absorption. Since MCT does not provide essential fatty acids, formulas must contain a mixture of MCT and LCT.

Research has not shown elemental formulas to be superior to semi-elemental formulas. Small peptides are absorbed just as well as free amino acids[106] and peptide containing formulas may have greater nitrogen absorption compared to free-amino acid formulas.[107,108] Additionally, the osmolality of elemental formulas is much higher. Elemental formulas cost significantly more than semi-elemental formulas.

Evidence is also lacking to recommend semi-elemental or elemental formulas over polymeric formulas. Meta-analysis comparing semi-elemental formulas to standard formulas in critically ill patients did not find a significant difference in mortality, infection, or diarrhea. The *E.S.P.E.N. Guidelines for Enteral Nutrition* found no difference when using semi-elemental or standard formulas in patients with Crohn's disease.[109] Semi-elemental formulas have traditionally been used in patients with AP due to the presumed reduction of pancreatic stimulation compared to polymeric formulas. However, multiple studies have shown polymeric formulas can be safely fed through small bowel feeding tubes to patients with AP.[110–112] A meta-analysis found polymeric formulas did not increase feeding intolerance, infections, or mortality in AP as compared to semi-elemental enteral formulas.[113]

13.5.8   Modular Products

Modular products are available to provide additional protein, fiber (soluble and insoluble), carbohydrate, MCT oil, arginine, and glutamine (Table 13.5). Protein modulars are the most popularly used and can provide 7–15 g protein per serving. Modulars designed for wound healing may contain a combination of arginine, glutamine, and additional vitamins and minerals.

TABLE 13.5

Summary of the Macronutrient Content of Select Modular Products

Product	Serving Size	Calories per Serving	Protein g per Serving	Carbohydrate g per Serving	Fat g per Serving	Other Ingredients per Serving
Arginaid[a]	9.2 g packet	25	4.5	2	0	4.5 g arginine, vitamin C, and vitamin E
Benecalorie[a]	44 mL	330	7	0	33	
Beneprotein[a]	7 g packet	25	7	0	0	
Glutasolve[a]	22.5 g packet	90	15	7	0	15 g glutamine
Juven[b]	24 g packet	80	14	8	0	7 g arginine 7 g glutamine
Liquigen[c]	15 mL	68	7.5	0	0	
MCT Oil[b]	15 mL	116	0	0	7.5	
Nutrisource Fiber[a]	4 g packet	15	0	4	0	3 g soluble fiber
ProMod Liquid Protein[b]	30 mL	100	10	14	0	
Pro-Stat Sugar Free[c]	30 mL	100	15	10	0	
Pro-Stat Sugar Free AWC[c]	30 mL	100	17	0	7	3.3 g arginine, vitamin C, and zinc
Super Soluble Duocal[c]	5 g scoop	25	3.6	3.6	1.1	

[a] Nestlé Nutrition.
[b] Abbott Nutrition.
[c] Nutricia.

13.5.9 FOOD ALLERGIES AND INTOLERANCES

It is important to consider possible allergies when selecting an enteral formula. Enteral formulas may contain common allergens including milk, soy, corn, or egg products. A complete nutrition assessment should include questions about any possible food allergies or intolerances. Fortunately, most enteral formulas are now gluten free and lactose free.

13.5.10 ENTERAL COMPLICATIONS AND MONITORING

Although EN is the preferred method of nutrition support, it is not without some challenges. Complications of EN can be classified as mechanical, GI, metabolic, and infectious as summarized in Table 13.6.[114–116] It is possible to avoid some complications with careful monitoring and evaluation of signs of intolerance (Table 13.7).

TABLE 13.6
Possible Complications of EN

Gastrointestinal

Nausea and/or vomiting

Abdominal distention, bloating, or cramping

Diarrhea

Constipation

Pulmonary aspiration

Metabolic

Refeeding syndrome

Electrolyte imbalances

Dehydration or fluid overload

Glucose intolerance/hyperglycemia

Mechanical

Tube misplacement

Tube displacement or migration

Tube obstruction

Tube deterioration

Nasal/esophageal ulceration or irritation

EN misconnection

Leakage from stoma site

Infectious

Stoma site infection

Contamination of formula or administration set

TABLE 13.7
Parameters for Monitoring EN

Routine physical assessment and abdominal exam

Evaluating signs of dehydration or fluid retention

Recording fluid intake and output

Trending weight changes

Recording stool output—consistency and frequency

Evaluating laboratory data—serum electrolytes, blood urea nitrogen, creatinine, glucose, triglycerides

Review of medications

Evaluating adequacy of enteral intake

13.6   GI COMPLICATIONS

13.6.1   Diarrhea

GI complications are the most commonly reported of the described EN complication; the incidence varies greatly from 6% in a general hospital population to 63% in the critically ill.[116,117] Diarrhea is the most frequently reported GI complication, but the reported frequency also varies greatly.[118,119] This may attributed to lack of a consistent definition of diarrhea. Diarrhea is often defined as greater than 200 g of stool per day or three or more liquid stools per day.[120] EN itself is often blamed as the cause of diarrhea, but in most instances other etiologies exist including antibiotic therapy, preexisting GI conditions, hyperosmolar medications, pancreatic insufficiency, and bacterial contamination.[118,119,121]

Infectious processes should be considered, and stool samples tested for *Clostridium difficile*, especially in patients recently on antibiotic therapy. *Clostridium difficile*-associated diarrhea has been reported in 9%–50% of patients on EN with diarrhea.[122–124] Current medical conditions such as inflammatory bowel disease, radiation enteritis, pancreatic insufficiency, previous gastric and small bowel resections, short bowel syndrome, fat or bile acid malabsorption, celiac sprue, and intestinal malignancies, and sepsis or critical illness may predispose a patient to EN-related diarrhea.[119] The use of a semi-elemental formula, a high percentage MCT formula, and/or the addition of pancreatic enzymes could be considered if GI medical condition is suspected of causing malabsorption, or pancreatic insufficiency is present. Antidiarrheal medications can also be used in the case of malabsorption to slow transit time and allow for greater nutrient and water absorption.[119] Medications should be reviewed, and any magnesium-containing antacids, sorbitol-containing elixirs, prokinetics agents, stool softeners, laxatives, or cathartics agents should be reduced or eliminated if possible.[119,125] Medications have been shown to be responsible for up to 61% cases of diarrhea.[123] Lastly, in patients on long-term EN or with a history of constipation, impaction should be considered as a potential cause of diarrhea as impaction may present as diarrhea from the seepage of liquid stool around the site of impaction.[116]

The type of enteral formula and mode of administration should also be considered in the treatment of diarrhea if other causes have been ruled out. High fat and fiber-free formulas have been suggested to cause diarrhea.[119,126] Changing to a fiber containing formula or adding supplemental fiber may reduce diarrhea.[127–129] Although not well supported by the literature, switching to a lower osmolarity or less concentrated formula may also be beneficial.[130] However, dilution of enteral formulas with water in an attempt reduce diarrhea is not recommended and may only delay the delivery of adequate calories and protein.[131,132] Additionally, too rapid of an infusion rate or the provision of bolus feeds may cause diarrhea in some individuals.[133] Lowering the infusion rate or providing feedings over a longer period of time may improve tolerance.

Microbial contamination of the enteral formula can also cause diarrhea.[134,135] Ensuring the cleanliness during the preparation and administration of EN is very important. Any unused formula that has been opened should be refrigerated and discarded after 24 h.[119] Do not exceed recommended hang times for open- and closed-system feeding bags (24–48 h), and change the feeding bag and tubing per manufacturing recommendations.[118,119]

Most cases of E-related diarrhea are treatable and do not require withholding EN. However, EN should be held for severe diarrhea that is refractive to treatment and results in weight loss, dehydration, pressure ulcer formation, or severe abdominal pain.[136] In these rare cases, patients may require PN until the diarrhea resolves.[119,125,137]

13.6.2 CONSTIPATION

Constipation is another possible complication of EN, usually occurring in patients on long-term EN.[119] The definition of constipation is not well defined, and the expected stool frequency can vary based on the EN formula used, the patients' medical conditions and historical bowel elimination pattern.[119] Constipation is frequently caused by inadequate fluid intake, inadequate or excessive fiber intake, decreased bowel motility, medications, and inactivity.[125,133–139] Enteral formulas may not provide adequate fluid intake and additional fluid boluses via syringe or feeding pump may be required to aid regular bowel movements, especially in those patients receiving fiber containing formulas.[119] A minimum of 1 mL of fluid per kcal has also been suggested to prevent constipation.[139] In patients, who are fluid restricted for medical conditions (e.g., congestive heart failure, end-stage renal disease, end-stage liver failure), a stool softener and/or laxative should be considered.[119]

Frequency of bowel movements should be closely monitored as impaction can occur in severe cases of constipation and in some cases require endoscopic or surgical intervention. In addition to adjustments in fluid intake, fiber intake, and physical activity, patients may require stool softeners, laxatives, prokinetic agents, and/or enemas to treat constipation and prevent impaction.[119]

13.6.3 NAUSEA AND VOMITING

Nausea and vomiting are often the second most commonly reported GI complication in patients who receive EN (12%–20%).[116,140,141] Multiple etiologies exist for the presence of nausea and vomiting in the hospitalized patient including delayed gastric emptying, pancreatitis, ileus, peptic ulcer disease, cholecystitis, inflammation, fever, pain, and medications.[119] Often nausea and vomiting can be resolved by reducing the feeding rate, changing to a low fat formula, administering antiemetics or prokinetics, and/or advancing the feeding tube to the small bowel.[119,125]

Abdominal distention, bloating, and cramping may present with or without nausea and vomiting. Abdominal distention has been found in up to 13% of critically ill patients.[117] The presence of abdominal distention is not automatic indication to hold EN but could be a sign of GI ileus, obstruction, obstipation, ascites, or diarrheal illness. If any of these conditions are suspected, radiological evaluation may be warranted. Other causes of abdominal distention include the infusion of a cold formula, rapid infusion of a bolus or intermittent feeding, delayed gastric emptying, malabsorption and fermentation, usage of a high fiber formula, and intake of narcotics.[119] Ensure that the enteral formula is at room temperature prior to infusion. Consider intermittent or continuous feedings for patients intolerant to bolus feeds. Consider semi-elemental formulas for in patients with bloating and additional signs of malabsorption. In some cases, a low fiber formula may be indicated. Reduce or discontinue narcotic medications when possible.

13.6.4 GASTRIC RESIDUAL VOLUME

Delayed gastric emptying, which occurs in up to 39% of critically ill patients, is another possible cause of nausea and vomiting in patients receiving EN.[140] Slowed gastric emptying is closely monitored in the hospitalized patient as vomiting or regurgitation of EN is thought to increase the risk of pulmonary aspiration, pneumonia, and sepsis, especially in the critically ill and minimally responsive patient.[119] Traditionally, delayed gastric emptying and the risk for regurgitation and subsequent aspiration of EN has been monitored by measuring gastric residual volume (GRV); EN has often been held in patients with a "high" GRV. However, procedures for checking gastric residuals and the definition of a high GRV are not standardized. Furthermore, there is evidence indicating that the presence of elevated GRVs is not correlated to regurgitation, gastric emptying, vomiting, pneumonia or mortality.[142–146]

In recent years, multiple randomized control trials (RTC) and observational studies have called into question the efficacy of monitoring GRV. In 2010 RCT, Montejo et al.[147] did not find any significant difference in the incidence of aspiration when EN was held for GVR >200 mL versus >500 mL in a medical ICU population.[147] Similarly, a 2013 RCT by Reignier et al.[148] failed to find an increased frequency of ventilation-associated pneumonia when GRV were not checked, and EN was held only for vomiting compared to holding EN for GRVs >250 mL. In a 2013 review of six RCTs and six prospective observational studies, the authors concluded that monitoring of GRV may be unnecessary in medical ICU patients.[149] The practice of withholding GRV may benefit patients by decreasing interruptions in feedings and allowing patients to reach goal EN rates faster and receive a significantly greater provision of goal calories and protein.[150] However, in surgical ICU patients monitoring of GRV and maintaining a low threshold for holding EN (GRV>200 mL) may still be indicated.[151]

The current *A.S.P.E.N.'s Enteral Nutrition Practice Guidelines* recommend checking GRV every 4 h after initiating EN, adding a promotility agent for two consecutive GRVs of >250 mL, and holding EN for GRV >500 mL.[151,152] The Canadian Clinical Practice Guidelines, which were updated in 2013, found insufficient data to make a recommendation for GRV threshold for feeding but stated that a volume somewhere between 250 and 500 mL was acceptable.[153] A.S.P.E.N. also recommends keeping the head of the bed at 30–45° and considering feeding past the ligament of Treitz in patients with GRVs persistently >500 mL.[151] Stable patients who have demonstrated tolerance of EN do not need GRV checked as frequently, and patients on long-term EN at home may not need to check GRVs unless they exhibit signs of intolerance (e.g., abdominal distention or severe nausea).

Additional tests to detect pulmonary aspiration of enteral feedings have been studied, but a feasible and reliable test has not been found. The use of blue dye to tint enteral formulas to reveal aspiration by the presence of blue tinted tracheal aspirates was found to be ineffective.[154] Additionally, the use of blue dye has been largely abandoned after a 2003 FDA Public Health Advisory reported the use of FD and C Blue No. 1 dye in some patients followed was by refractory hypotension, metabolic acidosis, and death.[155] Using glucose oxidase strips to detect glucose in tracheal aspirates is also not recommended as this test was shown to have positive results in unfed patients.[156]

13.6.5 Metabolic Complications

Metabolic complications are less common and may be associated with the patient's underlying medical condition rather than the EN formula. Patients at risk for complications should be identified and closely monitored. These patients often include those patients with severe malnutrition, excessive GI losses, organ dysfunction, fluid restriction, and glucose intolerance.[119] These complications include refeeding syndrome, hyperglycemia, fluid and electrolyte imbalances, acid–base disturbances, and nutrient deficiencies. Possible causes and treatments of metabolic complications are reviewed in Table 13.8.[119,157–159]

13.6.6 REFEEDING SYNDROME

Refeeding syndrome is often the most feared metabolic complication, and patients should be evaluated for their risk of developing refeeding syndrome prior to initiating EN. Possible risk factors for refeeding syndrome are noted in Table 13.9.[157–159] Refeeding syndrome occurs in response to changing the body's fuel source from fat during starvation to carbohydrate in the fed patient.[158] The shift to carbohydrate metabolism can lead to potentially dangerously low serum electrolyte levels of phosphorus, potassium and magnesium, and depletion of thiamine.[157] Other complications of refeeding syndrome include fluid retention and respiratory, cardiac dysfunction, and neuromuscular dysfunction.[159]

Once a patient has been identified at risk for refeeding syndrome serum electrolytes levels should be closely monitored, and any abnormalities corrected before initiating EN. Additional thiamine should be considered, especially those with a history of alcohol abuse. EN should be started slowly (15–20 kcal/kg) and advanced to the goal over a period of several days.[119] Labs should continue to be monitored daily until serum levels become stable after reaching goal EN rate. Refeeding syndrome usually occurs within the first few days of initiating EN, but the presentation of symptoms can be delayed in some patients, including those with renal dysfunction.

13.6.7 FLUID AND ELECTROLYTE IMBALANCES

Electrolyte imbalances can be caused by medical conditions or therapies unrelated to refeeding syndrome. Potassium, magnesium, phosphorus, and sodium can be lost in the output from stool, ostomies, fistulae, NG tubes or emesis, urine, skin, and wounds. Certain medications including antibiotics and chemotherapy agents can cause depletion of some electrolytes. Furthermore, electrolytes are utilized in during anabolism and protein synthesis. In contrast, renal insufficiency can lead to potassium, magnesium, and phosphorus to be retained and serum levels to rise.

Alterations in fluid status from dehydration or overhydration can cause electrolyte imbalances. Signs of dehydration include increasing sodium, BUN (blood urea nitrogen), or BUN/creatinine ratio. Patients should be monitored for adequate fluid provision, which is often estimated to be 1 mL/kcal of formula or 30–40 mL/kg in the adult populations.[119] Calculations of estimated fluid needs may be adjusted for medical conditions causing fluid losses or retention. Although most standard enteral formulas are 80%–85% water, many patients will require additional fluid orally, via feeding tube, or from intravenous (IV) fluids. Patients with renal failure or congestive heart disease may require a concentrated formula to prevent overhydration. Overhydration, hyponatremia, and edema can also occur in patients receiving both

TABLE 13.8

Summary of Metabolic Complications, Causes, and Possible Treatments

Complication	Possible Cause	Possible Treatment
Hypokalemia	Refeeding syndrome Diuretics or other medications Catabolic stress Excessive potassium losses from diarrhea or NGT Insulin therapy Metabolic alkalosis Volume overload	Replete potassium prior to initiating EN Reduce initial calorie provision if refeeding syndrome risk Supplement potassium Monitor serum potassium levels Replete serum magnesium if low
Hyperkalemia	Renal failure Excessive potassium intake Metabolic acidosis Acute dehydration Poor perfusion from CHF Potassium sparing medications	Changing to a renal formula Decreasing potassium intake from IV fluids or oral foods Treating underlying condition Provide kayexalate, glucose, and/or insulin
Hypophosphatemia	Refeeding syndrome Anabolism Insulin therapy Phosphate binding antacids Calcium carbonate supplements	Replete phosphorus prior to initiating EN Reduce calorie provision initially if refeeding syndrome risk Supplement phosphorus as needed Adjust/discontinue medications as appropriate Monitor serum phosphorus level
Hyperphosphatemia	Renal failure	Consider phosphate binder Change to renal formula
Hypomagnesemia	Refeeding syndrome High output ostomy or fistula	Reduce calorie provision initially if refeeding syndrome risk Supplement magnesium
Hyponatremia	Excessive free water Fluid overload Excessive production of antidiuretic hormone (SIADH) Abnormal sodium loss Renal, cardiac, or hepatic insufficiency	Decrease/discontinue water boluses or IV fluids Change to concentrated formula Replace sodium losses Consider diuretics as indicated Monitor fluid intake and output Monitor weight Monitor serum sodium level
Hypernatremia	Inadequate fluid provision Excessive fluid losses from NGT output, diarrhea, ostomy output, fistula output, fevers, or increased urine output Diabetes insipidus High protein intake	Increase free water bolus Add or increase IV fluids Monitor fluid intake and output Monitor serum sodium, serum osmolality, BUN, and BUN/creatinine ratio Monitor weight

(Continued)

TABLE 13.8 (*Continued*)
Summary of Metabolic Complications, Causes, and Possible Treatments

Complication	Possible Cause	Possible Treatment
Hyperglycemia	Diabetes mellitus	Monitor serum glucose
	Refeeding syndrome	Provide oral hypoglycemia agents or
	Insulin resistance	insulin
	Excessive CHO (carbohydrates) provision	Consider insulin drip as needed
		Avoid overfeeding
	Hypercatabolism	Treat underlying condition
	Stress or trauma	Consider higher fat and/or fiber formula
	Sepsis	
	Inflammation	
	Infection	
	Corticosteroids	
Hypoglycemia	Sudden discontinuation of EN	Monitor serum glucose
		Provide IV fluids with D10 if EN stopped after long acting insulin given
		Treat hypoglycemia with IV glucose or enteral glucose via feeding tube

IV fluids and EN. IV fluids should be adjusted when EN is initiated and potentially discontinued when goal EN rate has been achieved.

13.6.8 HYPERGLYCEMIA

Hyperglycemia is a potential complication of EN and can occur in patients without diabetes mellitus. Sepsis, catabolism, trauma, stress, corticosteroids, insulin resistance, and inflammatory diseases can lead to hyperglycemia in the acutely ill patient. In some cases, hyperglycemia can also be a sign of overfeeding in a stable patient. As previously noted, the use of diabetic enteral formula may not improve glucose control, especially in the acutely ill patients.[81] Oral hypoglycemic agent and/or insulin

TABLE 13.9
Patients at Risk for Refeeding Syndrome

Chronic malnutrition
Anorexia nervosa
Chronic alcoholism
Oncology patients
Postoperative patients
Morbid obesity with massive weight loss
Patients not fed for >7 days
Prolonged vomiting and diarrhea
Uncontrolled diabetes mellitus
Elderly patients with depression

therapy may be required to keep serum glucose levels within an acceptable range. If EN is abruptly stopped in patients on insulin or oral hypoglycemic medications, hypoglycemia may occur. Medications should be reviewed and adjusted before discontinuing EN.

13.6.9 ACID–BASE DISTURBANCES

Metabolic acidosis from elevated blood levels of CO_2 is a possible complication of EN, occurring most often in the ventilated patient or patients with COPD who retain CO_2. As previously discussed in the section on pulmonary formulas, hypercarbia was initially thought to be related to excessive carbohydrate provision since CO_2 is a by-product of carbohydrate metabolism. However, research has shown that excessive caloric provision has a greater effect on CO_2 production and overfeeding should be avoided.[99]

13.6.10 MICRONUTRIENT DEFICIENCIES

Micronutrient deficiencies are now relatively rare in the enterally fed patient as most commercial products provide 100% of DRI per 1000–1500 kcal. However, patients receiving <1500 kcals/day, using blenderized/homemade formulas, or diluting commercial formulas may not receive 100% of the DRI. Additionally, patients who are malnourished prior to starting EN may have preexisting deficiencies that may require supplemental amounts of micronutrients to achieve normal levels. Patients with malabsorption, excessive GI losses, or medications with drug–nutrient interactions, may also need additional supplementation.[119] Patients should be assessed for possible micronutrient deficiencies when EN is initiated and periodically reassessed in patients at risk for deficiency.

13.6.11 MECHANICAL COMPLICATIONS

Mechanical complications of EN include misplacement during insertion, tube migration, tube deterioration, tube occlusion, and nasal pharyngeal or esophageal irritation.[160] NG tubes can become accidentally dislodged, fall out, or be pulled out by patients after placement. Many of the complications related to feeding tubes and feeding tube placement were discussed in an earlier section on enteral access.

Feeding tube occlusion is one of the most common mechanical complications and can lead to interruptions in feeding and in some cases require replacement of the feeding tube. Many common practices can increase the risk of tubes becoming clogged: inadequate routine water flushes during feeding and after feedings are stopped, administering crushed or powdered medications through the feeding tube, administering acidic or alkaline medication through the feeding tube, the using small bore feeding tubes, and checking GRV.[160–163] The use blenderized or homemade formulas also increase the risk of occlusion.

Providing adequate water flushes is the primary method of prevention of feeding tube occlusions. Feeding tubes should be flushed with water every 4–6 h during continuous feeds, before and after bolus feeds, whenever feedings are stopped, and before and after medication administration.[119] Liquid medications may help reduce the risk of a clogged tube but will, not prevention occlusion as acidic, alkaline, and viscous elixir medications can cause formulas to clump or thicken.[161,162] If possible, administration of medications via J-tubes or other small bore feeding tubes should be avoided.

The use of soft drinks, juices, and other liquids are often thought to be useful in unclogging feeding tubes, but these liquids can increase the risk of future occlusion by leaving a sticky residue and can cause degradation of the feeding tube.[160] Furthermore irrigation of the feeding tube with warm water has been shown to be significantly more effective than juice or soda and does not leave any residue.[164] Commercially available pancreatic enzyme and sodium bicarbonate "cocktails" can be used as a second line option if warm water alone failed to clear the obstruction.[165] Endoscopy brushes and stylets used for tube placement are sometimes used to physically break up the obstruction, but caution must be used to avoid perforation of the tube or the GI tract.[160] Stiff wires should be avoided. If the occlusion is still not resolved to dislodge it after multiple attempts, the feeding tube may need to be replaced.

13.6.12   EN MISCONNECTIONS

An enteral misconnection is a possible life threating complication of EN when the distal end of the feeding set is connected to an intravascular catheter or another medical tubing. The occurrence of these misconnections is rare, and the risk of occurrence has been reduced by the introduction of enteral feeding sets incompatible with luerlock or IV connections and the use of enteral pumps for feeding instead of IV pumps.[166] Enteral connections are also being color coded and labeled "not for IV use" to provide a visual reminder to clinicians that it is not an IV connection. Syringes for oral or enteral use should also be used instead of luerlock syringes to draw up and deliver medications into the enteral feeding system.

13.6.13   HOME EN

EN delivered in the home setting is a common practice both in the United States and globally. There is no central U.S. database for the collection of the home enteral nutrition (HEN) practice. A 2005 epidemiologic analysis was performed in Italy on 655 HEN patients.[167] Approximately 27% of patients had neurovascular disease, 41% neurodegenerative disease, 10% abdominal cancer, 3% congenital abnormalities, 1.5% head injury and the rest an "other" diagnosis. Before the initiation of HEN, this group had lost on average 22.9% of their body weight. The prevalence rate for HEN was 308/1 million inhabitants, and the incidence rate for HEN was 380/1 million inhabitants. The mean length of HEN therapy was 196 days. The median survival rate was 9.1 months. Approximately 8% of patients returned to oral nutrition.

An 11-year HEN experience was reported on 416 pediatric patients in France.[168] The average age of patients was 5.4 years. Indications for HEN were digestive disorders (35%), neurologic and muscular disorders (35%), malignancy (11%), failure to thrive (8%), and miscellaneous (9%). A mechanical pump was used for delivery of EN in 98% of patients. The mean duration of HEN therapy was 595 ± 719 days.

One of the major questions regarding HEN patients is their outcomes in the home setting. This is especially true for feeding tube-related complications. A retrospective review was performed on 55 patients in Canada on HEN followed for 25.9 months.[169] Results were expressed as a percentage of total patients. Common feeding tube-related complications included granulation tissue formation (60%), stoma infection requiring antibiotics (45%), broken or leaking tube (56%), and leaking around the tube (60%). Health care resource utilization for problems related to feeding tubes included phone calls (69%), clinic visit (45%), ER visit (35%), and hospital admission (11%). The same authors subsequently reported on the prospectively recorded outcomes of HEN patients who were provided with a diary to record their problems.[170] These patients were followed for an average of 10.5 months. The most common tube-related complications included tube displacement (5/8), stoma discharge (6/8), pain at the stoma site (5/8), granulation tissue (5/8), bloody stoma (5/8), leakage (4/8), breakage (3/8), and occlusion (2/8). Unscheduled health care use for tube-related complications averaged 5.4 incidences/patient. Both of these studies demonstrate the need for patient and family education and dedicated follow-up of patients receiving enteral access for HEN.

13.6.13.1 Case Study

A 54-year-old male develops difficulty swallowing. He has a history of moderate to severe alcohol intake and 30-pack-a-year smoking history. He also has a history of insulin dependent diabetes mellitus and hypertension. An esophagram reveals no lesions in the esophagus. A modified barium swallow notes some delay in passage of a bolus of food from the oral cavity to the esophagus. A consult and exam by an otolaryngologist denotes a squamous cell carcinoma of the hypopharynx.

The patient underwent a localized surgical resection of the lesion and a series of radiation treatments. He now presents to the gastroenterologist with odynophagia and weight loss. He has had two emergency room visits for dehydration. An oral examination denotes severe mucositis. A discussion ensues, and the patient is told he needs a PEG for feeding access. After hearing about the procedure, he opts for a NG tube as an alternative.

An NG tube is placed in the office, and a radiograph confirms proper position. The tube is connected to the patient's nose by an adhesive fixation device. The patient is taught by the dietitian how to use a syringe for bolus feeding of 300 cc four times a day of a 1.5 cal/cc polymeric tube feeding formula.

Two days later the patient returns to the office for a "displaced" NG tube. A new NG tube is placed. Two days following this he states he wants the NG tube out because of worsening of his odynaphagia and the fact that he feels uncomfortable in public. He is scheduled for an upper endoscopy and PEG placement which occurs the next day. During the endoscopy candida, esophagitis is discovered, and the patient is treated with an antifungal agent.

The patient is sent home on bolus feedings again at 300 cc four times a day for a total of 1800 cal. After each bolus feeding, he feels distended and develops nausea. He refuses to instill four cans of tube feeding a day. Considering that the patient may have gastroparesis, you add a promotility agent with no success. You also decided to change the patient to continuous pump feedings at 75 cc/h. The patient notes he is

somewhat better but still has constant nausea and bloating. You get a gastric emptying scan which is grossly abnormal.

The patient is told that most likely he will need a jejunostomy tube. He will
require a J-tube through the existing PEG (PEG/J) or a new jejunostomy tube (surgical or a DPEJ). He opts for the PEG/J, and a 12 Fr J-tube is threaded through the
existing PEG during a repeat upper endoscopy. That upper endoscopy also revealed
no anatomical lesion responsible for the reduced gastric emptying.

The patient returns 3 weeks later with pain and leakage around the PEG site.
There is also a distinct foul odor. You examine the PEG tube and note that the external bolster was pushed tight against the abdominal wall resulting in stomal breakdown and an infection. You loosen the bolster to the point you can slide one finger
between it and the abdominal wall. You place the patient on oral antibiotic with a
wide spectrum of bacterial coverage and also prescribe wound cleansing two times
a day with soap and water.

The patient returns to the office 2 weeks later, and the PEG stomal site looks healed.
There is no more leakage. However, starting this morning you are told that he cannot
infuse his tube feeding through the J-tube. Upon questioning you are told he has been
using a powdered herbal supplement each morning passed through the J-tube in a
"honey" consistency when mixed with water. You reeducate the patient that only liquid medications or extremely well dissolved solid medications can be passed through
a J-tube in order to prevent tube clogging. The patient says his wife used Coca-Cola in
the J-tube to try to break up the occlusion. You let him know that soft drinks will not
work to break up a tube occlusion and may make the tube more "sticky" and further
increase the size of the occlusion. You take a 10 cc syringe filled with warm water and
with gentle pushing in and out of the J-tube by the syringe the occlusion passes. You
ask the patient to return in 1 month so you can follow his progress on his tube feeding
regimen and also monitor for any feeding tube-related complications.

REFERENCES

1. Kudsk, K. A., M. A. Croce, T. C. Fabian et al. Enteral versus parenteral feeding.
   Effects on septic morbidity after blunt and penetrating abdominal trauma. *Ann Surg*
   1992;215:503–511.
2. DeWitt, R. C. and K. A. Kudsk. The gut's role in metabolism, mucosal barrier function,
   and gut immunology. *Infect Dis Clin North Am* 1999;13:465–481.
3. Duszak, R., Jr. and M. R. Mabry. National trends in gastrointestinal access procedures:
   An analysis of Medicare services provided by radiologists and other specialists. *J Vasc
   Interv Radiol* 2003;14:1031–1036.
4. Burtch, G. D. and C. H. Shatney. Feeding jejunostomy (versus gastrostomy) passes the
   test of time. *Am Surg* 1987;5354–5357.
5. Neumann, D. A. and M. H. DeLegge. Gastric versus small-bowel tube feeding in the intensive care unit: A prospective comparison of efficacy. *Crit Care Med*
   2002;30:1436–1438.
6. McClave, S. A., M. T. DeMeo, M. H. DeLegge et al. North American Summit on aspiration in the critically ill patient: Consensus statement. *JPEN* 2002;26:S80-S85.
7. Cataldi-Betcher, E. L., M. H. Seltzer, B. A. Slocum, and K. W. Jones. Complications
   occurring during enteral nutrition support: A prospective study. *JPEN* 1983;7:546–552.

8. Zaloga, G. P. Bedside method for placing small bowel feeding tubes in critically ill patients. A prospective study. *Chest* 1991;100:1643–1646.
9. Ugo, P. J., P. A. Mohler, and G. L. Wilson. Bedside postpyloric placement of weighted feeding tubes. *Nutr Clin Pract* 1992;7:284–287.
10. Berger, M. M., M. D. Bollmann, J. P. Revelly et al. Progression rate of self-propelled feeding tubes in critically ill patients. *Intensive Care Med* 2002;28:1768–1774.
11. Kaffarnik, M. F., J. F. Lock, G. Wassilew, and P. Neuhaus. The use of bedside electromagnetically guided nasointestinal tube for jejunal feeding of critical ill surgical patients. *Technol Health Care* 2013;21:1–8.
12. Powers, J., M. Luebbehusen, T. Spitzer et al. Verification of an electromagnetic placement device compared with abdominal radiograph to predict accuracy of feeding tube placement. *JPEN J Parenter Enteral Nutr* 2011;35:535–539.
13. Whatley, K., W. W. Turner, Jr., M. Dey, J. Leonard, and M. Guthrie. When does metoclopramide facilitate transpyloric intubation? *JPEN* 1984;8:679–681.
14. Kalafrentzos, F., V. Alivizatos, K. Panagopoulos et al. Nasodudoenal intubation with the use of metoclopramide. *Nutr Support Serv* 1987;7:33–34.
15. Silva, C. C., H. Saconato, and A. N. Atallah. Metoclopramide for migration of nasoenteral tube. *Cochrane Database Syst Rev* 2004;1:1–15.
16. Lovell, M. A., M. Y. Mudaliar, and P. L. Klineberg. Intrahospital transport of critically ill patients: Complications and difficulties. *Anaesth Intensive Care* 2001;29:400–405.
17. Wiggins, T. F. and M. H. DeLegge. Evaluation of a new technique for endoscopic nasojejunal feeding-tube placement. *Gastrointest Endosc* 2006;63:590–595.
18. Gunn, S. R., B. J. Early, M. S. Zenati, and J. B. Ochoa. Use of a nasal bridle prevents accidental nasoenteral feeding tube removal. *JPEN* 2009;33:50–54.
19. Hirdes, M. M., J. F. Monkelbaan, J. J. Haringman et al. Endoscopic clip-assisted feeding tube placement reduces repeat endoscopy rate: Results from a randomized controlled trial. *Am J Gastroenterol* 2012;107:1220–1227.
20. Gauderer, M. W., J. L. Ponsky, and R. J. Izant, Jr. Gastrostomy without laparotomy: A percutaneous endoscopic technique. *J Pediatr Surg* 1980;15:872–875.
21. Jain, N. K., D. E. Larson, K. W. Schroeder, D. O. Burton et al. Antibiotic prophylaxis for percutaneous endoscopic gastrostomy. A prospective, randomized, double-blind clinical trial. *Ann Intern Med* 1987;107:824–828.
22. Duarte, H., C. Santos, M. L. Capelas, and J. Fonseca. Peristomal infection after percutaneous endoscopic gastrostomy: A 7-year surveillance of 297 patients. *Arq Gastroenterol* 2012;49:255–258.
23. Hogan, R. B., D. C. DeMarco, J. K. Hamilton, C. O. Walker, and D. E. Polter. Percutaneous endoscopic gastrostomy—To push or pull. A prospective randomized trial. *Gastrointest Endosc* 1986;32:253–258.
24. Martins, F. P., M. C. Sousa, and A. P. Ferrari. New "introducer" PEG-gastropexy with T fasteners: A pilot study. *Arq Gastroenterol* 2011;48:231–235.
25. Campoli, P. M., A. A. de Paula, L. G. Alves, and M. D. Turchi. Effect of the introducer technique compared with the pull technique on the peristomal infection rate in PEG: A meta-analysis. *Gastrointest Endosc* 2012;75:988–996.
26. Lin, L. F. and H. C. Shen. Unsedated transnasal percutaneous endoscopic gastrostomy carried out by a single physician. *Dig Endosc* 2013;25:130–135.
27. Marcuard, S. P., J. L. Finley, and K. G. MacDonald. Large-bore feeding tube occlusion by yeast colonies. *JPEN* 1993;17:187–190.
28. Kobak, G. E., D. T. McClenathan, and S. J. Schurman. Complications of removing percutaneous endoscopic gastrostomy tubes in children. *J Pediatr Gastroenterol Nutr* 2000;30:404–407.

29. DeLegge, M. H., P. Patrick, and R. Gibbs. Percutaneous endoscopic gastrojejunostomy with a tapered tip, nonweighted jejunal feeding tube: Improved placement success. *Am J Gastroenterol* 1996;91:1130–1134.
30. Taylor, S. J., R. Przemioslo, and A. R. Manara. Microendoscopic nasointestinal feeding tube placement in mechanically ventilated patients with gastroparesis. *Dig Dis Sci* 2003;48:713–716.
31. Adler, D. G., C. J. Gostout, and T. H. Baron. Percutaneous transgastric placement of jejunal feeding tubes with an ultrathin endoscope. *Gastrointest Endosc* 2002;55:106–110.
32. Shike, M., Y. N. Berner, H. Gerdes et al. Percutaneous endoscopic gastrostomy and jejunostomy for long-term feeding in patients with cancer of the head and neck. *Otolaryngol Head Neck Surg* 1989;101:549–554.
33. Mellert, J., M. B. Naruhn, K. E. Grund, and H. D. Becker. Direct endoscopic percutaneous jejunostomy (EPJ). Clinical results. *Surg Endosc* 1994;8:867–869; discussion 869–870.
34. Varadarajulu, S. and M. H. Delegge. Use of a 19-gauge injection needle as a guide for direct percutaneous endoscopic jejunostomy tube placement. *Gastrointest Endosc* 2003;57:942–945.
35. DeLegge, M. H. Enteral access—The foundation of feeding. *JPEN* 2001;25:S8–S13.
36. Fan, A. C., T. H. Baron, A. Rumalla, and G. C. Harewood. Comparison of direct percutaneous endoscopic jejunostomy and PEG with jejunal extension. *Gastrointest Endosc* 2002;56:890–894.
37. Stiegmann, G. V., J. S. Goff, D. Silas, N. Pearlman, J. Sun, and L. Norton. Endoscopic versus operative gastrostomy: Final results of a prospective randomized trial. *Gastrointest Endosc* 1990;36:1–5.
38. Scott, J. S., R. A. de la Torre, and S. W. Unger. Comparison of operative versus percutaneous endoscopic gastrostomy tube placement in the elderly. *Am Surg* 1991;57:338–340.
39. Munro, J. C. Abdominal surgery. In: W. W. Keen, Ed. *Keen's Surgery*. London, UK: WB Sunders; 1908. pp. 937–938.
40. Gerndt, S. J. and M. B. Orringer. Tube jejunostomy as an adjunct to esophagectomy. *Surgery* 1994;115(2):164–169.
41. Rombeau J. L. and J. Carnilo. Feeding by tube enterostomy. In: J. L. Rombeau and M. D. Caldwell, Eds. *Enteral Nutrition and Tube Feeding*, 2nd Edition. Philadelphia, PA: Saunders; 1990. pp. 230–249.
42. Rombeau J. L., M. D. Caldwell, L. Forlaw et al. *Atlas of Nutrition Support Techniques*. Boston, MA: Little Brown; 1989. pp. 167–174.
43. Myers, J. G., C. P. Page, R. M. Stewart, W. H. Schwesinger, K. R. Sirinek, and J. B. Aust. Complications of needle catheter jejunostomy in 2022 consecutive applications. *Am J Surg* 1995;170:547–550; discussion 550–551.
44. de Gottardi, A., L. Krahenbuhl, J. Farhadi, S. Gernhardt, M. Schafer, and M. W. Buchler. Clinical experience of feeding through a needle catheter jejunostomy after major abdominal operations. *Eur J Surg* 1999;165:1055–1060.
45. Haun, J. L. and J. S. Thompson. Comparison of needle catheter versus standard tube jejunostomy. *Am Surg* 1985;51:466–469.
46. Rosser, J. C., Jr., E. B. Rodas, J. Blancaflor, R. L. Prosst, L. E. Rosser, and R. R. Salem. A simplified technique for laparoscopic jejunostomy and gastrostomy tube placement. *Am J Surg* 1999;177:61–65.
47. Gedaly, R., P. Briceno, R. Ravelo, and K. Weisinger. Laparoscopic jejunostomy with an 18-mm trocar. *Surg Laparosc Endosc* 1997;7:420–422.
48. Woo, S. H., C. K. Finch, J. E. Broyles, J. Wan, R. Boswell, and A. Hurdle. Early vs delayed enteral nutrition in critically ill medical patients. *Nutr Clin Pract* 2010;25:205–211.

49. Smith-Choban, P. and M. H. Max. Feeding jejunostomy: A small bowel stress test? *Am J Surg* 1988;155:112–117.
50. Khalid, I., P. Doshi, and B. DiGiovine. Early enteral nutrition and outcomes of critically ill patients treated with vasopressors and mechanical ventilation. *Am J Crit Care* 2010;19:261–268.
51. Preshaw, R. M. A percutaneous method for inserting a feeding gastrostomy tube. *Surg Gynecol Obstet* 1981;152:658–660.
52. Ho, C. S. Percutaneous gastrostomy for jejunal feeding. *Radiology* 1983;149:595–596.
53. Spelsberg, F. W., R. T. Hoffmann, R. A. Lang et al. CT fluoroscopy guided percutaneous gastrostomy or jejunostomy without (CT-PG/PJ) or with simultaneous endoscopy (CT-PEG/PEJ) in otherwise untreatable patients. *Surg Endosc* 2013;27:1186–1195.
54. Ho, C. S. and E. Y. Yeung. Percutaneous gastrostomy and transgastric jejunostomy. *AJR Am J Roentgenol* 1992;158:251–257.
55. Petsas, T., P. Kraniotis, C. Spyropoulos, K. Katsanos, A. Karatzas, and F. Kalfarentzos. The role of CT-guided percutaneous gastrostomy in patients with clinically severe obesity presenting with complications after bariatric surgery. *Surg Laparosc Endosc Percutan Tech* 2010;20:299–305.
56. Power, S., L. N. Kavanagh, M. C. Shields, M. F. Given, A. N. Keeling, F. P. McGrath, and M. J. Lee. Insertion of balloon retained gastrostomy buttons: A 5-year retrospective review of 260 patients. *Cardiovasc Intervent Radiol* 2013;36:484–491.
57. Wollman, B. and H. B. D'Agostino. Percutaneous radiologic and endoscopic gastrostomy: A 3-year institutional analysis of procedure performance. *Am J Roentgenol* 1997;169:1551–1553.
58. Silas, A. M., L. F. Pearce, L. S. Lestina et al. Percutaneous radiologic gastrostomy versus percutaneous endoscopic gastrostomy: A comparison of indications, complications and outcomes in 370 patients. *Eur J Radiol* 2005;56:84–90.
59. Marian, M. and C. McGinnis. Overview of enteral nutrition, In: M.M. Gottschlich, Ed. The *A.S.P.E.N. Nutrition Support Core Curriculum: A Case-Based Approach—The Adult Patient*. Silverspring, MD: ASPEN; 2007. pp. 187–208.
60. Scolapio, J. S. A review of the trends in the use of enteral and parenteral nutrition support. *J Clin Gastroenterol* 2004;38:403–407.
61. McClave, S. A. and W. K. Chang. When to feed the patient with gastrointestinal bleeding. *Nutr Clin Pract* 2005;20:544–550.
62. American Society for Parenteral and Enteral Nutrition. Guidelines for the use of parenteral and enteral nutrition in adult and pediatric patients. *JPEN* 2002;26:SA1–SA138.
63. Zaloga, G. P. Parenteral nutrition in adult inpatients with functioning gastrointestinal tracts: Assessment of outcomes. *Lancet* 2006;367:1101–1111.
64. Magnotti, L. J. and E. A. Deitch. Burns, bacterial translocation, gut barrier function, and failure. *J Burn Care Rehabil* 2005;26:383–391.
65. Heyland, D. K., R. Dhaliwal, J. W. Drover, L. Gramlich, P. Dodek, and Canadian Critical Care Clinical Practice Guidelines Committee. Canadian clinical practice guidelines for nutrition support in mechanically ventilated, critically ill adult patients. *JPEN* 2003;27:355–373.
66. Dray, X. and P. Marteau. Crohn's disease: Nutrition should not be forgotten. *Gastroenterol Clin Biol* 2006;30:215–216.
67. Taylor, S. J., S. B. Fettes, C. Jewkes, and R. J. Nelson. Prospective, randomized, controlled trial to determine the effect of early enhanced enteral nutrition on clinical outcome in mechanically ventilated patients suffering head injury. *Crit Care Med* 1999;27:2525–2531.
68. Kudsk, K. A., G. Minard, M. A. Croce et al. A randomized trial of isonitrogenous enteral diets after severe trauma. An immune-enhancing diet reduces septic complications. *Ann Surg* 1996;224:531–540.

69. Kalfarentzos, F., J. Kehagias, N. Mead, K. Kokkinis, and C. A. Gogos. Enteral nutrition is superior to parenteral nutrition in severe acute pancreatitis: Results of a randomized prospective trial. *Br J Surg* 1997;84:1665–1669.

70. Farber, M. S., J. Moses, and M. Korn. Reducing costs and patient morbidity in the enterally fed intensive care unit patient. *JPEN* 2005;29(suppl 1):S62–S69.

71. Neumayer, L. A., R. J. Smout, H. G. Horn, and S. D. Horn. Early and sufficient feeding reduces length of stay and charges in surgical patients. *J Surg Res* 2001;95:73–77.

72. Lefton J., D. H. Esper, and M. Kochevar. Enteral formulations. In: M.M. Gottschlich, Ed. *The A.S.P.E.N. Nutrition Support Core Curriculum: A Case-Based Approach—The Adult Patient.* Silverspring, MD: ASPEN; 2007. pp. 209–232.

73. Boullata, J., L. N. Carney, and P. Guenter, Eds. *A.S.P.E.N. Enteral Nutrition Handbook.* Silverspring, MD: ASPEN; 2010.

74. Malone, A. Enteral formula selection: A review of selected product categories. *Pract Gastroenterol* 2005;24:44–74.

75. Schneider, S. M., F. Girard-Pipau, R. Anty et al. Effects of total enteral nutrition supplemented with a multi-fibre mix on fecal short-chain fatty acids and microbiota. *Clin Nutr* 2006;25:82–90.

76. Kagansky, M. and E. Rimon. Is there a difference in metabolic outcome between different enteral formulas? *JPEN* 2007;31:320–323.

77. McClave, S. A. and W. K. Chang. Feeding the hypotensive patient: Does enteral feeding precipitate or protect against ischemic bowel? *Nutr Clin Pract* 2003;18:279–284.

78. Pohl, M., P. Mayr, M. Mertl-Roetzer et al. Glycemic control in patients with type 2 diabetes mellitus with a disease-specific enteral formula: Stage II of a randomized, controlled multicenter trial. *JPEN* 2009;33:37–49.

79. León-Sanz, M., P. P. García-Luna, M. Planas et al. Glycemic and lipid control in hospitalized type 2 diabetic patients: Evaluation of 2 enteral nutrition formulas (low carbohydrate-high monounsaturated fat vs high carbohydrate). *JPEN* 2005;29:21–29.

80. Mesejo, A., J. A. Acosta, C. Ortega et al. Comparison of a high-protein disease-specific enteral formula with a high-protein enteral formula in hyperglycemic critically ill patients. *Clin Nutr* 2003;22:295–305.

81. McMahon, M. M., E. Nystrom, C. Braunschweig, J. Miles, C. Compher, and the American Society for Parenteral and Enteral Nutrition Board of Directors. ASPEN. Clinical guidelines: Nutrition support of adult patients with hyperglycemia. *JPEN* 2013;37:23–36.

82. U.S. Department of Agriculture and U.S. Department of Health and Human Services. *Dietary Guidelines for Americans*, 7th Edition. Washington, US: Government Printing Office; 2010.

83. Kopple, J. D. National kidney foundation K/DOQI clinical practice guidelines for nutrition in chronic renal failure. *Am J Kidney Dis* 2001;37:S66–S70.

84. Wooley, J. A., I. F. Btaiche, and K. L. Good. Metabolic and nutritional aspects of acute renal failure in critically ill patients requiring continuous renal replacement therapy. *Nutr Clinical Pract* 2005;20:176–191.

85. Dejong, C. H. C., M. C. G. van de Poll, P. B. Soeters et al. Aromatic amino acid metabolism during liver failure. *J Nutr* 2007;137:S1579–S1585.

86. Als-Nielsen, B., R. L. Koretz, L. L. Kjaergard, and C. Gluud. Branched-chain amino acids for hepatic encephalopathy. *Cochrane Database Syst Rev* 2003;(2):CD001939.

87. Schloerb, P. R. Immune-enhancing diets: Products, components, and their rationales. *JPEN* 2001;25:S3–S7.

88. Wischmeyer, P. E. Glutamine: Mode of action in critical illness. *Crit Care Med* 2007;35:S541–S544.

89. Vermeulen, M. A., M. C. van de Poll, G. C. Ligthart-Melis et al. Specific amino acids in the critically ill patient—Exogenous glutamine/arginine: A common denominator? *Crit Care Med* 2007;35:S568–S576.

90. Waitzberg, D. L., H. Saito, L. D. Plank, G. G. Jamieson et al. Postsurgical infections are reduced with specialized nutrition support. *World J Surg* 2006;30(8):1592–1604.

91. American Society for Parenteral and Enteral Nutrition. Consensus recommendations from the U.S. Summit on immune-enhancing enteral therapy. *JPEN* 2001;25:S61–S63.

92. Cresci, G. Targeting the use of specialized nutritional formulas in surgery and critical care. *JPEN* 2005;29:S92–S95.

93. McClave, S. A., R. G. Martindale, V. W. Vanek et al. Guidelines for the provision and aAssessment of nutrition support therapy in the adult critically ill patient: Society of critical care medicine (SCCM) and American Society for Parenteral and Enteral Nutrition (ASPEN). *JPEN* 2009;33:277–316.

94. Kreymann, K. G., M. M. Berger, N. E. Deutz et al. ESPEN guidelines on enteral nutrition: Intensive care. *Clin Nutr* 2006;25:210–223.

95. Dhaliwal, R., N. Cahill, M. Lemieux, and D. K. Heyland. The Canadian critical care nutrition guidelines in 2013: An update on current recommendations and implementation strategies. *Nutr Clin Pract* 2014;29:29–43.

96. van den Berg, B., J. M. Bogaard, and W. C. Hop. High fat, low carbohydrate, enteral feeding in patients weaning from the ventilator. *Intensive Care Med* 1994;20:470–475.

97. Angelillo, V. A., S. Bedi, D. Durfee, J. Dahl, A. J. Patterson, and W. J. O'Donohue, Jr. Effects of low and high carbohydrate feedings in ambulatory patients with chronic obstructive pulmonary disease and chronic hypercapnia. *Ann Intern Med* 1985;103:883–885.

98. Kuo, C. D., G. M. Shiao, and J. D. Lee. The effects of high-fat and high-carbohydrate diet loads on gas exchange and ventilation in COPD patients and normal subjects. *Chest* 1993;104:189–196.

99. Talpers, S. S., D. J. Romberger, S. B. Bunce, and S. K. Pingleton. Nutritionally associated increased carbon dioxide production. Excess total calories vs high proportion of carbohydrate calories. *Chest* 1992;102:551–555.

100. Gadek, J. E., S. J. DeMichele, M. D. Karlstad et al. Effect of enteral feeding with eicosapentaenoic acid, gamma-linolenic acid, and antioxidants in patients with acute respiratory distress syndrome. Enteral nutrition in ARDS study group. *Crit Care Med.* 1999;27:1409–1420.

101. Singer P., M. Theilla, H. Fisher, L. Gibstein, E. Grozovski E, and J. Cohen. Benefit of an enteral diet enriched with eicosapentaenoic acid and gamma-linolenic acid in ventilated patients with acute lung injury. *Crit Care Med* 2006;34:1033–1038.

102. Pontes-Arruda, A., A. M. Aragao, and J. D. Albuquerque. Effects of enteral feeding with eicosapentaenoic acid, gamma-linolenic acid, and antioxidants in mechanically ventilated patients with severe sepsis and septic shock. *Crit Care Med* 2006;34:2325–2333.

103. Stratton, R. J., A. Ek, M. Engfer et al. Enteral nutritional support in prevention and treatment of pressure ulcers: A systematic review and meta-analysis. *Ageing Res Rev* 2005;4:422–450.

104. Chernoff, R. S., K. Y. Milton, and D. A. Lipschitz. The effect of a high protein formula (replete) on decubitus ulcer healing in long-term tube fed institutionalized patients. *J Am Diet Assoc* 1990;90:A130.

105. Scholl, D. and B. Langkamp-Henken. Nutrient recommendations for wound healing. *J Intraven Nurs* 2001;24:124–132.

106. Freitas, O., J. E. Dos Santos, L. J. Greene, and J. E. Dutra de Oliveira. Biochemical basis of enteral nutrition. *Arch Latinoam Nutr* 1995;45:84–89.

107. Silk, D. B., P. D. Fairclough, M. L. Clark, J. E. Hegarty, T. C. Marrs, J. M. Addison, D. Burston, K. M. Clegg, and D. M. Matthews. Use of a peptide rather than free amino acid nitrogen source in chemically defined "elemental" diets. *JPEN* 1980;4:548–553.

108. Craft, I. L., D. Geddes, C. W. Hyde, I. J. Wise, and D. M. Matthews. Absorption and malabsorption of glycine and glycine peptides in man. *Gut* 1968;9:425–437.

109. Lochs, H., C. Dejong, F. Hammarqvist et al. ESPEN guidelines on enteral nutrition: Gastroenterology. *Clin Nutr* 2006;25:260–274.
110. Makola, D., J. Krenitsky, C. Parrish et al. Efficacy of enteral nutrition for the treatment of pancreatitis using standard enteral formula. *Am J Gastroenterol* 2006;101:2347–2355.
111. Windsor, A. C., S. Kanwar, A. G. Li, E. Barnes, J. A. Guthrie, J. I. Spark, F. Welsh, P. J. Guillou, and J. V. Reynolds. Compared with parenteral nutrition, enteral feeding attenuates the acute phase response and improves disease severity in acute pancreatitis. *Gut* 1998;42:431–435.
112. Pupelis, G., G. Selga, E. Austrums, and A. Kaminski. Jejunal feeding, even when instituted late, improves outcomes in patients with severe pancreatitis and peritonitis. *Nutrition* 2001;17:91–94.
113. Petrov, M. S., B. P. T. Loveday, R. D. Pylypchuk, K. McIlroy, A. R. J. Phillips, and J. A. Windsor. Systematic review and meta-analysis of enteral nutrition formulations in acute pancreatitis. *Br J Surg* 2009;96:1243–1252.
114. Bowling, T. E. and D. B. Silk. Enteral feeding—Problems and solutions. *Eur J Clin Nutr* 1994;48:379–385.
115. Stratton, R. J. and T. R. Smith. Role of enteral and parenteral nutrition in the patient with gastrointestinal and liver disease. *Best Pract Res Clin Gastroenterol* 2006;20:441–466.
116. Cataldi-Betcher, E. L., M. H. Seltzer, B. A. Slocum, and K. W. Jones. Complications occurring during enteral nutrition support: a prospective study. *JPEN* 1983;7:546–552.
117. Montejo, J. C., T. Grau, J. Acosta et al. Multicenter, prospective, randomized, single-blind study comparing the efficacy and gastrointestinal complications of early jejunal feeding with early gastric feeding in critically ill patients. *Crit Care Med* 2002;30:796–800.
118. Barrett, J. S., S. J. Shepherd, and P. R. Gibson. Strategies to manage gastrointestinal symptoms complicating enteral feeding. *JPEN* 2009;33:21–26.
119. Malone, A. M., D. S. Seres, and L. Lord. Complications of enteral nutrition. In: M.M. Gottschlich, Ed. *The A.S.P.E.N. Nutrition Support Core Curriculum: A Case-Based Approach—The Adult Patient.* Silverspring, MD: ASPEN; 2007. pp. 246–262.
120. Bliss, D. Z., P. A. Guenter, and R. G. Settle. Defining and reporting diarrhea in tube-fed patients—What a mess! *Am J Clin Nutr* 1992;55:753–759.
121. Eisenberg, P. G. Causes of diarrhea in tube-fed patients: A comprehensive approach to diagnosis and management. *Nutr Clin Pract* 1993;8:119–123.
122. Guenter, P. A., R. G. Settle, S. Perlmutter, P. L. Marino, G. A. DeSimone, and R. H. Rolandelli, Tube feeding-related diarrhea in acutely ill patients. *JPEN* 1991;15:277–280.
123. Edes, T. E., B. E. Walk, and J. L. Austin. Diarrhea in tube-fed patients: Feeding formula not necessarily the cause. *Am J Med* 1990;88:91–93.
124. Bliss, D. Z., S. Johnson, K. Savik, C. R. Clabots, K. Willard, and D. N. Gerding. Acquisition of clostridium difficile and clostridium difficile-associated diarrhea in hospitalized patients receiving tube feeding. *Ann Intern Med* 1998;129:1012–1019.
125. Lefton, J. Management of common gastrointestinal complications in tube-fed patients. *Support Line* 2002;24:19–25.
126. Gottschlich, M. M., G. D. Warden, M. Michel et al. Diarrhea in tube-fed burn patients: Incidence, etiology, nutritional impact, and prevention. *JPEN J Parenter Enteral Nutr* 1988;12:338–345.
127. Liebl, B. H., M. H. Fischer, S. C. Van Calcar, and J. A. Marlett. Dietary fiber and long-term large bowel response in enterally nourished nonambulatory profoundly retarded youth. *JPEN J Parenter Enteral Nutr* 1990;14:371–375.
128. Shankardass, K., S. Chuchmach, K. Chelswick et al. Bowel function of long-term tube-fed patients consuming formulae with and without dietary fiber. *JPEN J Parenter Enteral Nutr* 1990;14:508–512.

129. Zimmaro, D. M., R. H. Rolandelli, M. J. Koruda, R. G. Settle, T. T. Stein, and J. L. Rombeau. Isotonic tube feeding formula induces liquid stool in normal subjects: Reversal by pectin. *JPEN J Parenter Enteral Nutr* 1989;13:117–123.
130. Smith, C. E., L. Marien, C. Brogdon et al. Diarrhea associated with tube feeding in mechanically ventilated critically ill patients. *Nurs Res* 1990;39:148–152.
131. Keohane, P. P., H. Attrill, M. Love, P. Frost, and D. B. Silk. Relation between osmolality of diet and gastrointestinal side effects in enteral nutrition. *Br Med J (Clin Res Ed)* 1984;288:678–680.
132. Pesola, G. R., J. E. Hogg, N. Eissa, D. E. Matthews, and G. C. Carlon. Hypertonic nasogastric tube feedings: Do they cause diarrhea? *Crit Care Med* 1990;18:1378–1382.
133. Ciocon, J. O., D. J. Galindo-Ciocon, C. Tiessen, and D. Galindo. Continuous compared with intermittent tube feeding in the elderly. *JPEN* 1992;16:525–528.
134. Anderson, K. R., D. J. Norris, L. B. Godfrey, C. K. Avent, and C. E. Butterworth Jr. Bacterial contamination of tube-feeding formulas. *JPEN* 1984;8:673–678.
135. Okuma, T., M. Nakamura, H. Totake, and Y. Fukunaga. Microbial contamination of enteral feeding formulas and diarrhea. *Nutrition* 2000;16:719–722.
136. DeLegge, M. H. Enteral nutrition and gastrointestinal intolerance. When should we be concerned? *Clinical Nutrition Highlights: Science Supporting Better Nutrition* 2006;2:2–7.
137. Fuhrman, M. P. Diarrhea and tube feeding. *Nutr Clin Pract* 1999;14:83–84.
138. Vickery, G. Basics of constipation. *Gastroenterol Nurs* 1997;20:125–128.
139. Wong K. The role of fiber in diarrhea management. *Support Line* 1998;20:16–20.
140. Montejo, J. C. Enteral nutrition-related gastrointestinal complications in critically ill patients: A multicenter study. The nutritional and metabolic working group of the Spanish society of intensive care medicine and coronary units. *Crit Care Med* 1999;27:1447–1453.
141. Jones, B. J., R. Lees, J. Andrews, P. Frost, and D. B. Silk. Comparison of an elemental and polymeric enteral diet in patients with normal gastrointestinal function. *Gut* 1983;24:78–84.
142. McClave, S. A., J. K. Lukan, J. A. Stefater et al. Poor validity of residual volumes as a marker for risk of aspiration in critically ill patients. *Crit Care Med* 2005;33:324–330.
143. Tarling, M. M., C. C. Toner, P. S. Withington, M. K. Baxter, R. Whelpton, and D. R. Goldhill. A model of gastric emptying using paracetamol absorption in intensive care patients. *Intensive Care Med* 1997;23:256–260.
144. Cohen, J., A. Aharon, and P. Singer. The paracetamol absorption test: A useful addition to the enteral nutrition algorithm? *Clin Nutr* 2000;19:233–236.
145. Wolf, S. E., M. G. Jeschke, J. K. Rose, M. H. Desai, and D. N. Herndon. Enteral feeding intolerance: An indicator of sepsis-associated mortality in burned children. *Arch Surg* 1997;132:1310–1313; discussion 1313–1314.
146. Mentec, H., H. Dupont H, M. Bocchetti, P. Cani, F. Ponche, and G. Bleichner. Upper digestive intolerance during enteral nutrition in critically ill patients: Frequency, risk factors, and complications. *Crit Care Med* 2001;29:1955–1961.
147. Montejo, J. C., E. Minambres, L. Bordeje et al. Gastric residual volume during enteral nutrition in ICU patients: The REGANE study. *Intensive Care Med* 2010;36:1386–1393.
148. Reignier, J., E. Mercier, A. Le Gouge et al. Effect of not monitoring residual gastric volume on risk of ventilator-associated pneumonia in adults receiving mechanical ventilation and early enteral feeding: A randomized controlled trial. *JAMA* 2013;309:249–256.
149. Kuppinger, D. D., P. Rittler, W. H. Hartl, and D. Ruttinger. Use of gastric residual volume to guide enteral nutrition in critically ill patients: A brief systematic review of clinical studies. *Nutrition* 2013;29:1075–1079.
150. Poulard, F., J. Dimet, L. Martin-Lefevre et al. Impact of not measuring residual gastric volume in mechanically ventilated patients receiving early enteral feeding: A prospective before-after study. *JPEN* 2010;34:125–130.

151. Metheny, N. A., L. Schallom, D. A. Oliver, and R. E. Clouse. Gastric residual volume and aspiration in critically ill patients receiving gastric feedings. *Am J Crit Care* 2008;17:512–519; quiz 520.

152. Bankhead, R., J. Boullata, S. Brantley et al. Enteral nutrition practice recommendations. *JPEN* 2009;33:122–167.

153. Dhaliwal, R., N. Cahill, M. Lemieux, and D. K. Heyland. The Canadian critical care nutrition guidelines in 2013: An update on current recommendations and implementation strategies. *Nutr Clin Pract* 2014;29:29–43.

154. Metheny, N. A., T. E. Dahms, B. J. Stewart et al. Efficacy of dye-stained enteral formula in detecting pulmonary aspiration. *Chest* 2002;122:276–281.

155. FDA Public Health Advisory: Subject: Reports of Blue Discoloration and Death in Patients Receiving Enteral Feedings Tinted With The Dye, FD&C Blue No. 1. Available at: http://www.fda.gov/ForIndustry/ColorAdditives/ColorAdditivesinSpecificProducts/InMedicalDevices/ucm142395.htm. Published: September 29, 2003.

156. Metheny, N. A., T. E. Dahms, B. J. Stewart, K. S. Stone, P. A. Frank, and R. E. Clouse. Verification of inefficacy of the glucose method in detecting aspiration associated with tube feedings. *Medsurg Nurs* 2005;14:112–119, 121; discussion 120.

157. Kraft M. D., I. F. Btaiche, and C. S. Sacks. Review of the refeeding syndrome. *Nutr Clin Pract* 2005;20:625–633.

158. Marinella, M. A. Refeeding syndrome and hypophosphatemia. *J Intensive Care Med* 2005;20:155–159.

159. Stanga, Z., A. Brunner, M. Leuenberger et al. Nutrition in clinical practice-the refeeding syndrome: Illustrative cases and guidelines for prevention and treatment. *Eur J Clin Nutr* 2008;62:687–694.

160. McClave, S. A. and W. K. Chang. Complications of enteral access. *Gastrointest Endosc* 2003;58:739–751.

161. Cutie, A. J., E. Altman, and L. Lenkel. Compatibility of enteral products with commonly employed drug additives. *JPEN* 1983;7:186–191.

162. Estoup, M. Approaches and limitations of medication delivery in patients with enteral feeding tubes. *Crit Care Nurse* 1994;14:68–72, 77–79; quiz 80–81.

163. Nicholson, L. J. Declogging small-bore feeding tubes. *JPEN* 1987;11:594–597.

164. Wilson, M. F. and V. Haynes-Johnson. Cranberry juice or water? A comparison of feeding-tube irrigants. *Nutr Support Serv* 1987;7(7):23.

165. Marcuard, S. P. and K. S. Stegall. Unclogging feeding tubes with pancreatic enzyme. *JPEN* 1990;14:198–200.

166. Guenter, P., R. W. Hicks, and D. Simmons. Enteral feeding misconnections: An update. *Nutr Clin Pract* 2009;24:325–334.

167. Paccaquella A., C. Banruffi, D. Pizzalota et al. Home enteral nutrition in adults: A five year epidemiologic analysis. *Clin Nutr* 2008;27:378–385.

168. Debeluy W., D. Guimber, K. Mention et al. Home enteral nutrition in children: An 11-year experience with 416 patients. *Clin Nutr* 2004;24:48–54.

169. Crosby J., D. Duersksen. A retrospective survey of tube-related complications in patients receiving long-term home enteral nutrition. *Dig Dis Sci* 2005;50:1712–1717.

170. Crosby J., D. Duerksen. A prospective study of tube and tube feeding-related complications in patients receiving long-term home enteral nutrition. *J Parent Enteral Nutr* 2007;31:274–277.

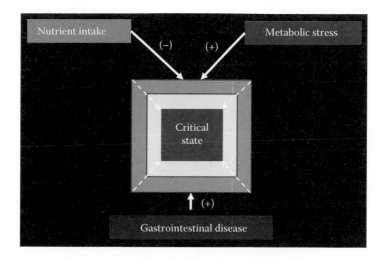

FIGURE 1.1   Interaction of factors influencing nutritional status.

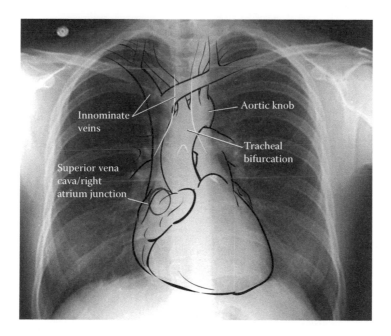

FIGURE 14.1   Anatomical landmarks for determining catheter tip location.

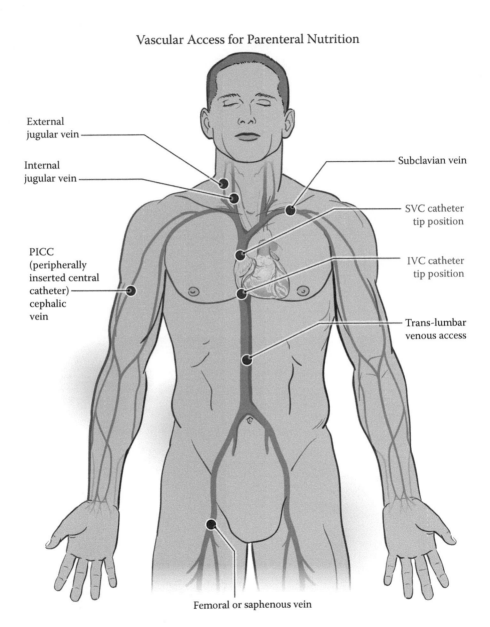

Vascular Access for Parenteral Nutrition

External jugular vein

Internal jugular vein

PICC (peripherally inserted central catheter) cephalic vein

Subclavian vein

SVC catheter tip position

IVC catheter tip position

Trans-lumbar venous access

Femoral or saphenous vein

FIGURE 14.2 Catheter insertion sites utilized in the hospital and home settings.

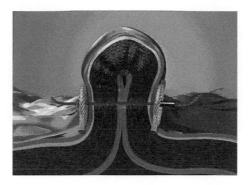

FIGURE 15.1 Plication of tissue using the incisionless operating platform. (From Espinós JC et al. *Obes Surg* 2013;23(9):1375–1383.)

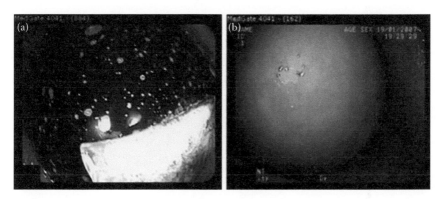

FIGURE 15.2 BioEnterics Intragastric Balloon (a) and Heliosphere BAG (b). (From Caglar E, Dobrucali A, Bal K. *Dig Endosc* 2013;25(5):502–507.)

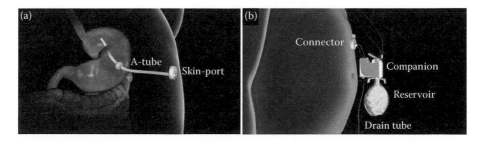

FIGURE 15.3 Aspire A-tube (a) and AspireAssist (b). (From Sullivan S et al. *Gastroenterology* 2013;145(6):1245–1252.e1-5.)

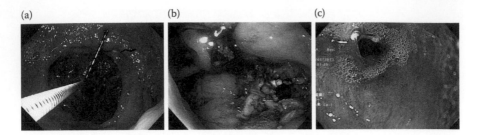

FIGURE 15.4 Gastrojejunal anastomosis before (a), immediately after (b), and six months after TORe using Apollo OverStitch (c). (From Kumar N and Thompson CC. *Gastrointest Endosc* 2014;79(6):984–989.)

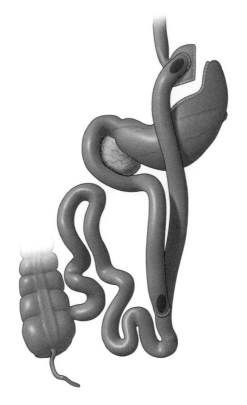

FIGURE 16.1 Roux-en-Y gastric bypass. (Copyright 2013, Brigham and Women's Hospital.)

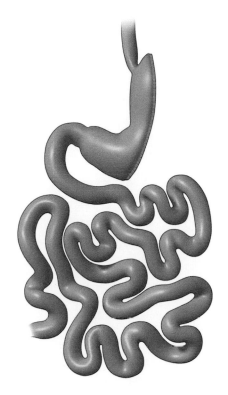

FIGURE 16.2 Sleeve gastrectomy. (Copyright 2013, Brigham and Women's Hospital.)

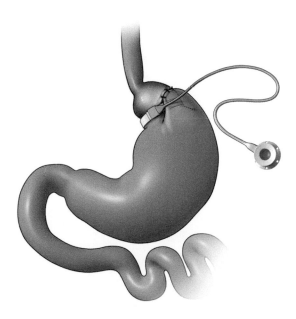

FIGURE 16.3 Adjustable band. (Copyright 2013, Brigham and Women's Hospital.)

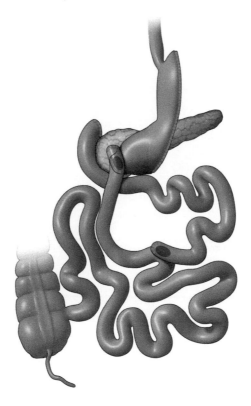

FIGURE 16.4 Biliopancreatic diversion with duodenal switch. (Copyright 2013, Brigham and Women's Hospital.)

14 Parenteral Nutrition

Indications, Access, Formula, Monitoring, and Complications

Mandy L. Corrigan and Ezra Steiger

CONTENTS

14.1 INTRODUCTION

Parenteral nutrition (PN) is a solution of chemically defined elemental nutrients delivered directly into the bloodstream that is customized to meet the unique and individual nutritional needs of each patient. The delivery of this therapy has evolved

321

over the past 5 decades following the successful infusion of PN by Dudrick and colleagues in the 1960s. PN has been a life sustaining therapy for patients with permanent intestinal failure, who would have otherwise died without PN. Use of PN is not without risk and requires appropriate patient selection, and careful monitoring and the expertise of an interdisciplinary team. This chapter on PN has been designed to target practicing clinicians with information on topics applying the use of PN in both the hospital and at home. Topics will include determining appropriate indications for the use of PN, selection of vascular access, basic components of PN formulas, monitoring PN, as well as preventing and treating PN complications.

14.2   PN INDICATIONS

The use of PN should not be routine and requires consideration of all other feeding routes before initiation as PN is not without risks. Appropriate candidates for PN are those with a nonfunctioning gastrointestinal (GI) tract that are unable to ingest or absorb adequate nutrients from the enteral route (either oral or by enteral tube feeding). Examples of conditions warranting PN include diffuse peritonitis, intestinal obstruction, intractable vomiting (refractory to pharmacological interventions or postpyloric enteral nutrition, EN), prolonged ileus, GI ischemia, malabsorption (from short bowel syndrome or radiation enteritis), high output enterocutaneous fistula (where enteral feedings distal are not possible), or pseudo-obstruction.[1-4] *Prolonged* inability to access the GI tract can be another possible indication; however, with advances in options for gaining access to the GI tract (electromagnetic guided tube placement, endoscopy, radiology, etc.) the use of PN for this reason should be rare.

The use of PN is contraindicated in the presence of a functional GI tract. Patients must also be hemodynamically stable, free of extreme electrolyte derangements, and able to tolerate fluid volumes to meet nutritional requirements. The use of PN in end-of-life care has not shown any improvements in outcomes and PN should not be initiated especially if aggressive care is not being pursued.

The timing of initiating PN is especially important in critically ill malnourished patients with a nonfunctional GI tract. This is best understood from two meta-analyses done by Heyland and Braunschweig, which are included in the Society for Critical Care Medicine and the American Society for Parenteral and Enteral Nutrition (ASPEN) Guidelines for critically ill patients.[5]

For intensive care unit (ICU) patients with malnutrition, where EN is not an option, early introduction of PN after resuscitation is appropriate. In the presence of malnutrition and a nonfunctional GI tract, the use of standard therapy (i.e., intravenous fluids [IVF] and no PN) lead to a higher risk of mortality and a trend toward higher rates of infection.

The early beneficial use of PN in malnourished patients cannot be generalized to all ICU patients with a nonfunctioning GI tract. When PN was delivered to patients *without* malnutrition, an increase in mortality and a trend toward increased rates of complications occurred. The use of IVF and avoidance of PN for 7 days is advised for patients *without* malnutrition and a nonfunctional GI tract.

The timing of initiating PN has clearly been linked to outcomes and is determined by the patient's nutritional status upon arrival to the ICU. When the GI tract is functional and EN is possible, EN should be initiated as early as possible regardless of the patient's nutritional status.

14.2.1 PREOPERATIVE PN IN SURGICAL PATIENTS

The use of PN preoperatively has shown reductions in postoperative complications in select malnourished patients that can safely have surgery delayed for 5 to 7 days for the use of PN.[5] Malnourished patients undergoing planned major upper GI surgical procedures (esophagectomy, gastrectomy, pancreatectomy) are candidates for preoperative PN based on data showing a 10% decrease in risk of postoperative complications.[6]

14.3 PN VASCULAR ACCESS DEVICES

Clinicians caring for patients requiring PN infusions should be familiar with the type of vascular access device (VAD) the patient has, available types of VADs, indications for use by type, VAD-associated complications, and how to monitor for, prevent, and treat VAD complications. Assessment of the VAD is not strictly the duty of nursing, but a shared responsibility of the interdisciplinary team and the patient.

VADs are divided into two groups: peripheral VADs and central vascular access devices (CVADs). The important factor that dictates the VAD as central or peripheral is not the site of insertion, but the location of the tip of the catheter. For a catheter to be considered a CVAD, the tip must reach the high blood flow of the superior vena cava (SVC) or inferior vena cava. Optimal catheter tip position is in the SVC adjacent to the right atrium.[7] Other acceptable tip locations for delivery of central PN include the middle and lower thirds of the SVC. Catheter tips outside these locations should be considered peripheral VADs. See Figure 14.1 for anatomical landmarks for determining catheter tip location. Catheter tips in the right atrium may lead to arrhythmias and thrombosis and should be placed near the cavoatrial junction to avoid these risks.

The risk of thrombosis is increased when the tip of the catheter is in the upper third of the SVC.[8–10] Cadman retrospectively reviewed tunneled catheter tip placement in oncology patients and showed a thrombosis rate of 41.7% corresponded to catheter tips in the upper third of the SVC versus 2.6% in the lower SVC ($p < 0.0005$).[9]

Catheter tip placement is also associated with catheter malfunction. Petersen and colleagues retrospectively evaluated oncology patients with tunneled catheters and implanted ports to determine potential factors for malfunction. When the tip of the catheter was >4 cm superior to the junction of the right atrium and SVC, a significant increase in complications was observed ($p = 0.003$). No other factors were found to be significant and malfunctions were minimal when the catheter tip was placed in the right atrium.[10]

14.3.1 SELECTION OF VADs

CVADs are further subdivided as short- and long-term catheters based on their intended length of use. CVADs intended for short-term use (i.e., length of treatment

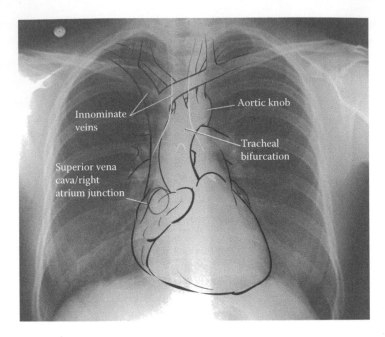

Innominate veins

Aortic knob

Tracheal bifurcation

Superior vena cava/right atrium junction

FIGURE 14.1   **(See color insert.)** Anatomical landmarks for determining catheter tip location.

ranging from days to weeks) include peripherally inserted central catheters (PICC) and temporary nontunneled central venous catheters (CVC). CVADs for long-term use are tunneled subcutaneously, have a subcutaneous cuff, and are intended for use for months to years. Implanted ports are also an option for use over months to years.

Nontunneled, noncuffed temporary CVC and PICCs are frequently used for short-term PN in the hospital setting. The subclavian site is preferred over the jugular (internal or external) and femoral sites to minimize risk of infection.[11] Additionally, femoral placement has been associated with higher risk of DVT compared to subclavian and jugular sites.[11]

When home PN (HPN) is needed for more than a few weeks, tunneled catheters offer multiple benefits to patients including: allowing the patient to serve as his/her own caregiver (having two hands free for catheter dressing changes and site care), decreased risk of infection compared to PICCs, a cuff to reduce dislodgment and prevent infection, potential to salvage the catheter in cases of catheter sepsis, nonsurgical removal when the catheter is no longer needed, and the ability to swim in a chlorinated pool (after the catheter in place for at least 1 month). See Figure 14.2 for catheter insertion sites utilized in hospital and home settings. Note that use of femoral catheters is discouraged due to infection potential[11] and the use of transhepatic and translumbar sites are rare (only when no other locations are available). CVADs are available in one, two, or three lumens, but selecting the catheter with the fewest number of lumens essential for care is prudent to minimize risk of infection.[11]

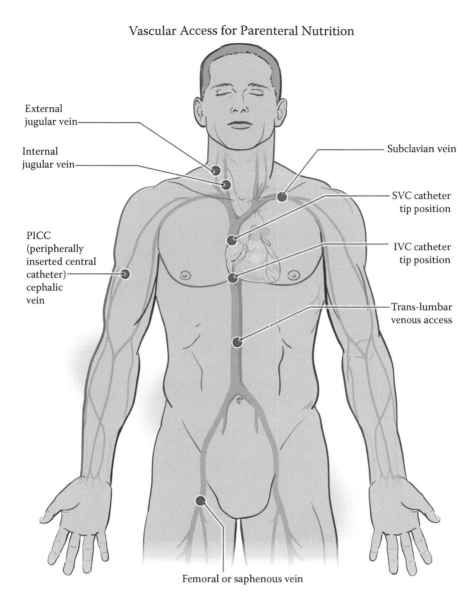

FIGURE 14.2 **(See color insert.)** Catheter insertion sites utilized in the hospital and home settings.

14.4 FORMULATIONS

14.4.1 Macronutrients and Micronutrients

Amino acids, dextrose, intravenous fat emulsion (IVFE), micronutrients, (vitamins, minerals, trace elements, and electrolytes) and sterile water are the basic components that make up PN solutions.

Amino acids are delivered as crystalline amino acids which are manufactured in a variety of concentrations (e.g., 8.5%, 10%, 15%, 20%) that contain both essential and nonessential amino acids. Amino acids provide 4 cal/g. Concentrated amino acid products (i.e., 15% or 20% amino acids) should be utilized for fluid restricted patients.

Dextrose for intravenous use contains 3.4 cal/g (dextrose monohydrate) and 70% dextrose is most often utilized for PN compounding.

IVFEs are available in 10%, 20%, and 30% concentrations and the only IVFEs in the United States are composed of long-chain fatty acids. Recommendations are to limit IVFE to 1 g/kg/day.[7,12] Essential fatty acid deficiency (EFAD) can be prevented with providing 2%–4% of calories as linoleic and linolenic acids.[7] Delivery of 1000 cal of soybean based IVFE weekly will satisfy this amount and prevent EFAD from developing.[13] Often 500 mL of soy based 20% IVFE will be delivered once weekly as part of the PN solution to prevent EFAD. Table 14.1 lists different types of IVFEs. Of note, omega-3-based IVFE solutions have been successful in treating and reversing PN-associated liver disease (PNALD) in pediatric patients.[14,15]

Multivitamins and trace elements should be added to PN solutions daily. The intravenous multiple vitamins were last changed in 2000 and the notable change was the inclusion of 150 mcg of vitamin K. This small and consistent daily dose of vitamin K should not interfere with anticoagulation regimens. Trace element preparations available in the United States contain chromium, copper, manganese, selenium, and zinc. These are also available as single trace element products. Refer to Table 14.2 for dosing recommendations. In recent years intermittent shortages of commercially available vitamin and trace element additives have made optimal fluid formulation more difficult.

Although iron is an essential micronutrient, it is not routinely added to PN solutions. If oral iron supplementation is not effective, iron dextran can only be added to PN solutions that do not contain IVFE.[16] Iron has great potential to destabilize IVFE

TABLE 14.1
Types of Intravenous Fat Emulsions

IVFE	Composition
Soybean (LCT)[a]	100% soybean oil
MCT/LCT	MCT and soybean oil
Structured lipids	MCT/LCT (soybean or coconut oils)
Olive oil/soy	MUFA, PUFA
Fish oil	Omega-3 PUFA
SMOF	Soybean oil, MCT, olive oil, fish oil

Source: Vanek VW, Seidner DL, Allen P et al. *Nutr Clin Pract* 2012;27(2):150–192.
Note: MCT = medium chain triglyceride, LCT = long chain triglyceride, MUFA = monounsaturated fatty acids, PUFA = polyunsaturated fatty acids.
[a] Only available type in the United States.

TABLE 14.2
Vitamin and Trace Element Daily Requirements

Vitamin Component	Requirement
Thiamin	6 mg
Riboflavin	3.6 mg
Niacin	40 mg
Folic acid	600 mcg
Pantothenic acid	15 mg
Pyridoxine	6 mg
Cyanocobalamin	5 mcg
Biotin	60 mcg
Ascorbic acid	200 mg
Vitamin A	3300 IU
Vitamin D	200 IU
Vitamin E	10 IU
Vitamin K	150 mcg
Trace Element Component	
Chromium	10–15 mcg
Copper	60–100 mcg
Manganese	60–100 mcg
Selenium	20–60 mcg
Zinc	2.5–5 mg

Source: American Medical Association Department of Foods and Nutrition. Guidelines for essential trace element preparations for parenteral use. A statement from an expert panel. *JAMA* 1979;241:2051–2054; Federal Register. 2000;65:21200–21201.

and therefore safety concerns prevents the use of iron dextran with IVFE. A test dose of iron dextran is required due to the potential for allergic reactions before it can be safely added to the PN solution. Iron and ferritin levels should be monitored at least every 3 months to evaluate response to therapy and for any dosing changes that may be required. There are many intravenous iron preparations, such as sodium ferric gluconate or iron sucrose, which can be infused separately from PN which avoids problems with compatibility.

Electrolytes are added to PN solutions in varying amounts individualized to the patient's clinical condition. Suggested ranges for electrolyte components are listed in Table 14.3. Available electrolyte salts for PN include calcium (gluconate), magnesium (sulfate or chloride), phosphorus (potassium phosphate or sodium phosphate), potassium (phosphate, chloride, or acetate), and sodium (chloride or acetate). The two components responsible for acid–base balance are acetate (base) and chloride (acid). Bicarbonate cannot be used in PN solutions because it forms a solid precipitate.

TABLE 14.3
Electrolyte Starting Point Recommended Ranges for PN

Component	Amount
Sodium	1–2 mEq/kg
Potassium	1–2 mEq/kg
Chloride	Balanced with acetate for acid–base balance
Acetate	Balanced with acetate for acid–base balance
Magnesium	10–30 mEq
Phosphorus	10–40 mmol
Calcium	10–20 mEq
	(at least 15 mEq for long-term HPN patients)

Source: Adapted from Taskforce for the revision of safe practices for parenteral nutrition, Mirtallo J et al. *JPEN J Parent Enteral Nutr* 2004;28(6):S39–S70.

14.4.2 MEDICATIONS AND ADDITIVES

Medications such as insulin, octreotide, or H-2 blockers are frequently and safely added to PN solutions. While other medications, such as corticosteroids, can be added, there are drawbacks to this practice. If the PN solution is suddenly stopped for any reason (such as electrolyte abnormalities, hyperglycemia >400 mg/dL, etc.), the patient will not receive the full dose of the medication. The pharmacy should be consulted before considering addition of other drugs to the PN solution.

14.4.3 SOLUTION COMPOSITION AND COMPATIBILITY

When using customized solutions, the basic macronutrient components can be combined in two different ways. PN solutions can either be delivered as a 2-in-1 solution which contains two macronutrients: amino acids and dextrose with a separate delivery of IVFE or as a 3-in-1 solution (containing all three macronutrients: amino acids, dextrose, and IVFE in one bag). Premixed PN solutions are available in various standardized concentrations and may be appropriate for facilities with low usage of PN or for short-term PN delivery. Customized solutions allow the clinician to individually tailor the PN solution to the patient's requirements with the ability to adjust the delivery of each individual component.

When 3-in-1 solutions are used stability (stability and compatibility often are interchangeably used terms) issues are at the forefront of ensuring safe delivery of the formula. Two types of precipitations can occur. A solid precipitate forms when incompatible salts are combined or a liquid precipitate when IVFEs separates from solution.[7] The emulsifier of the IVFE can destabilize when excess cations (calcium^{+2}, magnesium^{+2}, any amount of iron^{+3}) are added to the solution. Manufacturer guidelines for the products used in compounding the PN solution should be followed for known stability ranges. Refer to Table 14.4 for compatibility ranges used by the Cleveland Clinic.

TABLE 14.4
Compatibility for 3-in-1 PN Solutions

Additive	Acceptable Range
Amino acid	20–60 g/L
Dextrose	40–250 g/L
Intravenous fat emulsion	20–60 g/L
Divalent cations (Mg + Ca)	≤20 mEq/L
Calcium phosphorus product	<200
(mEq calcium/L × mEq phosphorus/L)	

Calcium and phosphate solubility is an important consideration for every PN solution regardless if it is delivered as a 2-in-1 or as a 3-in-1 solution. Factors influencing calcium phosphate solubility include amino acid, type and amount of calcium salt, amount of phosphorus, temperature, pH, fluid volume, and the order of compounding the PN solution.[7,17] Calcium phosphate curves exist for each amino acid product and/or a simple calculation clinicians can use is ensuring the calcium phosphorus product is <200 by the equation: mEq calcium/L*mEq phosphate/L.

14.4.4 PERIPHERAL PARENTERAL NUTRITION VERSUS CENTRAL PN

The distinction between peripheral parenteral nutrition (PPN) or central PN depends on the characteristics of the solution that is in turn dictated by the VAD tip location. When the tip of the catheter does *not* reach the middle third of the SVC, lower third of the SVC, cavoatrial junction, or the right atrium, PPN must be infused. The osmolarity of PPN is limited to 900 mOsm to minimize peripheral vein damage. PPN is most frequently delivered as a 3-in-1 solution because IVFE contributes the least to osmolarity while providing the most concentrated source of calories.[18] PPN solutions are not indicated in volume restricted patients, generally are not used beyond 2 weeks, and rarely delivered in excess 3 L.

When the VAD tip is within the middle third of the SVC, lower third of the SVC, cavoatrial junction, or the right atrium, a central PN solution can be used. Central PN solutions do not have osmolarity restrictions due to high blood flow and can be delivered as a 2-in-1 or 3-in-1.

14.4.5 INFUSION SCHEDULE

Most often in the hospital setting, PN is infused continuously over 24 h to achieve glycemic control and stable electrolyte and fluid balance while slowly increasing calories to meet energy requirements. For home going, patients free of cardiopulmonary compromise can be cycled to reduce the number of infusion hours. The cycling process reduces the infusion hours by 4–6 h daily until a 10–12-h cycle is achieved (i.e., decrease from 24 to 18 h, then 18 to 12 h). Reducing the infusion rate during the final hour of the cycle is clinically utilized to prevent rebound hypoglycemia that can potentially be seen with the sudden stop of the highly concentrated dextrose infusion.

14.4.6 SOLUTION CONSIDERATIONS FOR HEART/KIDNEY FAILURE

Patients with heart and kidney failure that require PN can be challenging to manage and often require manipulations to the PN solution to prevent fluid overload, electrolyte abnormalities, and metabolic complications. To limit volume, concentrated amino acid products (i.e., 15% or 20%) can be used. Physical assessment should closely monitor for the presence of edema, ascites, or pulmonary rales. Sodium is frequently limited with careful monitoring for dysnatremias.

Patients with kidney disease have increased lipolysis and an impaired ability to clear serum lipids. Triglyceride levels should be monitored and IVFE withheld when serum triglyceride levels are >400 mg/dL.[7] Often paints with renal disease have a chronic metabolic acidosis and PN solutions can maximize the acetate in the solution to assist with acid–base balance. Electrolytes that are dependent on renal clearance (including potassium, magnesium, and phosphorus) should be closely monitored. Patients with renal failure requiring hemodialysis or renal replacement therapies have increased protein needs and protein restriction is not warranted. If peritoneal dialysis or renal replacement contains dextrose, the total caloric load of the PN solution should be adjusted to account for these calories and prevent overfeeding.

14.5 MONITORING PN

As part of ensuring safe delivery of PN solutions monitoring is a continuous process and includes evaluating a variety of factors including vital signs, biochemical studies, weight status, fluid balance, the VAD, and for ongoing appropriateness of PN.

Laboratory studies that should be evaluated include a basic metabolic panel, magnesium, phosphorus, hepatic aminotransferases, complete blood count, and point of care blood sugar tests. If the patient is being prepared for HPN, baseline trace elements (copper, chromium, selenium, whole blood manganese, and zinc) are suggested, but there are no practice guidelines that suggest frequency of reevaluation. No studies have evaluated the effectiveness of monitoring these values as there are no gold standard measurements lending some concern about reliability. When trace element labs are ordered it is critical to obtain these when patients are free of acute illness. Correlating trace element laboratory values to the patient's underlying disease, indication for HPN, type of GI losses, and nutrition focused physical examination findings is prudent. During the acute care stay labs are often drawn daily. In the home setting labs may be weekly at the time of initial discharge, but the frequency over time can be reduced to monthly once stabilized (frequency varies based on the individual patient).

Intake and output (I/O) records completed daily by the patient at home are helpful tools in assessing fluid status. One study found I/O data to be consistent with signs and symptoms of dehydration 80% of the time.[23] Daily weights can aid in assessing fluid changes, but monitoring weight trends over time will be helpful to direct adjustments to caloric delivery. Determining a goal weight is helpful to direct the goals of HPN care (i.e., weight gain, weight loss, weight maintenance).

While in the acute care setting, the VAD should be assessed daily by a clinician and the patient can be trained to monitor the site daily when HPN is required. Transparent dressings allow for visualization of the catheter site to monitor for any redness, drainage, and swelling. Dressings should be changed on a schedule according to their type and anytime they become loose, wet, or soiled. Transparent dressings should be changed weekly and gauze dressings every 48 h.

Monitoring the patient's response to PN therapy includes the above data, but consideration to the patient's changes in functional status, quality of life, and coping with HPN therapy are also important. Social workers and patient-centered foundations for nutrition support patients, such as the Oley Foundation, are excellent resources.

Weaning of PN solutions differs between the hospital and home settings. In the hospital, calories and/or volume are reduced until the patient transitions off PN. Once the patient is taking 60% of nutritional needs via the enteral route PN can be discontinued. While calories and volume can be reduced this way at home, HPN is typically reduced by the number of days the patient infuses. For example, a patient would reduce from 7 to 6 days per week of HPN then have labs drawn the following week with evaluation of I/O and weight status. If the patient is able to maintain adequate hydration, enteral intake, and electrolytes then further reduction in days of HPN infusions can be attempted. Three days of HPN per week is usually the minimum for insurance reimbursement (see reimbursement section). One advantage to weaning HPN infusion days is allowing the patient to be free from the infusion pump which has potential to impact the quality of life.

14.6   COMPLICATIONS

While PN can be a life sustaining therapy, it is not without potential for both short- and long-term risks. Careful selection of patients for PN therapy can assist in maximizing the benefits while minimizing risks. Complications of PN can be divided into three main categories including: (1) metabolic complications, (2) infectious complications, and (3) noninfectious catheter-related complications.

14.6.1   METABOLIC COMPLICATIONS

There are no best practices for management of blood sugars for patients receiving PN and each patient requires an individualized regimen. Achieving acceptable glycemic control, often blood glucose below 150 mg/dL in PN patients, can be challenging. The dextrose content of PN is typically limited to 150–200 g on the first day of PN and capillary blood sugar is checked every 6 h.[7] Advancement of dextrose calories should be gradual to prevent hyperglycemia, but when blood glucose levels are consistently above 200 mg/dL, further advancement should be delayed until improved glycemic control is achieved. Clinicians frequently will add a portion (66%–100%) of the insulin the patient received subcutaneously into the PN solution for the next day. After calories have been advanced to goal most hospitalized patients will be prepare the patient for discharge by cycling PN over a shorter number of hours. Hyperglycemia is the most common adverse event associated with cycling PN. In one study, 71% of the patients necessitated addition of insulin or an increase in insulin dose during the PN cycling process.[19] Cycled PN should be tapered off slowly to prevent rebound hypoglycemia. After patients are discharged on a stable HPN solution urine glucose testing can take the place of finger sticks. One drawback to urine glucose testing is the inability to detect hypoglycemia. Hypoglycemia can occur for reasons such as too much insulin via the PN solution or if PN is suddenly stopped (rebound hypoglycemia).

Refeeding syndrome, or the intracellular shift of electrolytes and fluids upon the reintroduction of feeding in patients with prolonged inadequate energy delivery, is usually observed 2–5 days after the reintroduction of nutrition.[20–22] Gradual advancement of calories (as dextrose) via PN and careful monitoring of serum phosphorus, potassium, and magnesium with correction of any abnormalities is prudent. Patients may develop electrolyte abnormalities along their course of therapy that is not related to refeeding syndrome. PN solutions can be adjusted when mild abnormalities occur, but any severe values should be corrected outside of PN. Electrolytes should be stable in the hospitalized setting before patients are discharged home with HPN. When dealing with electrolyte abnormalities in HPN patients it is important to assess the underlying contributors of the altered lab value (recent changes to electrolyte content of HPN, change in patient's baseline GI losses, change in renal function, lab inaccuracies due to hemolysis, changes in medications, change in HPN infusion schedule, changes in fluid status) to direct changes in management.

Many patients requiring PN or HPN have the potential to develop dehydration due to high volume GI losses and inadequate bowel length to correct dehydration through the enteral route. The incidence of dehydration in HPN patients is unclear, but one study identified 201 episodes of dehydration among 308 patients in one calendar year with successful treatment at home in 84% of the cases.[23] Monitoring for dehydration is a joint effort of the patient/caregiver (physical signs such as excessive thirst, increased GI losses compared to baseline, negative I/O records, decreased volume or darker colored urine, decreased weight, cramping in extremities, lightheadedness) and clinician monitoring of lab values and I/O records. Careful attention should be made to preventing repeated episodes of dehydration to preserve kidney function.

Whereas primary renal failure due to PN has not been documented, a decrease in glomerular filtration has been observed in both adult and pediatric patients receiving long-term PN. The etiology remains unknown, but the work of Lauverjat suggests chronic dehydration.[24–26]

EFAD can develop within 2–4 weeks of fat-free PN (when no other sources of enteral fat are delivered/absorbed). Presenting symptoms include dry scaly skin, poor wound healing, decreased platelet function, and hair loss.[7] Refer to the section on PN formulations for prevention strategies. Withholding of IVFE due to hepatobiliary abnormalities may lead to EFAD and should be closely monitored. A phospholipid fatty acid level (comparing the triene:tetraene ratio) can biochemically confirm the diagnosis. Alternatively, linoleic fatty acid concentrations can be measured.

Metabolic bone disease (MBD) describes abnormalities in bone metabolism, density, and strength.[27] The causes of MBD are likely multifactorial and are poorly understood including the contribution of PN.[28] Patients receiving long-term PN should have a DEXA scan after 1 year of PN to screen for MBD. PN solutions for long-term HPN patients should avoid the use of potassium phosphate salts (due to increased aluminum contamination), adequate amounts of magnesium and phosphates, at least 15 mEq calcium, adjust acid–base composition in PN to prevent acidosis, and limit protein to 0.8–1 g/kg/day (excess protein contributes to hypercalcuria) after the patient is nutritionally repleted.[27,28]

Many factors are thought to influence the development of PNALD, which is most often steatosis or steatohepatitis in adults and a chlolestatic picture in pediatrics. PN is frequently suggested to be the cause whenever hepatic aminotransferase concentrations increase, but any rapid and sudden incline in these tests warrants an investigation of other potential contributors such as sepsis, obstruction, bacterial overgrowth, hepatotoxic medications, etc. (see Table 14.5).

Serum hepatic aminotransferase concentrations are not considered good surrogate markers of liver disease.[29,30] One study compared results of liver biopsies to liver tests at the time of biopsy, 6 months before biopsy, and 12 months before biopsy. Serum liver tests showed no correlation to the stage of fibrosis seen on the liver biopsy.[30]

The incidence of PNALD differs between reports. Cavicchi and colleagues report associations between longer exposure to PN and higher prevalence of complicated liver disease. After 17 months of HPN therapy, clinical manifestations occurred, but histologic evidence did not occur until after 27 months of HPN.[12] The high incidence of severe liver disease in the Cavicchi report is thought to be associated with giving large amounts of IVFE.

Salvino, in a report from the Cleveland Clinic, showed 154 of 162 (89%) long-term HPN patients had abnormal LFTs, but only 7 (4.5%) experienced severe abnormalities (total bilirubin >3 mg/dL, albumin <2.8 mg/dL, PT > 19 s).[31] The low incidence

---

TABLE 14.5
Strategies to Troubleshoot Hepatobiliary Abnormalities

PN Solution Strategies	Non-PN Solution Strategies
Start enteral nutrition	Investigate for underlying history of liver disease
Evaluate ability to wean or discontinue PN	Rule out sepsis/infection
Assess for overfeeding	Rule out EFAD
1. Decrease dextrose or fat calories if overfeeding present	
IVFE evaluation	Evaluate medications (enteral and intravenous)
1. If no signs of fat malabsorption with established tolerance of enteral fat source, discontinue IVFE	1. Any medications with known hepatobiliary side effects
2. Decrease to <1 g/kg/day	2. Herbal supplements
3. Limit lipids to 100 g (500 mL of 20% IVFE) weekly	3. Antisecretory agents that may promote cholestasis
4. Only use 3-in-1 PN if required to achieve glycemic control	
Cycle PN	Assess for clinical symptoms of small bowel bacterial overgrowth
Evaluate trace elements that are eliminated via the biliary route	Imaging studies
1. If whole blood manganese is elevated, omit manganese from PN	Hepatology consultation
2. If serum copper elevated, omit from PN	

Note: IVFE = Intravenous fat emulsion.

of severe liver disease in the Salvino report is thought to be associated with low amounts of IVFE administered.

Manganese is part of multiple trace element preparation as well as a contaminant of amino acids, dextrose, and electrolytes used to compound PN. There are no known cases of manganese deficiency, but manganese toxicity has been well documented, especially in long-term HPN patients despite removal of multiple trace element products from HPN solutions. Manganese collects in the basal ganglia which can be viewed on magnetic resonance imaging and causes symptoms including tremors, muscle rigidity, confusion, and headaches.[32,33] Manganese is excreted via the biliary route and monitoring of erythrocyte manganese or whole blood manganese is recommended regardless of the presence or absence of hepatobiliary abnormalities.

Choline deficiency may also play a role in PNALD as the pathway to synthesize choline from methionine may be impaired in PN patients.[29] Choline is not routinely included in PN solutions in the United States due to unavailability of a commercial product.

14.6.2 Infectious Catheter-Related Complications

It is estimated there is an excess of 250,000 cases of catheter associated infections annually in the United States with costs ranging from $30,000 to $56,167 per episode.[34] The significant morbidity and mortality associated with catheter infections make this a key target area of prevention for any patients with intravascular devices and those receiving PN. Catheter-associated blood steam infection (CRBSI) is the most common infectious complication among HPN patients and can lead to hospital readmissions, loss of venous access, and potentially a decreased quality of life. See Table 14.6 for common presenting symptoms, prevention, and treatment.

A definitive diagnosis of CRBSI is by either quantitative blood cultures (cultures taken from the catheter and the peripheral venous blood) or differential time to positivity cultures taken before initiation of antimicrobial therapies[35] (see Table 14.6). Culturing only one lumen of a triple lumen catheter has only a 60% chance of detecting colonization of an organism[36] and therefore blood cultures should be obtained from each lumen of multiple lumen catheters.

Migration of skin organisms at the catheter entrance site is the source of CRBSI for short-term catheters whereas intraluminal hub contamination is most often the route in long-term tunneled CVADs.[11,35] The goal with long-term catheters is to salvage the catheter when possible if the patient is hemodynamically stable by use of systemic antibiotics to clear the infection. Removal of long-term catheters is recommended with the following causative organisms: *Staphylococcus aureus*, *Pseudomonas aeruginosa*, *Mycobacteria*, and fungemia.[35] Septic thrombophlebitis and endocarditis are other reasons to remove venous access devices.[35] Retaining the CVAD in cases of fungemia has been associated with increased risk of death leading to recommendations for catheter removal within 72 h of suspected or confirmed fungemia.[34] Fungemia also warrants evaluation by ophthalmology to exclude endophthalmitis. Fungemia, recurrent, or persistent CRBSIs warrant transesophageal echo (TEE) to exclude endocarditis.[35]

TABLE 14.6
Infectious Central Catheter Complications

Complication	Signs and Symptoms	Treatment	Prevention
CRBSI Clinical definition	• Fever (>101 F/38.3 C) and rigors when HPN infusing/catheter in use, elevated white blood cells (WBCs) • No other source of infection identified • Quantitative blood cultures—central catheter culture is at least three fold greater colony count than peripheral blood culture. • Differential time to positivity • Growth detected from cultures drawn via catheter 2 h before growth on cultures drawn from peripheral site	• Infectious disease consultation to evaluate salvage versus removal of long-term tunneled catheters • IV antibiotics per infectious disease • Catheter replacement after infection cleared	Maximal barrier protection and aseptic technique during insertion Hand hygiene policy Prompt removal of central lines that are no longer necessary Education on line maintenance (inpatient staff, homecare staff, patients/caregivers) Hub disinfection with every access Ethanol lock
Tunnel infection (only tunneled catheters)	• Erythema, tenderness, swelling along the skin following along the track of the tunnel	• Catheter removal • IV antibiotics • Catheter replacement at another site	• Aseptic line care • Routine site care with chlorhexidine
Exit site infection	• Drainage localized to catheter site (exit site for tunneled catheters; insertion site for PICC), redness, tenderness	• Site culture • Oral antibiotics • Stitch removal (tunneled catheters only) • Increase frequency of dressing change (avoid transparent dressing)	• Aseptic line care • Routine site care with chlorhexidine • Clean and dry dressing

Source: Centers for Disease Control and Prevention/National Healthcare and Safety Network. Central line associated blood stream infections. July 2013. Available at: http://www.cdc.gov/nhsn/pdfs/pscmanual/4psc_clabscurrent.pdf. Accessed August 16, 2013.

Patients with CRBSI from *Staph aureus* are at risk for septic thrombophlebitis, endocarditis, and venous thrombosis. Crowley and colleagues studied a cohort of 48 patients with *Staph aureus* with an ultrasound of the internal jugular, subclavian, and brachial veins. Imaging uncovered definite or probable thrombosis in 71%

of patients where physical exam did not identify any thrombosis.[37] Routine venous imaging to rule out thrombosis in patients with *Staph aureus* CRBSI seems prudent. Additionally, many infectious disease experts suggest a TEE to evaluate for endocarditis in patients with *Staph aureus* CRBSI.

Prevention of catheter associated infections begins with basic measures such as hand washing, good catheter care, and aseptic technique when connecting to HPN and during preparation of additives to the bag. Risk factors for CRBSI specifically in adult HPN patients has been associated with delivery of IVFE more than twice weekly, blood draws from the CVAD, and use of the catheter for non-HPN therapies.[38] Suggested countermeasures include infusing IVFE less than twice weekly (see section on PN formulations), obtain blood samples peripherally, and to avoid multiple manipulations of the CVAD with non-PN medications.

Another method for prevention of CRBSI in HPN patients is use of ethanol lock therapy with silicone CVADs. Although the ideal dwell time, strength of ethanol, or dose has not been determined, many HPN providers caring for adult patients are instilling 3 mL of 70% ethanol lock into the lumen of the silicone CVAD when PN is not infusing (typically 10–12 h) and then flushing with 10 mL of 0.9% NaCl before starting the next cycled HPN infusion. Ethanol is a good catheter locking solution due to its inherent bactericidal and fungicidal properties, low cost, no potential for resistance (ethanol denatures proteins), and low risk for side effects. Ethanol lock has been shown as safe and efficacious in prevention of CRBSI in numerous adult and pediatric HPN cohort studies. A significant decrease in catheter sepsis hospital readmissions has been observed with use of ethanol lock as a preventative agent.[39–42]

Exit site infections are characterized by drainage, redness, and tenderness. The exudates can be cultured to determine the causative organism. The VAD does not require removal in the majority of exit site infections and can be successfully treated with oral antibiotics for 7–10 days. If the VAD is tunneled, the stitch should be removed in the presence of a site infection. In rare cases, the VAD must be removed such as if an exit site infection is left untreated for an extended period of time and then progresses to a tunnel infection. Tunnel infections present with erythema, tenderness, swelling along the skin following the track of the tunnel. The VAD must always be removed in tunnel infections, treated with IV antibiotics, and the VAD is then replaced at an alternate site.

14.6.3   Noninfectious Catheter-Related Complications

Noninfectious catheter complications include catheter occlusions, malposition of the catheter tip, SVC syndrome, catheter-associated thrombosis, exposed cuff, break, and air embolism. See Table 14.7 for an overview of these complications, prevention measures, and suggested treatment strategies.

14.7   OTHER CONSIDERATIONS

14.7.1   Reimbursement

Before hospital discharge, the case manager plays an important role in serving as a liaison between the provider and the insurance company to determine benefits

TABLE 14.7

Noninfectious Central Catheter Complications

Complication	Signs and Symptoms	Treatment	Prevention
Occlusion	Inability to withdraw or resistance to infusing	*Dictated based on cause* *Precipitate* • Lipid: ethanol • Drug: 0.1 normal hydrogen chloride or sodium bicarbonate *Fibrin sleeve* • Thrombolytic agent (i.e., t-PA) in patients free of fever/infection *Pinch off syndrome* • Remove catheter	Flush with 0.9% NaCl after each IV infusion • Volume of flush to be twice the volume of the catheter If blood back up occurs, promptly • Flush with 0.9% NaCl • Change the end cap Placement of catheters on the right side when possible
Air embolism	Sudden onset chest pain, cough, shortness of breath caused by air entry	Clamp catheter Lay patient on the left side awaiting urgent medical assessment	• Clamp catheter when not in use • Clamp catheter during routine endcap change • If catheter integrity compromised (i.e., hole), clamp between body and the hole until repaired
Catheter-associated deep vein thrombosis	Swelling of arms or neck on the same side as the catheter, warmth, discoloration/redness	Anticoagulation if no contraindications exist	• Prophylactic, low dose anticoagulation with catheter placement
Superior Vena Cava syndrome	Swelling to the shoulders, neck, or face on the same side as the catheter, enlarged chest veins, sore throat, cough, excessive tearing/rhinorrhea	Ultrasound or CT evaluation Thrombolytics and/or anticoagulation Vascular surgery consultation • Evaluation for endovascular interventions	• Proper catheter tip placement • Prophylactic anticoagulation in patients with previous thrombosis
Malposition (high risk for nontunneled or noncuffed catheters)	Catheter dislodged/migration of catheter tip, asymptomatic or chest pain on infusion	Catheter replacement	• Routine CXR with hospital admissions to check catheter tip position (especially with PICCs)
Exposed cuff (only cuffed catheters)	Cuff visible on the outside of the skin	Catheter replacement	• Delay removal of sutures after catheter placement until cuff has adhered in tunnel
Break/hole	Visible damage Fluid leaking from catheter with flush/infusion	Clamp catheter (between break and the body) Replace catheter Repair catheter (possible if tunneled catheter depending on location of break)	• Rotate location where catheter is clamped when not in use

for HPN. Medicare has specific criteria that must be met for HPN coverage to be provided. The patient must require at least 90 days of HPN and have an inability to maintain weight though other methods such as enteral feedings or pharmaceutical interventions. The patient must also have one of the following diagnoses that involves the small bowel (or exocrine gland) that affects absorption of nutrients or a motility disorder that impairs transport of nutrients though the GI tract including: a massive small bowel resection in the last 3 months (≤5 feet of small bowel distal to the ligament of Treitz), short bowel syndrome, pancreatitis, Crohn's exacerbation, enterocutaneous fistula (where distal enteral feeding tube placement is not possible), small bowel obstruction, severe fat malabsorption, or a motility disorder.

Many of the Medicare HPN criteria require the patient to demonstrate 10% weight loss over 3 months and have a serum albumin below 3.4 g/dL. Through a joint effort of ASPEN and the Academy of Nutrition and Dietetics, the definition and diagnostic criteria, and etiology based nomenclature for malnutrition have been developed.[43,44] The new malnutrition diagnostic criteria do not include use of any hepatic proteins such as albumin for diagnosis of malnutrition. Medicare utilizes albumin in part for determination of nutritional status and criteria for reimbursability of HPN therapy. New ICD-10 codes are planned to incorporate the new malnutrition etiology based nomenclature and Medicare definitions/guidelines should be monitored for future changes regarding nutritional status.

HPN formulas are billed based off codes that correspond to the grams of amino acid and IVFE. Estimates on the annual cost of HPN in 1992 were $140,000, but most likely are higher now.[45] Of note, reimbursement is received by the compounding homecare pharmacy and not the ordering physician.[46]

14.7.2 Outcomes

Nutrition support literature contains multiple case studies and single center cohort studies from HPN centers highlighting patient longevity and outcomes with HPN support, however; no recent data exists on a national level about safety, effectiveness, or outcomes associated with HPN. In 2011, ASPEN developed Sustain™, a national patient registry for nutrition care. This prospective, longitudinal registry was developed to evaluate the effectiveness and outcomes of HPN therapy with the ability to benchmark institutional data to the aggregated national data.[47] The first phase of the registry is seeking providers to voluntarily provide information on patients receiving HPN therapy.

14.8 CONCLUSION

PN is a complex therapy and requires careful monitoring in the hospital and home settings. While PN can be a life sustaining therapy, it is not without risk for short-term and long-term complications. Careful patient selection, clinical monitoring, vascular access selection, and strategies to minimize complications require the nutrition support clinician to oversee many facets of the patient's nutritional care.

14.9 CASE STUDY

A 54-year-old male with Crohn's disease s/p lysis of adhesions and a 15 cm small bowel resection at an OSH presents to the ER 5 days after discharge from an OSH with a leak confirmed by CT scan. He is taken to surgery and requires a proximal diverting jejunosotomy.

Current anatomy: 75 cm of small bowel to the jejunostomy and 175 cm of small bowel out of continuity, 50% of colon, rectum and anus
Past medical history: Crohn's disease, vitamin B_{12} deficiency, small bowel resections, cholecystectomy, enterocutaneous fistula s/p repair
Social history: married with three children

The plan is to send the patient home with PN and to restore intestinal continuity in 3 months' time. The nutrition support team (NST) has evaluated the patient with the following findings:

58 kg, 6′ BMI: 17.3
Usual body weight (UBW) 3 months ago: 65 kg
7 kg weight loss in 3 months (10.7% of body weight)

Nutrition focused physical exam:

- Loss of subcutaneous fat (orbital and overlying the ribs)
- Loss of muscle (temporal wasting, squared shoulders)
- No edema

Patient reports decreased PO intake due to pain (50% meals for 2 months)
Current hospital diet:
1. Serving of starch thrice daily

1 L of oral rehydration solution daily
Medications: 1000 mcg vitamin B_{12} once monthly intramuscular (IM), Imodium 2 caps 30 min before meals 4 times daily
Intake and output records
Oral 240   Urine 1600
IV 3600   Ostomy 2400

Estimated nutritional needs: 2300 cal, 115 g protein
Nutritional assessment: severe malnutrition
Current VAD: right 1 L PICC with tip in the lower third of the SVC on chest x-ray (CXR).

The NST physician approves of the usefulness of HPN and agrees to HPN management (Figure 14.8). The casemanager/discharge planner is consulted to verify insurance benefits and to arrange for home infusion pharmacy and homecare nursing

TABLE 14.8
PN Solution Advancement and Monitoring for Case Study

Plan	PN Solution (Order Due 1700, PN Start at 2200)	Blood Sugars	Labs (0400 Daily)	
Day 1 PN 1/2 cal, full protein	115 g AA 200 g dextrose 3.4 L at 141 mL/h Ca 10 mEq Mg 24 mEq NaPhos 30 mEq KAce 65 mEq NaCl 160 mEq NaAce 45 mEq MVI 10 mL MTE 5C 1 mL	Order to start point of care testing q 6 h	Na 138 mmol/L K 4.6 mmol/L Cl 103 mmol/L CO_2 6 mEq/L BUN 8 mg/dL Cr 0.5 mg/dL Glu 108 mg/dL	Magnesium 1.5 mg/dL Phosphorus 2.5 mg/dL WBC 8.0 K/UL AST 20 units/L ALK Phos 80 units/L T. Bilirubin 0.3 mg/dL Albumin 2.3 mg/dL
Day 2 Increase calories	115 g AA 350 g dextrose 3.4 L at 141 mL/h Ca 10 mEq Mg 24 mEq NaPhos 40 mEq KAce 90 mEq NaCl 180 mEq NaAce 25 mEq MVI 10 mL MTE 5C 1 mL	2400:110 mg/dL 0600:120 mg/dL 1200:107 mg/dL 1800:118 mg/dL	Na 138 mmol/L K 4.1 mmol/L Cl 105 mmol/L CO_2 27 mEq/L BUN 25 mg/dL Cr 0.6 mg/dL Glu 135 mg/dL	Magnesium 1.6 mg/dL Phosphorus 2.3 mg/dL Calcium 8.1 mg/dL
Day 3 Increase calories to goal	115 g AA 500 g dextrose 100 g IVFE 1 day/week 3.4 L at 141 mL/h Ca 10 mEq Mg 24 mEq NaPhos 40 mEq KAce 90 mEq NaCl 180 mEq NaAce 25 mEq MVI 10 mL MTE 5C 1 mL	2400:145 mg/dL 0600:178 mg/dL 1200:188 mg/dL 1800:157 mg/dL	Na 137 mmol/L K 4.3 mmol/L Cl 104 mmol/L CO_2 26 mEq/L BUN 27 mg/dL Cr 0.5 mg/dL Glu 155 mg/dL	Magnesium 1.9 mg/dL Phosphorus 2.6 mg/dL Calcium 8.2 mg/dL

TABLE 14.8 (Continued)
PN Solution Advancement and Monitoring for Case Study

Plan	PN Solution (Order Due 1700, PN Start at 2200)			Blood Sugars	Labs (0400 Daily)			
Day 4 Cycle to 18 h	115 g AA	Ca	10 mEq		Na	139 mmol/L	Magnesium	1.7 mg/dL
	500 g dextrose	Mg	30 mEq		K	4.4 mmol/L	Phosphorus	2.8 mg/dL
	100 g IVFE 1 day/week	NaPhos	44 mEq	*With 18 h cycle*	Cl	105 mmol/L	Zinc ↓	50 mcg/dL
	3.4 L over 18 h	KAce	90 mEq	2400:176 mg/dL	CO$_2$	27 mEq/L	Copper	99 mcg/dL
	100 mL/h × 1 h	NaCl	180 mEq	0600:215 mg/dL	BUN	26 mg/dL	Chromium	0.5 mcg/dL
	200 mL/h × 16 h	NaAce	25 mEq	1500:93 mg/dL	Cr	0.5 mg/dL	Selenium	100 mcg/dL
	100 mL/h × 1 h	MVI	10 mL		Glu	188 mg/dL	Manganese	0.3 mcg/dL
		MTE 5C	1 mL					
		Insulin	10 Units					
Day 5 Cycle to 12 h	115 g AA	Ca	10 mEq		Na	138 mmol/L	Magnesium	1.9 mg/dL
	500 g dextrose	Mg	30 mEq		K	4.4 mmol/L	Phosphorus	3 mg/dL
	100 g IVFE 1 day/week	NaPhos	44 mEq	*With 12 h cycle*	Cl	105 mmol/L	Calcium	8.2 mg/dL
	3.4 L over 12 h	KAce	90 mEq	2400:143 mg/dL	CO$_2$	26 mEq/L		
	155 mL/h × 1 h	NaCl	180 mEq	0600:148 mg/dL	BUN	26 mg/dL		
	309 mL/h × 10 h	NaAce	25 mEq	1100:108 mg/dL	Cr	0.5 mg/dL		
	155 mL/h × 1 h	MVI	10 mL		Glu	150 mg/dL		
		MTE 5C	1 mL					
		Zinc	5 mg					
		Insulin	20 Units					

services. The NST RN (registered nurse) and MD (doctor/physician) discuss long-term VADs with the patient and caregiver. It was jointly decided that a single lumen Hickman would be ideal and an order for the line to be placed in Interventional Radiology was entered into the electronic medical record. A one lumen catheter is deemed appropriate and the patient and NST RN select and mark a location for the catheter in an easily visible area on the chest that will allow for self-care and visualization of the exit site. The following day a right internal jugular single lumen Hickman is placed and the tip is visualized under fluoroscopy to be in the cavo-atrial junction. Meanwhile the PN solution is initiated and adjusted according to Table 14.8. While the PN solution is being advanced and cycled in preparation for discharge, the NST RN educates the patient and his wife on HPN procedures. The patient and his wife are both trained to monitor the following:

- Daily weight and temperature
- Intake and output records
- Testing for presence of glucose in the urine
- Catheter care and catheter complications
- Signs and symptoms of hypo/hyperglycemia, dehydration, over hydration, hypo/hyper-kalemia
- How and when to reach the NST 24 h/day

The patient was cycled to a 12-h infusion and stabilized on the home going HPN formula with acceptable blood sugars. Once cleared by the surgical team, the patient was discharged home. The NST MD ordered the patient receive ethanol lock (3 mL of 70% ethanol) daily to dwell in the line for 12 h when PN was not infusing. Homecare nursing continues the education received in the hospital over twice daily visits for the first 3 days home and then weekly visits thereafter until the patient and wife are independent with catheter care and PN procedures. The NST MD and HPN service enroll the patient into Sustain™ A.S.P.E.N.'s National Patient Registry for Nutrition Care. The patient is scheduled for follow-up with the NST MD and HPN clinician 1 month after discharge (see Table 14.8).

REFERENCES

1. American Society for Parenteral and Enteral Nutrition Board of Directors. Guidelines for the use of parenteral and enteral nutrition in adult and pediatric patients. *JPEN J Parenter Enteral Nutr* 2002;26:1SA–138SA.
2. DiBaise JK, Scolapio JS. Home parenteral and enteral nutrition. *Gastroenterol Clin North Am* 2007;36(1):123–144.
3. Mirtallo J, Patel M. Overview of parenteral nutrition. In: Mueller CM, Ed. *The ASPEN Adult Nutrition Support Core Curriculum*, 2nd Edition. Silver Spring: ASPEN; 2012. pp. 234–244.
4. Skipper A. Principles of parenteral nutrition. In: Matarese LE, Gottschlich MM, Eds. *Contemporary Nutrition Support Practice*, 2nd Edition. St Louis: Saunders; 2003. pp. 227–242.
5. McClave SA, Martindale RG, Vanek VW et al. Guidelines for the provision and assessment of nutrition support therapy in the adult critically ill patient: Society of critical care medicine and American society for parenteral and enteral nutrition. *JPEN J Parenter Enteral Nutr* 2009;33(3):277–316.

6. Klein S, Kinney J, Jeejeebhoy K et al. Nutrition support in clinical practice: Review of published data and recommendations for future research directions. *JPEN J Parenter Enteral Nutr* 1997;21:133–156.
7. Taskforce for the revision of safe practices for parenteral nutrition, Mirtallo J, Canada T, Johnson D, Kumpf V, Petersen C, Sacks G, Seres D, Guenter P. Safe practices for parenteral nutrition. *JPEN J Parent Enteral Nutr* 2004;28(6):S39–S70.
8. Steiger E. Dysfunction and thrombotic complications of vascular access devices. *J Parent Enteral Nutr* 2006;30(1):S70–S71.
9. Cadman A, Lawrence JA, Fitzsimmons L, Spencer-Shaw A, Swindell R. To clot or not to clot? That is the question in central venous catheters. *Clin Radiol* 2004;59(4):349–355.
10. Petersen J, Delaney JH, Brakestad MT, Rowbotham RK, Bagley CM Jr. Silicone venous access devices positioned with their tips in the superior vena cava are more likely to malfunction. *Am J Surg* 1999;178(1):38–41.
11. O'Grady NP, Alexander M, Burns LA et al. Guidelines for the prevention of intravascular catheter-related infections. *Clin Infect Dis* 2011;52:1087–1099.
12. Cavicchi M, Beau P, Crenn P et al. Prevalence of liver disease and contributing factors in patients receiving home parenteral nutrition for permanent intestinal failure. *Ann Intern Med* 2000;132:523–532.
13. Jeppesen PB, Hoy CE, Mortensen PB. Essential fatty acid deficiency in patients requiring home parenteral nutrition. *Am J Clin Nutr* 1998;68:126–133.
14. Diamond IR, Sterescu A, Pencharz PB et al. Changing the paradigm: Omegaven for the treatment of liver failure in pediatric short bowel syndrome. *J Pediatr Gastroenterl Nutr* 2009;48:209–215.
15. Gura KL, Lee S, Valim C et al. Safety and efficacy of a fish-oil-based fat emulsion in the treatment of parenteral nutrition associated liver disease. *Pediatrics* 2008;121:e678–e686.
16. Kumpf VJ. Update on parenteral iron therapy. *Nutr Clin Pract* 2003;18:318–326.
17. Allwood MC, Kearney MC. Compatibility and stability of additives in parenteral nutrition admixtures. *Nutrition* 1998;14(9):697–706.
18. Gura KM. Is there still a role for peripheral parenteral nutrition? *Nutr Clin Pract* 2009;24(6):709–717.
19. Suryadevara S, Celestin J, DeChicco R et al. Type and prevalence of adverse events during the parenteral nutrition cycling process in patients being prepared for discharge. *Nutr Clin Pract* 2012;7(2):268–273.
20. Solomon SM, Kirby DF. The refeeding syndrome: A review. *JPEN J Parenter Enteral Nutr* 1990;14(1):90–97.
21. Kraft MD, Btaich IF, Sacks GS. Review of refeeding syndrome. *Nutr Clin Pract* 2005;20:625–633.
22. Skipper A. Refeeding syndrome or refeeding hypophosphatemia: A systematic review of cases. *Nutr Clin Pract* 2012;27(1):34–40.
23. Konrad D, Corrigan ML, Hamilton C, Steiger E, Kirby DF. Identification and early treatment of dehydration in home parenteral nutrition and intravenous fluid patients prevents hospital admissions. *Nutr Clin Pract* 2012;27(6):802–807.
24. Buchman AL, Moukarzel A, Ament ME et al. Serious renal impairment is associated with long-term parenteral nutrition. *JPEN J Parenter Enteral Nutr* 1993;17(5):438–444.
25. Moukarzell AA, Ament ME, Buchman A, Dahlstrom KA, Vargas J. Renal function of children receiving long-term parenteral nutrition. *J Pediatr* 1991;119(6):864–868.
26. Lauverjat M, Hadj Aissa A, Vanhems P, Bouletreau P, Fouque D. Chronic dehydration may impair renal function in patients with chronic intestinal failure on long-term parenteral nutrition. *Clin Nutr* 2006;25:75–81.
27. Hamilton C, Seidner DL. Metabolic bone disease in the patient on long term home parenteral nutrition. *Pract Gasteroenterol* 2008;32:18–32.

28. Kumpf VJ, Gervasio J. Complications of parenteral nutrition. In: Mueller CM, Ed. *The ASPEN Adult Nutrition Support Core Curriculum*, 2nd Edition. Silver Spring, MD: ASPEN; 2012. pp. 284–297.

29. Buchman AL. Choline deficiency during parenteral nutrition in humans. *Nutr Clin Pract* 2003;18:353–358.

30. Porter MJ, Parekh NR, Soliman M et al. Liver functions tests may not represent a reliable marker of intestinal failure liver disease. *JPEN J Parenter Enteral Nutr* 2010;34:176–177.

31. Salvino R, Ghanta R, Seidner DL, Mascha E, Xu Y, Steiger E. Liver failure is uncommon in adults receiving long-term parenteral nutrition. *JPEN J Parenter Enteral Nutr* 2006;30(3):202–208.

32. Btaiche IF, Carver PL, Welch KB. Dosing and monitoring of trace elements in long-term home parenteral nutrition patients. *JPEN J Parenter Enteral Nutr* 2011;35(6):736–747.

33. Abdalian R, Saqui O, Fernandes G, Allard JP. Effects of manganese from a commercial multi-trace element supplement in a population sample of Canadian patients on long-term parenteral nutrition. *JPEN J Parenter Enteral Nutr* 2013;37(4):538–543.

34. Raad I, Hanna H, Maki D. Intravascular catheter-related infections: Advances in diagnosis, prevention, and management. *Lancet Infect Dis* 2007;7:645–657.

35. Mermel LA, Allon M, Bouza E et al. Clinical practice guidelines for the diagnosis and management of intravascular catheter-related infection: 2009 update by the infectious diseases society of America. *CID* 2009;49:1–45.

36. Dobbins BM, Catton JA, Kite P, McMahon MJ, Wilcox MH. Each lumen is a potential source of central venous catheter related blood stream infection. *Crit Care Med* 2003;31:2385–2390.

37. Crowley AL, Peterson GE, Benjamin DK Jr et al. Venous thrombosis in patients with short-and long-term central venous catheter-associated staphylococcus aureus bacteremia. *Crit Care Med* 2008;36(2):385–390.

38. Buchman AL, Opilla M, Kwasny M, Diamantidis TG, Okamoto R. Risk factors for the development of catheter-related bloodstream infections in patients receiving home parenteral nutrition. *JPEN J Parenter Enteral Nutr* 2013. Available online first at: http://pen.sagepub.com/content/early/2013/06/04/0148607113491783.full.pdf+html. Accessed August 15, 2013.

39. John BK, Khan MA, Speerhas R et al. Ethanol lock therapy in reducing catheter-related blood stream infections in adult home parenteral nutrition patients: Results of a retrospective study. *JPEN J Parenter Enteral Nutr* 2012;36(3):603–610.

40. Opilla MT, Kirby DF, Edmond MB. Use of ethanol lock therapy to reduce the incidence of catheter related blood stream infections in home parenteral nutrition patients. *JPEN J Parenter Enteral Nutr* 2007;31:302–305.

41. Metcalf SC, Chambers ST, Pithie AD. Use of ethanol locks to prevent recurrent central line sepsis. *J Infect* 2004;49:20–22.

42. Cober MP, Kovacevich DS, Teitelbaum DH. Ethanol lock therapy for the prevention of central venous access device infections in pediatric patients with intestinal failure. *JPEN J Parenter Enteral Nutr* 2011;35(1):67–73.

43. Jensen GL, Compher C, Sullivan DH, Mullin GE. Recognizing malnutrition in adults: Definitions and characteristics, screening, assessment, and team approach. *JPEN J Parenter Enteral Nutr* 2013. Available online first at: http://pen.sagepub.com/content/early/2013/08/22/0148607113492338. Accessed August 22, 2013.

44. White JV, Guenter P, Jensen G, Malone A, Schofield M. Consensus statement of the academy of nutrition and dietetics/American society for parenteral and enteral nutrition: Characteristics recommended for the identification and documentation of adult malnutrition (undernutrition). *J Acad Nutr Diet* 2012;112:730–738.

45. Howard L. Home parenteral nutrition: survival, cost, and quality of life. *Gastroenterology* 2006;130(2):S52–S59.

46. Hendrickson E, Corrigan ML. Navigating reimbursement for home parenteral nutrition. *Nutr Clin Pract* 2013;28(5):566–571.

47. Guenter P, Robinson L, Dimaria-Ghalili RA, Lyman B, Steiger E, Winkler MF. Development of sustain: ASPEN's national patient registry for nutrition care. *JPEN J Parenter Enteral Nutr* 2012;36(4):399–406.

48. Vanek VW, Seidner DL, Allen P et al. A.S.P.E.N. Position paper: Clinical role for alternative intravenous fat emulsions. *Nutr Clin Pract* 2012;27(2):150–192.

49. American Medical Association Department of Foods and Nutrition. Guidelines for essential trace element preparations for parenteral use. A statement from an expert panel. *JAMA* 1979;241:2051–2054.

50. Federal Register. 2000;65:21200–21201.

51. Centers for Disease Control and Prevention/National Healthcare and Safety Network. Central line associated blood stream infections. July 2013. Available at: http://www.cdc.gov/nhsn/pdfs/pscmanual/4psc_clabscurrent.pdf. Accessed August 16, 2013.

15 Medical and Endoscopic Therapy of Obesity

Nitin Kumar and Christopher C. Thompson

CONTENTS

15.1 INTRODUCTION

Obesity has become a global epidemic, afflicting hundreds of millions worldwide.[1] Additionally, associated comorbidities, including type 2 diabetes mellitus and cardiovascular disease, inflict considerable morbidity and mortality.[2] Although bariatric surgery is effective, novel pharmacologic and endoscopic technologies have the potential to treat obesity in patients unwilling to undergo surgery, patients with a BMI too low to qualify for bariatric surgery, patients who need optimization for bariatric surgery, and patients with metabolic disease. Pharmacologic therapy offers a noninvasive option complementary to diet and lifestyle modification. Endoscopic procedures may offer lower invasiveness, reversibility, repeatability, and lower cost than bariatric surgery.

15.2 MEDICAL THERAPY

Medical therapies offer the potential to augment weight loss achieved by modification of diet and lifestyle. These therapies can suppress appetite via central action or act peripherally to alter caloric balance. The Food & Drug Administration has recently approved drugs in both of these categories.

15.2.1 ORLISTAT

Orlistat is a lipase inhibitor approved for weight loss or weight maintenance in patients on a low-calorie diet. The medication, which should be taken with each meal, prevents hydrolysis of dietary fat into fatty acids and monoacylglycerols.[3] Approximately 30% of dietary fat intake is not absorbed. Placebo-subtracted weight loss in randomized double-blinded placebo-controlled trials has been 2.7–3.2 kg after 1–2 years.[4] More patients on orlistat lose >10% of total body weight (34% versus 16%). Tolerability is good, as the medication is minimally absorbed from the gastrointestinal tract. Reported adverse events include fecal leakage, urgency, and frequent bowel movements. These generally diminish as patients modify their intake to include less fat. Orlistat is available in an over-the-counter dose and a higher prescription dose.

15.2.2 LORCASERIN

Lorcaserin is a serotonin type 2C receptor agonist approved for weight loss. The medication specifically targets this receptor while avoiding serotonin type 2A and 2B receptors, which previously resulted in withdrawal of the medication fenfluramine.[5] Lorcaserin has been evaluated in randomized double-blinded placebo-controlled trials. The BLOOM trial included 3182 patients with a BMI of 30–45 kg/m², or a BMI of 27–45 kg/m² with at least one comorbidity.[6] Patients in the therapy group received lorcaserin 10 mg twice daily. The BLOSSOM trial included 4008 patients with a BMI of 30–45 kg/m², or a BMI of 27–30 kg/m² with at least one comorbidity.[7] In addition to placebo, lorcaserin was evaluated at 10 mg daily and 10 mg twice daily. A meta-analysis of five randomized controlled trials resulted in weight loss of 3.2 kg and BMI loss of 1.2 kg/m² compared to placebo.[8] Additionally, study of lorcaserin in overweight or obese patients with type 2 diabetes already on sulfonylurea or metformin (BLOOM-DM) found total body weight gain of 1.5% on placebo versus weight loss of 5.0% on lorcaserin 10 mg once daily and weight loss of 4.5% on lorcaserin 10 mg twice daily.[9] Lorcaserin should be discontinued if 5% weight loss is not achieved by 12 weeks, as continued treatment will likely be ineffective. Reported adverse events include incidences of blurry vision, dizziness, somnolence, headache, and nausea. There was no significant difference between valvulopathy rates between lorcaserin and placebo. Lorcaserin is contraindicated during pregnancy due to risk of teratogenicity. Furthermore, animal studies found increased incidence of mammary fibroadenoma in female rats at all doses and increased incidence of mammary adenocarcinoma at very high doses.

15.2.3 PHENTERMINE/TOPIRAMATE

The combination of phentermine and extended-release topiramate has been approved for weight loss. Phentermine is a nonselective stimulator of synaptic noradrenaline, dopamine, and serotonin release. It is an effective appetite suppressant.[10] Topiramate is an anticonvulsant medication which has been shown to induce weight loss.[11] However, it has not been used as monotherapy due to cognitive and psychiatric effects.[12] The combination of these medications allows use of lower doses of each medication. Three doses of the combination were evaluated: phentermine/topiramate 3.75/23, 7.5/46, and 15/92 mg.

The EQUIP trial, a placebo-controlled trial comparing placebo with the 3.75/23 and 15/92 mg doses, enrolled 1267 patients with a BMI over 35 kg/m^2.[13] The placebo group lost a mean 1.6% of weight, while the 3.75/23 mg group lost 5.1% of weight and the 15/92 mg group lost 10.9% of weight after 56 weeks. The CONQUER trial included 2487 patients with a BMI of 27–45 kg/m^2 (or any BMI in patients with type 2 diabetes) and two weight-related comorbidities.[14] Patients were randomized to placebo, 7.5/46 mg, or 15/92 mg. Weight loss at 56 weeks was 1.4 kg in the placebo group, 8.1 kg in the medium-dose group, and 10.2 kg in the high-dose group. The average weight loss was 9.8% in the high-dose group versus 1.2% in the placebo group. 70% of patients in the high-dose group lost at least 5% of total body weight, versus 21% of the placebo group. The incidence of commonly reported side effects in the high-dose group were dry mouth (21%), paresthesia (21%), constipation (17%), insomnia (10%), dizziness (10%), and dysgeusia (10%). These were somewhat less prevalent in the medium dose group. At the end of a second year of treatment, reported in the 676-patient SEQUEL study, patients on the medium dose maintained a weight loss of 9.3% below baseline, and patients on the high dose maintained a weight loss of 10.7% below baseline.[15]

Phentermine/topiramate should be initiated at a dose of 3.75/23 mg daily for two weeks. At that time, the dose can be doubled. After two weeks, the dose can be increased to 7.5/46 mg daily. If 3% of total body weight is not lost from the baseline by 12 weeks, the drug should be discontinued or escalated to 11.25/69 mg daily for two weeks and then 15/92 mg daily. If weight loss of 5% from the baseline is not reached after 12 weeks of this dose, the drug should be discontinued. Notable adverse events, other than those reported in the CONQUER trial, can include palpitations, metabolic acidosis, renal calculi, headache, hypokalemia, acute myopia, and secondary angle closure glaucoma.[16] Cognitive dysfunction, including attention disturbances, language and memory difficulty, and confusion may develop and warrant cessation of driving and cessation of the medication. Monoamine oxidase inhibitors should not be used concurrently. Additionally, teratogenicity is a concern, and women of childbearing potential must have a negative pregnancy test prior to starting the medication, and a negative pregnancy test monthly while on the medication. Pregnancy requires immediate discontinuation. Finally, the medication has not been studied in patients with unstable or recent cardiovascular or cerebrovascular disease.

15.2.4 GLP-1 RECEPTOR AGONISTS

Although GLP-1 receptor agonists are currently approved for treatment of diabetes mellitus, they have demonstrated effectiveness for induction of weight loss in both diabetics and nondiabetics. A meta-analysis of 21 trials (6411 subjects) including overweight or obese patients (with or without diabetes) showed greater weight loss in the GLP-1 agonist group than in controls. The magnitude of the weight difference was 2.9 kg.[17] A randomized trial of liraglutide in 564 adults with a BMI between 30 kg/m^2 and 40 kg/m^2 compared liraglutide with orlistat and placebo.[18] Diet and exercise counseling was provided. The liraglutide 3.0 mg group lost 5.8 kg more than the placebo group and 3.8 kg more than the orlistat group during the first year. At 2 years, the liraglutide group lost 3.0 kg more than the orlistat group. The prevalence of metabolic syndrome decreased by 59% over 2 years. The SCALE trial examined the effectiveness of liraglutide in weight maintenance in patients who had lost at least 5% of total body weight with a low-calorie diet.[19] Patients were randomly assigned to liraglutide 3.0 mg daily or to placebo for 56 weeks; diet and exercise counseling were provided throughout. During this period, patients on liraglutide lost 6.1% more weight than the placebo group, whose weight remained stable. During these trials, patients experienced nausea and vomiting, which were usually transient. Concern has been raised about the relationship between GLP-1 agonists and pancreatitis, pancreatic cancer, and thyroid cancer.[20]

15.3 ENDOSCOPIC PROCEDURES

Current endoscopic procedures for weight loss are restrictive, malabsorptive, space-occupying, or aspiration therapy. Restrictive procedures include restrictive implants and endoscopic gastroplasty. Malabsorptive devices preclude caloric absorption by the small intestine. Space-occupying devices include the intragastric balloon. Additionally, endoscopic procedures are being used to address the growing population of patients with weight regain after gastric bypass. These procedures will be discussed below.

15.3.1 RESTRICTIVE PROCEDURES

Restrictive procedures reduce gastric volume using suturing or tissue anchors. These procedures continue to evolve.

The TransOral GAstroplasty (TOGA) system (Satiety, Palo Alto, CA) is a flexible stapler for full-thickness tissue apposition. The device has been used for endoscopic gastroplasty. Vacuum suction is used to appose the gastric walls. A partition is then created parallel to the lesser curvature. The device must be removed, reloaded, and reinserted. TOGA was studied in 21 patients with an average BMI of 43.3 kg/m^2.[21] Although vomiting, pain, nausea, and transient dysphagia were reported, no serious adverse events occurred. A partially or fully intact stapled sleeve was found in each patient at six months, although 13 patients had gaps. The average weight loss was 12 kg after six months (24.4% excess weight loss). A subsequent study of TOGA was performed using a second-generation device in 11 patients.[22] Retreatment was performed to create additional distal restrictions when necessary. No serious adverse events were reported. The average weight loss after three months was 17.5 kg, and after six months was 24.0 kg. BMI decreased from a mean of 41.6–33.1 kg/m^2 at six months. A subsequent multicenter study of 67 patients (with follow-up in 53 patients) reported 52.2% excess weight loss in patients with a BMI ≥40 and 41.3% excess weight loss in patients with a BMI <40 kg/m^2.[23] The hemoglobin A1c decreased from 7.0% to 5.7%, and there were significant improvements in HDL and triglyceride levels. However, respiratory insufficiency was reported in one case and asymptomatic pneumoperitoneum was reported in another. Twenty-nine patients with an average BMI of 41.7 kg/m^2 had TOGA at a single center.[24] At 2 years, the average BMI had fallen to 35.5 kg/m^2, with a 14.9% total body weight loss and an average loss of 16.8 kg.

The EndoCinch (Bard Davol, Murray Hill, NJ) is a superficial-thickness suturing device. The device has a hollow capsule at the endoscope tip, which is used to suction mucosa and trap tissue. A needle is then passed through the tissue. The EndoCinch has been used to perform endoscopic gastroplasty in multiple studies including both adolescents and adults. A study of 64 patients by Fogel et al. (not IRB-approved) with an average BMI of 39.9 kg/m^2 categorized participants into three groups.[25] Group 1 had BMI ≥40 kg/m^2 (33 patients), Group 2 had BMI 35–40 kg/m^2 (19 patients), and Group 3 had BMI of <35 kg/m^2 (12 patients). No serious adverse events were reported, and no patients required overnight observation. 94.1% of patients were available for 1-year follow-up. Patients lost an average 39.6% ± 11.3% of excess weight at three months, and 58.1% ± 19.9% of excess weight at 1 year. A subsequent study was made of 21 adolescents (aged 13–17) with mean BMI of 36.2 kg/m^2.[26] Weight loss was 63.8% of EWL at six months, 67.3% of EWL at 12 months, and 61.5% of EWL at 18 months.

The RESTORe Suturing System, a modified version of the EndoCinch, is capable of both suture reloading without removal of the endoscope and full-thickness suturing. A two-site trial of endoscopic gastroplasty included 18 patients at two sites.[27] An average six plications were created, with an average procedure time of 125 ± 23 min. No significant adverse events were reported. The average 1-year weight loss was 11.0 ± 10 kg, or 27.7 ± 21.9% excess weight loss. Half of the study group lost more than 30% of excess weight. Waist circumference decreased by 12.6 ± 9.5 cm on average. There was a significant decrease in blood pressure (15.2 mm Hg systolic, 9.7 mm Hg diastolic). Despite the improvements over the EndoCinch, partial or complete release of plications was found in 13/18 patients on follow-up endoscopy.

TERIS (Trans-oral Endoscopic Restrictive Implant System, Barosense, Menlo Park, CA) is a diaphragm with a 10 mm orifice. The diaphragm is stapled into the gastric cardia. A study of 13 patients reported 12 successful placements, with one unsuccessful procedure due to gastric perforation.[28] Additionally, pneumoperitoneum was reported in two patients. As a result of these events, the procedure was modified; no further complications occurred. Procedure time was 142 min on average. At three-month follow-up, the median BMI fell from 42.1 kg/m^2 to 37.9 kg/m^2. The three-month weight loss was 16.9 kg, or 22.2% of excess weight.

Apollo OverStitch (Apollo Endosurgery, Austin, TX) can place interrupted or running stitches under direct endoscopic visualization using a curved needle driver and catheter-based anchor. This device has been used to perform endoscopic sleeve gastroplasty. Initial human cases were performed in a three-center international study: a pilot study of 5 patients to demonstrate safety and feasibility, followed by 23 cases in patients with an average BMI of 34.2 ± 1.1 kg/m^2.[29] Running stitches were placed in a triangular configuration starting in the antrum and moving proximally. These were reinforced with interrupted stitches. After 1 year, the average BMI had decreased to 29.4 kg/m^2. The procedure was also studied in a single-center pilot trial including four patients.[30] Two parallel rows of interrupted plications were created to fashion a gastric sleeve. Patients were placed on a four-week liquid diet and two-week pureed diet.

Incisionless Operating Platform (USGI Medical, San Clemente, CA) is capable of performing full-thickness tissue plication. The IOP contains multiple channels: a 4.9 mm endoscope is passed through one channel for endoscopic visualization, and a tissue grasper and a tissue approximator are passed through two other channels. The tissue grasper is used to acquire tissue, and then the tissue approximator is used to drive a needle through the tissue. Plications are cinched using tissue anchors (Figure 15.1). The device has been used to perform the Primary Obesity Surgery Endolumenal (POSE) procedure. Eight to nine plications are created in the gastric fundus and 3–4 in the distal gastric body. A study of 45 patients (mean BMI 36.7 ± 3.8 kg/m^2) reported weight loss of 16.3 ± 7.1 kg or $15.5 \pm 6.1\%$ of total weight at six months.[31] The BMI fell by 5.8 ± 2.5 kg/m^2. Adverse events associated with the procedure included low-grade fever, chest pain, abdominal pain, sore throat, and nausea; there was no device-related morbidity.

15.3.2 Malabsorptive Procedures

Bypass of the small intestine is part of many bariatric surgical procedures, such as Roux-en-Y gastric bypass, and is considered to play a fundamental role in the metabolic benefits seen after these surgeries. Endoluminal devices have been developed to bypass contact between oral intake and the mucosa of the small intestine.

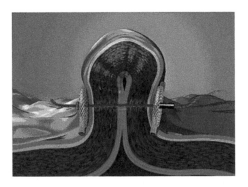

FIGURE 15.1   **(See color insert.)** Plication of tissue using the incisionless operating platform. (From Espinós JC et al. *Obes Surg* 2013;23(9):1375–1383.)

The EndoBarrier duodenal–jejunal bypass liner (DJBL, GI Dynamics, Lexington, MA) comprises an implant and a sleeve. The implant is a self-expanding nickel–titanium device which attaches to a 60 cm polymer tube extending into the jejunum. Although oral intake of nutrients is precluded from contact with the mucosa of the small intestine, biliary and pancreatic secretions are able to travel along the outside of the sleeve into the jejunum. A multicenter randomized trial including 41 patients assigned 30 patients (BMI 48.9 kg/m^2) to DJBL and 11 patients (BMI 47.4 kg/m^2) to diet control.[32] Of the 30 DJBL patients, four required device removal after migration, obstruction, pain, or anchor dislocation. No serious adverse events were reported. At a three-month follow-up, the DJBL group had a BMI decrease of 5.5 kg/m^2, versus 1.9 kg/m^2 in control patients. Seven of eight diabetics in the DJBL group had an improvement in diabetes. A subsequent open-label multicenter randomized trial of 25 patients reported successful DJBL placement in 21 patients.[33] Implantation failed in patients with small duodenal bulb size. Of 21 patients successfully implanted, seven patients experienced adverse events requiring device removal. Three of seven patients experienced bleeding presenting as hematemesis. Three-month weight loss was significantly higher in patients with DJBL: 8.2 ± 1.3 kg versus 2.0 ± 1.1 kg. Another randomized trial enrolled 25 patients in the DJBL group and 14 patients in the control group.[34] Patients in both groups had baseline diet and lifestyle counseling. 12-week follow-up revealed 22% excess weight loss in the DJBL group, versus 5% excess weight loss in the control group. Adverse events, including bleeding, migration, and obstruction, were reported in 20% of patients.

A modified DJBL with a 4 mm restrictive orifice was studied in 10 patients (average BMI 40.8 kg/m^2).[35] Three-months weight loss was 16.7 ± 1.4 kg. Of 10 patients in the trial, eight developed abdominal pain, nausea, and vomiting, requiring balloon dilation of the restrictive orifice. Delayed gastric emptying was noted in 84% of patients at three months, but improved in most cases after device removal.

Longer-term outcomes after DJBL implantation were studied in a 1-year prospective open-label trial.[36] Thirty-nine patients (average BMI 43.7 ± 5.9 kg/m^2) had DJBL placement; a short duodenal bulb precluded implantation in three patients. Of 39 implanted patients, 15 required premature removal due to anchor movement (in eight patients), device obstruction (in three patients), abdominal pain (in two patients), acute cholecystitis (in one patient), and patient request (in one patient). The average weight loss in the 24 patients with the device in place for 1 year was 22.1 ± 2.1 kg, with a BMI loss of 9.1 ± 0.9 kg/m^2, and excess weight loss of 47.0 ± 4.4%. There was a significant decrease in waist circumference, from 120.5 ± 6.8 to 96.0 ± 2.6 cm. Additionally, statistically significant improvements in blood pressure, hemoglobin A1c, total cholesterol, LDL, triglycerides, and in the prevalence of metabolic syndrome were reported.

A randomized trial of patients with type II diabetes (an average hemoglobin A1c of 9.2%, and an average BMI of 38.9 kg/m^2) assigned 12 patients to DJBL or to sham endoscopy.[37] Diet and lifestyle counseling was provided to all patients, with a controlled low-calorie diet during the follow-up period. Self-monitoring of glucose levels was required, and patients on sulfonylurea medications were advised to cut the dose in half when the device was implanted. The hemoglobin A1c fell by 2.4 ± 0.7% in the DJBL patients at six months, versus a fall of 0.8 ± 0.4% in the sham arm. The result did not reach significance, although postprandial plasma glucose did decrease significantly more in the DJBL group after one week (19% versus 11%).

15.3.3 SPACE-OCCUPYING DEVICES

Space-occupying devices include balloons and polymers. These devices displace volume and can induce gastric distention; they may also alter gastric motility and hormone levels.[38] The intragastric balloon has been approved for use in the United States since 1985. Despite its noninvasiveness, the technology has not achieved broad use in the United States during the past 30 years. Currently, intragastric balloons are primarily in use in Europe, where they have found a role as a bridge to definitive therapy.

The BioEnterics Intragastric Balloon (BIB, Allergan, Irvine, CA) is an endoscopically implanted silicone elastomer device.[38] Once placed in the stomach, it is filled with saline. The injection of a methylene blue dye changes the color of urine if the balloon leaks. The device is resistant to the effects of gastric acid for six months.

Compared with other endoscopic weight loss technologies, the BIB has been studied in a large number of patients. A meta-analysis including 3698 patients found a six-month average weight loss of 14.7 kg, 32.1% of excess weight, and decrease in BMI by 5.7 kg/m^2.[39] The device was removed early in 4.2% of patients, and complications included nausea, vomiting, bowel obstruction (0.8%), and gastric perforation (0.1%). A retrospective study of the balloon including 2515 patients (average BMI 44.4 kg/m^2) reported six-month decrease in BMI of 9.0 kg/m^2.[40] There was significant improvement in comorbidities, including blood pressure, lipid profile, and fasting glucose. Of the 488 diabetic patients in the series, 87.2% had significant decrease in or normalization of the hemoglobin A1c level. Notably, there were two mortalities after BIB placement, both in patients who had had prior gastric surgery.

A prospective study of 130 patients (average BMI 43.1 kg/m^2) reported metabolic changes after BIB placement.[41] Patients were maintained on 1000–1200 kcal daily during the six-month follow-up period. The result was a weight loss of 13.1 kg at six months, and a decrease in class IV obesity from 23% to 8% of patients. Significant metabolic improvements included a decrease in hyperglycemia from 50% to 12%, and a decrease in hypertriglyceridemia from 58% to 19%. In patients with a BMI decrease greater than 3.5 kg/m^2, the prevalence of severe hepatic steatosis decreased from 52% to 4%. Early balloon removal was required in ten patients, of which six were due to intolerance, abdominal pain, or vomiting. During the follow-up period after BIB removal (median 22 months), 50% of patients regained some weight.

Dietitian counseling after BIB placement has been studied in 28 patients with a mean BMI of 32.4 ± 3.7 kg/m^2.[42] After six months, the average BMI had decreased to 28.5 ± 3.7 kg/m^2. While the BIB was in place, patients saw the dietitian in follow-up weekly for two weeks, every two weeks for one month, and then monthly. Patients were classified as having good adherence if they appeared for 50% of scheduled visits. Responders were patients who achieved at least 20% excess weight loss. At the time of balloon removal, 20 patients were classified as responders and 8 were classified as nonresponders. Of the responders, 85% had good adherence versus 25% of nonresponders.

Histologic improvement in nonalcoholic steatohepatitis after placement of the BIB was studied in a prospective single-blinded clinical trial.[43] 11 patients were randomized to BIB placement, and 10 patients were randomized to sham endoscopy with instillation of 500 mL of saline into the stomach. All patients were on the American Heart Association diet. Three of 11 patients in the BIB group required early removal of the balloon due to epigastric discomfort and vomiting. At the end of treatment, BMI had decreased by 1.6 kg/m^2 in the BIB group, versus a decrease 0.8 kg/m^2 in controls. Furthermore, the NAFLD activity score was significantly lower in the BIB group (2 versus 4). However, there was no change in histologic characteristics of median lobular inflammation, hepatocellular ballooning, or fibrosis. Additionally, serum ALT and AST measurements did not change significantly in either group.

The effect of BIB therapy on depression was studied in 100 consecutive female patients.[44] Patients were characterized as depressed (65 patients) or nondepressed (35 patients) using the Beck Depression Inventory score. Other characteristics of the groups were similar. Weight loss of 39.3% of excess weight was reported in the depressed group, similar to the 36.1% excess weight loss in the nondepressed group. However, the depressed group experienced a marked improvement in depression score (20.3 ± 8.5 to 7.9 ± 5.6) at the time of BIB removal. 70.8% of the depressed patients had resolution of depression, and the prevalence of severe depression declined (27.7%–1.5%).

The efficacy of repeat BIB insertion was studied in 118 patients.[45] Of this group, eight patients underwent immediate BIB reinsertion, 11 patients underwent BIB placement after a balloon-free interval, and 99 patients did not have repeat BIB placement. Patients with a second BIB placement after a balloon-free interval regained an average 13.6 kg during the balloon-free interval. The second BIB placement was less effective than the first BIB placement, with significantly less weight loss (9.0 kg weight loss after the second BIB versus 14.6 kg weight loss after the first BIB). There was also significantly less excess weight loss (18.2% after the second BIB versus 49.3% after the first BIB) with the second BIB therapy. The complication rate was higher with the second BIB (26% versus 11%), although this did not reach significance. By the third year of follow-up, weight loss was no different in patients who had had a second BIB placement. Additionally, the second BIB placement had no effect on the proportion of patients achieving ≥10% weight loss or in the rate of patients having bariatric surgery during the post-BIB follow-up period. Another study of 112 patients undergoing a second BIB placement (within one month of removing the first BIB) found that mean BMI loss was 6.5 kg/m^2 after the first BIB, versus 2.5 kg/m^2 with the second BIB.[46]

A study of long-term weight loss in 500 patients after BIB removal (initial BMI 43.7 kg/m^2) defined success as excess weight loss of at least 20%.[47] 83% of patients met this threshold at the time of BIB removal; these patients had an average weight loss of 23.9 ± 9.1 kg and an average BMI loss of 8.3 kg/m^2. 41% of the original cohort was available for a 5-year follow-up; this group had an average weight loss of 7.3 ± 5.4 kg and an average BMI loss of 2.5 kg/m^2. At 5 years, 23% of patients maintained a weight loss of at least 20% of excess weight.

The BIB has been studied as a bridge to RYGB in 60 consecutive super-super obese patients (mean BMI of 66.5 ± 3.4 kg/m^2).[48] Twenty-three patients had BIB placement, while 37 patients did not. In the BIB group, the device was left in place for 155 ± 62 days. The BIB group experienced BMI loss of 5.5 ± 1.3 kg/m^2 at the time of surgery, as well as significant decrease in both systolic blood pressure and gamma-glutamyl transpeptidase. The operative time for performance of Roux-en-Y gastric bypass was significantly shorter in the BIB group (146 ± 47 versus 201 ± 81 min). Additionally, there were significantly fewer major adverse events (defined as conversion to laparotomy, ICU stay longer than two days, and total hospital stay longer than two weeks) in the BIB group—2 versus 13. Weight loss was similar between groups at 1 year after gastric bypass.

The Heliosphere BAG, which is filled with 950 mL of air, has been compared with the BIB, which is filled with 500 mL of saline.[49] Both balloons are shown in Figure 15.2. Thirty patients (average BMI 46.3 kg/m^2) were randomized to each device. The Heliosphere group experienced a decrease in BMI of 4.2 kg/m^2, versus 5.7 kg/m^2 in the BIB group. The Heliosphere group experienced significantly longer procedure time for extraction, and significantly more discomfort during the extraction procedure. A nonrandomized study compared the Heliosphere BAG with the BIB in patients who did not respond to six months of medical and diet therapy.[50] The Heliosphere BAG was placed in 13 patients (mean BMI 45.0 ± 8 kg/m^2), while the BIB was placed in 19 patients (BMI 45.6 ± 9 kg/m^2). The Heliosphere BAG was not as effective as the BIB, with a weight loss of 13.0 kg versus 19.0 kg. However, one patient in the BIB group required removal at one month for persistent nausea and vomiting. Another patient in the BIB group died 13 days after placement after having a cardiac arrest related to the aspiration of gastric contents.

The Duo (Reshape, San Clemente, CA) contains two silicone spheres filled with 900 mL of saline. Deflation of one balloon will not result in device migration. Reports from the company disclose that patients have had loss of one-third of excess weight at six months. A prospective trial studied the Duo in 30 patients (21 Duo and 9 control) at three centers.[51] Both groups were provided with counseling regarding

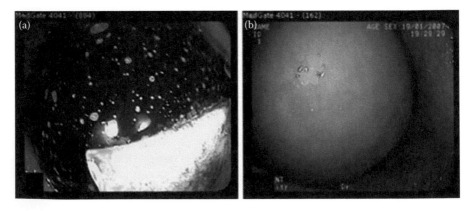

FIGURE 15.2 **(See color insert.)** BioEnterics Intragastric Balloon (a) and Heliosphere BAG (b). (From Caglar E, Dobrucali A, Bal K. *Dig Endosc* 2013;25(5):502–507.)

diet and lifestyle measures. Four of 21 Duo patients required readmission for nausea, and two patients had gastritis at balloon removal. After 48 weeks, 30% of the Duo patients had lost 25% of excess weight, compared with 25% of the control patients.

The Transpyloric Shuttle (BAROnova, Goleta, CA) is made from a large spherical bulb and a smaller cylindrical bulb connected by a flexible tether. The spherical bulb is too large to traverse the pylorus, while the cylindrical bulb is designed to enter the duodenal bulb during peristalsis. The device reduces gastric emptying rate by intermittently occluding the pylorus. The Transpyloric Shuttle is delivered transorally via catheter, but it must be removed endoscopically. An open-label prospective study of 20 patients at a single center (average BMI of 36.0 kg/m^2) found a weight loss of 8.9 ± 5.2 kg, or $31.3 \pm 15.7\%$ of excess weight, at three months.[52] At six months, the weight loss was 14.6 ± 5.7 kg, or $50.0 \pm 26.4\%$ of excess weight. Early removal of the device due to persistent ulcers was necessary in two patients.

The SatiSphere (Endosphere, Columbus, OH) is made from a preformed memory wire that conforms to the shape of the duodenum, anchoring itself in the distal stomach and in the duodenum. The SatiSphere slows the travel of food through the duodenum, which can alter satiety hormone levels and glucose metabolism. A trial including 31 patients (average BMI 41.3 kg/m^2) compared 21 SatiSphere patients with 10 control patients.[53] Migration of the SatiSphere was reported in 10 of 21 implanted patients. Emergency surgery was necessary in two patients. At three months, the SatiSphere patients lost an average 6.7 kg, versus 2.2 kg in the control group. Additionally, the device was found to delay absorption of glucose, delay secretion of insulin, and to change GLP-1 kinetics.

15.3.4 ASPIRATION THERAPY

A modified percutaneous endoscopic gastrostomy tube can be placed for the purpose of aspirating a portion of ingested caloric intake from the stomach.[54] The device comprises a large-bore gastrostomy tube with holes in the intragastric portion, a skin port including a valve placed at the skin, a connector, and a 600 mL reservoir that allows flushing and aspiration of the stomach (A-tube and AspireAssist, Aspire Bariatrics, King of Prussia, PA). The device is shown in Figure 15.3. The device was studied in a randomized trial of 18 patients, with 11 patients randomized to receive the device and seven patients in the control group. All patients had lifestyle therapy consisting of a 15-session diet and behavioral education program. 10/11 Aspire patients and 4/7 control patients completed 1 year of follow-up. Weight loss in the Aspire group was $18.6 \pm 2.3\%$ of total body weight versus $5.9 \pm 5.0\%$ in the control group. 7/10 of the Aspire patients who completed follow-up did an additional year, with maintenance of $20.1 \pm 3.5\%$ total body weight loss. There was no evidence of compensation manifested by increased intake to replace aspirated food. The most common adverse events were abdominal pain at the A-tube site (which improved after a device redesign), infection in three patients that resolved with topical medication or oral antibiotics, and persistent fistula in one of the four patients who had tube removal (the fistula eventually closed spontaneously).

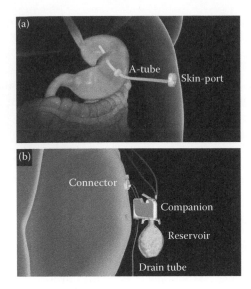

FIGURE 15.3 (**See color insert.**) Aspire A-tube (a) and AspireAssist (b). (From Sullivan S et al. *Gastroenterology* 2013;145(6):1245–1252.e1-5.)

15.3.4.1 Weight Regain

15.3.4.1.1 Gastric Bypass

Roux-en-Y gastric bypass is currently the most common postsurgical anatomy in bariatric surgery patients with weight regain.[55,56] Gastric bypass typically results in excess weight loss between 56.7% and 66.5% during the 24 months after surgery. There is commonly improvement in or resolution of comorbidities, including hypertension in 68%, diabetes in 84%, obstructive sleep apnea in 81%, and improvement in hyperlipidemia in 97%.[55–59] Although the multiple mechanisms responsible for postoperative weight loss and improvements in comorbidities have not been fully elucidated, it is postulated that part of the effect is due to a restrictive effect caused by the small gastric pouch size and gastrojejunal anastomotic aperture.

15.3.4.1.2 Postoperative Weight Regain

Weight regain can result in the recurrence of comorbidities, decreased quality of life, and adverse effects on mental health. After initial rapid weight loss, patients who have had a gastric bypass reach a stable weight once caloric intake and expenditure reach an equilibrium, typically 12–18 months after surgery.[60,61] Approximately one-fifth of patients fail to lose more than 50% of excess weight within 1 year after surgery. Approximately 30% of patients have regained weight by 18–24 months after surgery, and regain of an average 18 kg has been reported at 2 years.[62,63] Patients with a BMI >50 kg/m² do not reach a BMI of less than 35 kg/m² in 60% of cases.[64,65] Long-term results after RYGB are affected by many factors, including preoperative BMI and postoperative adherence to dietary and lifestyle recommendations.[66]

Additionally, neuroendocrine-metabolic dysregulation can induce a starvation-like response, resulting in elevated appetite and decreased metabolic rate.[67,68] Loss of restriction can also result from larger pouch size and larger diameter of the gastrojejunal anastomosis, which has been shown to correlate with increased weight regain after RYGB.[69–72]

15.3.5 TREATMENT OF WEIGHT REGAIN

Although several surgical procedures are available to address post-RYGB weight regain, including reconstruction of the gastrojejunal anastomosis and placement of an adjustable gastric band over the gastric pouch, few patients with weight regain undergo surgical revision.[73] Surgeons are faced with older patients, altered anatomy, and adhesions.[74] Complication and mortality rates are higher than that of the primary surgery.[75,76] Endoluminal revision to reduce gastrojejunal anastomosis diameter may be a better option in this patient set. Endoscopic sclerotherapy, tissue plication, and endoscopic suturing are discussed below.

15.3.5.1 Sclerotherapy

Endoscopic sclerotherapy is performed by injecting a sclerosant around the margin of the gastrojejunal anastomosis. The use of sodium morrhuate as a sclerosant has been reported in multiple studies. The procedure can be performed under conscious sedation. First, a test dose is injected at the rim of the anastomosis, and the patient is monitored for an adverse reaction. Approximately 2 mL of the sclerosing agent should be injected into the submucosa at the margin of the gastrojejunal anastomosis until a bleb forms. Several injections should be performed around the anastomosis, for a total injection of 10–25 mL.[77] Overinjection can cause dark red or black discoloration, followed by overt bleeding. Prophylactic ciprofloxacin should be given intravenously prior to the procedure, and a five-day course of liquid ciprofloxacin or trimethoprim-sulfamethoxazole after the procedure. The patent should remain *nil per os* for one day postprocedure, and then advance from a liquid diet to a regular diet during the month after the procedure. The procedure should be repeated every three to six months until the anastomosis aperture has decreased to 12 mm. Two or three sessions are typically required.[78] The anastomotic aperture should be measured at the start of the subsequent sclerotherapy procedure, as the aperture at the end of the procedure is temporarily reduced due to edema.[77] After multiple sclerotherapy procedures, the development of scar tissue can make submucosal injection difficult.

Endoscopic sclerotherapy has proven effective to treat post-RYGB weight regain. An early study reported weight loss in 15/20 patients within eight weeks.[78] A study of 28 patients reported a loss of greater than 75% of the regained weight in 64% of patients. Two or three sessions were required on average. Patients with an anastomotic diameter larger than 15 mm did not benefit.[79] Another study of 32 patients reported arrest or reversal of weight regain in 91.6% of the patients after 1 year.[77] A study of 71 patients reported weight maintenance or loss in 72% of the patients after 1 year.[79]

15.3.5.1.1 Endoscopic Suturing and Plication

Endoscopic suturing has been studied for revision of dilated gastric pouch and gastrojejunal anastomosis after RYGB. The EndoCinch Suturing System, StomaphyX, Incisionless Operating Platform, and Overstitch are discussed below.

15.3.5.2 EndoCinch Suturing System

The EndoCinch Suturing System is a superficial-thickness suturing device, which uses suction to trap mucosa within a hollow cylinder at the endoscope tip. A needle is then passed through the tissue. The EndoCinch has been used to perform a transoral outlet reduction (TORe), or an endoscopic revision of the gastric bypass. The aperture of the gastrojejunal anastomosis can be reduced by the placement of interrupted stitches at the anastomotic margin. First, the entire gastric margin of the anastomosis is treated with argon plasma coagulation. Sutures are placed across the anastomosis and then cinched, reducing the diameter of the anastomosis. The volume of the gastric pouch can be reduced by creating ridges and suturing them together.

The use of the EndoCinch to perform TORe was first reported in 2004.[80] The first study to be published included eight patients with an average anastomotic diameter of 25 mm.[81] The average weight regain was 24 kg from nadir postoperative weight. An average of two interrupted stitches was placed to reduce anastomotic size to an average of 10 mm. No significant adverse events occurred. Six of the eight patients lost weight; the average weight loss at four months was 10 kg. Three patients had repeat TORe; two of these had a weight loss of 19 kg and 20 kg by five months after the procedure. The average BMI fell from 40.5 kg/m² to 37.7 kg/m².

RESTORe, a randomized sham-controlled double-blinded multicenter trial, resulted in level 1 evidence for the effectiveness of endoscopic suturing for the revision of gastric bypass.[82] 77 patients with a gastrojejunal anastomosis aperture larger than 20 mm were included. The average BMI was 47.6 kg/m². The anastomotic aperture was reduced to <10 mm in 89% of subjects undergoing TORe. There were no perforations, and there was no difference in the rate of adverse events between groups. The TORe patients lost an average 3.8% of body weight, versus a loss of 0.3% in the sham group in intent-to-treat analysis ($p = 0.02$). 96% of TORe patients achieved weight loss or stabilization during the six-month follow-up period.

15.3.5.3 StomaphyX

StomaphyX (EndoGastric Solutions, Redmond, WA) passes polypropylene H-fasteners through tissue to create full-thickness plications. Endoscopic reduction of the gastrojejunal anastomosis aperture can be performed by applying approximately 20 fasteners circumferentially around the margin of the anastomosis. A study of 39 patients (average BMI 39.8 kg/m²) reported 13.1% EWL after three months and 19.5% EWL after 1 year; there were no significant adverse events.[83] A subsequent study of 64 patients (average BMI 39.5 kg/m²) reported placement of 23 plications and concomitant reduction of anastomotic diameter from 22 mm to 9 mm.[84] Procedure time was an average of 50 min. One patient had bleeding that did not require transfusion. There were no other significant adverse events. The average weight loss was 7.6 kg at the end of the follow-up period (average 5.8 months).

15.3.5.4   Incisionless Operating Platform

Incisionless Operating Platform (USGI Medical, San Clemente, CA) is capable of performing full-thickness tissue plication. The device contains multiple channels. A 4.9 mm diameter endoscope passes through one channel for endoscopic visualization. A tissue grasper and a tissue approximator are passed through two other channels. The tissue grasper is used to acquire tissue, and the tissue approximator is then used to drive a needle through the tissue. The tissue is plicated together using tissue anchors.[85]

IOP has been studied for the reduction of the dilated gastric pouch and gastrojejunal anastomosis in a prospective study called Revision Obesity Surgery Endolumenal (ROSE). 20 patients with weight regain were included; technical success was achieved in 85% of patients, with a reduction of the anastomotic aperture by 65% and a reduction of gastric pouch length by 36%. At the end of the procedure, the mean anastomotic aperture was 16 mm. The average weight loss was 8.8 kg at three months. The device has been improved subsequently. One subsequent iteration was studied in five patients, with resulting weight loss in all five (average weight loss of 7.8 kg).[86] A prospective multicenter study including 116 patients with a dilated gastrojejunal anastomosis and gastric pouch reported technical success in 97% of patients.[87] The gastrojejunal anastomosis aperture was reduced by an average of 50%, and gastric pouch length was reduced by an average 44%. No procedural complications occurred. Patients with an anastomotic aperture of less than 10 mm at the end of the procedure experienced loss of 24% of excess weight. During the six-month follow-up period, the entire group lost 32% of the weight regained after RYGB.

15.3.5.5   Apollo OverStitch

OverStitch (Apollo Endosurgery, Austin, TX) uses a curved needle driver and catheter-based anchor to place interrupted or running stitches under direct endoscopic visualization. OverStitch is capable of placing full-thickness sutures, and it does not need to be removed to reload sutures. The device is designed to be used with a double-channel endoscope. A helical tissue retraction accessory can be used through the empty channel of the double-channel endoscope. Transoral outlet reduction can be performed using a pursestring technique, with placement of a pursestring suture around the gastrojejunal anastomosis. Argon plasma coagulation or endoscopic mucosal resection can be performed around the margin of the anastomosis for preparation. A controlled radial expansion balloon can be passed through the second channel of the endoscope and inflated to 8–10 mm. The pursestring can be tightened around this balloon, allowing precise control over final anastomotic aperture. Two pursestrings can be placed around the anastomosis. The change in anastomotic aperture is demonstrated in Figure 15.4.

OverStitch has proven effective for endoscopic revision of gastric bypass in a study of 25 patients.[88] The average gastrojejunal anastomosis aperture was reduced from 26.4 to 6 mm, and no significant adverse events were noted. Patients lost 69.5% of the regained weight during the six-month follow-up period, with an average weight loss of 11.7 kg.

Endoscopic revision of gastric bypass using the superficial-thickness EndoCinch and full-thickness OverStitch devices have been compared directly in a matched

(a)   (b)   (c)

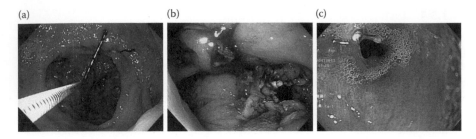

FIGURE 15.4 (See color insert.) Gastrojejunal anastomosis before (a), immediately after (b), and six months after TORe using Apollo OverStitch (c). (From Kumar N and Thompson CC. *Gastrointest Endosc* 2014;79(6):984–989.)

cohort study.[89] A total of 118 patients (59 in each group) were matched sequentially by gastrojejunal anastomosis aperture, then BMI, and then age. After six months, the average weight loss was 4.4 ± 0.8 kg in the EndoCinch group versus 10.6 ± 1.8 kg in the OverStitch group ($p < 0.01$). Weight loss after 1 year was 2.9 ± 1.0 kg in the EndoCinch group versus 8.6 ± 2.5 kg in the OverStitch group ($p < 0.01$).

15.4 CONCLUSION

Despite the availability of dietary counseling, exercise programs, lifestyle modification, and bariatric surgery, the reach of the global obesity epidemic has continued to expand. New pharmacologic therapies and endoscopic bariatric therapies will potentially play an important role in the treatment of obesity in the near future. Additionally, endoscopic procedures are proving their safety and efficacy for the treatment of weight regain after gastric bypass.

15.5 CASE STUDY

A 53-year-old-female with history of open Roux-en-Y gastric bypass 8 years prior presents with weight regain. She had a BMI of 51.1 kg/m^2 prior to the procedure and reached a low BMI of 38 kg/m^2 within 18 months of gastric bypass. Since then, she has regained weight steadily. She has attempted multiple diets without success. Exercise is limited by bilateral osteoarthritis in her knees. Although diabetes mellitus, hypertension, and obstructive sleep apnea resolved after the procedure, her hemoglobin A1c has now increased to 7.8%.

This patient was referred for endoscopy to examine the gastric pouch for gastrogastric fistula and to measure the pouch length and the gastrojejunal anastomosis aperture. Although no fistula was found, the gastric pouch was wide and the anastomosis was dilated to 35 mm (10 mm is ideal). The Apollo OverStitch was used to reduce the anastomotic aperture to 10 mm around a controlled radial expansion balloon. She lost 12 kg in the six months after the procedure.

REFERENCES

1. Finucane M, Stevens G, Cowan M et al. National, regional, and global trends in body-mass index since 1980: Systematic analysis of health examination surveys and epidemiological studies with 960 country-years and 9.1 million participants. *Lancet* 2011;377:557–567.
2. Whitlock G, Lewington S, Sherliker P et al. Body-mass index and cause-specific mortality in 900,000 adults: Collaborative analyses of 57 prospective studies. *Lancet* 2009;373:1083–1096.
3. Lucas KH and Kaplan-Machlis B. Orlistat—A novel weight loss therapy. *Ann Pharmacother* 2001;35:314–328.
4. Rucker D, Padwal R, Li SK et al. Long term pharmacotherapy for obesity and over-weight: Updated meta-analysis. *BMJ* 2007;335:1194–1199.
5. Fiorella D, Helsley S, Lorrain D, Rabin R, and Winter J. The role of the 5-HT2A and 5-HT2C receptors in the stimulus effects of hallucinogenic drugs. III: The mechanistic basis for supersensitivity to the LSD Stimulus following serotonin depletion. *Psychopharmacology (Berl)* 1995;121:364–372.
6. Smith S, Weissman N, Anderson C et al. Multicenter, placebo-controlled trial of lorcaserin for weight management. *N Engl J Med* 2010;363:245–256.
7. Fidler M, Sanchez M, Raether B et al. A one-year randomized trial of lorcaserin for weight loss in obese and overweight adults: The BLOSSOM trial. *J Clin Endocrinol Metab* 2011;96:3067–3077.
8. Chan E, He Y, Chui C, Wong A, Lau W, and Wong I. Efficacy and safety of lorcaserin in obese adults: A meta-analysis of 1-year randomized controlled trials (RCTs) and narrative review on short-term RCTs. *Obes Rev* 2013;14:383–392.
9. O'Neil P, Smith S, Weissman N et al. Randomized placebo-controlled clinical trial of lorcaserin for weight loss in type 2 diabetes mellitus: The BLOOM-DM study. *Obesity (Silver Spring)* 2012;20:1426–1436.
10. Ryan D and Bray G. Pharmacologic treatment options for obesity: What is old is new again. *Curr Hypertens Rep* 2013;15:182–189.
11. Astrup A, Caterson I, Zelissen P et al. Topiramate: Long term maintenance of weight loss induced by a low calorie diet in obese subjects. *Obes Res* 2004;12:1658–1669.
12. Nathan P, O'Neill B, Napolitano A, and Bullmore E. Neuropsychiatric adverse effects of centrally acting antiobesity drugs. *CNS Neurosci Ther* 2011;17:490–505.
13. Allison D, Gadde K, Garvey W et al. controlled release phentermine/topiramate in severely obese adults: A randomized controlled trial (EQUIP). *Obesity (Silver Spring)* 2012;20:330–342.
14. Gadde K, Allison D, Ryan D et al. Effects of low-dose controlled-release phentermine plus topiramate combination on weight and associated comorbidities in overweight and obese adults (CONQUER): A randomised placebo-controlled phase 3 trial. *Lancet* 2011;377:1341–1352.
15. Garvey WT, Ryan DH, Look M et al. Two-year sustained weight loss and metabolic benefits with controlled-release phentermine/topiramate in obese and overweight adults (SEQUEL): A randomized, placebo-controlled, phase 3 extension study. *Am J Clin Nutr* 2012;95(2):297–308.
16. Manning S, Pucci A, and Finer N. Pharmacotherapy for obesity: Novel agents and paradigms. *Ther Adv Chronic Dis* 2014;5(3):135–148.
17. Vilsboll T, Christensen M, Junker A, Knop F, and Gluud L. Effects of glucagon-like peptide-1 receptor agonists on weight loss: Systematic review and meta-analyses of randomised controlled trials. *BMJ* 2012;344:d7771.
18. Astrup A, Carraro R, Finer N et al. Safety, tolerability and sustained weight loss over 2 years with the once-daily human GLP-1 analog, liraglutide. *Int J Obes (Lond)* 2012;36(6):843–854.

19. Wadden TA, Hollander P, Klein S et al. Weight maintenance and additional weight loss with liraglutide after low-calorie-diet-induced weight loss: The SCALE Maintenance randomized study. *Int J Obes (Lond)* 2013;37(11):1443–1451.

20. Butler PC, Elashoff M, Elashoff R, and Gale EA. A critical analysis of the clinical use of incretin-based therapies: Are the GLP-1 therapies safe? *Diabetes Care* 2013;36(7):2118–2125.

21. Deviere J, Ojeda Valdes G, Cuevas Herrera L et al. Safety, feasibility and weight loss after transoral gastroplasty: First human multicenter study. *Surg Endosc* 2008;22:589–598.

22. Moreno C, Closset J, Dugardeyn S et al. Transoral gastroplasty is safe, feasible, and induces significant weight loss in morbidly obese patients: Results of the second human pilot study. *Endoscopy* 2008;40:406–413.

23. Familiari P, Costamagna G, Blero D et al. Transoral gastroplasty for morbid obesity: A multicenter trial with a 1-year outcome. *Gastrointest Endosc* 2011;74(6):1248–1258.

24. Nanni G, Familiari P, Mor A et al. Effectiveness of the Transoral Endoscopic Vertical Gastroplasty (TOGa®): A good balance between weight loss and complications, if compared with gastric bypass and biliopancreatic diversion. *Obes Surg* 2012;22(12):1897–1902.

25. Fogel R, De Fogel J, Bonilla Y et al. Clinical experience of transoral suturing for an endoluminal vertical gastroplasty: 1-year follow-up in 64 patients. *Gastrointest Endosc* 2008;68:51–58.

26. Fogel R and De Fogel J. Trans-oral vertical gastroplasty as a viable treatment for childhood obesity—A study of 21 adolescents with up to 18 months of follow-up. *Gastrointest Endosc* 2009;69(5):AB169–AB170.

27. Brethauer SA, Chand B, Schauer PR, and Thompson CC. Transoral gastric volume reduction as intervention for weight management: 12-month follow-up of TRIM trial. *Surg Obes Relat Dis* 2012;8(3):296–303.

28. de Jong K, Mathus-Vliegen EM, Veldhuyzen EA et al. Short-term safety and efficacy of the trans-oral endoscopic restrictive implant system for the treatment of obesity. *Gastrointest Endosc* 2010;72(3):497–504.

29. Kumar N, Sahdala HN, Shaikh S et al. Endoscopic sleeve gastroplasty for primary therapy of obesity: Initial human cases. *Gastroenterology* 2014;146(5):S571–S572.

30. Abu Dayyeh BK, Rajan E, and Gostout CJ. Endoscopic sleeve gastroplasty: A potential endoscopic alternative to surgical sleeve gastrectomy for treatment of obesity. *Gastrointest Endosc* 2013;78(3):530–535.

31. Espinós JC, Turró R, Mata A, Cruz M, da Costa M, Villa V, Buchwald JN, and Turró J. Early experience with the Incisionless Operating Platform™ (IOP) for the treatment of obesity: The Primary Obesity Surgery Endolumenal (POSE) procedure. *Obes Surg* 2013;23(9):1375–1383.

32. Schouten R, Rijs CS, Bouvy ND et al. A multicenter, randomized efficacy study of the EndoBarrier gastrointestinal liner for presurgical weight loss prior to bariatric surgery. *Ann Surg* 2010;251(2):236–243.

33. Gersin KS, Rothstein RI, Rosenthal RJ et al. Open-label, sham-controlled trial of an endoscopic duodenojejunal bypass liner for preoperative weight loss in bariatric surgery candidates. *Gastrointest Endosc* 2010;71(6):976–982.

34. Tarnoff M, Rodriguez L, Escalona A et al. Open label, prospective, randomized controlled trial of an endoscopic duodenal-jejunal bypass sleeve versus low calorie diet for pre-operative weight loss in bariatric surgery. *Surg Endosc* 2009;23(3):650–656.

35. Escalona A, Yáñez R, Pimentel F, Galvao et al. Initial human experience with restrictive duodenal-jejunal bypass liner for treatment of morbid obesity. *Surg Obes Relat Dis* 2010;6(2):126–131.

36. Escalona A, Pimentel F, Sharp A et al. Weight loss and metabolic improvement in morbidly obese subjects implanted for 1 year with an endoscopic duodenal-jejunal bypass liner. *Ann Surg* 2012;255(6):1080–1085.

37. Rodriguez L, Reyes E, Fagalde P et al. Pilot clinical study of an endoscopic, removable duodenal-jejunal bypass liner for the treatment of type 2 diabetes. *Diabetes Technol Ther* 2009;11(11):725–732.
38. Evans JT and DeLegge MH. Intragastric balloon therapy in the management of obesity: Why the bad wrap? *JPEN J Parenter Enteral Nutr* 2011;35:25–31.
39. Imaz I, Martínez-Cervell C, García-Alvarez EE et al. Safety and effectiveness of the intragastric balloon for obesity. A meta-analysis. *Obes Surg* 2008;18(7):841–846.
40. Genco, BT, Doldi B et al. BioEnterics intragastric balloon: The Italian experience with 2515 patients. *Obes Surg* 2005;15:1161–1164.
41. Forlano R, Ippolito AM, Iacobellis A et al. Effect of the BioEnterics intragastric balloon on weight, insulin resistance, and liver steatosis in obese patients. *Gastrointest Endosc* 2010;71(6):927–933.
42. Tai CM, Lin HY, Yen YC et al. Effectiveness of intragastric balloon treatment for obese patients: One-year follow-up after balloon removal. *Obes Surg* 2013;23(12):2068–2074.
43. Lee YM, Low HC, Lim LG et al. Intragastric balloon significantly improves nonalcoholic fatty liver disease activity score in obese patients with nonalcoholic steatohepatitis: A pilot study. *Gastrointest Endosc* 2012;76(4):756–760.
44. Deliopoulou K, Konsta A, Penna S et al. The impact of weight loss on depression status in obese individuals subjected to intragastric balloon treatment. *Obes Surg* 2013;23(5):669–675.
45. Dumonceau JM, François E, Hittelet A et al. Single vs repeated treatment with the intragastric balloon: A 5-year weight loss study. *Obes Surg* 2010;20(6):692–697.
46. Lopez-Nava G, Rubio MA, Prados S et al. BioEnterics intragastric balloon (BIB). Single ambulatory center Spanish experience with 714 consecutive patients treated with one or two consecutive balloons. *Obes Surg* 2011;21(1):5–9.
47. Kotzampassi K, Grosomanidis V, Papakostas P et al. 500 intragastric balloons: What happens 5 years thereafter? *Obes Surg* 2012;22(6):896–903.
48. Zerrweck C, Maunoury V, Caiazzo R et al. Preoperative weight loss with intragastric balloon decreases the risk of significant adverse outcomes of laparoscopic gastric bypass in super-super obese patients. *Obes Surg* May 2012;22(5):777–782.
49. Giardiello C, Borrelli A, Silvestri E et al. Air-filled vs water-filled intragastric balloon: A prospective randomized study. *Obes Surg* 2012;22(12):1916–1919.
50. Caglar E, Dobrucali A, and Bal K. Gastric balloon to treat obesity: Filled with air or fluid? *Dig Endosc* 2013;25(5):502–507.
51. Ponce J, Quebbemann BB, and Patterson EJ. Prospective, randomized, multicenter study evaluating safety and efficacy of intragastric dual-balloon in obesity. *Surg Obes Relat Dis* 2013;9(2):290–295.
52. Marinos G, Eliades C, Muthusamy V et al. First clinical experience with the TransPyloric shuttle device, a non-surgical endoscopic treatment for obesity: Results from a 3-month and 6-month study. *Surg Endosc* 2013;27(1):505.
53. Sauer N, Rösch T, Pezold J et al. A new endoscopically implantable device (SatiSphere) for treatment of obesity-efficacy, safety, and metabolic effects on glucose, insulin, and GLP-1 levels. *Obes Surg* 2013;23(11):1727–1733.
54. Sullivan S, Stein R, Jonnalagadda S, Mullady D, and Edmundowicz S. Aspiration therapy leads to weight loss in obese subjects: A pilot study. *Gastroenterology* 2013;145(6):1245–1252.e1-5.
55. Pratt GM, Learn CA, Hughes GD et al. Demographics and outcomes at American Society for Metabolic and Bariatric Surgery Centers of Excellence. *Surg Endosc* 2009;23:795–799.
56. Buchwald H, Avidor Y, Braunwald E et al. Bariatric surgery. A systematic review and meta-analysis. *JAMA* 2004;13:1724–1737.
57. Schauer PR, Burguera B, Ikramuddin S et al. Effect of laparoscopic Roux-en Y gastric bypass on type 2 diabetes mellitus. *Ann Surg* 2003;238:467–485.

58. Maggard MA, Shugarman LR, Suttorp M et al. Meta-analysis: Surgical treatment of obesity. *Ann Intern Med* 2005;142:547–559.
59. Elder KA and Wolfe BM. Bariatric surgery: A review of procedures and outcomes. *Gastroenterology* 2007;132:2253–2271.
60. Mitchell JE, Lancaster KL, Burgard MA et al. Long-term follow-up of patients' status after gastric bypass. *Obes Surg* 2001;11:464–468.
61. Sjostrom L, Lindroos AK, Peltonen M et al. Lifestyle, diabetes, and cardiovascular risk factors 10 years after bariatric surgery. *N Engl J Med* 2004;351:2683–2693.
62. Powers PS, Rosemurgy A, Boyd F et al. Outcome of gastric restriction procedures: Weight, psychiatric diagnoses, and satisfaction. *Obes Surg* 1997;7:471–477.
63. Hsu LK, Benotti PN, Dwyer J et al. Nonsurgical factors that influence the outcome of bariatric surgery: A review. *Psychosom Med* 1998;60:338–346.
64. Christou NV, Look D, and MacLean LD. Weight gain after short- and long-limb gastric bypass in patients followed for longer than 10 years. *Ann Surg* 2006;244(5):734–740.
65. Prachand V, DaVee R, and Alverdy J. Duodenal switch provides superior weight loss in the super-obese (BMI > 50 kg/m^2) compared with gastric bypass. *Ann Surg* 2006;244:611–619.
66. Malone M and Alger-Mayer S. Binge status and quality of life after gastric bypass surgery: A one-year study. *Obesity Res* 2004;12:473–481.
67. Flier JS. Clinical review 94: What's in a name? In search of leptin's physiologic role. *J Clin Endocrinol Metab* 1998;83:1407–1413.
68. Ahima RS, Prabakaran D, Mantzoros C et al. Role of leptin in the neuroendocrine response to fasting. *Nature* 1996;382:250–252.
69. Muller MK, Wildi S, Scholz T et al. Laparoscopic pouch resizing and redo of gastro-jejunal anastomosis for pouch dilatation following gastric bypass. *Obes Surg* 2005;15:1089–1095.
70. Gagner M, Gentileschi P, de Csepel J et al. Laparoscopic reoperative bariatric surgery: Experience from 27 consecutive patients. *Obes Surg* 2002;12:254–260.
71. Dayyeh BK, Lautz DB, and Thompson CC. Gastrojejunal stoma diameter predicts weight regain after Roux-en-Y gastric bypass. *Clin Gastroenterol Hepatol* 2011;9(3):228–233.
72. Gumbs AA, Pomp A, and Gagner M. Revisional bariatric surgery for inadequate weight loss. *Obes Surg* 2007;17:1137–1145.
73. Behrns K, Smith C, Kelly K et al. Reoperative bariatric surgery—Lessons learned to improve patient selection and results. *Ann Surg* 1993;218:646–653.
74. Ryou M, Ryan MB, and Thompson CC. Current status of endoluminal bariatric procedures for primary and revision indications. *Gastrointest Endosc Clin N Am* 2011;21(2):315–333.
75. Coakley BA, Deveney CW, Spight DH et al. Revisional bariatric surgery for failed restrictive procedures. *Surg Obes Relat Dis* 2008;4:581–586.
76. Dapri G, Cadiere GB, and Himpens J. Laparoscopic conversion of adjustable gastric banding and vertical banded gastroplasty to duodenal switch. *Surg Obes Relat Dis* 2009;5:678–683.
77. Spaulding L, Osler T, and Patlak J. Long-term results of sclerotherapy for dilated gastro-jejunostomy after gastric bypass. *Surg Obes Relat Dis* 2007;3:623–626.
78. Catalano MF, Rudic G, Anderson AJ et al. Weight gain after bariatric surgery as a result of a large gastric stoma: Endotherapy with sodium morrhuate may prevent the need for surgical revision. *Gastrointest Endosc* 2007;66:240–245.
79. Loewen M and Barba C. Endoscopic sclerotherapy for dilated gastrojejunostomy of failed gastric bypass. *Surg Obes Relat Dis* 2008;4:539–542.
80. Thompson CC, Carr-Locke DL, Saltzman J et al. Peroral endoscopic repair of staple-line dehiscence in Roux-en-Y gastric bypass: A less invasive approach [abstract]. *Gastroenterology* 2004;126(suppl 2):A.

81. Thompson CC, Slattery J, Bundga ME et al. Peroral endoscopic reduction of dilated gastrojejunal anastomosis after Roux-en-Y gastric bypass: A possible new option for patients with weight regain. *Surg Endosc* 2006;20:1744–1748.

82. Thompson CC, Chand B, Chen YK et al. Endoscopic suturing for transoral outlet reduction increases weight loss after Roux-en-Y gastric bypass surgery. *Gastroenterology* 2013;145(1):129–137.

83. Mikami D, Needleman B, Narula V et al. Natural orifice surgery: Initial US experience utilizing the StomaphyX device to reduce gastric pouches after Roux-en-Y gastric bypass. *Surg Endosc* 2010;24:223–228.

84. Letiman IM, Virk CS, Avgerinos DV et al. Early results of trans-oral endoscopic placation and revision of the gastric pouch and stoma following Roux-en-Y gastric bypass surgery. *JSLS* 2010;14:217–220.

85. Seaman DL, Gostout CJ, de la Mora Levy JG, and Knipschield MA. Tissue anchors for transmural gut-wall apposition. *Gastrointest Endosc* 2006;64:577–581.

86. Ryou MK, Mullady DK, Lautz DB, and Thompson CC. Pilot study evaluating technical feasibility and early outcomes of second-generation endosurgical platform for treatment of weight regain after gastric bypass surgery. *Surg Obes Relat Dis* 2009;5(4):450–454.

87. Horgan S, Jacobsen G, Weiss GD et al. Incisionless revision of post-Roux-en-Y bypass stomal and pouch dilation: Multicenter registry results. *Surg Obes Relat Dis* 2010;6:290–295.

88. Jirapinyo P, Slattery J, Ryan MB et al. Evaluation of an endoscopic suturing device for transoral outlet reduction in patients with weight regain following Roux-en-Y gastric bypass. *Endoscopy* 2013;45(7):532–536.

89. Kumar N and Thompson CC. Comparison of a superficial suturing device with a full-thickness suturing device for transoral outlet reduction (with videos). *Gastrointest Endosc* 2014;79(6):984–989.

16 Surgical Management of Obesity and Associated Complications

Travis J. McKenzie and Scott A. Shikora

CONTENTS

16.1 INTRODUCTION

Obesity is of epidemic proportions in the United States and in the world. In 2009–2010, 35.5% of adult males and 35.8% of adult females in the United States met the criteria for obesity (body mass index, BMI > 30 kg/m²).[1] Furthermore, the estimated annual U.S. health care expenditure related to the management of obesity and related diseases in 2010 is staggering at $168 billion dollars, accounting for approximately 16.5% of total health care cost.[2] Given the magnitude of this problem, physicians, surgeons, and scientists are working diligently to effectively prevent and treat obesity.

It is apparent that the overall health risk of obesity is substantially improved with weight loss. Thus the aim of both medical and surgical therapy is to achieve both meaningful and durable weight loss. Unfortunately, it has been consistently demonstrated that the nonoperative management of obesity fails to accomplish substantial, durable weight loss.[3] However, in most patients, the surgical management of weight loss has proven to be effective at achieving clinically significant and sustainable weight loss and comorbidity resolution with low risk of complications. Furthermore, studies have demonstrated reduction in total mortality following bariatric surgery.[4] In addition, patients after bariatric surgery have significantly higher rates of resolution of comorbid conditions such as diabetes mellitus, dyslipidemia, and hypertension compared to nonoperative obese subjects.[5]

Since bariatric surgery achieves these excellent outcomes with relatively low morbidity, it is not surprising that it is now considered more acceptable by potential candidates, their families, and their clinicians. As a result, the number of cases performed yearly has dramatically increased since the early 1990s.[6] With more and more of these operative procedures being performed, bariatric surgical patients will present in increasing numbers to nonbariatric physician offices and clinics. It is therefore, essential that all clinicians caring for these patients have a better understanding of the characteristics of these operations and their relevant potential complications. This chapter will aim to provide an overview of the surgical management of obesity and related comorbidities. It will include a review of the history and evolution of bariatric surgery, a description and comparison of the commonly performed bariatric procedures and a synopsis of their likely outcomes and potential complications.

16.2   EVOLUTION OF BARIATRIC SURGERY

Surgery for obesity and metabolic disease has undergone substantial evolution over the past half century. This evolution has its origins in the recognition of obesity as a disease associated with a multitude of life-threatening comorbid conditions. Surgical intervention for obesity began in the 1950s. Kremen et al.[7] from the University of Minnesota, performed the first intestinal bypass, the jejunoileal bypass (JIB) in a human in 1954. The JIB involved transecting the proximal jejunum and anastomosing it with the distal ileum, thereby bypassing a substantial portion of the small intestine. The procedure was initially considered successful in regard to excess weight loss and increased in popularity over the next 20 years. Over the years, many variants were also performed. The success and popularity of these procedures were not to last, as they often resulted in late complications such as profound malabsorption, protein deficiencies, chronic diarrhea, electrolyte abnormalities, dehydration, hepatic dysfunction, and micronutrient and vitamin deficiencies. Furthermore, the long blind limb promoted bacterial overgrowth resulting in symptoms of abdominal bloating and cramping, arthralgias and myalgias. These complications often required surgical reversal for correction. Although intestinal bypass eventually fell out of favor and was abandoned, it paved the way for further techniques in bariatric surgery and helped promote the concept of malabsorption for weight loss and comorbidity amelioration.[8]

In 1966, Mason and Ito[9] from the University of Iowa first introduced the concept of gastric restriction for the promotion of weight loss after observing that patients lost weight after partial gastrectomy for ulcer disease. Their initial procedure essentially mimicked a Billroth II gastrectomy with a transection of the stomach perpendicular to its axis and the anastomosis of the remaining gastric segment to a loop of the small intestine. However, this procedure was plagued by bile reflux gastritis which ultimately prompted reconstruction with a roux limb instead of a loop. Further refinements by Mason included creating a much smaller gastric pouch to promote better food restriction and to reduce the incidence of marginal ulceration. Shortly after Mason published his results with the gastric bypass, surgeons began developing various simpler forms of gastric partitioning procedures collectively known as gastroplasty. These procedures involved stomach partitioning without connection to the small intestine. It was believed that gastroplasty would achieve similar food restriction with a less complex procedure that avoided some of the complications of gastric bypass.[10,11] However, such procedures ultimately failed due to dilation of the gastric pouch or the pouch outlet. The vertical banded gastroplasty (VBG) was developed to combat this problem.[12,13] This procedure created a small gastric pouch by vertically stapling the stomach in combination with a reinforcement of the outlet to prevent dilatation. This reinforcement included wrapping prolene suture, fixed bands or rings around the gastric outlet. Due to problems with erosion, the suture was replaced with a silastic ring. The VBG rose in popularity due to its greater simplicity and safety and was the prominent bariatric surgical procedure in the 1980s. However, the VBG eventually fell out of favor due to inferior weight loss compared with the gastric bypass. This was demonstrated to be secondary to a high incidence of pouch dilatation, staple line breakdown, or the maladaptive eating patterns that often developed as a result of solid food intolerance created by fixed bands and rings.

In an attempt to simplify operative intervention for obesity and eliminate the need for staple lines, Wilkinson developed a gastric band in 1981, which consisted of wrapping a nonadjustable mesh band around the proximal stomach, thereby creating a small gastric pouch and a fixed outlet.[14] Many variations of fixed gastric banding were subsequently employed. However, the use of a fixed size and non-adjustable band resulted in failure from both technical complications related to inappropriate band sizing as well as erosion, and band slippage. Furthermore, many patients experienced severe dysphagia with solid food intolerance that often resulted in maladaptive eating and weight loss failure. Adjustable bands consisting of a band with an inner inflatable balloon connected to a subcutaneous port were eventually introduced. These newer bands could be inflated to allow titration of outlet restriction. Adjustable bands proved superior to their nonadjustable counterparts in both efficacy and complication rates.

In 1979, Scopinaro et al.[15] developed, in a dog model, the biliopancreatic diversion (BPD) as a combined malabsorptive and restrictive procedure. The BPD was a modified intestinal bypass created to utilize malabsorption for weight loss without the deleterious effects of the original intestinal bypass procedures. This procedure involves a distal gastrectomy anastomosed to a very long limb intestinal bypass. The BPD was later modified by Hess and Hess in 1998 and Marceau et al. in 1999 and involved a sleeve gastrectomy (SG) instead of a horizontal gastric transection to preserve the pylorus. The bowel anastomosis was made to the duodenum not the stomach pouch.[16,17] They named the procedure, the BPD with duodenal switch (BPD-DS) or just simply, the duodenal switch (DS). Ultimately, the SG as a stand-alone procedure arose out of the BPD-DS experience in patients in whom a staged approach was planned—the SG would be performed first and the remainder of the BPD-DS at a later date. It was noted that after SG alone and prior to performing BPD, many patients refused to have the second stage as they had achieved significant weight loss and the comorbidity amelioration was generally excellent. Further follow up of these patients confirmed that the results were durable and thus, the SG was now considered to be a viable surgical option.

A significant event in the specialty of bariatric surgery was the introduction of laparoscopic (minimally invasive) surgical approaches for conventional bariatric surgery. In 1992, Broadbent performed the first minimally invasive bariatric procedure when he laparoscopically placed a gastric band.[18] Wittgrove and Clark[19] are credited with performing the first laparoscopic RYGBP in 1993, and later publishing their results again in 2000. Shortly thereafter, all bariatric procedures were successfully performed laparoscopically and in time, by the majority of bariatric surgeons. The development and widespread utilization of laparoscopy has led to a dramatic increase in the number of bariatric surgical procedures performed as patients, their families and their clinicians find laparoscopic bariatric surgery to be more acceptable. Laparoscopic bariatric surgery has been proven to be associated with decreased length of hospital stay, quicker return to normal activity, less wound complications, and better cosmesis while maintaining the excellent outcomes seen with open surgery.[20] The minimally invasive approach has become the preferred method due to these proven advantages.

16.3   CURRENT BARIATRIC PROCEDURES AND ASSOCIATED COMPLICATIONS

16.3.1   OVERVIEW

Bariatric surgical procedures most commonly performed today include the RYGBP, SG, laparoscopic adjustable gastric banding (LAGB), and BPD-DS as well as revisional operations for failed weight loss or complications after a primary bariatric procedure. Classically, procedures were categorized by presumed mechanism(s) of action such as either purely restrictive (LAGB, VBG), purely malabsorptive (JIB), or combined (RYGBP, BPD/DS). However, it has become apparent that these categories do not encompass the myriad of physiologic alterations that occur following bariatric surgery. There is an increasingly recognized metabolic and hormonal component to many of these operations that have varying degrees of influence on the overall success of the bariatric surgical procedure for achieving both weight loss and improvements of the associated medical comorbid conditions. Each bariatric procedure can result in unique complications, both surgical and medical. The next section will not cover all of the potential complications but will highlight the most significant.

Bariatric surgery has proven to be both safe and effective. The refinement of minimally invasive surgical techniques and the introduction of new technologies have resulted in safer surgery. However, as with any surgical procedure, there are inherent risks on which patients should be educated. Complications that are generalizable to all bariatric procedures are discussed below and include those of general anesthesia, enteric leak, venous thromboembolism (VTE), gastrointestinal bleeding (GIB), intra-abdominal bleeding, wound complications, and complications of malnutrition and vitamin deficiencies.

One of the most feared complications of bariatric surgery is enteric leak, most commonly occurring from an anastomosis or staple line. Depending on the particular bariatric procedure, intestinal leak can occur in various locations. The most commonly described leak occurs at the gastrojejunostomy after gastric bypass with an incidence of 0%–5.6% in large series.[21] The precepts of management include wide drainage, control of sepsis, and nutritional support. However, the approach to treatment of the patient with intestinal leak depends on the patient's clinical status, which can range from subclinical signs and symptoms to life-threatening septic shock. Stable patients can potentially be approached with radiologic guided drainage and antibiotics, while unstable patients may require return to the operating room. It should be noted that endoscopic stent placement is an increasingly common option for gastric pouch, sleeve or gastrojejunostomy leaks in hemodynamically stable patients. It is important to emphasize that the bariatric surgical patient does not consistently present with pain and peritonitis that are more readily appreciated with the nonobese population with abdominal sepsis. Therefore, a high index of suspicion is always warranted.

Venous thromboembolism (VTE) events such as deep venous thrombosis (DVT) and pulmonary embolism (PE) are rare, but possibly lethal complications. VTE and gastrointestinal leak are the top two causes of mortality in the perioperative period.[22] The reported incidence of VTE is 0.12%–3.8% after RYGBP.[23] The incidence is likely to be similar after the other operative procedures. The increased risk of VTE in this patient population is multifactorial and includes the increased abdominal pressure seen with obesity and the abdominal insufflation with laparoscopy, the decreased venous return with patient positioning on the operating room table, the limited mobility postoperatively, and the possible hypercoagulable state of obesity. While VTE prophylaxis is generally encouraged, there is no clear consensus on the type, dose, or duration of VTE prophylaxis. However, most bariatric surgeons employ some form of prophylaxis in the pre and postoperative period including graded compression stockings, pneumatic compression boots, and chemical prophylaxis in the form of either unfractionated or low molecular weight heparin. Many surgeons practice combination therapy. Although controversial, the use of extended duration chemical prophylaxis postoperatively is becoming increasingly employed in high risk patients. However, the dosage and duration of therapy have yet to be determined.

GIB may occur after any bariatric procedure in which the viscera are cut (RYGBP, Sleeve, BPD/DS). The risk of GIB is reported to be 1.1%–4% in most series.[24] Bleeding can occur at any staple line or anastomosis. Bleeding in the postoperative period is most often managed with fluid and blood product resuscitation, correction of coagulation parameters, maintenance of euthermia, and possibly endoscopic intervention. GIB can almost always be managed with these conservative measures. However, profound hemorrhage resulting in hemodynamic instability or an ongoing transfusion requirement may mandate operative intervention.

Intraabdominal hemorrhage is a rare complication that can potentially occur with any bariatric surgical procedure with an incidence that is less than 1% in most surgical series. Postoperative intraabdominal bleeding can range from minor bleeding in an otherwise stable patient to life threatening hemorrhage requiring transfusion and operative reexploration. Bleeding can occur from several possible sources including the liver, spleen, the mesenteries, the trocar wounds, and so on. Like GIB, intraabdominal bleeding which results in hemodynamic instability, ongoing transfusion requirements, or other symptoms may require surgical intervention.

Wound complications including infection and incisional hernia have been dramatically reduced and rarely occur with the utilization of preincisional prophylactic antibiotics and the evolution from large open incisions to the multiple small incisions characteristic of laparoscopic surgery. The incidence of trocar site hernia is generally less than 1%.

16.3.2 Roux-en-Y Gastric Bypass

Roux-en-Y gastric bypass is currently considered the gold standard by which other bariatric procedures are compared. This procedure, currently predominantly performed laparoscopically, entails division of the proximal stomach yielding a small gastric pouch (approximately 15 mL) connected to a 100–150 cm segment of small intestine referred to as the "roux limb" (Figure 16.1). Ingested food bypasses the remnant stomach, duodenum, and proximal jejunum before entering a long common intestinal channel where the mixing of food with bile and digestive enzymes occur. The mechanism of action leading to weight loss and comorbidity amelioration is multifactorial. Creation of a very small gastric pouch results in nutrient restriction.

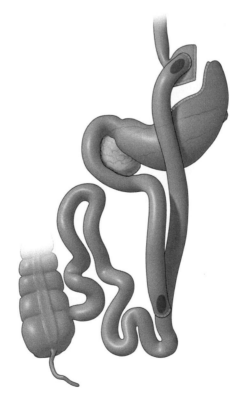

FIGURE 16.1   (See color insert.) Roux-en-Y gastric bypass. (Copyright 2013, Brigham and Women's Hospital.)

The gastric fundus (which is responsible for receptive relaxation upon eating) and the antrum are purposefully excluded. The patient can therefore only tolerate very small amounts of food at any given time. Bypassing the duodenum and proximal jejunum lends a small component of malabsorption of micro- and macronutrients. However, given the long common enteric channel, malabsorption plays a lesser role with gastric bypass than with the BPD and BPD/DS. In addition to the mechanical causes of weight loss (restriction and malabsorption due to intestinal bypass), RYGBP results in hormonal changes that are currently being investigated. These include a reduction in the secretion of an appetite hormone, ghrelin and the stimulation of incretin hormones such as GLP-1 (glucagon like peptide 1) and PYY (polypeptide YY).

Complications specific to RYGBP include anastomotic stenosis or marginal ulceration at the gastrojejunostomy, internal hernia, and gastrogastric fistula. Mortality has dramatically fallen over the past few decades with the conversion from open surgery to laparoscopic. Mortality after RYGBP is generally reported as 0.2%.[25] Although rare, the major contributors to mortality following RYGBP are intestinal leak and pulmonary embolism.

Anastomotic stenosis is a narrowing of the gastrojejunal anastomosis such that patients cannot tolerate eating and vomit frequently. Symptoms include nausea, emesis, dysphagia, and odynophagia. This complication is reported to occur in 5%–27% of cases and typically occurs in the first few months following surgery.[26] The rate of stenosis varies with surgical technique and is generally less with hand-sewn versus stapled anastomoses.[27] The diagnosis is made with the use of contrast enhanced upper gastrointestinal fluoroscopy and upper endoscopy. Therapeutic upper endoscopy with gentle balloon dilation of the anastomosis is first line therapy and often successful in relieving symptoms, thereby allowing patients to tolerate oral intake.

Marginal ulceration of the unprotected jejunal mucosa at the gastrojejunostomy occurs in 1%–16% of patients.[28] The cause of ulceration is often multifactorial such as the presence of a gastrogastric fistula (abnormal luminal communications between the gastric pouch and the remnant fundus), large pouch size (presence of acid secreting parietal cells), ischemia, tension, nonsteroidal anti-inflammatory drugs (NSAIDs) use, and smoking. The symptoms of marginal ulceration include pain in the epigastrium radiating to the back, nausea, vomiting, and food intolerance. The diagnosis is made by visualization of the ulcer endoscopically. If there is concern for a gastrogastric fistula with retrograde acid flow, upper gastrointestinal contrast radiography may be helpful in securing the diagnosis. For marginal ulceration, the treatment includes the use of proton pump inhibitors (PPIs) and sucralfate in combination. If the ulcer is secondary to an irritant such as tobacco or NSAIDs, the use of these substances must be ceased. If the patient is found to have a gastrogastric fistula or a significantly enlarged pouch, surgical takedown of the fistula and pouch volume reduction respectively, can be performed. Revision of the gastrojejunostomy may be necessary for medically refractory ulceration, ulceration secondary to chronic ischemia, or marginal ulceration complicated by hemorrhage or perforation.

Intestinal obstruction after RYGBP is often caused by internal hernia though one of the three possible hernia defects created with gastric bypass anatomy. The incidence is less than 2%.[29] A patient with internal hernia will generally present with abdominal pain and obstructive symptoms. These symptoms may be acute in onset and persistent or may be of recurrent nature indicating a hernia that self-reduces. A high level of suspicion is warranted as findings by computed tomography (CT) can be nonspecific. Intestinal obstruction may also be secondary to other causes such as adhesions, intussusception, impaction, or intraperitoneal (or luminal) blood clots. The correct treatment of intestinal obstruction caused by internal hernia or other etiologies is early surgical exploration. Conservative therapies are usually not indicated and may lead to intestinal infarction. Intestinal obstruction in a RYGBP patient is considered a surgical emergency as internal herniation may result in bowel ischemia and necrosis potentially requiring long length intestinal resection and short-gut syndrome. Therefore cramping abdominal pain and obstructive symptoms in a patient with RYGBP anatomy should be evaluated by contrast enhanced CT scan and potentially by laparoscopic abdominal exploration for suspicious clinical signs or CT findings concerning for obstruction. Furthermore, if the index of suspicion of internal hernia is high, the surgeon should proceed with exploration even in the absence of abnormal CT findings.

16.3.3 SLEEVE GASTRECTOMY

SG was initially described as the restrictive portion of the BPD/DS. Due to the complexity of this procedure, and the high morbidity when performed in high risk and superobese patients, Regan et al.[30] proposed dividing the procedure into two distinct operative stages. The DS would be performed first. The intestinal bypass stage would be performed at a later date after the patient lost significant weight and reduced their operative risk. In their initial series, Regan et al. reported that patients did achieve substantial weight loss and comorbidity resolution with the SG. It was noted, however, that some patients were satisfied with the SG and refused to undergo the second stage. When it was observed that these patients maintained excellent results, the SG was then adopted as a stand-alone procedure.

Since that time, SG had gained popularity among bariatric surgeons and patients as a stand-alone procedure for both for its excellent short-term results as well as its perceived comparative ease of performance as a surgical procedure. The technique of SG involves removing the entire greater curvature of the stomach thereby creating a narrow tubular-shaped gastric sleeve (Figure 16.2). The sleeve is fashioned with a calibration bougie in place along the lesser curve of the stomach. This bougie is of varying size (32–40 French) depending on surgeon preference. The mechanism of action of the SG may also be multifactorial. First, it involves nutrient restriction from the creation of a narrow gastric lumen with small capacity. Second, the resection of the fundus results in a lack of receptive relaxation. Additionally, SG removes the region of the stomach where the majority of the Ghrelin production takes place—the fundus. Furthermore, there may be a component of up-regulation of incretin secretion from the distal small bowel secondary to a more rapid transit of nutrients through the gastrointestinal (GI) tract. These mechanisms have yet to be fully elucidated.

The SG is a technically less complex procedure than the RYGBP and therefore it can result in fewer late perioperative complications. However, creation of a SG entails formation of the longest staple line of any bariatric procedure. This staple line, like that of the RYGBP or DS may leak. The incidence of leak is less than 2% in most series.[31,32] Proximal leak, the most common location for leak, occurs near the

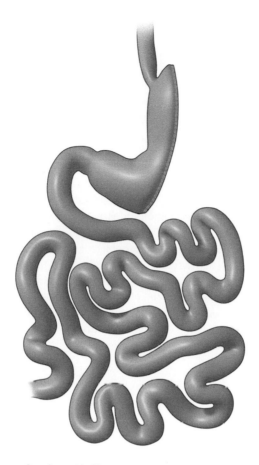

FIGURE 16.2 (See color insert.) Sleeve gastrectomy. (Copyright 2013, Brigham and Women's Hospital.)

esophagogastric junction near the angle of His. The leak may occur if the final stapling of the sleeve impinges upon the abdominal esophagus. The esophagus, unlike the stomach and intestines does not have an outer fibrous serosal layer and is therefore more prone to leak. Proximal leaks can also be result from "blow out" secondary to a distal sleeve obstruction or stenosis. A leak at the distal staple line is usually due to staple line failure. The gastric antrum is much thicker than other regions of the stomach. If the tissue is too thick for the chosen staple height, the staples will not deploy correctly and the staple line would be prone to fail. The management principles of a sleeve leak are similar to that of RYGBP, including wide drainage and nutritional support. Endoluminal stenting has been utilized for proximal leaks in small series of highly selected patients and may prove beneficial, but requires ongoing study.[33] Unstable patients should undergo emergent surgery with wide drainage.

Sleeve stenosis or stricture occurs in 1%–2% of cases and results in food intolerance with nausea and emesis. Although, the sleeve is constructed over a calibration tube, creating the sleeve too tightly against the tube can result in a narrowing. This most commonly occurs at a region of the stomach known as the incisura which is just proximal to the gastric antrum. At this location, the stomach changes orientation from vertical to more transverse. Sleeve stenosis can be managed endoscopically, although mechanical spiraling of the gastric sleeve due to an uneven staple line may require revision to a RYGBP. Late complications following SG are rare. There is no potential anatomic space created during SG and therefore no potential of internal hernia. The perioperative mortality of SG was 0.19% in a series of 2570 patients.[34]

16.3.4 LAPAROSCOPIC ADJUSTABLE GASTRIC BAND

Laparoscopic placement of a restrictive adjustable gastric band around the proximal stomach was first used in the mid-1980s. Since that time, these bands have undergone major refinement in both technology as well as technique of placement. The procedure involves placement of the adjustable band around the proximal stomach approximately 3 cm distal to the gastroesophageal junction resulting in a 15–20 cc pouch (Figure 16.3). The gastric fundus is plicated around the anterolateral side of the band to prevent the complication of gastric prolapse. The band consists of an outer ring and inner inflatable reservoir connected to a subcutaneous port thereby allowing variable levels of gastric outlet restriction with inflation of the reservoir with saline. The mechanism of action leading to weight loss after banding is purely restrictive.

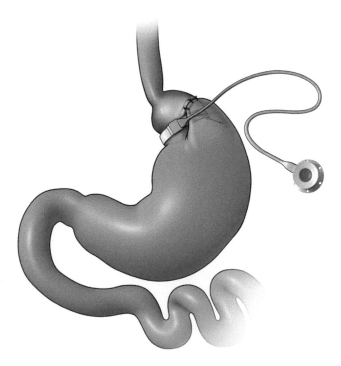

FIGURE 16.3 **(See color insert.)** Adjustable band. (Copyright 2013, Brigham and Women's Hospital.)

Since the LAGB is a foreign body, it is prone to unique complications not encountered with the other described procedures. These complications include band erosion, band prolapse, and port complications such as leakage, flipping or infection.

The band may erode into the underlying stomach or esophagus over time. The incidence of erosion is 0%–5.5% in most series.[35] Diagnosis is made by upper endoscopy although the diagnosis may be suggested by upper gastrointestinal contrast fluoroscopy. It may also be suspected if the patient presents with a late port infection. Erosion generally presents with the feeling of a loss of restriction, abdominal pain, or heartburn. It always requires surgical removal. However, endoscopic removal has been described.[36]

Gastric band prolapse (also called band slippage) describes a condition where the stomach below the band herniates through it resulting in a tilted band and a large proximal gastric pouch. Prolapse usually presents as new onset heartburn and reflux but can result in complete proximal gastric obstruction, which is a surgical emergency. If left untreated, gastric necrosis and perforation may occur. The diagnosis is made on upper GI fluoroscopy. Initial management entails deflation of the balloon. However, if the patient continues to be symptomatic, surgical band repositioning, or even band removal may be necessary.

Novel band and port complications may also occur. These include leakage of fluid from the band, tubing, or port. Band infection, although rare, may necessitate removal.

The perioperative mortality is 0.03%, which is the lowest of the various bariatric procedures.[37]

16.3.5 BILIOPANCREATIC DIVERSION WITH DUODENAL SWITCH

BPD-DS is a modification of the operation originally described by Scopinaro called the BPD. The modification involves creation of a SG followed by transection of the duodenum just distal to the pylorus with Roux-en-Y reconstruction to the distal small intestine creating a proximal ileoduodenostomy and distal ileoileostomy. This leaves approximately 50–100 cm of common channel for nutrient absorption (Figure 16.4). The mechanism of action of the BPD/DS is multifactorial. Creation of a SG results in gastric restriction and alteration in Ghrelin production as previously described. Furthermore, the short common channel that characterizes the BPD/DS is largely malabsorptive. However, much like the RYGBP, there is likely a substantial hormonal component to weight loss and comorbidity amelioration that has yet to be fully described. BPD/DS is the most technically complicated procedure and carries the highest perioperative risk. In addition, this procedure can be complicated by malnutrition and micronutrient deficiency due to the substantial malabsorptive mechanism. It does however, result in the greatest weight loss and best comorbid condition amelioration of all of the bariatric procedures.

Complications of BPD/DS include those previously described for RYGBP including VTE, intestinal leak, and internal hernia. The described perioperative mortality for laparoscopic BPD/DS is 2.5% and may be higher for the superobese.[38] As previously mentioned, this procedure employs a highly malabsorptive mechanism, so nutritional complications such as dehydration, protein malnutrition and macro—and micronutrient deficiencies can occur.

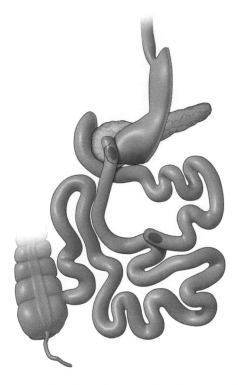

FIGURE 16.4 (See color insert.) Biliopancreatic diversion with duodenal switch. (Copyright 2013, Brigham and Women's Hospital.)

16.4 COMPARISON OF WEIGHT LOSS AMONG BARIATRIC PROCEDURES

There are no randomized controlled data suggesting that a single procedure is superior to others for all patients. Recommendations, therefore, are individualized to the patient's particular needs including presence and severity of comorbid conditions, dietary habits, and degree of adiposity rather than simply the desire for weight loss. It is readily accepted, and demonstrated in multiple randomized trials, that laparoscopic RYGBP compares favorably with its open counterpart.[39,40] Benefits of the laparoscopic approach include decreased wound complications, better cosmesis, less pain, and earlier return to activities without compromise of efficacy. These benefits can be reasonably extrapolated to the other bariatric procedures, all of which are performed laparoscopically preferentially.

It is possible to generalize published data with regard to percent excess weight loss (%EWL) after bariatric surgery. Patients after BPD/DS can be expected to have the greatest weight loss (70%–80%). This is followed by RYGBP (60%–70%), SG (50%–60%), and LAGB (45%–50%).[41,42] However, individual studies vary widely in regard to %EWL, and certainly these percentages may vary from program to program and patient group to patient group. In addition, an estimated %EWL does not necessarily mean that every patient will lose the desired amount of weight. There will be patients that fail to lose meaningful weight or will regain back lost weight. A recent meta-analysis of six randomized control trials compared the weight loss of RYGBP, SG, and LAGB with 6 months to 3 years follow up. %EWL after LAGB was 28.7%–48%, SG was 40%–90%, and RYGBP was 62.1%–94.4%.[43]

16.5 NUTRITIONAL COMPLICATIONS FOLLOWING BARIATRIC SURGERY

Nutritional deficiencies can occur to varying degrees after all of the commonly performed bariatric surgical procedures. As a general guideline, the risk of nutritional deficiency varies in direct proportion to the success of the procedure when defined as %EWL. As such, the spectrum of increasing risk of nutritional complications starts with the LAGB, SG, and followed by RYGBP and BPD/DS. An alternative way of viewing this spectrum is that the risk increases with increasing malabsorption. As LAGB and SG are largely restrictive, the risk of nutritional complication is much lower. However, this risk increases with RYGBP and BPD/DS, which employ the bypass of a variable length of small intestine yielding a substantial malabsorptive component. This is particularly true of BDP/DS which bypasses the greatest length of intestine and has the shortest common channel (approximately 100 cm).

Nutritional complications can involve deficiency in one or a combination of macro- and micronutrients. Macronutrients include protein, carbohydrate, and lipids. Micronutrients include essential minerals such as calcium and iron, fat and water-soluble vitamins, and trace elements such as zinc and chromium.

A multidisciplinary approach to the prevention, diagnosis, and treatment of nutritional deficiency in the post bariatric surgical patient is vital to success. This multidisciplinary team should include surgeons, endocrinologists, and dietary/nutritional specialists. Regular follow up is necessary to continued success.

Following bariatric surgery, and particularly after malabsorptive procedures, protein is the major macronutrient deficiency encountered, particularly with BPD-DS. Carbohydrate and lipid malnutrition is of lesser concern. Current guidelines recommend a minimum of 60 g of ingested protein daily.[44] However, many postbariatric surgical patients struggle to meet this minimum guideline, and even when an appropriate amount of protein is ingested, malabsorption can further compound the risk of protein malnutrition. Protein malnutrition rarely occurs after gastric banding but can occur in patients that have chronic vomiting and poor oral intake resulting from food intolerance or anatomic conditions such as inappropriate tightness of the band. Protein malnutrition can also occur in patients with psychiatric conditions or fear of weight gain. After SG this complication can occur in patients with sleeve stricture, psychiatric issues, or poor dietary intake. Protein malnutrition as evidence by hypoalbuminemia occurs in approximately 1.3% of patients after RYGBP and can be as high as 18% after BPD/DS.[45,46] Inciting factors include limited gastric capacity, malabsorption secondary the intestinal bypass, and intolerance to high protein foods. Gastric restriction can lead to an inability to tolerate many high protein foods, such as red meat. Recurrent emesis can compound the risk of this complication. Bypass of the duodenum and varying lengths of jejunum may yield a relatively short common channel where digestive enzymes are insufficiently in contact with ingested protein. This results in a lack of protein digestion and therefore lack of absorption of amino acids. Signs of protein malnutrition include emaciation, edema, and alopecia. Biochemical evidence is usually seen late and includes anemia and hypoalbuminemia.

Calcium is essential to normal cellular function. Calcium is actively absorbed largely in the duodenum and secondarily by a passive mechanism in the proximal jejunum and elsewhere in the distal gastrointestinal tract. Therefore, procedures that bypass the duodenum and/or the proximal jejunum, such as the RYGBP and BPD/DS are at the greatest risk for calcium malabsorption and its consequences. Furthermore, calcium absorption occurs most efficiently following exposure to a low pH environment. However, RYGBP creates a small pouch that is largely void of acid producing parietal cells.[47] SG may also result in reduction of parietal cell mass and therefore reduced acid production. Problems with malabsorption and deficiency of calcium are compounded by the concurrent vitamin D deficiency that is discussed below. Symptoms of hypocalcemia may be subclinical or vague, including myalgia and arthralgia, but rarely result in tetany. Ultimately chronic calcium and vitamin D deficiency can result in secondary hyperparathyroidism which has downstream effects such as bone loss. To combat this calcium and vitamin D deficiency, the American Society for Metabolic and Bariatric Surgery (ASMBS) recommends supplementing 1.5–2 g/day of oral calcium with vitamin D in divided doses.[48] This guideline should be followed in all bariatric surgical patients, including all types of bariatric procedures.

Iron deficiency leading to anemia is a common complication of bariatric procedures with a malabsorptive component and to a lesser extent with restrictive procedures. Anemia is present in approximately 36% of patients one year or more after RYGBP.[49] Bypass of the stomach as occurs with RYGBP or parietal cell debulking that occurs with SG can result in a relatively high pH environment, which results in suboptimal iron absorption. Bypass of the proximal small intestine can compound this problem, leading to further iron deficiency and resultant anemia. Iron deficiency following bariatric surgery should be treated with iron supplementation including 150 mg/day of oral ferrous gluconate. The use of oral supplementation may be insufficient in some patients, who may require parenteral iron.

Fat-soluble vitamin deficiencies (vitamins A, D, E, and K) have been observed, particularly after procedures with a large malabsorptive component, such as BPD/DS and distal RYGBP, both of which yield a short common channel.

Deficiency of vitamin D exacerbates the problems encountered with calcium malabsorption and deficiency. Vitamin D plays a vital role in the regulation of calcium homeostasis, having effect on calcium absorption in the intestine. Vitamin D deficiency following bariatric surgery can result in secondary hyperparathyroidism with rates exceeding 30%.[50,51] Secondary hyperparathyroidism can result in bone loss thereby making patients prone to fracture. Supplementation is recommended for all bariatric surgical patients and generally includes oral calcium/vitamin D. Vitamin D levels in the form of 25-hydroxyvitamin D should be monitored.

Deficiency of vitamins A, E, and K following bariatric procedures are much less common and poorly studied. Vitamin A deficiency may result in poor night vision and pruritus. Oral supplementation is generally adequate. Deficiency of vitamin E has not been studied. Deficiency of vitamin K has not been formally described in the literature. However, the authors have noted supratheraputic INR elevation following RYGBP in patients taking warfarin preoperatively. This may be due to the fact that the turnover of vitamin K is relatively rapid so the total body amount of vitamin K is not large enough to prevent subclinical deficiency after bariatric surgery, particularly malabsorptive procedures.

In contrast to fat-soluble vitamins, water-soluble vitamins including thiamine, folate, cobalamin, and vitamin C have limited body stores. For example, the human body has enough thiamine for approximately 20 days. Although water-soluble vitamin deficiency is uncommon, symptoms of deficiency can occur relatively rapidly due to inadequate stores. Notable deficiencies include that of thiamine (B_1), resulting in neuropsychiatric and cardiac symptoms (beriberi). Folate and cobalamin (B_{12}) deficiency can result in macrocytic anemia in the postbariatric surgical population. Deficiency of folate is rare. In contrast, B_{12} deficiency is common following RYGBP (12%–33%) in the absence of supplementation.[48] Inadequate vitamin C can result in inadequate collagen synthesis and poor tissue integrity leading to symptoms of scurvy.

Trace element deficiency can occur after bariatric surgery (particularly malabsorptive procedures such as BPD-DS) in the setting of prolonged malnutrition. These deficiencies are rare, and potentially include zinc, copper, selenium, and chromium.

16.6 RECOMMENDED NUTRITIONAL SUPPLEMENTATION AND SCREENING FOR DEFICIENCY FOLLOWING BARIATRIC SURGERY

The American Society for Metabolic and Bariatric Surgery guidelines for nutritional supplementation following bariatric surgery include a high potency multivitamin containing 100%–200% of the daily recommended value for all patients.[48] This multivitamin should include iron. All postbariatric patients should receive oral calcium and vitamin D supplementation in the form of calcium citrate/D_3 at a dose of 1500–2000 mg of elemental calcium daily in divided doses. Additional vitamin B_{12} is recommended for RYGBP patients specifically. Recommended method of delivery includes either oral (500 µg/day) or injectable intramuscular (1000 µg/mo) formulations. Additional elemental iron at a dose of 18–27 mg/day (in addition to that provided in the multivitamin) is recommended for those patients prone to anemia such as menstruating women. Of special concern, patients following BPD-DS should be supplemented with fat soluble vitamins (A, D, E, K) as well as an optional B-complex multivitamin.

In general, nutritional laboratory values should be reviewed annually for life following bariatric surgery. Furthermore, specific laboratory values may be checked more frequently as indicated by symptomatic clinical presentation.

16.7 CONCLUSION

In the face of the growing obesity epidemic, bariatric surgery has provided clinicians with a safe and effective tool to combat obesity and its related comorbid conditions.

Bariatric surgery is now a widely accepted treatment modality for type-2 diabetes that has compared favorably to optimal medical management in randomized controlled trials. With the increasing trend towards the utilization of this powerful tool, clinicians that may encounter postbariatric surgical patients should be familiar with the various procedures performed today and the relevant short- and long-term complications that may occur, including nutritional deficiency. Close life-long interdisciplinary follow up is a necessary component for continued success after bariatric surgery.

16.8   CASE STUDY

A 32-year-old female with 12 year history of obesity (current BMI 42 kg/m^2) is referred for consideration of bariatric surgery. The patient has a 3-year history of type-2 diabetes (Hgb A1C 7.5% on metformin and low dose insulin) and gastro-esophageal reflux disease (GERD) on maximal PPI therapy with current esophagitis by endoscopy. After a 6-month period of preoperative evaluation and education including visits with endocrinology, psychology, nutrition, and surgery, the patient elects to pursue surgical therapy for the treatment of her obesity and related comorbid conditions. RYGBP is chosen in this patient in order to maximize both weight loss and amelioration of diabetes while limiting the risk of exacerbating GERD. The patient undergoes an uncomplicated laparoscopic RYGBP and is discharged to home on postoperative day 2 with blood sugars in the normal range off insulin and metformin. She is discharged on a daily multivitamin including iron, calcium citrate with vitamin D, and monthly B$_{12}$ injections. At 1-year follow up, the patient has 60% EWL with current BMI 31.8 kg/m^2. She continues to have normal blood sugars with Hgb A1C of 6.0% off all previous diabetic medications. She has likewise discontinued PPI therapy and has no symptoms of GERD.

REFERENCES

1. Flegal K, Carroll M, Kit B et al. Prevalence of obesity and trends in the distribution of body mass index among US adults, 1999–2010. *JAMA* 2012;307(5):491–497.
2. Cawley J, Meyerhoefer C. The medical care costs of obesity: An instrumental variables approach. *J Health Econ* 2012;31(1):219–230.
3. Goodrick G, Poston W, Foreyt J. Methods for voluntary weight loss and control: Update 1996. *Nutrition* 1996;12:672–676.
4. Adams T, Gress R, Smith S et al. Long-term mortality after gastric bypass surgery. *N Engl J Med* 2007;357:753–761.
5. Adams T, Pendleton R, Strong M et al. Health outcomes of gastric bypass patients compared to nonsurgical, nonintervened severely obese. *Obesity* 2010;18:121–130.
6. Steinbrock R. Surgery for severe obesity. *N Engl J Med* 2004;350(11):1075–1079.
7. Kremen A, Linner J, Nelson C. An experimental evaluation of the nutritional importance of proximal and distal small intestine. *Ann Surg* 1954;140:439–444.
8. Buchwald H, Rucker R. The rise and fall of jejunoileal bypass. In: Nelson RL, Nyhus LM, Eds. *Surgery of the Small Intestine*. Norwalk, CT: Appleton Century Crofts; 1987. pp. 529–541.
9. Mason E, Ito C. Gastric bypass in obesity. *Surg Clin North Am* 1967;47(6):1345–1351.

10. Gomez C. Gastroplasty in the surgical treatment of morbid obesity. *Am J Clin Nutr* 1980;33:406–415.
11. Pace W, Martin E, Tetirick T et al. Gastric partitioning for morbid obesity. *Ann Surg* 1979;190:392–400.
12. Long M, Collins J. The technique and early results of high gastric reduction for obesity. *Aust N Z J Surg* 1980;50:146–149.
13. Mason E. Vertical banded gastroplasty for obesity. *Arch Surg* 1982;117:701–706.
14. Wilkinson L, Peloso O. Gastric (reservoir) reduction for morbid obesity. *Arch Surg* 1981;116:602–605.
15. Scopinaro N, Gianetta E, Civalleri D et al. Bilio-pancreatic bypass for obesity: An experimental study in dogs. *Br J Surg* 1979;66:613–617.
16. Hess DS, Hess DW. Biliopancreatic diversion with a duodenal switch. *Obes Surg* 1998;8:267–282.
17. Marceau P, Hould F, Potvin M et al. Biliopancreatic diversion (duodenal switch procedure). *Eur J Gastroenterol Hepatol* 1999;11:99–103.
18. Broadbent R, Tracy M, Harrington P. Laparoscopic gastric banding: A preliminary report. *Obes Surg* 1993;3:63–67.
19. Wittgrove A, Clark G. Laparoscopic gastric bypass, Roux-en-Y 500 patients: Technique and results, with 3–60 month follow-up. *Obes Surg* 2000;10:233–239.
20. Westling A, Gustavsson S. Laparoscopic vs. open Roux-en-Y gastric bypass: A prospective, randomized trial. *Obes Surg* 2001;11:284–292.
21. Fernandez A, DeMaria E, Tichansky D et al. Experience with over 3000 open and laparoscopic bariatric procedures: Multivariate analysis of factors related to leak and resultant mortality. *Surg Endosc* 2004;18:193–197.
22. Sapala J, Wood M, Schuhknecht M et al. Fatal pulmonary embolism after bariatric operations for morbid obesity: A 24-year retrospective analysis. *Obes Surg* 2003;13:819–825.
23. Escalante-Tattersfield T, Tucker O, Fajnwaks P et al. Incidence of deep vein thrombosis in morbidly obese patients undergoing laparoscopic Roux-en-Y gastric bypass. *Surg Obes Relat Dis* 2008;4:126–130.
24. Nguyen N, Longoria M, Chalifoux S et al. Gastrointestinal hemorrhage after laparoscopic gastric bypass. *Obes Surg* 2004;14:1308–1312.
25. Longitudinal Assessment of Bariatric Surgery (LABS) Consortium et al. Perioperative safety in the longitudinal assessment of bariatric surgery. *N Engl J Med* 2009; 361(5):445–454.
26. Ryskina K, Miller K, Aisenberg J et al. Routine management of stricture after gastric bypass and predictors of subsequent weight loss. *Surg Endosc* 2010;24:554–560.
27. Gonzalez R, Lin E, Venkatesh K et al. Gastrojejunostomy during laparoscopic gastric bypass: Analysis of 3 techniques. *Arch Surg* 2003;138:181–184.
28. Rasmussen J, Fuller W, Ali M. Marginal ulceration after laparoscopic gastric bypass: An analysis of predisposing factors in 260 patients. *Surg Endosc* 2007;21:1090–1094.
29. Brolin R, Kella V. Impact of complete mesenteric closure on small bowel obstruction and internal mesenteric hernia after laparoscopic Roux-en-Y gastric bypass. *Surg Obes Relat Dis* 2013;9:850–854.
30. Regan J, Inabnet W, Gagner M et al. Early experience with two-stage laparoscopic Roux-en-Y gastric bypass as an alternative in the super-super obese patient. *Obes Surg* 2003;13:861–864.
31. Rubin M, Yehoshua R, Stein M et al. Laparoscopic sleeve gastrectomy with minimal morbidity early results in 120 morbidly obese patients. *Obes Surg* 2008;18:1567–1570.
32. Nocca D, Krawczykowsky D, Bomans B et al. A prospective multicenter study of 163 sleeve gastrectomies: Results at 1 and 2 years. *Obes Surg* 2008;18:560–565.
33. Casella G, Soricelli E, Rizzello M et al. Nonsurgical treatment of staple line leaks after laparoscopic sleeve gastrectomy. *Obes Surg* 2009;19:821–826.

34. Brethauer S, Hammel J, Schauer P. Systematic review of sleeve gastrectomy as staging and primary bariatric procedure. *Surg Obes Relat Dis* 2009;5:469–475.
35. Cherian P, Goussous G, Ashori F et al. Band erosion after laparoscopic gastric banding: A retrospective analysis of 865 patients over 5 years. *Surg Endosc* 2010;24:2031–2038.
36. Neto M, Ramos A, Campos J et al. Endoscopic removal of eroded adjustable gastric band: Lessons learned after 5 years and 78 cases. *Surg Obes Relat Dis* 2010;6:423–427.
37. Nguyen N, Hohmann S, Nguyen X et al. Outcome of laparoscopic adjustable gastric banding and prevalence of band revision and explantation at academic centers: 2007–2009. *Surg Obes Relat Dis* 2012;8:724–727.
38. Ren C, Patterson E, Gagner M. Early results of laparoscopic biliopancreatic diversion with duodenal switch: A case series of 40 consecutive patients. *Obes Surg* 2000;10:514–523.
39. Westling A, Gustavsson S. Laparoscopic vs. open Roux-en-Y gastric bypass: A prospective, randomized trial. *Obes Surg* 2001;11:284–292.
40. Nguyen N, Goldman C, Rosenquist C et al. Laparoscopic versus open gastric bypass: A randomized study of outcomes, quality of life, and costs. *Ann Surg* 2001;234:279–289.
41. Colquitt J, Picot J, Loveman E et al. Surgery for obesity. *Cochrane Databases Syst Rev* 2009;2:CD003641.
42. Maggard M, Sugarman L, Suttorp M et al. Meta-analysis: Surgical treatment of obesity. *Ann Intern Med* 2005;142:547–559.
43. Trastulli S, Desiderio J, Guarino S et al. Laparoscopic sleeve gastrectomy compared with other bariatric surgical procedures: A systematic review of randomized trials. *Surg Obes Relat Dis* 2013;9:816–829.
44. Heber D, Greenway F, Kaplan L et al. Endocrine and nutritional management of the post-bariatric surgery patient: An endocrine society clinical practice guideline. *J Clin Endocrinol Metab* 2010;95:4823–4843.
45. Skroubis G, Sakellaropoulos G, Pouggouras K et al. Comparison of nutritional deficiencies after Roux-en-Y gastric bypass and after biliopancreatic diversion with Roux-en-Y gastric bypass. *Obes Surg* 2002;12:551–558.
46. Dolan K, Hatzifotis M, Newbury L et al. A clinical and nutritional comparison of biliopancreatic diversion with and without duodenal switch. *Ann Surg* 2004;240:51–56.
47. Sipponen P, Härkönen M. Hypochlorhydric stomach: A risk condition for calcium malabsorption and osteoporosis? *Scand J Gastroenterol* 2010;45:133–138.
48. Aills L, Blankenship J, Buffington C et al. ASMBS allied health nutritional guidelines for the surgical weight loss patient. *Surg Obes Relat Dis* 2008;4(Suppl 5):S73–S108.
49. Cable C, Colbert C, Showalter T et al. Prevalence of anemia after Roux-en-Y gastric bypass surgery: What is the right number? *Surg Obes Relat Dis* 2010;7:134–139.
50. Signori C, Zalesin K, Franklin B et al. Effect of gastric bypass on vitamin D and secondary hyperparathyroidism. *Obes Surg* 2010;20:949–952.
51. Youssef Y, Richards W, Sekhar N et al. Risk of secondary hyperparathyroidism after laparoscopic gastric bypass in obese women. *Surg Endosc* 2007;21:1393–1396.

17 Nutrition Counseling and Nutrition Tidbits

Laura E. Matarese, Eslam Ali, and Hossam M. Kandil

CONTENTS

17.1 INTRODUCTION

Nutritional intake can affect the immediate health and symptoms of patients as well as impact the incidence and severity of many long-term complications. Although many health care professionals have an innate ability to empathize and listen to their patients, they often lack the knowledge, skills, and techniques to affect change in the behaviors of their patients. Change is difficult, especially when it involves something as personal as diet. Except for a few circumstances, what a patient eats and drinks is an independent decision which may be based on habit, previous learning, or practices deep rooted in family, religion, and culture. Changing or modifying these behaviors in an effort to improve the nutritional health of patients is difficult and complex.

17.2 CHANGING BEHAVIORS

Behaviors can be changed with the use of education and counseling interventions. Both nutrition education and nutrition counseling are used to impart information and to a certain degree, motivation. But they differ in their scope and level of intensity. Nutrition education involves a transmission of knowledge which can be individualized or delivered in a group setting; the focus is usually more preventative than therapeutic. Nutrition counseling is generally used on an individual basis during medical nutrition therapy to help individuals make meaningful changes in their dietary behaviors in order to affect a positive therapeutic outcome. At the most basic level, good nutrition counseling requires communication which is grounded in empathetic and skillful provider–patient exchange. Realistically, before a change can be made, the client must be made aware that a change is needed; the rationale for that change and the motivational impetus to make the change.

There are a number of factors that determine the likelihood of changing a particular behavior. These determinants can be classified as either internal or external factors. Internal factors include the client's knowledge about health risk factors and risk reduction and literacy level; attitudes, beliefs and core values, which are often rooted in culture and religion; social and life adaptation skills; as well as their psychological, emotional and physiological disposition. Some of the external factors affecting ability to change include the client's capacity to afford nutrition counseling or the capability to buy food; safe and adequate transportation and a stable living environment are key issues in affecting change. All of these can be barriers to achieving nutritional health. Because dietary habits are difficult to change, counseling is most likely to be successful when recommendations are consistent with the cultural background, personal food preferences, religious and cultural beliefs and the economic status of the individual.

The counseling session begins with a detailed history to assess dietary intake patterns, food preferences, eating patterns, exercise, and lifestyle habits. This establishes a basis for the advice on how to alter the diet to affect change. The goal is to take the nutrition prescription and translate this into diet, that is, food which is habitually consumed.

It is important to consider all aspects of the patient and their care when planning a nutrition intervention. For example, if pain is not well controlled, the ability to eat will be compromised. If the patient is unable to buy food either due to finances or transportation issues, their compliance to the dietary intervention will be impacted.

17.3   TOOLS OF THE TRADE

Essential to changing behavior is the use of tools which can aid in identification of behaviors and self-monitoring of progress for the patient. A food diary also referred to as a food log or journal can be as simple as a piece of paper or as elaborate as an Internet-based web site in which the patient records everything they eat and drink as well as the amounts during the day. Additionally, it is helpful to have them include all activities which are performed during the day especially as they relate to eating. For example, do they eat in front of the television? Or, do they eat when they feel nervous or anxious? The patient must be able to determine the triggers in their lives that cause them to eat indiscriminately. This allows the patient to increase their awareness of activities and habits, which may be leading to poor dietary choices. It also aids the clinician in determining where and what types of interventions are required. It should be noted however, that the very process of recording what one is about to eat may change that behavior and cause the client to refrain from consuming the particular food item.

In some circumstances it may be advantageous to engage the client with the use of a contract in which all expectations are clearly defined. The patient commits to the plan and is aware of all responsibilities. This reinforces the seriousness of the nutrition intervention and the importance of compliance.

The interaction with the patient does not end at the completion of the counseling session. Compliance to the diet is best achieved and maintained if the patient receives adequate education and long-term monitoring. Follow-up sessions will ensure adequate knowledge of the diet, compliance, as well as the opportunity to modify the plan or meal patterns to optimize the therapy.

17.4 NUTRITION COUNSELING IN SPECIFIC GI DISORDERS

17.4.1 INFLAMMATORY BOWEL DISEASE

Many patients believe that anxiety, depression, and psychological stress worsen their inflammatory bowel disease (IBD) and will result in a flare up. Although the exact cause of IBD remains unknown it appears to involve a complex interaction between the individual's genotype and multiple environmental factors. Consumption of refined sugar, food additives (carrageenan), and cow's milk have been proposed as factors which predispose an individual to Crohn's disease, but the evidence to support these theories is limited.[1] There is a link between anxiety, depression, and psychological stress, and IBD. These individuals are frequent consumers of health care resources. Both Crohn's disease and ulcerative colitis share some clinical characteristics, including diarrhea, fever, weight loss, anemia, numerous food intolerances, malnutrition, and growth failure. Many will often voluntarily restrict oral intake in order to prevent abdominal pain or uncontrolled diarrhea or ostomy output. Due to the increased risk and incidence of malnutrition in this patient population, the first priory in the nutritional care of someone with IBD is to restore and maintain the nutritional status. Food, dietary and micronutrient supplements, enteral and parenteral nutrition may be used to accomplish this. Due to the chronic and changing nature of this disease oral diet and other means of nutrition interventions may change during remissions and exacerbations of the disease. One of the aspects of this disease that makes nutrition counseling so challenging is that this group of patients is very heterogeneous and will have numerous and various food intolerances. Not only is there intervariability but also intravariability in food tolerances. The patient should be counseled on dealing with a changing environment, that is, they may tolerate certain foods on one day but not the next. Individuals with IBD often have fears and misconceptions regarding GI symptoms and the role of food. There is no single dietary regimen for reducing symptoms or decreasing the flare ups in IBD. An individualized plan must be developed after a careful and detailed dietary history. Although the degree of malabsorption is variable and somewhat unpredictable in this patient population, most will benefit from daily multivitamin supplementation.

17.4.2 SHORT BOWEL SYNDROME

Short bowel syndrome (SBS) is one of the most common forms of intestinal failure. Patients with SBS typically experience severe diarrhea, steatorrhea, nutrient deficiencies, electrolyte disturbances, dehydration, malnutrition, and weight loss.[2] Diet is the foundation of therapy for these patients. Because of the heterogeneous nature of the patient population defining the diet prescription is difficult and should be individualized based on remnant GI anatomy and health of the mucosa. The SBS diet should be rich in complex carbohydrates with limited disaccharides, which create a high osmotic load to the gut leading to diarrhea or increase ostomy output.[3] Patients with colon in continuity can salvage up to 1000 additional calories per day through colonic bacterial fermentation of unabsorbed carbohydrates into absorbable SCFAs.[4–6] In general, protein should comprise 20% of dietary intake.[7] Although the optimal amount of fat to be consumed varies based on remnant anatomy (Table 17.1), all patients should be encouraged to consume fats high in essential fatty acids (EFAs) to prevent EFA deficiencies.[8] Patients with a remnant colon should minimize dietary fat as increased fat intake may result in increased diarrhea and loss of electrolytes and minerals.[9–10]

Patients with SBS with a colon in circuit are at risk of oxalate stones. There are two ways to address this potential problem. A low-oxalate diet will reduce oxalate absorption. Alternatively, the patient can consume additional oral calcium supplementation to absorb oxalate.[11–12] A low-oxalate diet can be restrictive and in our experience, most patients will choose to take additional oral calcium.

Fermentable fibers have a theoretical advantage for those individuals with a colon. The bacteria in the colon ferment the undigested fibers into short-chain fatty acids, which can be used as an energy substrate and enhance water absorption.[13,14] These fibers can prolong intestinal transit.[15] In our experience, the incorporation of these fermentable fibers is best achieved with foods in the diet. The use of fiber supplements is generally reserved for those individuals with more than 3 L of output. Fiber

---

TABLE 17.1
Diet Prescription for Patients with SBS

	Colon	No Colon
Carbohydrate	50%–60% of total calories (limit simple sugars)	40%–50% of total calories (restrict simple sugars)
Protein	20%–30% of total calories	20%–30% of total calories
Fat	20%–30% of total calories primarily as essential fats	30%–40% of total calories primarily as essential fats
Fluid	Isotonic or hypo-osmolar fluids	Isotonic, high-sodium oral rehydration solutions
Soluble fiber	5–10 g/day (if stool output is >3 L/day)	5–10 g/day (if stool output is >3 L/day)
Oxalates	Limit intake	
Meals/snacks	5–6 meals/day	4–6 meals/day

Source: Adapted from Byrne TA, Veglia L, Camelio M et al. *Nutr Clin Pract* 2000;15:306–311.

supplements can be used in those with an ostomy in order to gelatinize the ostomy effluent. The patient starts out with a small amount of fiber supplement and slowly titrates up to a dose, which produces the desired effect. It should be noted that sometimes the use of fiber supplements actually increases output.

Most patients with SBS will experience adaptive hyperphagia and will consume five to six small meals and snacks each day.[16] They are instructed that "grazing" and "snacking" is good for them. This should be encouraged and is preferable to consumption of two to three large meals.

Training the patient to consume the appropriate oral fluids can be challenging. Both hypo- and hyper-osmolar beverages should be avoided.[17–19] Patients with jejunostomies will benefit from oral rehydration solutions that are isotonic, high sodium (90 mmol/L or greater), glucose-containing solutions. Because the colon absorbs sodium against a steep electrochemical gradient[10] the composition of the oral fluids is not as critical in patients with a colon in circuit. Consumption of hyper-osmolar beverages (e.g., regular sugar-containing soda, fruit juice) are not well tolerated particularly in large volumes and when consumed rapidly. These should be avoided. Patients must be instructed to sip the rehydration fluids throughout the day. Although most find the fluids more palatable if they are cold, the patient should be instructed not to put them over ice. As the ice melts, it will dilute the solution and therefore change the concentration of the salts. An alternative is to place these fluids in an ice cube tray, which allows the patient to consume these slowly and at a very cold temperature. For those individuals who simply will not drink the oral rehydration solutions, an alternative is to provide salt tablets. The absorption is not as good but it may work for some patients.[20] Salt enhances absorption in patients with SBS. The patients will often comment that they crave salt. They should be encouraged to generously salt their foods.

Vitamin and mineral supplementation is another consideration. Even with the dietary modifications to improve absorption and minimize output, SBS patients generally require additional vitamin and mineral supplementation (Table 17.2). These are best taken with food. Many of these patients have osteopenia or osteoporosis due to long-term malabsorption and use of steroids. Therefore, additional calcium supplementation is generally warranted. The absorption of calcium citrate is superior to calcium carbonate. Calcium carbonate is a relatively insoluble compound. Absorption of calcium carbonate can be improved if the patient is instructed to take this with meals. Patients often require magnesium supplementation since they lose magnesium via ostomy effluent and diarrhea. Unfortunately, magnesium tends to produce more diarrhea. Consequently, the choice of supplementation is important. Although magnesium oxide contains the highest percentage of magnesium, it is also a strong cathartic. Magnesium supplementation can be maximized with the use of magnesium lactate or magnesium gluconate. The patient should be instructed to take magnesium supplementation 1 h prior to meals in order to maximize absorption.

Nutrition intervention for patients with SBS is complex. Translating the nutrition prescription into diet is intricate and must include a variety of components. First, a detailed diet history is performed in order to determine foods and behaviors which contribute to malabsorption. This also aids in determining the relationship of oral intake to stomal or stool output. Consideration must be given to the patient's lifestyle

TABLE 17.2

Vitamin and Mineral Supplementation for Patients with SBS

Nutrient	Strength	Dose
General multivitamin		1–3 daily
Vitamin A	25,000 IU	1 tablet PO daily
Vitamin B$_{12}$	1000 µg	Injection once monthly
Vitamin D	1000 IU	1 tablet PO daily
Vitamin E	400 IU	1 tablet PO daily
Calcium citrate	500- to 600-mg tablet	1–2 tablets PO tid
Magnesium lactate	8-mg tablet	1–2 tablets PO tid
Magnesium gluconate	1000-mg tablet (or liquid)	1–3 tablets PO tid
Potassium chloride	20-mg tablet	1–2 tablets PO daily
Phosphate (NeutraPhos)	250-mg package	1 package PO tid
Sodium bicarbonate	650-mg tablet	1 tablet PO tid
Chromium	100-µg tablet	1–2 tablets PO tid
Copper	3-mg tablet	1–2 tablets PO daily
Selenium	200-µg tablet	1 tablet PO daily
Zinc sulfate	220-mg tablet	1–3 tablets PO daily

Source: Adapted with permission from Matarese LE. *Nutricion Enteral y Parenteral.* 2nd Edition. New York, NY: McGraw-Hill; 2012:484–496.

Note: IU, International Unit; PO, by mouth; tid, 3 times daily.

so that the diet can be initiated to conform to the lifestyle rather than having the patient change lifestyle to make the diet fit. A strong and intense educational component is required. It is also helpful to provide the patient with "cheating" guidelines. For example, it is acceptable to occasionally indulge in a small sliver of cake after consuming a meal with complex carbohydrates and protein. But it is not acceptable to eat a large piece of cake as a meal replacement along with a glass of sugar-containing cola. We have also found it helpful to provide the patient with a one- to three-week menu cycle which exhibits the appropriate foods and amounts as well as timing to fulfill the requirements of the diet modification. It is also important to establish realistic goals with the patient and modify the goals as the patient progresses and the bowel adapts.

This patient population suffers from numerous barriers to oral intake. These barriers are often learned but can be difficult to overcome. For patients suffering from oral aversions, treat symptoms with medications as needed (e.g., antidiarrheals, H$_2$ blockers, etc.). Provide support and positive reinforcement. Start with small amounts of "safe foods" for example, white bread and then progress to higher fiber foods such as oatmeal bread and eventually whole wheat bread. The same approach can be used with advancing textures. For example, the patient can be started with carrot puree and then advanced to soft cooked carrots and finally raw carrots. Introducing fermentable (insoluble) fiber into the diet can be challenging. The patient can be started with unsweetened applesauce, advanced to a peeled fresh apple and eventually to a fresh apple with skin as tolerated. Advancing amounts can be done using the same techniques, for example, start with 1 or 2 sections of fresh orange, then 1/4 orange and eventually 1/2 orange. Set patient goals and involve the patient in the decision making. Eating is social and the patient should be encouraged to eat with family members so that the diet interventions seem less "therapeutic."

Anorexia and early satiety can be overcome with the use of small frequent meals, appetite stimulants, and prokinetic agents. If necessary, augment oral intake with nocturnal tube feeding or oral supplements. Dysgeusia is common in the SBS patient and is often associated with zinc deficiency and some medications. There are some adults who never learned to eat appropriately, especially if they were sick as a child. New foods should be introduced slowly. Cognitive restructuring to change beliefs and perceptions of food may be necessary. Individuals with SBS often suffer from numerous psychosocial issues such as depression and fear of eating. Empowering the patient in order to change dependency to independence is important. They will benefit from the support of other patients and family. A multidisciplinary approach using cognitive-behavioral therapy is also helpful.

Those individuals with eating disorders in addition to their SBS are especially challenging. It is important to set patient goals, use contracts and food diaries. Ultimately, it may require intervention from a psychiatrist, psychologist, or social worker.

17.4.3 IRRITABLE BOWEL SYNDROME

Irritable bowel syndrome (IBS) is characterized by chronically recurring abdominal discomfort, flatulence, and altered bowel habits. In the past these patients were counseled on a high fiber diet, unfortunately, without successful achievement of relief of symptoms. Recently, a diet low in fermentable oligo-, di-, and monosaccharides and polyols (FODMAPs) has been shown to be useful in this patient population.[21] This is a fairly complex elimination diet and involves cooperation from the patient. In our experience, most of these patients have suffered for years and are not only willing but anxious to try the diet in order to get relief. Many of these individuals have become so anxious about food, GI distress (bloating, flatulence), and social embarrassment that they become unnecessarily restrictive in their food selection. This group of individuals also tends to have exacerbation of their symptoms when stressed. Thus, along with the diet instruction, patients are counseled on methods to reduce stress including exercise and provided with support and reassurance through thorough workup and patient–health provider interaction.

17.4.4 CELIAC DISEASE

Lifelong, strict adherence to a gluten-free diet is the only known treatment for celiac disease (CD). The gluten-free diet diminishes the autoimmune process, and the intestinal mucosa usually reverts to normal or near normal. Within two to eight weeks of starting the gluten-free diet, most patients report abatement of their clinical symptoms. Histologic, immunological, and functional improvement may take months to years, depending on the duration of the disease, age of the client, and degree of dietary compliance. With strict dietary control, levels of the specific antibodies usually become undetectable within three to six months in most individuals. Because of the seriousness of dietary noncompliance in this disorder, the patient must be counseled so that there is a complete understanding of the implications of noncompliance. In our experience, most patients with CD are compliant with the dietary modifications but will admit to occasional noncompliance with the diet. Inadvertent gluten intake is the most common problem in this group of patients. In the past, this diet had limited food choices and was expensive to follow. There has been an increase in the number of gluten-free products available in local grocery stores although they remain more expensive than gluten-containing foods.

17.4.5   NONALCOHOLIC FATTY LIVER DISEASE

Nonalcoholic fatty liver disease is a spectrum of liver disease ranging from steatosis to steatohepatitis. It is commonly associated with obesity, diabetes mellitus, dyslipidemia, and insulin resistance. Some patients with NAFLD may progress to nonalcoholic steatohepatitis (NASH), which may then progress to cirrhosis. A dietary regimen for weight loss can lead to histologic improvement in NASH patients.[22] When combined with exercise and behavior modification, diet interventions aimed at weight loss have been shown to result in improved NASH disease activity, steatosis, inflammation, and ballooning.[23] Yet sudden weight loss can worsen liver injury.[24] Thus slow controlled weight loss is the goal with a moderate calorie restriction of 100–500 kcal/day to achieve 5%–10% body weight reduction over one year. The best diet to achieve this weight loss has been debated. Various diets (low CHO or low fat) are equally effective for long-term weight loss.[25] However, it should be noted that high protein, low carbohydrate diets such as Atkins and South Beach may cause rapid weight loss during the induction phase which in turn, may be deleterious in NAFLD and NASH and result in increased steatosis. Additionally, Atkins, Zone and South Beach may be deleterious in patients with hyperuricemia or kidney dysfunction due to the high protein content. On the other hand, excessive carbohydrate and fat could play a role in increasing blood glucose, free fatty acids, and insulin concentrations, independently or together which may be harmful to the liver. Patients with NASH have higher postprandial triacylglycerol response and increased production of VLDL; decreased total fat consumption may lead to decrease in postprandial lipemia. Smaller meals low in total fat may be beneficial in NAFLD. It is important to note that not all patients respond the same way to diet intervention. Therefore, the diet should be individualized based on a thorough assessment of the individual metabolic, physiologic, and nutritional status. In addition to diet, the patient should be counseled about general lifestyle changes. Aerobic exercise has been shown to reduce steatosis without weight change.[26] For many patients the implementation of an exercise program will be simply by walking and gradually increasing the duration and intensity. Once again, the seriousness of the disease process needs to be stressed to the patient and that dietary intervention may reverse this.

There are several other nutrients which have been shown to be beneficial for these patients. Vitamin E, 800 IU daily has been shown to decrease inflammation in nondiabetic NASH.[27] Fish oils promote oxidation of fatty acids and downregulate fatty acid synthesis. Although it is premature to recommend omega-3 fatty acids for the specific treatment of NAFLD or NASH, they may be considered as the first-line agents to treat hypertriglyceridemia in patients with NAFLD.[28]

17.4.6 CHRONIC LIVER DISEASE AND CIRRHOSIS

Protein calorie malnutrition (PCM) has been described in 50%–100% of patients with decompensated cirrhosis and at least 20% with compensated cirrhosis.[29–33] PCM is associated with a number of complications including development of variceal bleeding and ascites, increased surgical morbidity and mortality, reduced survival, and worsening hepatic function.[34–40] Patients with advanced cirrhosis may also have micronutrient deficiencies. Recognition of macro- and micronutrient deficiencies is important since supplemental nutrition has been associated with a reduction in the risk of infection and in-hospital mortality and has improved liver function parameters.[41–44]

The pathogenesis of malnutrition in cirrhosis is multifactorial.[33] Protein, carbohydrate, and lipid metabolism are all affected by liver disease. Other factors include inadequate dietary intake, impaired digestion and absorption, and altered metabolism. Anorexia, nausea, encephalopathy, gastritis, ascites, a sodium restricted diet and concurrent alcohol consumption can all contribute to a reduction in dietary intake. Malabsorption and maldigestion of nutrients can result from bile salt deficiency, bacterial overgrowth, altered intestinal motility, portal hypertensive changes to the intestine, mucosal injury, and increased intestinal permeability.[45–49] Cirrhosis represents an accelerated state of starvation and as such, fuels other than glucose that include lipids and proteins are used. There is an overall loss of protein from reduced synthesis of urea and hepatic proteins, reduced intestinal protein absorption, and increased urinary nitrogen excretion. Liver disease is associated with a lowered ratio of branched-chain to aromatic amino acids.

This group of patients is prone to malnutrition and nutritional intervention is often required to reverse the malnourished state. It is very important to refer such patients to a dietitian for proper intervention particularly when it involves the use of diet. General guidelines have been developed to guide nutrition management in patients with chronic liver disease and cirrhosis.[50] Patients with alcoholic steatohepatitis tend to be malnourished or at least at risk of malnutrition due to alcohol ingestion combined with poor oral diet. The assessment of nutritional status is best achieved with the use of simple bedside methods such as the Subjective Global Assessment (SGA) or anthropometry to identify patients at risk of under nutrition. The patient should be instructed to consume a well-balanced diet with complete cessation of all alcohol. Energy intake should be in the range of 35–40 kcal/kg/day and protein intake of 1.2–1.5 g/kg/day. The use of supplementary enteral nutrition in the form of oral supplements or tube feedings may be necessary when patients cannot meet their caloric requirements with normal food. Percutaneous endoscopic gastrostomy (PEG) tube placement is associated with a higher risk of complications and is not recommended. Whole protein formulas are generally recommended. Consider using more concentrated high-energy formulas in patients with ascites. The use branch chain amino acid (BCAA)-enriched formulas during enteral nutrition may be helpful in patients with hepatic encephalopathy. The use of oral BCAA supplements can improve clinical outcomes in advanced cirrhosis.[50]

There is some data to suggest that diets in which the protein source is derived from vegetables and casein may improve mental status compared with meat proteins. Vegetables are low in methionine and ammoniagenic amino acids, but rich in BCAA. The high-fiber content of a vegetable–protein diet may also aid in the excretion of nitrogenous compounds. Casein-based diets are lower in AAAs and higher in BCAA than meat-based diets. There have been a number of trials which have compared vegetable protein-based and meat protein-based diets in this group of patients.[51] In the majority of these studies, improved nitrogen balance and a reduction in hepatic encephalopathy was demonstrated with the use of vegetable protein when compared to meat protein. However, it should be noted that most of the studies had small sample sizes, varying clinical conditions and methods of assessment of encephalopathy, as well as differences in the diets used. Despite these shortcomings, a trial of a vegetable protein diet combined with optimum lactulose therapy is worthwhile in cirrhotic patients with chronic encephalopathy. It may be difficult to convince some patients to convert to a plant-based diet. One approach that we have found successful is to have the patient consume smaller amounts of meat protein while increasing the vegetables, fruits, grains, and dairy in the diet. The meat should be thought of as a "garnish" on the plate rather than the main component.

Sodium retention is central to the formation of ascites. The typical North American diet is high in sodium, containing 3–4 g sodium/day. Those patients with ascites should have a dietary sodium restriction of 2 g/day. These individuals will require counseling regarding the importance of a low-sodium diet as well as the implementation. In some instances it may be necessary to impose more severe limitations but this will also reduce the palatability of the diet. Since the sodium content of the diet comes from numerous sources and is often hidden in prepared and processed foods, the patient will require a strong educational component and referral to a dietitian will be essential.

Both probiotics and prebiotics have been used to treat the cognitive impairment experienced by some of these patients. Probiotics are live microorganisms which are thought to exert health benefits beyond those of basic nutrition. Prebiotics are nondigestible food ingredients that beneficially affect the host by selectively stimulating the growth and/or activity of the gut microbiota. Prebiotics and symbiotics have been shown to decrease endotoxemia resulting in improved encephalopathy. It may be beneficial to instruct the patient on methods of increasing the fermentable fiber content of the diet.[52]

The recommendations for patients prior to transplantation or surgery are the same as those for patients with cirrhosis. Additionally, normal food/enteral nutrition would be initiated within 12–24 h after liver transplantation and other surgical procedures. Use nasogastric tubes or catheter jejunostomy for early enteral nutrition. Whole protein formulas are generally recommended. In patients with ascites, concentrated high-energy formulas are preferred due to issues with fluid balance. Use BCAA-enriched formulas in patients with hepatic encephalopathy arising during enteral nutrition. If the liver patient has ascites, the patient should be placed on low salt diet consisting of less than 2 g daily. This is where referral to a dietitian would be most beneficial for instruction of oral intake as well as reading food labels.

For adults with heavy alcohol use, supplementation with a multivitamin that contains a minimum of thiamine 100 mg daily, vitamin B_6 2 mg daily, and folic acid 400 mcg to 1 mg daily is recommended. Heavy alcohol use is considered to be more than four drinks per day or more than 14 drinks per week for men and more than three drinks per day or more than seven drinks per week for women.

17.4.7 CHRONIC PANCREATITIS

Chronic pancreatitis evolves insidiously over many years. These individuals are at risk for malnutrition due to pancreatic insufficiency and poor oral intake. The objective of the nutrition intervention is to prevent further destruction of the pancreas, decrease the number of attacks, alleviate pain, decrease steatorrhea, and correct any existing malnutrition. Paramount to the effective nutrition intervention is to ensure the patient abstains from further alcohol ingestion. This may require the assistance of substance abuse counselors. Oral dietary intake should be as liberal as possible but modification may be necessary to alleviate pain. Overall, the diet should be low in fat, consisting primarily of vegetable-based oils. The patient should be instructed to reduce or eliminate *trans* fats from the diet. Patients who are taking pancreatic enzyme replacement should be instructed that these need to be taken with the meal and that the dose is dependent on the size of the meal. These patients may also benefit from vitamin and mineral supplementation particularly if the diet will be limited due to pain.

17.4.8 OBESITY AND WEIGHT MANAGEMENT

The greatest threat to global health is obesity. The real problem is not adiposity but the comorbidities which significantly increase mortality rates. Programs that combine diet, exercise, and behavioral modification have been the cornerstone of therapy but have lacked long-term success. Obesity is a complex disease and there are numerous factors influencing weight loss. These factors are interrelated and dynamic. For example, adding exercise can change metabolic rate and insulin sensitivity. Low glycemic index and low carbohydrate diets can beneficially impact resting energy expenditure and total energy expenditure.[53,54] Selecting the best weight loss program can be challenging. The program must be individualized for each patient with consideration given to lifestyle and metabolic parameters. For example, individuals who are insulin resistant may have better weight loss and maintenance with a low carbohydrate diet compared to low fat.[55] A "calorie" is not always a "calorie." Calories from foods that are less satiating can lead to overconsumption. Therefore, the macronutrient distribution can impact satiety. Diets high in protein and low in carbohydrates tend to be more satiating.[56] Thus, the selection of the appropriate weight loss diet intervention must be individualized considering the degree of obesity and comorbidities; metabolic status (insulin resistance/sensitivity); medications affecting appetite; food intake and physical activity; type of dietary approach the patient might adhere to; the patient's readiness to change and the degree of literacy. Ultimately, the best diet is the one the patient will follow and incorporate into their daily lives for life long maintenance of a healthy body weight.

Achievement and maintenance of a healthy body weight with the use of bariatric surgery is considered to be one of the most successful methods of weight loss and for the resolution of comorbidities. Four major bariatric operations are now commonly performed: (1) adjustable gastric banding (AGB), (2) sleeve gastrectomy (SG), (3) Roux-en-Y gastric bypass (RYGB), and (4) biliopancreatic bypass with duodenal switch (DS). The registered dietitian nutritionist is a vital component of the bariatric surgery process. Nutrition assessment and dietary management in surgical weight loss have been shown to correlate with success.[57,58] A comprehensive nutrition assessment should be conducted preoperatively to identify the patient's nutritional, educational, psychological, social, and financial needs. Appropriate interventions for correction are then instituted. Presurgical dietary interventions designed to induce a small amount of weight loss can reduce postoperative risk, abdominal adiposity, and the size of the liver.[59,60] The interventions may include a variety of weight loss diets or the use of commercial protein-sparing modified fasts. Vitamin and trace mineral deficiencies are common in this patient population.[61] Therefore, care should be taken to identify and correct nutrient deficiencies prior to surgical intervention. After weight loss surgery, the diet will require permanent changes, both in how much food is consumed and in the types of foods chosen. Meal replacements consisting of calorie- and portion-controlled shakes and bars are often promoted as a weight-loss strategy, particular for those patients who struggle with making appropriate food choices and controlling portion sizes and intake. Following surgery, the patient's oral intake progresses over several weeks to months through various stages of textures and food groups until solid foods are consumed (Table 17.3).[62] Although the dietitian will counsel the patient to consume a healthy and balanced diet within the limitations created by the surgical procedure, patients will require supplementation following bariatric surgery (Table 17.4). Most nutrient deficiencies associated with bariatric surgery are due to altered absorption or poor dietary intake.

17.4.9 MOTILITY DISORDERS

From a nutrition intervention perspective, motility disorders can be broadly categorized as accelerated emptying such as observed in dumping syndrome or delayed emptying as in gastroparesis. Dumping syndrome is a complex gastrointestinal (GI) and vasomotor response to the presence of large quantities of food and/or hypertonic foods and liquids.[63] It may occur as a result of surgical interventions such as total or partial gastrectomy, fundoplication, vagotomy, and bariatric procedures for obesity. The symptoms can be divided into early, intermediate and late stages of dumping of food into the small intestine. Early dumping is characterized by both GI and vasomotor symptoms in which the patient experiences abdominal fullness and nausea within 10–30 min of consuming a meal. In the intermediate stage patients may experience abdominal discomfort, bloating, flatulence and diarrhea. This is likely to occur from 20 min to 1 h after eating and may be related to the malabsorption of carbohydrates with subsequent fermentation by gut microbiota. Late dumping generally occurs from 1 to 3 h after a meal and is characterized by vascular symptoms

TABLE 17.3

Diet and Texture Progression Following Bariatric Surgery

Stage	Length	Goals	Typical Foods
1. Clear liquids	1–2 days	Restoration of gut motility	Water, sugar-free gelatin, bouillon
2. Full liquids	10–14 days	60–80 g protein 64 oz. fluids non-caffeinated, noncarbonated, minimal calories	Protein shakes, skim milk, soy milk. Low-fat yogurts, nonfat Greek style yogurt; fat-free or 1% cottage cheese, fat-free ricotta cheese, sugar-free or fat-free pudding, fat-free/low-fat cream soups made with skim milk
3. Pureed and mechanically soft	4–6 weeks	60–80 g protein; 64 oz. fluids noncaffeinated, noncarbonated, minimal calories Introduction of soft moistened protein foods; pureed, chopped, ground, and mashed foods	Ground meat >93% fat free (beef, chicken, pork, turkey), fish (sole, haddock, halibut, salmon, tuna) Chicken or turkey breast without skin; turkey chili, scrambled liquid egg substitute, tofu, beans (kidney, black refried)
4. High-protein, low-fat, low-sugar	8–10 weeks from date of surgery	60–80 g protein; 64 oz. fluids noncaffeinated, noncarbonated, minimal calories; introduction of one new food at each meal Goal: 3 serving of fruits/vegetables per day Goal: 2–3 servings of whole grains per day	Proteins from pervious states 1/4 cup berries 1/2 banana 1 small apple 1/4 cup green beans 1/4 cup salad 1/2 of 8" whole wheat pita pocket 1/4 cup brown rice

related to reactive hypoglycemia including flushing, tachycardia, lightheadedness, perspiring, and shaking. The basic guidelines for dumping syndrome include the consumption of small, frequent meals, which include complex carbohydrates and the elimination of simple sugars and disaccharides. Patients will need to be instructed on portion sizes as well as the composition of foods and liquids. It may also be helpful to separate solids from liquids by 30 min.

The dietary interventions for gastroparesis are more complex and can be divided into three stages depending on the patient's symptoms. In all cases, the importance of adequate mastication of food should be stressed. Food should be chewed slowly and thoroughly. In general, fat slows down gastric emptying but many can consume some fat especially in the form of liquids (as part of beverages such as whole milk, milkshakes, nutritional supplements, etc.) Fiber may act to slow gastric emptying and can result in the formation of bezoars. Those individuals with severe gastroparesis

TABLE 17.4

Routine Vitamin and Mineral Supplementation Following Bariatric Surgery

Supplement	Comment	AGB	RYGB	BPD-DS
Multivitamin-mineral supplement	A high-potency vitamin Begin with chewable or liquid; progress to whole tablet/capsule as tolerated Avoid time-released and enteric coating Choose a complete formula with at least 18 mg iron, 400 mcg folic acid, plus selenium and zinc Avoid children's formulas that are incomplete Take with food to improve GI tolerance Do not mix multivitamin containing iron with calcium (take at least 2 h apart) Specialized bariatric formulations are available but not required	100% daily value	200% daily value	200% daily value
B$_{12}$ (cobalamin)	Available as sublingual tablets, liquid drops, mouth spray, or nasal gel/spray Intramuscular injection Oral tablets	Oral 350–500 mcg/day	Sublingual or injections 1000 mcg/day Oral 350–500 mcg/day	Oral 350–500 mcg/day
Elemental calcium	Calcium citrate plus vitamin D$_3$ Chewable for the first 6–12 months Progression to tablets as tolerated Split into 500–600 mg doses and space doses evenly throughout the day Do not mix multivitamins with iron with calcium	1500 mg/day	1500–2000 mg/day	1800–2400 mg/day
Elemental Iron	Chewable for the first 6–12 months Progression to tablets as tolerated Avoid enteric coating Do not mix iron and calcium supplements, take 2 h apart Vitamin C may enhance absorption of nonheme iron sources	18–27 mg/day elemental Some may require 50–100 mg elemental	18–27 mg/day elemental Some may require 50–100 mg elemental	18–27 mg/day elemental Some may require 50–100 mg elemental
Vitamin D	Chewable for the first 6–12 months Progression to tablets as tolerated Intake of 2000 IU vitamin D$_3$ may be achieved with careful selection of multivitamin and calcium supplements Typically patients end up taking an additional 1000 IU of vitamin D$_3$ supplement	1600–2000 IU/day	1600–2000 IU/day	

Note: RYGB, Roux-en-Y gastric bypass; AGB, adjustable gastric banding; BPD-DS, biliopancreatic diversion with duodenal switch.

or who have had a bezoar should avoid fiber from foods and medications. Those individuals with diabetes mellitus should keep the blood sugar under 180 mg/dL to prevent a delay in gastric emptying.

The diet intervention for gastroparesis is broken down into three levels. Level 1 consists primarily of clear liquids with some saltine crackers as tolerated. It is inadequate in all nutrients except sodium and potassium and should not be continued for more than three days without additional nutrition support. This level is used when the patient is experiencing nausea. As symptoms resolve the patient can advance to the next level which incorporates full liquids and soft foods into the diet. The fat content is slowly increased as symptoms resolve. Level 3 incorporates more solid but soft cooked foods. Patients with gastroparesis may experience some variation in tolerance from day to day and they should be instructed to maximize oral intake on the days they are feeling well.

17.5 WORKING WITH A REGISTERED DIETITIAN NUTRITIONIST: WHEN TO REFER

Dietary management of most GI disorders is sufficiently complex to refer to a registered dietitian nutritionist (RDN). Simply supplying the patient with a brochure containing a diet or series of menus is not likely to be as effective as individualized counseling particularly for complicated elimination diets. The role of the RDN is to translate the nutrition prescription into a diet that the patient can consume and adhere to while maintaining a nutritiously sound intake. They possess a unique knowledge of the composition of foods. This is important as the food supply has changed significantly. There have been major changes in how food is grown, processed, cooked, served, and marketed resulting in confusion and misinformation often provided by unqualified individuals. The RDN can provide accurate information about nutrients, calories, serving sizes, food groups, labels, marketing tactics, food ingredients, allergies, and potential interactions. The RDN will also ensure that the diet fits into the patient's lifestyle rather than forcing the patient to make their lifestyle fit the diet.

Many gastroenterology practices employ RDNs. In some instances, a referral may be made to an RDN. The Academy of Nutrition and Dietetics' Find a Registered Dietitian Nutritionist online referral service allows individuals to search a national database of academy members for the exclusive purpose of finding a qualified registered dietitian nutritionist. This service is available at http://www.eatright.org/programs/rdfinder/.

17.6 SUMMARY

Changing or modifying behaviors in an effort to improve the nutritional health of patients is difficult and complex. Behaviors can be changed with the use of education and counseling interventions. These interventions must take into account numerous factors including the client's knowledge about health risk factors and risk reduction; literacy level; attitudes, beliefs and core values which are often rooted in culture and religion; social and life adaptation skills; as well as their psychological, emotional, and physiological disposition. Although there is overlap in the approach to these patients, each GI disorder has specific nutrition interventions which must be accomplished in order to affect change. The nutrition interventions required for the management of most GI disorders is sufficiently complex to justify referral to an RDN in order to maximize positive change with the best clinical outcomes.

REFERENCES

1. Rajendran N, Kumar D. Role of diet in the management of inflammatory bowel disease. *World J Gastroenterol* 2010;16:1442–1448.
2. Thompson JS, Weseman R, Rochling FA, Mercer DF. Current management of the short bowel syndrome. *Surg Clin North Am* 2011;91:493–510.
3. Matarese LE, O'Keefe SJ, Kandil HM et al. Short bowel syndrome: Clinical guidelines for nutrition management. *Nutr Clin Pract* 2005;20:493–502.
4. Royall D, Wolever TM, Jeejeebhoy KN. Evidence for colonic conservation of malabsorbed carbohydrate in short bowel syndrome. *Am J Gastroenterol* 1992;87:751–756.
5. Bond JH, Currier BE, Buchwald H, Levitt MD. Colonic conservation of malabsorbed carbohydrate. *Gastroenterology* 1980;78:444–447.
6. Nordgaard I, Hansen BS, Mortensen PB. Importance of colonic support for energy absorption as small-bowel failure proceeds. *Am J Clin Nutr* 1996;64:222–231.
7. Byrne TA, Veglia L, Camelio M et al. Beyond the prescription: Optimizing the diet of patients with short bowel syndrome. *Nutr Clin Pract* 2000;15:306–311.
8. Jeppesen PB, Hoy CE, Mortensen PB. Deficiencies of essential fatty acids, vitamin A and E and changes in plasma lipoproteins in patients with reduced fat absorption or intestinal failure. *Eur J Clin Nutr* 2000;54:632–642.
9. Woolf GM, Miller C, Kurian R, Jeejeebhoy KN. Diet for patients with a short bowel: High fat or high carbohydrate? *Gastroenterology* 1983;84:823–828.
10. Lennard-Jones JE. Practical management of the short bowel. *Aliment Pharmacol Ther* 1994;8:563–577.
11. Liebman M, Chai W. Effect of dietary calcium on urinary oxalate excretion after oxalate loads. *Am J Clin Nutr* 1997;65:1453–1459.
12. Curhan GC, Willett WC, Rimm EB, Stampfer MJ. A prospective study of dietary calcium and other nutrients and the risk of symptomatic kidney stones. *N Engl J Med* 1993;328:833–838.
13. Rombeau JL, Kripke SA. Metabolic and intestinal effects of short-chain fatty acids. *JPEN J Parenter Enteral Nutr* 1990;14:181S–185S.
14. Atia A, Girard-Pipau F, Hebuterne X et al. Macronutrient absorption characteristics in humans with short bowel syndrome and jejunocolonic anastomosis: Starch is the most important carbohydrate substrate, although pectin supplementation may modestly enhance short chain fatty acid production and fluid absorption. *JPEN J Parenter Enteral Nutr* 2011;35:229–240.
15. Meier R, Beglinger C, Schneider H et al. Effect of a liquid diet with and without soluble fiber supplementation on intestinal transit and cholecystokinin release in volunteers. *JPEN J Parenter Enteral Nutr* 1993;17:231–235.
16. Crenn P, Morin MC, Joly F et al. Net digestive absorption and adaptive hyperphagia in adult short bowel patients. *Gut* 2004;53:1279–1286.
17. MacMahon RA. The use of the World Health Organization's oral rehydration solution in patients on home parenteral nutrition. *JPEN J Parenter Enteral Nutr* 1984;8:720–721.
18. Griffin GE, Fagan EF, Hodgson HJ, Chadwick VS. Enteral therapy in the management of massive gut resection complicated by chronic fluid and electrolyte depletion. *Dig Dis Sci* 1982;27:902–908.

19. Spiller RC, Jones BJ, Silk DB. Jejunal water and electrolyte absorption from two proprietary enteral feeds in man: Importance of sodium content. *Gut* 1987;28:681–687.

20. Nightingale JMD, Lennard-Jones JE, Wlaker ER et al. Oral salt supplements to compensate for jejunostomy losses: Comparison of sodium chloride capsules, glucose electrolyte solution, and glucose polymer electrolyte solution. *Gut* 1992;33:759–761.

21. Halmos EP, Power VA, Shepherd SJ et al. A diet low in FODMAPs reduces symptoms of irritable bowel syndrome. *Gastroenterology* 2012;146:67–74.

22. Huang MA, Greenson JK, Chao C et al. One-year intense nutritional counseling results in histological improvement in patients with non-alcoholic steatohepatitis: A pilot study. *Am J Gastroenterol* 2005;100:1072–81.

23. Promrat K, Kleiner DE, Niemeier HM et al. Randomized controlled trial testing the effects of weight loss on nonalcoholic steatohepatitis. *Hepatology* 2010;51:121–129.

24. Luyckx FH, Desaive C, Thiry A et al. Liver abnormalities in severely obese subjects: Effect of drastic weight loss after gastroplasty. *Int J Obes Relat Metab Disord* 1998;22:222–226.

25. Zivkovic AM, German JB, Sanyal AJ. Comparative review of diets for the metabolic syndrome: Implications for nonalcoholic fatty liver disease. *Amer J Clin Nutr* 2007;86:285–300.

26. Johnson NA, Sachinwalla T, Walton DW et al. Aerobic exercise training reduces hepatic and visceral lipids in obese individuals without weight loss. *Hepatology* 2009;50:1105–1112.

27. Sanyal AJ, Chalasani N, Kowdley KV et al. Pioglitazone, vitamin E, or placebo for nonalcoholic steatohepatitis. *N Engl J Med* 2010;362:1675–85.

28. Chalasani N, Younossi Z, Lavine JE et al. The diagnosis and management of nonalcoholic fatty liver disease: Practice Guideline by the American Gastroenterological Association, American Association for the Study of Liver Diseases, and American College of Gastroenterology. *Gastroenterology* 2012;142:1592–1609.

29. Crawford DH, Shepherd RW, Halliday JW et al. Body composition in nonalcoholic cirrhosis: The effect of disease etiology and severity on nutritional compartments. *Gastroenterology* 1994;106:1611–1617.

30. Lautz HU, Selberg O, Körber J et al. Protein-calorie malnutrition in liver cirrhosis. *Clin Investig* 1992;70:478–486.

31. DiCecco SR, Wieners EJ, Wiesner RH et al. Assessment of nutritional status of patients with end-stage liver disease undergoing liver transplantation. *Mayo Clin Proc* 1989;64:95–102.

32. Hehir DJ, Jenkins RL, Bistrian BR, Blackburn GL. Nutrition in patients undergoing orthotopic liver transplant. *JPEN J Parenter Enteral Nutr* 1985;9:695–700.

33. Cheung K, Lee SS, Raman M. Prevalence and mechanisms of malnutrition in patients with advanced liver disease, and nutrition management strategies. *Clin Gastroenterol Hepatol* 2012;10:117–125.

34. Siriboonkoom W, Gramlich L. Nutrition and chronic liver disease. *Can J Gastroenterol* 1998;12:201–207.

35. Plauth M, Merli M, Kondrup J et al. ESPEN guidelines for nutrition in liver disease and transplantation. *Clin Nutr* 1997;16:43–55.

36. Møller S, Bendtsen F, Christensen E, Henriksen JH. Prognostic variables in patients with cirrhosis and oesophageal varices without prior bleeding. *J Hepatol* 1994;21:940–946.

37. Porayko MK, DiCecco S, O'Keefe SJ. Impact of malnutrition and its therapy on liver transplantation. *Semin Liver Dis* 1991;11:305–314.

38. Shaw BW Jr, Wood RP, Gordon RD et al. Influence of selected patient variables and operative blood loss on six-month survival following liver transplantation. *Semin Liver Dis* 1985;5:385–393.

39. Manguso F, D'Ambra G, Menchise A et al. Effects of an appropriate oral diet on the nutritional status of patients with HCV-related liver cirrhosis: A prospective study. *Clin Nutr* 2005;24:751–759.

40. Cabré E, Gassull MA. Nutritional and metabolic issues in cirrhosis and liver transplantation. *Curr Opin Clin Nutr Metab Care* 2000;3:345–354.

41. Cabre E, Gonzalez-Huix F, Abad-Lacruz A et al. Effect of total enteral nutrition on the short-term outcome of severely malnourished cirrhotics. A randomized controlled trial. *Gastroenterology* 1990;98:715–720.

42. de Lédinghen V, Beau P, Mannant PR et al. Early feeding or enteral nutrition in patients with cirrhosis after bleeding from esophageal varices? A randomized controlled study. *Dig Dis Sci* 1997;42:536–541.

43. Kearns PJ, Young H, Garcia G et al. Accelerated improvement of alcoholic liver disease with enteral nutrition. *Gastroenterology* 1992;102:200–205.

44. Fan ST, Lo CM, Lai EC et al. Perioperative nutritional support in patients undergoing hepatectomy for hepatocellular carcinoma. *N Engl J Med* 1994;331:1547–1552.

45. Vlahcevic ZR, Buhac I, Farrar JT et al. Bile acid metabolism in patients with cirrhosis. I. Kinetic aspects of cholic acid metabolism. *Gastroenterology* 1971;60:491–498.

46. Bode JC. Alcohol and the gastrointestinal tract. *Ergeb Inn Med Kinderheilkd* 1980;45:1–75.

47. Bode C, Bode JC. Effect of alcohol consumption on the gut. *Best Pract Res Clin Gastroenterol* 2003;17:575–592.

48. Dinda PK, Leddin DJ, Beck IT. Histamine is involved in ethanol-induced jejunal microvascular injury in rabbits. *Gastroenterology* 1988;95:1227–1233.

49. Sarfeh IJ, Aaronson S, Lombino D et al. Selective impairment of nutrient absorption from intestines with chronic venous hypertension. *Surgery* 1986;99:166–169.

50. Plauth M, Cabré E, Riggio O et al. ESPEN guidelines on enteral nutrition: Liver disease. *Clin Nutr* 2006;25:285–294.

51. Amodio P, Caregaro L, Patteno, E et al. Vegetarian diets in hepatic encephalopathy: Facts or fantasies? *Dig Liver Dis* 2001;33:492–500.

52. Liu Q, Duan ZP, Ha DK et al. Symbiotic modulation of gut flora: Effect on minimal hepatic encephalopathy in patients with cirrhosis. *Hepatology* 2004;39:1441–1449.

53. Pereira MA, Swain J, Goldfine AB et al. Effects of a low-glycemic load diet on resting energy expenditure and heart disease risk factors during weight loss. *JAMA* 2004;292:2482–2490.

54. Ebbeling CB, Swain JF, Feldman HA et al. Effects of dietary composition on energy expenditure during weight-loss maintenance. *JAMA* 2012;307:2627–2634.

55. Cornier MA, Donahoo WT, Pereira R et al. Insulin sensitivity determines the effectiveness of dietary macronutrient composition on weight loss in obese women. *Obes Res* 2005;13:703–709.

56. Boden G, Sargrad K, Homko C et al. Effect of a low-carbohydrate diet on appetite, blood glucose levels, and insulin resistance in obese patients with type 2 diabetes. *Ann Intern Med* 2005;142:403–411.

57. Cottam DR, Atkinson JA, Anderson A et al. A case-controlled matched-pair cohort study of laparoscopic Rouxen- Y gastric bypass and Lap-Band® patients in a single U.S. center with three-year follow-up. *Obes Surg* 2006;16:534–540.

58. Cummings DE, Shannon MH. Ghrelin and gastric bypass: Is there a hormonal contribution to surgical weight loss? *J Clin Endocrinol Metab* 2003;88:2999–3002.

59. Alami RS, Morton JM, Schuster R et al. Is there a benefit to preoperative weight loss in gastric bypass patients? A prospective randomized trial *Surg Obes Relat Dis* 2007;3:141–145.

60. Colles SL, Dixon JB, Marks P et al. Preoperative weight loss with a very-low energy diet: Quantitation of changes in liver and abdominal fat by serial imaging *Am J Clin Nutr* 2006;84:304–331.
61. Madan AK, Whitney SO, Tichansky DS, Ternovits CA. Vitamin and trace mineral levels after laparoscopic gastric bypass. *Obes Surg* 2006;16:603–606.
62. Allied Health Sciences Section Ad Hoc Nutrition Committee. Aills L, Blankenship J, Buffington C et al. ASMBS Allied Health Nutritional Guidelines for the Surgical Weight Loss Patient. *Surg Obes Relat Dis* 2008;4:S73–S108.
63. Ukleja A. Dumping syndrome: Pathophysiology and treatment. *Nutr Clin Pract* 2005;20:517–525.

Index

A

AA, *see* Amino acids (AA); Arachidonic acid (AA)
AAAs, *see* Aromatic amino acids (AAAs)
AAD, *see* Antibiotic associated diarrhea (AAD)
ABC, *see* ATP-binding cassette (ABC)
ACC, *see* Anterior cingulated cortex (ACC)
Acid–base disturbances, 309; *see also*
      Gastrointestinal complications
Acquired disease, 32
Acute lung injury (ALI), 299
Acute pancreatitis (AP), 264, 272; *see also* Chronic
      pancreatitis (CP); Enteral feeding
  feeding influence on trypsin secretory
      response, 267
  ileal brake, 264–265
  immunonutrition, 272
  inflammation pathophysiology, 265
  management, 265
  nutritional support, 266
  pancreatic rest, 265–266, 267
  parenteral feeding, 271–272
  probiotics in, 272
  secretion physiology, 264–265
Acute respiratory distress syndrome (ARDS),
      265, 299
Acute urticaria, 65
Adjustable gastric banding (AGB), 398
Adverse reactions to food (ARF), 63
AGB, *see* Adjustable gastric banding (AGB)
Aggravating foods, 162
Aggressive nutritional support, 148; *see also*
      Nutrition and gastrointestinal cancer
  chemoradiated patients, 149
  malnourished patient, 148–149
AICR, *see* American Institute for Cancer
      Research (AICR)
ALI, *see* Acute lung injury (ALI)
Alpha 1 antitrypsin, 44; *see also* Malabsorption
      diagnosis
α-gal, *see* Galactose-α-1, 3-galactose (α-gal)
Alternative dietary source; *see also* IgE-mediated
      food allergy
  of milk nutrients, 70
  of wheat nutrients, 72
American Institute for Cancer Research
      (AICR), 139
American Society for Metabolic and Bariatric
      Surgery (ASMBS), 382; *see also*
      Bariatric surgery

American Society for Parenteral and Enteral
      Nutrition (ASPEN), 299
Amino acids (AA), 20; *see also* Protein digestion
      and absorption
  absorption of, 21
  transporter classification systems, 22
Amylase trypsin inhibitors (ATI), 179
Anastomotic stenosis, 375; *see also* Roux-en-Y
      gastric bypass (RYGB)
Angioedema, 65
Anorexia, 147; *see also* Nutrition and
      gastrointestinal cancer
  agents to combat, 149–150
  cannabinoids, 150
ANS, *see* Autonomic nervous system (ANS)
Anterior cingulated cortex (ACC), 212
Anthropometric measurements, 275
Anthropometry, 3; *see also* Nutritional status
      parameters
Antibiotic associated diarrhea (AAD), 117, 122–123
AP, *see* Acute pancreatitis (AP)
Apolipoprotein A1 (ApoA1), 25
Apolipoprotein B (ApoB), 25
Apollo OverStitch, 351–352, 361–362; *see also*
      Restrictive procedures; Weight
      regain—treatment
Arachidonic acid (AA), 299
ARDS, *see* Acute respiratory distress syndrome
      (ARDS)
ARF, *see* Adverse reactions to food (ARF)
Arginine, 298
Aromatic amino acids (AAAs), 298
Ascorbic acid (vitamin C), 141; *see also*
      Gastric cancer
ASMBS, *see* American Society for Metabolic
      and Bariatric Surgery (ASMBS)
ASPEN, *see* American Society for Parenteral and
      Enteral Nutrition (ASPEN)
Aspiration therapy, 357–358; *see also* Obesity
      endoscopic procedures
ATI, *see* Amylase trypsin inhibitors (ATI)
ATP-binding cassette (ABC), 25
Autonomic nervous system (ANS), 210; *see also*
      Irritable bowel syndrome (IBS)
  dysfunction, 212

B

Bacteroidetes, 113
BAD, *see* Bile acid diarrhea (BAD)